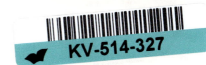

Immunological Diagnosis of Sexually Transmitted Diseases

CLINICAL AND BIOCHEMICAL ANALYSIS

A series of monographs and textbooks

EDITOR

Morton K. Schwartz

Chairman, Department of Biochemistry
Memorial Sloan-Kettering Cancer Center
New York, New York

ADDITIONAL VOLUMES IN PREPARATION

Immunological Diagnosis of Sexually Transmitted Diseases

edited by

Hugh Young
*Edinburgh University
Medical School
Edinburgh, Scotland*

Alexander McMillan
*The Royal Infirmary
Edinburgh, Scotland*

MARCEL DEKKER, INC.   New York and Basel

Library of Congress Cataloging-in-Publication Data

Immunological diagnosis of sexually transmitted diseases.

   (Clinical and biochemical analysis ; 23)
   Includes index.
   1. Serum diagnosis. 2. Sexually transmitted diseases--
Diagnosis. 3. Antibodies, Monoclonal--Diagnostic use.
I. Young, Hugh. II. McMillan, Alexander. III. Series.
[DNLM: 1. Antibodies, Monoclonal--diagnostic use.
2. Immunologic Technics. 3. Sexually Transmitted
Diseases--diagnosis. WI CL654 v.23 / WC 140 I33]
RC200.55.S4I46 1987   616.95'107561   87-20080
ISBN 0-8247-7808-1

MARCEL DEKKER, INC.
270 Madison Avenue, New York, New York 10016

Current printing (last digit):
10 9 8 7 6 5 4 3 2 1

PRINTED IN THE UNITED STATES OF AMERICA

Foreword

It is gratifying to be invited to write a foreword to this significant book. The editors are colleagues whom we greatly respect; their collaboration is another rewarding example of the constructive association that our departments have enjoyed over the years.

It is now more important than ever that clinicians engaged in the diagnosis and the management of sexually transmitted diseases should have close links with their colleagues in medical microbiological work. The daunting expansion of the range of recognized sexually transmitted diseases has called for very significant development of related laboratory expertise. Moreover, our increasing ability to offer specific and effective treatment to many patients increasingly obliges us to make a definitive diagnosis as promptly as possible and to have continuing liaison with the laboratory in the follow-up work that is often necessary. This relates to the continuing management of the patient and to our joint commitment to epidemiological surveillance.

To some extent, clinical bacteriologists have tended to rely unduly on cultural methods for the identification of pathogens, although *Treponema pallidum* remains elusive and still obliges us to rely heavily on indirect methods of laboratory diagnosis to identify syphilis. The advances made in our serological diagnostic work in the recent past indicate how much progress can be made when new technical methods become available. With the more recent development of immunological diagnostic methods, and with many other advances in our clinical and laboratory sciences, we are entering a new era in which the sensitive and specific detection of early antibody may be rivaled by elegant procedures to detect antigen. This optimistic view is endorsed by the quality and the range of the contributions that make this book.

The editors are to be congratulated on recruiting such an authoritative team. The book is a mine of information; it brings together up-to-date accounts of accepted practice and careful assessments of the potential value of new approaches to the diagnosis of sexually transmitted diseases. We join in wishing the book the success that it clearly deserves.

J. G. Collee
Head, Department of Bacteriology
Edinburgh University Medical School
Edinburgh, Scotland

D. H. H. Robertson
Head, Department of Genito-Urinary Medicine
Edinburgh University and The Royal Infirmary
Edinburgh, Scotland

Preface

Sexually transmitted diseases represent a major communicable disease problem on a global scale. The extent of their morbidity and mortality is now known to range from uncomplicated local genital infection to the lethal consequences of the acquired immunodeficiency syndrome (AIDS). Between these extremes lies their significant impact on infertility resulting from pelvic inflammatory disease, the health and well-being of the fetus and neonate, and the possible viral etiology of genital malignancy, particularly cervical carcinoma.

It is now clearly recognized that the control of sexually transmitted diseases requires the highly coordinated and collaborative efforts of many groups of health care personnel, including physicians, nurses, microbiologists, and epidemiologists, as well as those with responsibility for health education. Those in the forefront of health care have been fortunate in being supported by a cadre of enthusiastic and able researchers who have studied the basic biology of the pathogens, the pathophysiology of the diseases, and the development and application of new diagnostic methods.

It is this background that allowed the rapid exploitation of the pioneering work of George Köhler and Cesar Milstein on the production of individual mono-clonal antibodies of precise specificity by cloned hybrid cells. The diagnostic

potential of selecting monoclonal antibodies of required specificity was quickly
appreciated, thus underlining the particularly close relationship among diagnosis,
therapy, and epidemiology of sexually transmitted diseases. Because effective
management depends on a specific organismic diagnosis from within a broad spectrum of diverse infectious agents, a wide range of diagnostic methods is employed.
These include direct microscopy of exudates, conventional culture and identification, immunological detection of antigen, and the detection of specific antibodies. The rate of progress has been such that monoclonal antibodies have made
a major impact on each type of method and are already used routinely in the
diagnosis of gonococcal, chlamydial, and herpesvirus infections.

In this text we have not attempted to include every possible sexually transmissible infection but have selected a team of internationally renowned contributors to cover those areas where the monoclonal antibody technology is most advanced and where the development of monoclonal antibodies might be most
helpful. We have considered the role of immunological methods in the overall
diagnostic strategy and assessed the utility of monoclonal antibody reagents
already in routine use, as well as outlining current developments and future applications. We have striven throughout to provide appropriate background information on the choice of antigens and the selection and characterization of monoclonal antibodies, thus allowing the more specialized reader a full appreciation
of the significance and diagnostic implications of monoclonal antibody reagents.
Therefore, not only will the book be of interest to researchers, microbiologists,
and physicians directly involved in the management of patients with sexually
transmitted diseases, but by increasing the awareness of improved diagnostic capabilities it should be of value to all professional groups who may also deal with
such patients. We hope that we have provided a sound understanding and frame-
work of knowledge into which subsequent advances can be easily assimilated.

Circumstances have necessitated the omission of the chapter on the new and
complex issues arising from infection with the human immunodeficiency viruses
and AIDS, but we hope that our readers will nevertheless appreciate the focus of
the text on other major sexually transmissible viral, bacterial, and protozoal
causes of disease.

We are grateful to our expert contributors from many countries who produced texts that were a pleasure to edit. Thanks are also due to Paul Dolgert and
William Cary of Marcel Dekker, Inc., who have given us expert advice and guidance throughout this project. Finally, we are indebted to Mrs. Marilyn Cole for
dedicated secretarial support.

Hugh Young
Alexander McMillan

Contributors

John P. Ackers, D.Phil. Senior Lecturer, Department of Medical Protozoology, London School of Hygiene and Tropical Medicine, London, England

Sharon A. Baker-Zander, M.S. Department of Medicine, Division of Infectious Diseases, University of Washington, School of Medicine, Seattle, Washington

Janice E. Boyd, Ph.D.* Research Fellow, Department of Surgery, Edinburgh University Medical School, Edinburgh, Scotland

Solgun M. Bygdeman, M.D., Ph.D. Assistant Professor, Department of Clinical Bacteriology, Karolinska Institute, Huddinge University Hospital, Huddinge, Stockholm, Sweden

*Current affiliation: Cell Culture Development Manager, Damon Biotech Ltd., Kirkton Campus, Livingston, Scotland.

Charles S. F. Easmon, M.D., Ph.D., M.R.C.Path. Professor, Department of Medical Microbiology, Wright Fleming Institute, St. Mary's Hospital Medical School, London, England

Elizabeth E. Edmond, M.B.Ch.B., F.R.C.Path.[†] Senior Lecturer and Honorary Consultant, Department of Bacteriology, Edinburgh University Medical School, Edinburgh, Scotland

Edward A. C. Follett, Ph.D., M.R.C.Path. Head, Hepatitis Reference Laboratory, Regional Virus Laboratory, Ruchill Hospital, Glasgow, Scotland

Ian W. Halliburton, Ph.D. Senior Lecturer, Department of Microbiology, MRC Herpesvirus Research Group, University of Leeds, Leeds, England

Helena F. Hart, Ph.D. Manager, Research and Development, Bioscot Ltd., Edinburgh, Scotland

Catherine A. Ison, Ph.D., F.I.M.L.S. Research Assistant, Department of Medical Microbiology, Wright Fleming Institute, St. Mary's Hospital Medical School, London, England

Keith James, Ph.D., D.Sc., F.R.C.Path., F.R.S.E. Reader, Department of Surgery, Edinburgh University Medical School, Edinburgh, Scotland

Cho-chou Kuo, M.D., Ph.D. Professor, Department of Pathobiology, University of Washington, Seattle, Washington

Anton F. H. Luger, Dr. Med. Hofrat, Professor and Head, Ludwig Boltzmann Institut für Dermato-Venerologische Serodiagnostik, University of Vienna, Vienna, Austria

Sheila A. Lukehart, Ph.D. Research Associate Professor, Division of Infectious Diseases, University of Washington, School of Medicine, Seattle, Washington

Alexander McMillan, M.D., F.R.C.P. (Ed.) Consultant Physician, Department of Genito-Urinary Medicine, The Royal Infirmary, Edinburgh, Scotland

Mary Norval, Ph.D., D.Sc. Lecturer, Department of Bacteriology, Edinburgh University Medical School, Edinburgh, Scotland

John F. Peutherer, M.D., F.R.C.Path., M.R.C.P. (Ed.) Senior Lecturer, Department of Bacteriology, Edinburgh University Medical School, Edinburgh, Scotland

---

[†]Deceased.

Katherine G. Reid, Ph.D.   Assistant Microbiologist, Protein Fractionation Centre, Scottish Blood Transfusion Service, Edinburgh, Scotland

Eric G. Sandström, M.D., Ph.D.   Associate Professor, Department of Dermato-venereology, Karolinska Institute, Stockholm, Sweden

Isabel W. Smith, Ph.D.   Senior Lecturer, Department of Bacteriology, Edinburgh University Medical School, Edinburgh, Scotland

Richard S. Stephens, Ph.D., M.P.H.*   Research Immunologist, Department of Biomedical and Environmental Health Sciences, School of Public Health, University of California, Berkeley, California

Hiroshi Takahashi, M.D., Ph.D.   Research Fellow, Gastrointestinal Unit, Massachusetts General Hospital, Boston, Massachusetts

Milton R. Tam, Ph.D.   Program Manager, Department of Microbiology, Genetic Systems Corporation, Seattle, Washington

Jack R. Wands, M.D.   Associate Physician, Gastrointestinal Unit, Massachusetts General Hospital, Boston, Massachusetts

Hugh Young, Ph.D., M.R.C.Path.   Senior Lecturer, Department of Bacteriology, Edinburgh University Medical School, Edinburgh, Scotland

Alexander Yule, Ph.D.   Research Fellow, Department of Medical Protozoology, London School of Hygiene and Tropical Medicine, London, England

---

*Current affiliation: Assistant Adjunct Professor, Department of Pharmaceutical Chemistry, University of California, San Francisco, California.

Contents

Immunological Diagnosis of Sexually Transmitted Diseases

ONE

Development of Monoclonal Antibodies

Janice E. Boyd* and Keith James
Edinburgh University
Medical School
Edinburgh, Scotland

*Current affiliation: Damon Biotech Ltd., Kirkton Campus, Livingston, Scotland.

I. INTRODUCTION

Hybridoma technology has advanced enormously in the decade since Köhler and Milstein (1975) announced the production of a specific antibody-secreting hybrid cell line derived from immune mouse spleen cells. Such monoclonal antibodies (MAbs) are a pure form of a single antibody, each molecule in the preparation having identical structure, specificity, and avidity.

As most of the MAbs discussed in subsequent chapters are of murine origin, the basic steps involved in the production of these antibodies are shown in Fig. 1.

A rodent hybridoma is made by fusion of antibody-forming cells of the spleen or lymph node of an immunized animal with a myeloma cell line. Unfused spleen cells survive only about 2 weeks in culture, whereas myeloma cell lines survive indefinitely, i.e., they are immortal. However, culture conditions are adjusted so that only the product of a fusion between a spleen cell and a myeloma cell survives. The method of selecting such hybrid cells is outlined in Fig. 1. This method depends upon the principle that cells can make DNA by two routes: namely by de novo synthesis of nucleotides or by a salvage pathway that uses preformed nucleotides. The drug aminopterin blocks de novo synthesis of purines and pyrimidines. In the presence of culture medium containing hypoxanthine, aminopterin, and thymidine (HAT), spleen cells that contain the enzyme hypoxanthine-guanine phosphoribosyl transferase (HPRT), can use the salvage pathway to synthesize DNA. However, myeloma cell lines such as NS-1 (Table 1) lack the HPRT enzyme and cannot grow in the presence of aminopterin. Thus only the fusion partnership combining the HPRT activity of the spleen cell with the immortality of the myeloma cell can survive. This method of obtaining hybrids is known as HAT selection. Hybrid supernatants are screened for the antibody of interest, and cloned cell lines are cultured in bulk to produce the required amounts of MAb.

A. Historical Background

1. Early Developments

Although antibodies were discovered in 1890 by von Behring and Kitazato, it was not until 1958 (Nossal and Lederberg) that a single antibody-producing cell was demonstrated to secrete only one specific antibody. During the 1950s, in vitro cell culture techniques were developed into routine laboratory procedures.

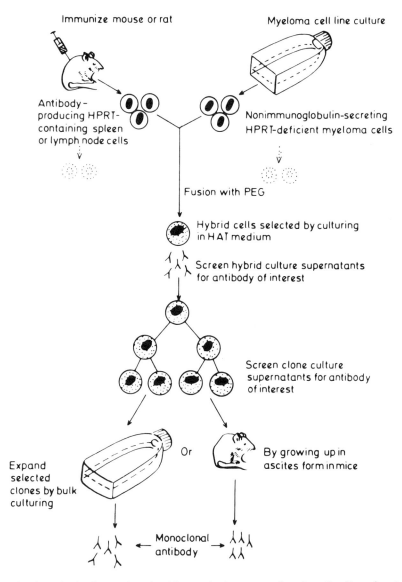

Fig. 1 Principal steps involved in producing monoclonal antibodies of rodent origin (*Source*: from James et al., 1984).

Table 1 Rodent Fusion Partners

Cell line	Derivation	Ig expression[a]	Reference
		A. *Mouse*	
4TO.2	45.6TG1.7	IgG_{2b} (κ)	Marguilies et al. (1976)
P3-X63/Ag8	P3K	IgG_1 (κ)	Köhler and Milstein (1975)
NSI/1.Ag4.1	P3-X63/Ag8	κ Nonsecretor	Köhler et al. (1976)
FOX-NY	NSI/1.Ag4.1	None	Taggart and Samloff (1983)
SP2/0	P3-X63/Ag8 hybrid	None	Schulman et al. (1978)
X63.Ag8.653	P3-X63/Ag	None	Kearney et al. (1979)
NSO/U	NSI/1.Ag4.1	None	Galfre and Milstein (1981)
		B. *Rat*	
Y3-Ag1.2.3	210.RCY3.Ag1	(κ)	Galfre et al. (1979)
YB2/3.0Ag20	Y3 X AO	None	Lachmann et al. (1980)
IR983F	Y3.Ag1.2.3	None	Bazin (1980)

[a]Ig expression: antibody isotype (light chain) secreted unless otherwise stated.

Spontaneous fusion of cultured mouse cells was observed (Barski et al., 1960) and the frequency enhanced using certain viruses (Okada and Tadokoro, 1962). However, separation of the fused cells from unfused cells was a problem until Littlefield (1964) solved it using enzyme-deficient cell lines followed by HAT selection, the same basic method that is used today.

This selection method stimulated the routine application of cell hybridization procedures, and because the resulting hybrids tended to be genetically unstable through preferential loss of chromosomes, the method was widely used to map genes to their individual chromosomes.

2. Myelomas

Researchers working on immunological tumors had discovered that multiple myeloma was a neoplasm of antibody-secreting cells and that each tumor was derived from a single clone (Cohn, 1967). This discovery permitted the isolation of large amounts of homogeneous antibodies for immunochemical studies. The artificial induction of myelomas in mice using mineral oil (Potter and Boyce, 1962), coupled with in vitro cell culture techniques, led to the development of large numbers of well-characterized immunoglobulin-secreting cell lines, although few appeared to react with identifiable antigens (Cohn, 1967; Potter et al., 1977).

3. Virus Transformation

Alternative methods were sought for immortalizing antibody-secreting cells, and a number of viruses were used to transform immune lymphocytes. Strosberg et al.

(1974) used simian virus 40 (SV40) to transform cells from a rabbit immunized with pneumococcal type III polysaccharide and isolated a line secreting small amounts of specific antibody. Baumal et al. (1971) used Epstein-Barr virus (EBV) to transform human lymphocytes from an immune donor. By this approach, several lymphoblastoid cell lines (LCL) were established that secreted large amounts of antibody, but none was specific for the immunizing antigen. However more recently, EBV transformation has been successfully used to produce a variety of human, specific antibody-secreting cell lines (see Sect. II.B).

4. Hybridization Studies

In the meantime, studies on the effects of fusing myeloma cells were being undertaken to analyze the expression of immunoglobulin genes. Spontaneous hybrid formation at frequencies of $1:10^6 - 10^7$ cells provided sufficient lines for these studies. Sendai virus promotion of fusion was largely unsuccessful, probably because most mouse myeloma cells lack virus receptors. However, Cotton and Milstein (1973) successfully fused rat with mouse myelomas by using Sendai virus and demonstrated that the hybrids continued to secrete both mouse heavy and light chains and rat light chains. At the same time, Schwaber and Cohen (1973) formed hybrids between human lymphocytes and mouse myeloma cells that secreted both human and mouse immunoglobulins (Igs).

Subsequent fusions of myeloma lines established a number of basic principles concerning hybrid expression of immunoglobulins. Crucially, hybrids continue to secrete all the Ig chains synthesized by the parent lines, irrespective of class or subclass of antibody (Marguilies et al., 1976; Milstein et al., 1976). Thus expression of Ig genes in hybrids is codominant, indicating that soluble mediators are not involved in their regulation. Furthermore, no new Igs are synthesized (Milstein and Köhler, 1977). Fusion of an antibody-secreting cell with a nonproducing variant does not extinguish Ig production (Köhler et al., 1976). Detailed studies of the Igs secreted by these hybrids indicated that many were mixed molecules containing heavy and light chains from both parents (Marguilies et al., 1976).

Continuation of this work was hampered by the low frequency of hybrid formation, thus when Davidson and Gerald (1976) reported polyethylene glycol (PEG)-promoted fusion of adherent cells, the method was quickly adapted for use with myeloma and spleen cells in suspension (Köhler and Milstein, 1976; Margulies et al., 1976). Further studies by Gefter et al. (1977) showed that optimum concentration and time of exposure considerably increased fusion frequencies.

5. Specific Antibody-Secreting Cells

All of these developments acquired greater importance when Köhler and Milstein (1975) fused a HAT-sensitive MOPC-21 myeloma with spleen cells derived from a mouse immunized with sheep red blood cells (SRBC) and produced several cloned hybrid lines secreting specific SRBC antibody. These cell lines could be grown as tumors in mice and thus were known as hybridomas. Further studies indicated that the hybrids produced were not a random representation of the initial spleen cell population because the percentage of Ig-secreting cells was increased from 5% in the spleen up to 95% in the hybrids, the latter figure depending upon the parent myeloma (Clark and Milstein, 1981). Thus, it appears that antibody-secreting cells are preferentially fused to form stable hybrids. It was also demonstrated that the antibodies secreted by the hybrids were generally representative of the antibodies secreted by the spleen cells. Therefore, when specific hybrids are required, it is important to ensure that a large proportion of spleen B cells have been antigen-stimulated before fusion.

II. PRODUCTION AND SELECTION

There is now a limited choice of species, namely mouse, rat, and man, in which to attempt the production of MAbs. Mice tend to be the first choice because they are convenient to handle and breed rapidly, although rats are a suitable alternative, offering similar advantages (Clark et al., 1983; Galfre et al., 1979). Human MAbs have many potential uses, in particular to replace the diagnostic and therapeutic antibodies currently derived from pooled immune plasma. One of the main considerations is the ability to induce a suitable immune response to the antigen in question. Second, there must be a method for immortalizing the immune lymphocytes so produced. Finally, the envisaged application may also influence the species used.

A. Rodent Cell Lines

1. Choice of Immunogen

Microorganisms are antigenically complex, and this complexity may lead to problems, because the response to individual components in a mixture will be variable, some antigens being immunodominant even when present in trace amounts. Nevertheless, a large number of MAbs have been raised against a variety of microorganisms (see Appendix) using different forms of immunogen. These include whole cells, cellular fractions, cell wall extracts, purified proteins or carbohydrates, in addition to bacterial products such as toxins and enzymes. In general, it appears that MAbs raised against whole bacterial cells are probably protective, either specificly or cross-reactively, whereas cell extracts induce the formation of highly specific MAbs. Antitoxin MAbs also are obviously potentially protective.

2. Immunization Schedule

There are many factors that can influence the immune response, and it may be necessary to try several immunization schedules and even different strains of animals before a suitable response is elicited (Boumsell and Bernard, 1980; Nussbaum et al., 1985). In general, bacterial extracts are highly immunogenic, and immunity can be achieved with two or three doses of antigen given over a short period of 3-4 weeks. Water-soluble proteins are usually given in the form of a water-in-oil emulsion, with or without heat-killed organisms of *Mycobacterium tuberculosis*, i.e., complete and incomplete Freund's adjuvant. Alternatively, protein antigens may be precipitated on alum, with or without the addition of killed *Bordetella pertussis* organisms. It should be noted, however, that many bacterial extracts contain traces of lipopolysaccharide, in itself a potent mitogen, which can act synergistically with complete Freund's adjuvant (CFA) with lethal consequences (Byars, 1984). The use of adjuvant can also influence the class of antibody elicited, as was demonstrated by Galloway et al. (1984) who immunized mice with toxin or toxoid plus adjuvant and produced IgG_1 MAbs, whereas infected mice yielded largely IgM MAbs.

The dose of antigen given can range from 1-100 μg and partly depends upon the purity of antigen as well as its likely immunogenicity. We have found that protein I extracts from *Neisseria gonorrhoeae* in 5 μg doses generated good responses and yielded a large number of specific MAbs with a range of isotypes—M, G_1, G_{2a}, G_{2b}, G_3. In contrast, pure protein antigens, such as hormones, produced an excellent response after one injection of 50-100 μg protein in CFA, followed 6 weeks later by the same amount in alum: the resultant hybrids were mainly of the IgG_1 isotype. Injections are normally given intraperitoneally, although subcutaneous administration over multiple sites can increase the response to less immunogenic antigens (Nussbaum et al., 1985). Gastric intubation has been used as a method for producing IgA-secreting hybrids (Colwell et al., 1982).

Intact bacterial cells, viable, heat-killed, or formalized, are highly immunogenic, and doses of 10^6 to 4-5 $\times$ 10^9 have been given intraperitoneally, subcutaneously, and intravenously (see Appendix).

The mice should always be rested for at least 1 month before the final antigenic boost. An intravenous boost with soluble protein will then ensure a vigorous blast-cell response. To increase this final response further, some authors recommend three to four daily injections before fusion (Cianfriglia et al., 1983; Stähli et al., 1980).

A novel method of immunization is to inject the antigen intrasplenically into an unimmunized mouse, followed by fusion of the spleen cells 3-4 days later (Spitz et al., 1984). Only minute amounts of antigen are required, and it is claimed that both IgG and IgM MAbs can be generated.

A variety of methods for enhancing production of antigen-specific hybrids has been explored. These include adoptive transfer of immune spleen cells into syngeneic, irradiated mice or in vitro culture of immunized cells with antigen (Fox et al., 1981). Nonimmune lymphocytes have also been stimulated in vitro with antigen plus additional factors such as thymocyte-conditioned medium

(Borrebaeck, 1983; Pardue et al., 1983; Reading, 1982), EL-4 thymoma-conditioned medium (Ma et al., 1984), or the adjuvant peptide N-acetylmuramyl-L-alanyl-D-iso-glutamine (Boss, 1984). Rathjen and Underwood (1985) observed that the limiting factor in stimulating nonimmune lymphocytes in vitro was the batch of young calf serum used.

3. Source of Lymphoid Cells

The spleen is the major source of immune cells from animals, yielding $2\text{-}3 \times 10^8$ cells of which 5% will be antibody-secreting. Draining lymph node cells can also be used and may yield a different spectrum of isotypes, depending upon the route of immunization.

Generally, no further manipulations of the immune cells are performed before fusion, but where the percentage of antigen-specific cells may be low, a number of enrichment procedures can be attempted. These are illustrated in Fig. 2 and can be broadly grouped into rosetting, panning, and the use of a cell separator.

4. Fusion Partners

There is a large choice of rodent myelomas that grow in culture, but not all of these make suitable fusion partners. To remove the risk of producing mixed antibody molecules, it is best to choose a cell line that is not only a nonsecretor but also a total nonproducer. The popular NS-1 line, for instance, synthesizes but does not secrete κ chains but its hybrids can produce MAbs containing two different light chains, the NS-1 κ chain secretion being reactivated in the presence of the spleen heavy chain (Milstein et al., 1976).

The main murine fusion partners are descendants of the MOPC-21 myeloma derived from a BALB/c mouse originally used by Cotton and Milstein (1973). Variants have been selected for loss of heavy and light chain synthesis and the X63.Ag8.653 and NSO lines are probably the most widely used. Sp2/0 is also a popular fusion partner and is itself a nonproducing hybrid (see Table 1).

The choice of rat myelomas is more restricted (see Table 1), but there are two nonproducers, one is an interstrain hybrid, YB2/0, whose hybrids must be grown in F_1 rats.

5. Fusion Procedures

Currently, there are three approaches for promoting the fusion of lymphoid cells: chemical, electrical, and antigen-driven. Chemical fusion is mediated by PEG, and electrical fusion requires a high-voltage pulse generator.

a. Polyethylene Glycol-Assisted. There are innumerable variables to this method, and a number of reports have described the principles and problems (Fazekas de St Groth and Scheidegger, 1980; Lane et al., 1984; Westerwoudt, 1985). The main variable appears to be the PEG itself, largely stemming from our ignorance of what factors in it are crucial for high fusion rates. Because PEG is toxic at the

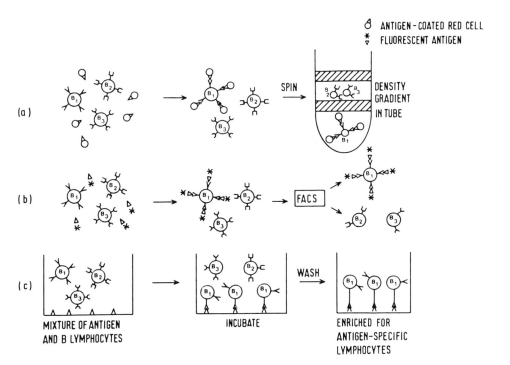

Fig. 2 Methods for isolating antigen-reactive lymphocytes: (a) rosetting with antigen-coated red cells and density gradient separation; (b) reaction with fluorescent antigen and separation by a cell sorter (FACS); (c) adsorption to antigen attached to plastic followed by elution of specific cells.

concentrations used for fusion (35-50%), successful hybridization is then the result of a fine balance between toxicity and no fusion. Variables include not only molecular weight (1000-4000), manufacturer, batch number, method of sterilization, diluent used, pH, and concentration, but also the addition of dimethylsulfoxide (DMSO), time and temperature of fusion, inclusion of a centrifugation step, and rate of dilution after fusion. The influence of some of these variables has been discussed previously (Fazekas de St Groth and Scheidegger, 1980; Lane et al., 1984).

In addition to fusing cells in suspension, other methods have been reported in which cells are fused as an adherent monolayer prepared by spinning the cell mixture onto a petri dish (McKearn, 1980) or a Millipore filter (Galfre and Milstein, 1981).

A further variable is the ratio of spleen to myeloma cells, the normal range being one to 10 spleen cells to one myeloma. For whole spleen cell suspensions we use a ratio of 3-4:1 but with antigen-enriched suspensions a ratio of 1:1 would be chosen.

b. Electrofusion. Cell fusion has been induced by electrical impulses to form hybridomas derived from both B lymphocytes (Zimmermann and Vienken, 1982) and T lymphocytes (Gravekamp et al., 1985). There are two stages to the process: first, an alternating electrical field brings the cells into close contact forming a "pearl chain," and second, fusion is induced by the application of a high-voltage pulse (3000-5000 V/cm) for a short time (10-50 μsec). Fusion occurs in a matter of seconds or minutes.

c. Antigen-Directed Fusion. Antigen-promoted cell fusion in which antigens were incorporated into the membranes of the fusion partner (P3 or Sp2/0) via a synthetic lipopolysaccharide carrier molecule without affecting their viability was reported in 1980 by Bankert et al. These cells were centrifuged with immune spleen cells and then plated out in HAT selection medium as before, except that no PEG was required. The percentage of antigen-specific hybrids was consistently greater than that yielded by PEG-mediated fusion, and in addition, the antibodies were less cross-reactive with analogues of the immunizing antigen.

This approach has been developed further by Lo et al. (1984) who used electrical impulses to promote cell fusion which generated MAbs of high affinity. The basic procedure is outlined in Fig. 3 and is based on the high affinity of avidin for biotin. Although the numbers of hybrid lines produced by this method are small, theoretically they should all be secreting specific antibody. With use of this method, MAbs with affinities 100 times greater than average have been reported.

6. Selection and Growth of Hybrids

a. Selection in Hypoxanthine, Aminopterin, Thymidine Medium. The basis for HAT selection has already been illustrated in Fig. 1. Some authors advocate a delay in initiation of HAT selection until 24 hr after fusion (Oi and Herzenberg, 1980); however, we have found that by this stage the myeloma cell numbers have doubled, thus increasing the amount of cell debris created when the unfused cells die.

Selection with HAT is continued until no viable myeloma cells are present in the appropriate control wells. However, hypoxanthine and thymidine (HT) continue to be supplied to the cells because of the lingering effects of aminopterin which is only slowly metabolized (Goding, 1983). Aminopterin is effective at a concentration of 10^{-9} M and because it is present in HAT at 4×10^{-7} M, its concentration must drop by more than 400-fold for the enzyme to regain its activity.

b. Other Selection Methods. Alternative selection methods include the strategy devised by Taggart and Samloff (1983) which is based on the Robertsonian (8.12)5

STEP 1   Label cells (a) Myeloma cell + NHS – biotin

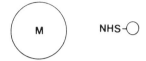

(b) B Lymphocyte + Avidin – antigen

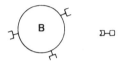

STEP 2   Mix labeled cells

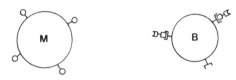

STEP 3   Specific adherence

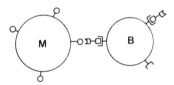

STEP 4   Apply voltage to fuse

NHS ─◯ Normal human serum – biotin
    └┘ Immunoglobulin
  Σ─□ Avidin – antigen

Fig. 3 Antigen-directed electrically mediated cell fusion. Myeloma cells are labeled with biotin. Soluble antigen is coupled covalently to avidin and binds specifically to lymphocytes. When mixed together, avidin binds to biotin thus holding the specific lymphocyte to a myeloma cell, and cells are fused by electrical discharge.

Bnr mouse in which the active heavy chain Ig locus on chromosome 12 is genetically linked to a selectable enzyme marker locus on chromosome 8 (adenosine phosphoribosyl transferase; APRT). Spleen cells from these mice were fused with a spontaneous mutant of NS-1, deficient in both HGPRT and APRT (FOX-NY). Those hybrids, which were capable of surviving in a medium requiring APRT activity, were also antibody-secreting because the two functions are linked.

Two selection procedures have been devised that do not require the use of drug-marked fusion partners. One used a fluorescent-activated cell sorter (FACS) to select fibroblastic hybrids (Jongkind et al., 1979). A similar strategy could be used in which, before fusion, myeloma cells are tagged with a fluorescein-lipid dye conjugate and spleen cells are tagged with rhodamine-lipid dye conjugate. After fusion, cells bearing both dyes and of the correct size for a hybridoma could be detected by the FACS and directed into wells of a microtiter plate (Shay, 1985).

In the second method, myeloma cells were pretreated with an irreversible biochemical inhibitor, such as iodoacetamide or diethylpyrocarbonate, which prevents the function of certain essential enzymes thereby leading to cell death (Wright, 1978). Fusion with a lymphocyte would restore the lost biochemical functions and provide the hybrid with a full complement of enzyme activity. However, although theoretically sound, in practice the drugs tended to leak from dead myeloma cells and poison the hybrids.

c. Feeder Cells and Factors.   Peritoneal macrophages are a useful addition in the culture well because they clear away cell debris created by the death of the unfused myeloma cells. They can increase the yield of hybridomas (Fazekas de St Groth and Scheidegger, 1980), perhaps by recycling nutrients within the culture (Reading, 1982). Thymocytes are often used as feeders, either as cells or in the form of thymocyte-conditioned medium (TCM) (Reading, 1982). Human endothelial culture supernatant (HECS) (Astaldi, 1983) and human umbilical cord serum (Westerwoudt et al., 1983) also contain factors that promote the growth of hybridomas.

7. Cloning

Hybrid cell lines must be cloned from an early stage for several reasons. It ensures true monoclonality of the product and overcomes the chromosomal instability inherent in hybrid cells. In addition, it prevents overgrowth by nonsecreting cells, which usually have a faster growth rate. Cloning should be repeated until $> 90\%$ of clones tested secrete specific antibody, this being used as an indicator of the stability of the line (Reading, 1982).

Because one successful fusion can create many hundreds of hybrids which could yield 10 times that number of clones, good record keeping then is vital. An essential part of this is to have a logical but simple numbering system for hybrids and clones. There is now no recognized standard method, but many laboratories identify a hybrid by its position on the microtiter plate, e.g., 1F11, whose clones may then be 1F11A3, 1F11C5. We have evolved what we feel to be a better system as follows: Each fusion is numbered, e.g., 121, and hybrids are numbered sequentially as their supernatants are tested, e.g., 121/44. Clones of each line are likewise numbered sequentially as they are tested, preceded by a point, e.g., 121/44.2 and subclones similarly, e.g., 121/44.2.1. No confusion can arise because each hybrid and its clones have a unique sequence of numbers. For publication purposes, and once a line has been characterized, it is given an ES number (Edinburgh, Surgery), e.g., 121/44.2.1 = ES10.

Cloning may be performed by several procedures including the following.

a. Limiting Dilution. Small numbers of cells are seeded into microtiter wells either by dilution in the range from 10 to 0.3 cells per well, or by micromanipulation when single cells are placed directly into each well (Gagnon and Raymond, 1985). Feeder cells, e.g., thymocytes or macrophages, may be added to the wells or factors such as TCM (Reading, 1982), HECS (Astaldi, 1983), human low-density lipoproteins (Mao and France, 1984), or macrophage-conditioned medium (Sugasawara et al., 1985) may be added to the culture medium.

b. Soft Agar. Small numbers of clump-free cells are suspended in a soft agar medium and poured into petri dishes which may contain feeder cells (Goding, 1980). However, growth of colonies in soft agar is not widely used because it requires an extra step of picking colonies at random and regrowing them in liquid medium before testing. However, the colonies may sometimes be screened for specific antibody in situ, e.g., by RBC lysis or immune precipitate formation. Davis et al. (1982) plated out the cell mixture immediately after fusion into methylcellulose that contained thymocytes and HAT. Separate hybrid colonies that grew up in this soft medium were assumed to be clonal and were grown on for testing without further cloning.

c. Cell Sorting. Antigen-specific hybrid cells can be identified by direct binding with fluorescent antigen or by antigen-coated fluorescent microspheres. Cells can then be analyzed by a FACS which directs labeled cells singly into wells of a microtiter plate (Parks et al., 1979). This could be a method for rescuing a small number of specific cells in an overgrown culture.

8. Freezing of Cell Lines

A sample of antigen-specific hybridoma cells should be stored in liquid nitrogen as soon as possible. This acts as a fallback should instability or contamination occur. Thereafter, cells should be stored on several occasions, ideally one from each batch being tested for recovery of the line, although this is time-consuming if many lines are being handled. We use as freezing medium 50% FCS, 45% RPMI 1640, 5% DMSO, and if cells spun out from 8-10 ml of a well-grown culture are resuspended in 0.5 ml freezing medium, there should be no problems in recovering viable cells. Vials are placed in polystyrene boxes overnight at −70°C before transfer to vapor phase liquid nitrogen storage. Records of cells and their clones must be kept meticulously and a computer program is available for aiding such record-keeping (Franklin, 1982). Wells and Price (1983) have devised a method for freezing whole 96-well plates of hybrids, while Harwell et al. (1984) freeze down some of the fusion mixture after 3 days in culture. These are both useful strategies for providing time to characterize the MAbs created, especially where a fusion has been highly successful.

B. Human Cell Lines

1. Methods Available

The production of cell lines secreting human MAbs has a much shorter history than that of their rodent counterparts. The first reports of human-human hybridomas were in 1980 (Croce et al.; Olsson and Kaplan), although previously Steinitz et al. (1977) had used EBV to transform human lymphocytes into specific antibody-secreting lines. Since then hybridization and EBV transformation have been developed and refined, even combined, to produce human MAbs with a wide range of specificities. Nevertheless, a considerable gap in our knowledge remains to be filled before the production of human MAbs becomes a routine procedure.

Looking to the future, there are exciting new approaches being developed in the field of genetic engineering. Immune mouse spleen cells have been transfected with human leukemia-derived DNA to form stable lines secreting specific antibody (Jonak et al., 1984) and a similar approach could be taken using human lymphocytes. Furthermore, murine Ig genes have been cloned and expressed in a nonproducing hybridoma line (Sp2/0) (Ochi et al., 1983). Comparable developments with human genes could lead to "genetic immunization" either by rescuing the genome of existing human hybrid cells or by the chemical synthesis of DNA to produce tailor-made antibodies.

2. Sources of Lymphoid Cells

Peripheral blood lymphocytes obviously are the most readily available from man but not necessarily the most suitable for the purpose. Other lymphoid organs can be obtained occasionally, e.g., tonsil, spleen, lymph nodes, bone marrow, although the donor may not be in a suitable state of immunity. Tumor-draining lymph nodes and tumors themselves are another potential source of specific immune lymphocytes. However, lymphocytes from different sources seem to vary in their ability to form hybrids, as several comparative studies have shown (Chiorazzi et al., 1982; Cote and Houghton, 1985; Glassy et al., 1983). Particularly disappointing were the poor fusion rates for peripheral blood lymphocytes (PBL), although fusion with murine partners did yield more hybrids. Interestingly, murine PBL are also difficult to fuse (Olsson et al., 1983). Because specific lymphocytes may be present in only small numbers, they may be enriched either without prior antigen boosting (Winger et al.,1983) or after further stimulation (see following discussion).

3. Immunization

a. *In Vivo.* Deliberate immunization of humans is limited to those vaccines currently in use. Even when donors can be boosted safely, specific antibody-producing cells appear only transiently in circulation and the optimum time for blood collection must be ascertained. In experiments with tetanus toxoid-boosted donors, blood was richest in specifically stimulated B cells at day 6, although memory cells capable of secondary activation in vitro were present for up to 2 months (Burnett et al., 1985). In addition to deliberate immunization, there are other situations in which immunization can occur, such as after infection, pregnancy, blood transfusion, growth of a tumor etc. On some occasions, boosting in vivo is possible (and ethical), e.g., for blood group antibodies.

b. *In Vitro.* Peripheral blood lymphocytes from an immune donor may be stimulated further in vitro, given the correct culture conditons. Olsson and Brams (1985) have adapted an in vitro priming method developed by van Ness et al. (1984) for murine lymphocytes, in which human thymocyte-conditioned medium was added to lymphocytes and monocytes, with the antigen complexed to silica beads. Although the fusion frequency was not altered, it did increase the percentage of specific hybrids by about 20-fold. Human serum has been shown to contain components necessary for the primary in vitro immunization of human lymphocytes. Several groups have successfully produced human hybridomas following incubation with both soluble and cellular antigens (Cavagnaro and Osband, 1983; Ho et al., 1985; Strike et al., 1984).

Mitogenic stimulation of lymphocytes in culture has sometimes increased the fusion efficiency (Olsson et al., 1983; Shoenfield et al., 1982), but in others such stimulation has made little difference (Burnett et al., 1985; Teng et al., 1985b). However, when pokeweed mitogen (PWM) stimulation was combined with antigen and endothelial cells, Astaldi et al. (1982) found a dramatic increase in positive hybrids.

Epstein-Barr virus also has been used as a polyclonal stimulator of B cells before fusion, with or without selection of antigen-specific cells. In comparative experiments, transformed cells fused 36 and 63 times more readily than unstimulated PBL from the same donors (Atlaw et al., 1985; Kozbor and Roder, 1984).

4. Fusion Partners

As previously outlined, myeloma cell lines of murine origin have been cultured in vitro and are now well-characterized. Human myeloma cells, however, have proved to be very difficult to establish in culture, and therefore lymphoblastoid cell lines (LCL) derived from Epstein-Barr virus-transformed B lymphocytes have

Table 2 Human Fusion Partners

Fusion partner	Original line	Cell type[a]	Antibody produced	Drug markers[b]	Reference
SKO-007	U-266	Myeloma	IgE (λ)	8-AG	Olsson and Kaplan (1980)
RPMI-8226	RPMI-8226	Myeloma	λ	8-AG	Abrams et al. (1983)
RH-L4	RH-L4	Lymphoma	IgG (κ) non-secretor	8-AG	Olsson et al. (1983)
GM-1500 6TG-A11	GM1500	LCL	IgG_2 (κ)	6-TG	Croce et al. (1980)
KR-4	GM1500 6TG-A11	LCL	IgG_2 (κ)	6-TG, OUA	Kozbor et al. (1982a)
GM4672	GM1500	LCL	IgG_2 (κ)	6-TG	Croce et al. (1980)
LICR-LON-HMy2	ARH77	LCL	IgG_1 (κ)	8-AG	Edwards et al. (1982)
H35.1.1	WI-L2	LCL	IgM (κ)	8-AG	Chiorazzi et al. (1982)
UC7296	WI-L2	LCL	IgM (κ)	6-TG	Glassy et al. (1983)
GM0467.3	PGLC33H	LCL	IgM (λ)	8-AG	Chiorazzi et al. (1982)
MC/MNS-2	MC/CAR	LCL	IgG_1 (κ)	8-AG	Ritts et al. (1983)
LTR228	LTR228	LCL	IgM (κ)	6-TG	Larrick et al. (1983)
GK-5	—	LCL	κ	6-TG	Satoh et al. (1983)
KR-12	KR-4 x RPMI-8226	Hybrid myeloma (human-human)	IgG_2 (κ, λ)	6-TG, OUA	Kozbor et al. (1984)
SHM-D3	U266 x X63Ag8.653	Hybrid myeloma (mouse-human)	non-secretor	6-TG, OUA, G418	Teng et al. (1983)
3HL	SHM-D3 x B lymphoma	Hybrid (mouse-human-human)	IgM (λ)	6-TG, OUA, G418	Teng et al. (1985b)

[a] LCL, lymphoblastoid cell line.
[b] 8-AG, 8-azaguanine; 6-TG, 6-thioguanine; OUA, ouabain.

been used as alternative fusion partners (Table 2). A comparative study of the phenotypic characteristics of myelomas and LCL relative to their suitability as fusion partners, concluded that other characteristics such as fusion frequency, cloning efficiency, and growth rate, were just as important as morphology (Kozbor et al., 1983).

Although many LCL have been rendered HAT-sensitive and compared for fusion frequency with a few myeloma lines, no cell line has consistently shown itself superior in forming stable human hybrids (Abrams et al., 1983; Cote and Houghton, 1985). Initially, hybridization experiments were conducted using mouse myeloma cells as fusion partners, the mouse lines being advantageous both because of their higher fusion frequency and the availability of nonsecretors (Butler et al., 1983; Cote et al., 1983; Gigliotti et al., 1984). However, chromosomal instability of the hybrids continued to be a problem, and therefore several groups set about constructing fusion partner lines with the desired characteristics.

Teng et al. (1983) formed hybrids between mouse myeloma cells and a human myeloma U-266 and selected hybrid clones were screened for suitability as fusion partners with human lymphocytes from various sources. In a similar approach, Kozbor et al. (1984) fused a HAT-sensitive, ouabain-resistant LCL (KR4) with RPMI 8226, a human plasmacytoma. The resultant hybrids grew as well as KR4 but were phenotypically similar to myeloma cells. Other potential fusion partners have been created along similar lines (Foung et al., 1984; Östberg and Pursch, 1983; Posner et al., 1983).

5. Fusion Procedures

The methods available for producing human hybrids are the same as those for mouse hybrids, although changes may be required in the conditions under which PEG-mediated fusion is optimal. We have found that a batch of PEG that gives excellent fusion of mouse cells is not necessarily as efficient in human fusions.

Even when the initial fusion of cell membranes has been accomplished, nuclear fusion must also occur during the next cell division so that the daughter cells contain chromosomes from both parents within their nucleus. This requires the lymphocyte parent to be in a state of cell division and may explain the poor fusibility of PBL if used without prior antigenic or mitogenic stimulation (Olsson et al., 1983). It should also be noted that EBV-transformed lymphocytes, which are actively dividing, fuse with much higher frequencies than their untransformed counterparts (see Sect. II.B.3.b). Electrofusion may be a more efficient method where small numbers of cells are involved, such as following in vitro stimulation, and some human hybrids have been prepared in this manner (Glassy and Hofmann, 1985).

The lymphocyte/partner cell ratio seems to be crucial, 1:1 or 2:1 gives better results than 5:1 or 10:1 (Cote et al., 1983; Massicotte et al., 1984). Cells may be fused in suspension or as a monolayer, the latter method apparently being superior for human cells (Truitt et al., 1984a).

6. Selection and Growth of Hybrids

When enzyme-deficient partner lines are used, selection for hybrids is effected by the use of HAT medium, although aminopterin may be replaced with azaserine (Edwards et al., 1982) to increase hybrid formation. Delaying the addition of HAT for 24 hr also seems to increase fusion efficiency (Olsson et al., 1983). Selection methods other than HAT have already been mentioned in Sect. II.A.6.

Feeder cells are often required, depending upon the fusion partner, and range from murine macrophages or spleen cells (Kozbor and Roder, 1984), to human monocytes (Brodin et al., 1983; Olsson et al., 1983), or fibroblasts (Evans et al., 1984). The recently identified B-cell growth factors may also play a role here (Butler et al., 1984; Gordon et al., 1984).

It has generally been felt that mouse-human hybrids were less stable than human-human hybrids. However, when Cote and Houghton (1985) compared 67 mouse-mouse hybrids with a large number of human hybrids derived from mouse and human partners, loss of Ig secretion was comparable throughout. The immunoglobulin production by these hybrids was examined and 70-75% produced between 1 and 10 μg/ml, while 25-30% secreted between 11 and 100 μg/ml. Hybrids derived from fusion with one of the mouse-human heteromyelomas were examined for chromosome segregation (Teng et al., 1985b). Some hybrids stabilized with only three to four human chromosomes and loss of Ig secretion, while others retained 10 or 12 human chromosomes and continued to secrete antibody. The mechanisms involved are not yet known and, obviously, bear further investigation.

Human hybrids tend to secrete lower amounts of Ig than mouse hybrids, and Olsson and Brams (1985) have attempted to increase secretion by treatment with 5-azacytidine which methylates DNA. Results were variable, but about 40% of hybrids had increased Ig secretion, while some 20% of nonsecretors could be induced to produce Ig.

7. Epstein-Barr Virus Transformation

Epstein-Barr virus (EBV) is a member of the herpesvirus group which infects only primate B lymphocytes. Infection can cause a transient stimulation of Ig production and, in a proportion of infected cells, a state of immortalization, leading to the formation of continuous lymphoblastoid cell lines (Tosato et al., 1985). B lymphocytes from the pre-B-cell stage through to B lymphoblasts, but not plasma cells, express the virus receptor and hence are susceptible to transformation (Hansson et al., 1983). Recent evidence suggests that this is the C3d complement receptor, a 140,000 dalton glycoprotein (Frade et al., 1985). Lymphocytes can be infected by incubation with culture supernatant from a marmoset line, B95-8, which secretes infectious virus (Miller and Lipman, 1973) or by cocultivation with HAT-sensitive virus-transformed, Epstein-Barr virus nuclear antigen (EBNA)-positive cells (cell-driven transformation) (Siadak and Lostrom, 1985). Because virus transformation is so efficient, it is particularly suitable when limited cell numbers are available, such as after enrichment for B cells or antigen-specific cells using the methods outlined in Sect. II.A.3 (Fong et al., 1981; Steinitz et al., 1979). If in vitro antigenic stimulation is attempted, however, the incubation time before EBV infection must be short because activated B cells cannot be infected.

Because 90% of the population have been infected by EBV, either clinically in the form of infectious mononucleosis or, more usually, subclinically, there will exist in the circulation suppressor T lymphocytes that can recognize and kill autologous EBV infected lymphocytes (Rickinson et al., 1979). T lymphocytes can be removed before infection by rosette formation (Kaplan et al., 1976), panning (Tsoi et al., 1982), or addition of cyclosporin A (Crawford et al., 1983b).

After virus infection, the cells can be plated at much lower densities than hybrids, 10^3 cells per round-bottomed microtiter well, producing 100% transformation, in our experience. Feeder cells are necessary at this density, and many cell types have been used, including fetal fibroblasts (Rosen et al., 1983), allogeneic PBL (Crawford et al., 1983a), cord blood cells (Stein and Sigal, 1983) and autologous T cells, all of which are usually X-irradiated before use.

Most EBV-transformed lines produce IgM antibodies, although IgG and even IgA-producing lines have been reported. This bias presumably reflects the preponderance of IgM-bearing cells in circulation, because no difference in EBV receptor density has been found between different B-cell subpopulations (Aman et al., 1984). Cell-driven transformation apparently induces a higher proportion of IgG-secreting lines, although the exact mechanism is unclear.

Reported Ig secretion rates vary from low levels of 10 ng/ml to around 20 μg/ml; antibody secretion may fall off shortly after transformation or continue for several months before waning, even if the lines are cloned as early as possible. This reduction in Ig secretion may be caused by gradual loss of light chain synthesis (Kozbor et al., 1982b). Nevertheless, a number of specific antibody-secreting lines have been reported as being stable in culture for 3 years and longer (Crawford et al., 1983a; 1983b; Steinitz et al., 1977; 1980).

8. Fusion of Epstein-Barr Virus Lines

In an attempt to stabilize Ig production by LCL, Kozbor et al. (1982b) fused a tetanus toxoid-specific line (B6) with HAT-sensitive mouse myeloma cells. They utilized the natural difference in sensitivity to ouabain between mouse and human cells to select for hybrids. Thus, ouabain killed unfused human LCL while aminopterin killed unfused myeloma cells. This approach has been widely used following the development of HAT-sensitive and ouabain-resistant human and mouse-human partner lines (Foung et al., 1984; Kozbor et al., 1982a).

9. Cloning

Cloning of human antibody-secreting lines is important for the same reasons as those for mouse hybridomas. Human-human and mouse-human hybrids tend to clone well at fewer than one cell per well, depending, to some extent, upon the characteristics of the fusion partner. However, LCL are especially difficult to grow at fewer than 10 cells per well, even in the presence of feeder cells. Given this difficulty, most workers clone LCL several times at 10 cells per well before attempting one cell per well. Generally, if a line is still stable at this stage, it tends to remain so. The same range of feeder cells are used as after hybridization or transformation, and again, growth factors such as B-cell growth factor (BCGF) may turn out to be useful in promoting clonal growth.

III. SCREENING AND CHARACTERIZATION

A. Initial Screening

One of the crucial steps in producing MAbs for a specific purpose is the initial screening assay, the results of which will decide the fate of each hybrid created. Consideration must be given to the ultimate purpose of the MAb because, for example, detection of antigen in liquid phase demands different properties of an antibody than immunohistochemical detection of antigen in Formalin-fixed tissue. Mierendorf and Dimond (1983) obtained MAbs with different characteristics by using two separate assays for initial screening. Furthermore, fine specificity is not the only criterion to be considered, but other properties, such as avidity, pH optimum, effect of salt concentration, biological activity, etc., may be of equal importance in the envisaged application. The speed with which results can be generated is also crucial because rapidly growing hybridoma cells will not remain viable in microtiter wells for several days while a complicated in vivo study is conducted on their supernatant. A maximum of 2 days can be allowed. In addition, the assay itself must have been well-characterized and standardized before fusions are attempted and must be capable of coping with a sudden rush of 200 or more samples, 3 days a week.

1. Sampling

Strategies for sampling cell culture supernatants fall into two types: individual testing of each well as hybrid growth dictates; and blanket testing of all plates at a set time after fusion. Individual sampling is time-consuming if a large number of plates have been set up, but it tests each hybrid at the optimum time, therefore risking nothing.

On the other hand, blanket screening at a fixed time will inevitably result in some wells being overgrown while others are not ready. However, samples can be taken rapidly, a row at a time, using a multiple-channel pipette. There are also commercially available probes that can be precoated with sterile antigen and, after incubation in supernatant, transferred to a fresh plate containing suitable reactants (Olsson et al., 1983; Scheinberg et al., 1983). Tests, if simple, could be carried out on each plate on several occasions to maximize the chance of picking out suitable hybrids.

2. Types of Assays

The types of assays used to screen culture supernatants have been as varied as the uses devised for MAbs, and basic methods have been refined and adapted to suit individual requirements. Assays can be broadly grouped into solid- or liquid-phased antigen (labeled/unlabeled). The remainder of this section will concentrate on those assays commonly used to screen antimicrobial MAbs (Fig. 4a,b,c).

a. Solid-Phased Antigen. Many screening assays use antigen attached to a solid support—wells, tubes, beads—the variations being in the method by which antibody binding is detected (Fig. 4a). Radiolabeled protein A or affinity-purified antimouse immunoglobulin (heavy-chain specific, if required) can be used in RIA-type assays. Protein A, however, does not bind IgM and IgA, but it is useful in identifying IgG MAbs and resolving them into their various isotypes (Lindmark et al., 1983). Alternatively, a second antibody, e.g., rabbit antimouse Ig, can be added before detection with protein A. The individual wells in a plate may be cut out and counted or an autoradiographic picture of the whole plate developed to detect positive supernatants (Goldstein et al., 1983; Nowak et al., 1984). The enzyme-linked immunosorbent assay (ELISA) developed by Engvall and Perlmann (1972) has been extended and modified. In principle, binding of antibody to solid-phased antigen is detected by an anti-Ig conjugated to an enzyme, the binding of which can be revealed by substrate conversion and quantitated by change in optical density (OD) (Fig. 4a). Enzymes in common use are alkaline phosphatase, peroxidase, β-galactosidase, and urease. There are several advantages to this type of system, including speed, expense, and stability of reagents; qualitative or quantitative results; automation and storage of antigen-coated plates. However, background enzyme activity can interfere if cells are used as targets, and there is a limited dynamic range because the OD scale maximum is 2.0. Fluorescent-labeled conjugates are occasionally used as are fluorescent substrates, but these require special equipment to detect substrate changes (Leaback and Creme, 1980).

The antigens used in detection systems have included proteins such as toxins (Galloway et al., 1984), lipids (Morrison-Plummer et al., 1983), polysaccharides (Callahan et al., 1979), fixed bacteria (Cannon et al., 1984), and viable cells (Feit et al., 1983). Binding of soluble antigen to plastic is often through nonspecific forces and can be optimized by choice of buffer and pH (bicarbonate buffer at pH 9.6 is commonly used), and specially treated plates are now available with high- or low-binding characteristics. A comparative study of commercial ELISA

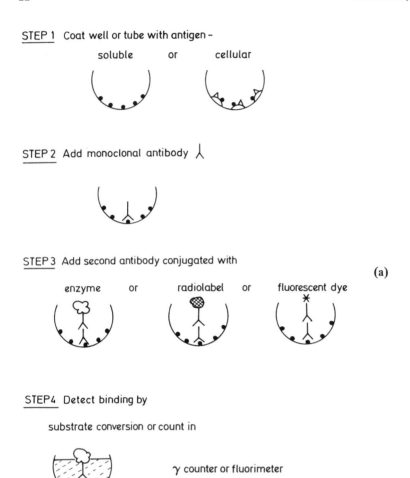

STEP 1   Coat well or tube with antigen –

soluble   or   cellular

STEP 2   Add monoclonal antibody λ

STEP 3   Add second antibody conjugated with   (a)

enzyme   or   radiolabel   or   fluorescent dye

STEP 4   Detect binding by

substrate conversion or count in

γ counter or fluorimeter

Fig. 4   Basic principles of assays for initial screening of monoclonal antibodies: (a) soluble or cellular antigens are adsorbed to wells/tubes. MAb binding can be detected by a second antibody conjugated with an enzyme followed by substrate conversion (ELISA), a radiolabel (RIA), or fluorescent dye (fluorimetry); (b) Radiolabeled soluble antigen is incubated with MAb and precipitated by binding to second antibody on solid phase; (c) anti-immunoglobulin on solid phase captures MAb. After reaction with unlabeled antigen, radiolabeled specific antibody is added and binds to complex.

STEP 1   Incubate radiolabeled antigen with MAb

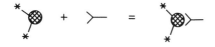

STEP 2   Add solid-phased anti-immunoglobulin   **(b)**

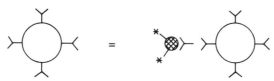

STEP 3   Counts bound to solid phase proportional
                to amount of MAb bound to antigen

STEP 1   Incubate solid-phased anti-immunoglobulin with MAb

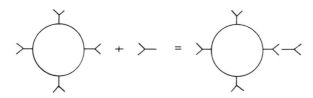

STEP 2   Add unlabeled antigen

STEP 3   Add labeled antibody specific for antigen

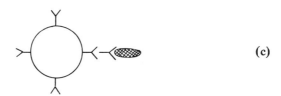

(c)

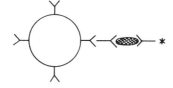

STEP 4   Counts bound to solid phase proportional to
          amount of MAb bound to antigen

plates has been undertaken by McCullough and Parkinson (1984). Terasaki microtest plates have been used in place of 96-well microtiter plates, thus reducing the amount of antigen required to less than 30 ng/well (Tanaka and Kurth, 1984).

Cells may adhere nonspecifically to wells/tubes or be encouraged by precoating with poly-L-lysine and subsequent fixation with gluteraldehyde (Kennett, 1980), although fixation may cause denaturation of surface antigens. Infected cells can be used as targets in wells or grown as coverslip cultures for direct examination using fluorescent conjugates to detect specifically bound MAb (Goldstein et al., 1983; Rosen et al., 1983).

b. Liquid Phase Antigen.   Double-antibody radioimmunoassay (RIA) can be used when the antigen is readily purified and can be labeled with ^{125}I without loss of antigenicity (Fig. 4b). Binding of MAb is detected by the addition of solid-phased antimouse Ig on Sephadex G-200 beads, and free labeled antigen is removed by a simple washing method in buffer containing sucrose (Wright and Hunter, 1982). Background counts are generally $<1\%$ total counts added. This method can be automated and is capable of handling several hundred samples at once, binding data being provided within 24 hr of sampling. Because antibody binding can be influenced by pH and salt concentration in the buffer used, a compromise must be reached for general screening, e.g., 0.25 M TRIS, pH 8.5. One further problem is that antibodies specific for the labeled sites in the antigen may be inhibited from binding. An alternative method (Fig. 4c) does not require a pure antigen preparation but uses a radiolabeled polyclonal antibody specific for the antigen and a solid-phased anti-Ig to capture the MAb (Hughes et al., 1984). Large glass beads are often used as solid phase, and washing steps are, therefore, greatly simplified.

c. Other Assays.   Some assays, such as the bacterial enzyme β-D-galactosidase (Frackelton and Rotman, 1980), bacterial toxins, or virus neutralization (see Appendix), can be used to measure a change in the biological activity of the antigen.

B. Isotyping

The isotype of an MAb can have important implications for its suitability for a particular purpose. For example, complement-mediated lysis cannot be effected by a noncomplement-fixing isotype, i.e., IgG_1 in the mouse. The initial screening test can be designed to discriminate for those isotypes desired or against those not desired. Our experience has been that soluble protein antigens tend to yield IgG_1 MAbs in mice, red cell antibodies are largely IgM (agglutinating antibodies), whereas bacterial cells or extracts produce MAbs with the whole spectrum of IgG subtypes as well as IgM. Immunoglobulin A MAbs tend to be much less common, perhaps because of the route of immunization and source of lymphoid cells.

Knowledge of the isotype of a MAb can influence the subsequent handling or expectations of it and is therefore an important part of characterization. It can also be a useful indicator about the monoclonality of the cell line if more than one isotype is detected.

There are a number of methods available in which heavy- and light-chain-specific antisera have been used to determine isotype: ELISA (Kozbor et al., 1982a; Smart and Koh, 1983); RIA (Price and Baldwin, 1984; Springer, 1983); adsorption to nitrocellulose strips (McDougal et al., 1983); by nephelometry (Miller and Gilbride, 1985); directly using fluorescent reagents (Crawford et al., 1983b; Kozbor et al., 1982a), or by the classic immunoprecipitation method of Ouchterlony (1958). The methods most widely used are probably the ELISA procedure and immunoprecipitation in agar, although some modification, such as the inclusion of PEG, may be necessary in the latter method for MAbs to form visible precipitation lines.

C. Further Evaluation

1. Purification

Standard methods employed for purification of Ig from serum are equally applicable to the purification of MAbs. Protein A, which is derived from the Cowan I strain of *Staphylococcus aureus*, binds certain isotypes that can then be eluted at a characteristic pH (Goding, 1978). Normal, mouse serum-derived isotypes elute at the following pH: $IgG_1 \cong 6.0, IgG_{2a} \cong 5.0, IgG_{2b} \cong 3.5, IgG_3 \cong 4.5$. However, MAbs can vary widely from these norms and will sometimes elute in a double peak when only a single isotype can be detected by other methods (Stephenson et al., 1984). In addition, protein A separation is widely used to characterize MAbs.

Purification and concentration can also be achieved by salt precipitation, freeze-drying, ion-exchange chromatography, or immunoaffinity purification using immobilized antigen or high-performance liquid chromatography (Carlsson et al., 1985; Clezardin et al., 1985; Goding, 1983).

2. Stability

Monoclonal antibodies exhibit considerable differences in stability, some being stable at 4°C for several years, whereas others are labile at this temperature but stable if frozen. Freeze-drying, often used to store polyclonal sera for long periods, can completely denature some MAbs. Immunoglobulin M MAbs, murine IgG_{2a}, and IgG_3 are particularly susceptible to freeze-thawing, whereas IgM and IgG_{2b} are sensitive to heat (Goding, 1983; Underwood and Bean, 1985).

Denaturation of antibody by protease action can occur in stored material, often because of microbial contamination which can be largely inhibited by the routine addition of sodium azide. Degradation can also occur in culture medium containing low serum levels, because they may contain insufficient serum-derived antiprotease activity. The MAbs vary in their susceptibility to proteases, and this seems to be related to isotype (Lamoyi and Nisonoff, 1983; Parham, 1983). Moreover, individual types of antibody inactivation may occur after iodination or binding to solid phase; some MAbs are particularly susceptible to this.

3. Identification of Antigen

It is necessary to determine the binding of a particular MAb to as wide a range of cells, tissues, bacteria, hormones, etc., as possible, depending upon the specificity and application. The distribution of reacting antigen, e.g., on a range of cell types, can often provide a great deal of information about its possible nature. Any MAbs that are to be used for direct diagnostic purposes, e.g., antibacterials, must be thoroughly tested for unwanted reactivity, particularly with nonpathogenic organisms that may be encountered at the sites to be examined.

More precise antigenic identification can be undertaken using a range of analytical methods, e.g., polyacrylamide gel (PAGE), two-dimensional electrophoresis, and peptide mapping (Goding, 1983; see also Kennett et al., 1980; Macario and Macario, 1985, for more specific examples). Blotting of separated peptides onto nitrocellulose followed by reaction with the MAb is often used, but one must be aware that the MAb may not react with sodium dodecyl sulfate (SDS)-denatured antigen. Mapping of reactive sites may be accomplished using synthetic peptides or other MAbs to inhibit binding. Antigens present in a mixture may be purified by affinity chromatography using the MAb prepared to absorb it out, after which further analysis can be undertaken. Ideally this analysis will result in the identification of the antigenic determinant (epitope) with which the MAb reacts.

IV. BULK PRODUCTION

The development of methods that are simple and inexpensive for producing MAbs in bulk quantities are increasingly necessary as worldwide requirements continue to grow. For example, the amount of MAb of a single specificity required for an assay may be tens or hundreds of grams per year, whereas for therapeutic use or immunoaffinity purification it is expected to be many kilograms per year. Of the two major options for bulk production, tissue culture methods are generally favored for a variety of reasons, although growth of the cells in ascites has advantages, depending upon the quantity and application.

A. Tissue Culture

The range of culture methods has recently been reviewed (Birch et al., 1985; Feder and Tolbert, 1983; Glacken et al., 1983). Cells may be grown in suspension or trapped in some way in static or circulated cultures. Volumes range from 250 ml to 10,000 L. Basic cell research has increased our understanding of the growth requirements of cells, thus leading both to novel methods of culture and to chemically defined media that reduce or remove the requirement for animal sera, an increasingly scarce and expensive commodity. Hybridoma cells, whether of rodent or human origin, tend to grow at lower densities in these serum-free media but secrete larger amounts of Ig (Cleveland et al., 1983; Cole et al., 1985; Fazekas de St Groth, 1983; Kawamoto et al., 1983; Murakami et al., 1981, 1982).

Purification of the MAb product from culture medium, particularly from serum-free, is a relatively simple process and one that can be scaledup to handle large volumes. Entrapment methods in gels or fibers can often produce increased antibody concentrations of 10- to 100-fold, equivalent to that produced in ascites but without contamination with mouse proteins (Berg, 1985; Duff, 1985; Nilsson et al., 1983). An important advantage of bulk culture is that most cell lines can be adapted to this method of growth, whereas not all cell lines, even of rodent origin, will grow satisfactorily as ascites tumors.

B. Ascites

Rodent hybridomas can be grown as ascites tumors in the appropriate strain to yield ascitic fluids containing milligram per milliliter amounts of MAb. Although the initiating dose of cells may have to be adjusted for each line, prior treatment of the rodent with pristane favors the growth of ascitic tumors (Brodeur et al., 1984; Hoogenraad et al., 1983). Typically, cell numbers of 1×10^5 to 5×10^5 per mouse are injected intraperitoneally (IP), and ascites collection usually begins 10-14 days later. Mice are tapped as required over the next 10-14 days, total volumes per mouse ranging from 3 to 13 ml, with an average of 10 ml and an average yield of antibody of 10 mg/mouse.

Some human hybridomas have been adapted to grow in mice in ascitic form. Bogard et al. (1985) used pristane-primed irradiated nude mice, and found that serial passage of cell lines in ascites form increased the efficiency of take and volume of ascites produced. Alternatively, human lines may be adapted by passage as a solid, subcutaneous tumor in irradiated mice (Kozbor et al., 1985; Truitt et al., 1984b) or grown in immunodeficient mice (Ware et al., 1985).

V. COMPARISON OF PROPERTIES OF POLYCLONAL AND MONOCLONAL ANTIBODIES

A. Polyclonal Antisera

Polyclonal antisera contain a mixture of antibodies that vary in their isotype, specificity, affinity, and cross-reactivity with the immunizing antigen. Thus antigen binding is a consensus of reactions and interactions within the mixture, and because the immune response is not a static process, each bleed from an animal or human must be treated as a separate reagent. However, several advantages can be gained from this heterogeneity. The effects of treatments such as iodination, freeze-thawing, or freeze-drying, may be small and reaction conditions such as salt concentration and pH, may have little effect over a wide range of values. In addition, minor antigenic changes, variant forms of bacteria, etc., may not affect binding. Nevertheless, specificity remains a major problem because it depends so much upon the purity of antigen used for immunization.

B. Monoclonal Antibodies

In contrast with polyclonal antisera, MAbs are a pure form of a single antibody, each molecule in the preparation having the same specificity and affinity and, therefore, also the same susceptibility to degradation. Hence, the reaction of an MAb to changes in its environment, such as freeze-drying, tends to be "all-or-none."

A major advantage of MAbs is the continuing supply of identical batches of antibody, facilitating direct comparisons of results from laboratories worldwide and allowing closer standardization of assays between laboratories. The single-affinity value of each MAb can be employed in specific situations, low-affinity antibodies being useful for immunoaffinity purification, whereas high-affinity antibodies can be used to remove contaminants, e.g., hepatitis B from serum (Marciniak et al., 1983).

However, these unique properties can be also be disadvantageous and can affect their use in a number of areas. Unexpected cross-reactions may result if the particular epitope with which the MAb reacts is represented on apparently unrelated organisms (reviewed by Lane and Koprowski, 1982). Reaction conditions, such as temperature, pH and salt concentration, can affect binding and must be optimized for each antibody. Because the binding site is small, even minor changes to it can alter binding. This is particularly relevant to genetic polymorphisms or variant strains of microorganisms, when pools of MAbs need to be prepared to cover all variants. However, MAbs often behave differently in mixtures and may react with higher affinity or greater neutralizing capacity than the individual MAbs (Ehrlich et al., 1982, 1983; Ichimori et al., 1985). Complement-mediated cell lysis or agglutination are often isotype-dependent, and therefore, MAbs must be screened by an appropriate assay if these properties are required (Neuberger and Rajewsky, 1981).

In addition to the physical stability mentioned earlier, chromosomal stability both of cellular secretion and secreted antibody can be a problem. Immunoglobulin secretion may be lost through physical loss of the appropriate chromosome(s) or through functional loss of chromosomal expression. Raison et al. (1982) used mitogen stimulation (lipopolysaccharide) of human-mouse hybrids to restore Ig secretion, thus demonstrating that rather than chromosome loss, some defect in regulation was present. Aberrant forms of antibody may occur in which whole domains are missing, frame shifts occur, or point mutations lead to loss of reactivity (see Köhler, 1985, for review). Therefore, occasional checks are necessary to ensure that such changes have not occurred.

VI. CURRENT AND POTENTIAL USES OF MONOCLONAL ANTIBODIES

Monoclonal antibodies can be used in diverse ways throughout many areas in science and medicine. Within the health care fields alone, they have enabled the introduction of new methodologies as well as improving the performance of existing tests. Their fine specificity can be used to advantage in those areas where cells or their products require identification, quantitation, isolation, or that their distribution be studied. Apart from diagnostic tests, MAbs could be useful for monitoring a variety of therapeutic agents, either in vivo or during production processes. In addition, MAbs are being explored as potential therapeutic agents, either with specific antimicrobial or antitumor activity or as a means to modulate the immune system.

A. Current Uses in Microbial Diagnosis

The range of bacteria and viruses against which MAbs have been created is given in the Appendix. Later chapters in this book will deal with MAbs against organisms causing sexually transmitted diseases (STD). For a more general discussion on MAbs in microbiology, the reader is referred to recent reviews by Macario and Macario (1984, 1985), Polin (1984), Porterfield and Tobin (1984), and Massey and Schochetman (1985).

One of the recently developed MAb-based assays is the immunoradiometric assay (IRMA) which is used at present to advantage in clinical chemistry laboratories (Hunter et al., 1982a) and has also been adopted as a sensitive detector for viral antigens (Goodall et al., 1981; Pizzocolo et al., 1985). The IRMAs use the fine specificity of MAbs to form a rapid, sensitive, and specific alternative to the conventional RIA. The basic principles are outlined in Fig. 5. Two MAbs are required, each reacting with a different epitope on the antigen, one being labeled with ^{125}I (or an enzyme) and the other being absorbed to Sephadex G-200 beads or some other solid-phased support.

Enzyme-linked immunosorbent assays (ELISAs) are widely used both for antigen and antibody detection and quantitation, and many sensitive assays have been developed with the use of MAbs. Examples include detection of group A meningococcal antigens in cerebrospinal fluid (Sugasawara et al., 1984), screening

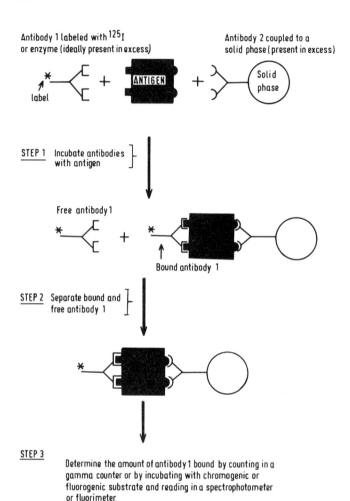

Antibody 1 labeled with ^{125}I
or enzyme (ideally present in excess)

Antibody 2 coupled to a
solid phase (present in excess)

label

ANTIGEN

Solid
phase

STEP 1   Incubate antibodies
        with antigen

Free antibody 1

+

Bound antibody 1

STEP 2   Separate bound and
        free antibody 1

STEP 3
        Determine the amount of antibody 1 bound by counting in a
        gamma counter or by incubating with chromogenic or
        fluorogenic substrate and reading in a spectrophotometer
        or fluorimeter.

Fig. 5 Basic principle of immunometric assays: Two MAbs reacting with different epitopes are necessary. One is labeled and the other adsorbed to solid phase,
capturing the antigen to be measured in between. These assays are very sensitive
and highly specific (*Source*: from James et al., 1984).

of food or stool cultures for *Salmonella* (Mattingly, 1984), and rapid detection of group B streptococcal antigens in pregnant women or neonates (Morrow et al., 1984). Serum antibodies against *M. tuberculosis* have been detected in a competitive inhibition assay using a panel of five MAbs directed against distinct determinants (Hewitt et al., 1982). This has the advantage of purified antigen not being required. A group of MAbs raised to *Legionella pneumophila* were shown to be useful for serotyping and for retrospective diagnosis by staining tissue sections (Miyazaki et al., 1985).

Fluorescent antibody (FA) staining is widely used to detect viral and other microbial antigens in culture or directly in patients' specimens. A major advantage of FA staining is rapidity. If such tests can be performed in the clinic in less than an hour the patient can usually wait. Fluorescent antibody tests using MAbs are available for the diagnosis of chlamydial infection (see Chap. 6), herpesvirus infection (see Chap. 12) and syphilis (see Chap. 7).

B. Future Uses in Microbial Diagnosis

It is unlikely that in the future we will see a major revolution in the methods used to diagnose disease. For one thing, it can be difficult for new technologies to be accepted in areas where present methods are reliable and well-characterized. However, there is no doubt that simple kits of reagents that can be used in the

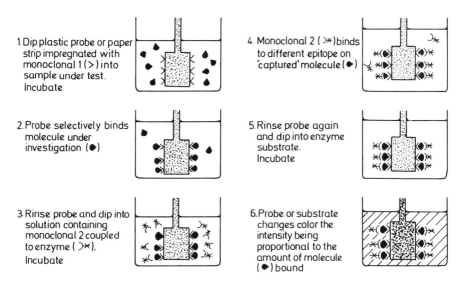

1. Dip plastic probe or paper strip impregnated with monoclonal 1 (>) into sample under test. Incubate

2. Probe selectively binds molecule under investigation (●)

3. Rinse probe and dip into solution containing monoclonal 2 coupled to enzyme ( )*). Incubate

4. Monoclonal 2 ( )*) binds to different epitope on 'captured' molecule (●)

5. Rinse probe again and dip into enzyme substrate. Incubate

6. Probe or substrate changes color the intensity being proportional to the amount of molecule (●) bound

Fig. 6   Future developments in monoclonal antibody diagnostics: Kits for clinic and home use.

clinic, in the physician's office, or at home will become more popular as commercial enterprises make them available at affordable prices. Many of these kits will have as their basis the type of "dipstick technology" outlined in Fig. 6 These types of assays will be particularly helpful when immediate treatment with the correct drug is dependent upon accurate identification of the causal organisms, e.g., in STD clinics. They could also simplify home monitoring of therapy.

To simplify matters further, mixed-molecule antibodies are being created with, for example, both antigen-binding and enzyme functions (Milstein and Cuello, 1983) or with dual specificities (Brennan et al., 1985). Thus far, reference has been made only to diseases in man, but it can be expected that the same advances will arise in the diagnosis of animal and even plant diseases.

C. Immunotherapy

Antibodies play a major role in the host defense against microorganisms and can affect them throughout their growth cycle. Viruses and many bacteria must adhere to cells or surfaces to initiate infection, and antibodies directed against the specific receptors can prevent this. Some bacteria invade tissues by secreting proteolytic enzymes, and the appropriate antibodies could protect against invasion. Protective antitoxin antibodies are also important in our defense against diseases such as tetanus.

Although there are effective vaccines for a variety of microbial infections, protective antibodies may not always be formed, especially in situations where the immune system is deficient through disease, treatment with drugs, or age (young and old). Passive immunization has been shown to be effective in some instances (McClelland and Yap, 1984), but current gamma-globulin preparations derived from pooled donor plasma are far from ideal, containing as they do only a small proportion of protective antibody. In addition, the problems of supply and batch control are formidable if a wide range of infections are to be catered for. The use of MAbs, and in particular those of human origin, has obvious application in this area, reducing the variability and increasing the specific activity of the treatment.

The range of bacterial diseases amenable to MAb prophylaxis or therapy has been discussed by Hunter (1985) and a wider range of applications for serotherapy has been reviewed by McClelland and Yap (1984). The specific MAbs generated in mouse, rat, or humans which either protect against infection in vivo or in vitro or neutralize the effect of toxins are given in the Appendix. It is to be hoped that the range of human MAbs will increase over the next few years as production problems are overcome.

An additional potential use for human MAbs has been suggested by Celis et al. (1985). They have shown potentiation of a T-lymphocyte response in vitro and antibody response in vivo to suboptimal amounts of hepatitis B virus surface antigen (HBsAg) in the presence of a human MAb directed against HBsAg. Other studies have found that hepatitis B infection in newborns of chronic carriers could be prevented by simultaneous use of vaccine and immune globulin (Wong et al., 1984). Thus, MAbs could be used both to stimulate the immune response and to reduce the amount of a particular vaccine required—both of which could be advantageous in Third-World countries.

In spite of all of the advantages cited for using human MAbs in vivo, there are a number of hurdles to be overcome, particularly concerning their safety. Products derived from virally transformed cells are, at present, unacceptable to the U.S. Food and Drug Administration. This rules out in vivo use of MAbs derived from EBV-transformed lines, whether the original LCL or a hybrid. Only MAbs from myeloma-derived hybridomas or transfected cell lines will be considered for clinical use. However, this could change in the future because the procedures used to purify MAbs have been shown to be effective (within the limits of detection) at excluding viral DNA (Crawford, 1983c). In addition, Teng et al. (1985b) found that one of their EBV-heteromyeloma hybrids had lost the chromosome containing the EBV genome and thus become EBNA negative. Perhaps a way of encouraging this to happen could ensure that EBV-hybrids continue to be a useful source of MAbs.

A further concern over viruses centers around the presence of retroviruses in many mouse cell lines, and secretion of C-type viruses has been observed in both mouse-mouse (Weiss, 1982) and mouse-human hybrids (Feliu et al., 1983). Although these viruses are infective for human cells in vitro, there is no evidence that cross-infection with retroviruses occurs between animals and man. Again, purification has been demonstrated as sufficient to remove these viruses (Levy et al., 1984).

A more serious consideration is the possibility of adverse reactions to human MAbs if administered over a period. It has been assumed that no anti-Ig response will be elicited, unlike those found in recipients of mouse MAbs. On the other hand, anti-idiotype and antiallotype responses could occur and consequently alter the immunoregulatory process. This assumes prolonged treatment with MAb, whereas it seems more likely in acute disease that only one or two treatments would be necessary. It would be anticipated that immunocompromised patients would not respond to prolonged treatments.

D. Other Uses

An additional aspect of protective MAbs is likely to be in their use to identify immunogenic fragments of organisms or their products with potential as vaccines. Most vaccines are now extremely crude preparations, the active component(s) of which have not been identified. Human MAbs will be particularly important in determining which of these components are necessary for an effective

immune response to be mounted. In addition, MAbs can be used in the purification of these vaccines, either from extracts of organisms or from culture broths
of genetically engineered bacteria synthesizing the required peptide. Monoclonal
antibodies against bacterial surface structures should also enable us to study metabolic processes. These studies, along with those on virulence antigens, should be
helpful in devising strategies to combat infection.

VII. DATA BANKS

The need to establish a centralized bank for both data and cell lines has been recognized by several organizations. The Hybridoma Data Bank (HDB) has been set
up as an international computerized data bank on cloned cell lines and their immunoreactive products. Information will be gathered and stored in three centers;
at the American Type Culture Collection (ATCC), at a center in Japan, and at
one in Europe (Bussard et al., 1985). Although the existence of a database of
this type could be useful, it is entirely dependent upon researchers being willing
to provide the necessary information. The ATCC itself acts as a repository for
cell lines, some of which are hybridomas. In addition, there is a European equivalent recently established at Porton Down, England (European Collection of Animal Cell Cultures).

An excellent source of information is Sheffield University Biomedical Information Service (SUBIS) that sends out monthly digests of the literature under
various headings including Monoclonal Antibodies.

In this chapter, we have attempted to give a broad insight into the principles
and problems of MAb technology and tried to relate them to the field of microbiology in general. The following chapters will deal in greater depth with the role
that MAbs can play within the area of sexually transmitted disease.

APPENDIX: MONOCLONAL ANTIBODIES SPECIFIC
FOR MICROORGANISMS

Bacteria

Organism	Species[a]	Immunogen	Action[b]	Ref.
Bacteroides fragilis	m	Outer membrane	NT	Linko-Kettunen et al. (1984)
B. gingivalis	m	Formalized whole cells	NT	Hanazawa et al. (1984)
Bordetella pertussis	m	Heat-killed whole cells	NT	Larsen et al. (1984)

Organism	Species[a]	Immunogen	Action[b]	Ref.
Chlamydia trachomatis	h	Infection	NT	Rosen et al. (1983)
C. trachomatis	m	Formalized EBs	NT	Caldwell and Hitchcock (1984)
C. trachomatis	m	Live organisms	p (in vitro)	Lucero and Kuo (1985)
C. trachomatis	m	Live organisms	NT	Wang et al. (1985)
Escherichia coli	m	K1 capsular polysaccharide	p (neonatal rat and mice)	Söderström et al. (1983)
E. coli	m	Whole pili	NT	Worobec et al. (1983)
E. coli	m	Heat-killed whole cells	p (mice)	Kirkland and Ziegler (1984)
E. coli	m	Formalized whole cells	NT	Peters et al. (1985)
E. coli	r	Viable whole cells	p (neonatal rat)	Pluschke and Achtman (1985)
E. coli	h	J5 LPS vaccine	p (mice)	Teng et al. (1985a)
Haemophilus influenzae	h	Infection	p (rat)	Hunter et al. (1982b)
H. influenzae	m	Outer membrane vesicles	NT	Robertson et al. (1982)
H. influenzae	h	Infection	p (neonatal rat)	Gigliotti et al. (1984)
Legionella pneumophila	m	Formalized whole cells	NT	Miyazaki et al. (1985)
Mycobacterium leprae	m	Antigens 10KP and 30KS	NT	Gillis and Buchanan (1982)
M. leprae	m	Soluble antigen	NT	Ivanyi et al. (1983)
M. leprae	h	Infection	NT	Atlaw et al. (1985)
Mycoplasma arthritidis	m	Arginine deaminase	NT	Thirkill et al. (1983)
M. pneumoniae	m	Whole cells	NT	Collier et al. (1983)
M. pneumoniae	m	Whole cells	NT	Hu et al. (1984)
Mycoplasma sp.	m	Whole cells	NT	Buck et al. (1982)

Organism	Species[a]	Immunogen	Action[b]	Ref.
Neisseria gonorrhoeae	m	Heat-killed whole cells	NT	Apicella et al. (1981)
N. gonorrhoeae	m	Viable whole cells	NT	Nachamkin et al. (1981)
N. gonorrhoeae	m	Protein I or formalized cells	NT	Tam et al. (1982)
N. gonorrhoeae	m	Outer membranes	p (in vitro)	Black et al. (1984)
N. gonorrhoeae	m	Outer membranes	NT	Cannon et al. (1984)
N. gonorrhoeae	m	Whole pili	NT	Edwards et al. (1984)
N. meningitidis	m	Formalized whole cells	NT	Sugasawara et al. (1983)
N. meningitidis	m	Outer membranes	p (mice)	Brodeur et al. (1985)
Pseudomonas aeruginosa	m	Infection	p (mice) p (in vitro)	Galloway et al. (1984)
P. aeruginosa	m	Formalized whole cells	p (mice)	Sawada et al. (1984)
P. aeruginosa	h	Infection	p (mice)	Sawada et al. (1985)
Salmonella typhimurium	m	Fixed whole cells	p (mice)	Colwell et al. (1984)
Streptococcus agalactiae	m	Viable whole cells	p (neonatal rat)	Shigeoka et al. (1984)
S. mutans	m	Surface antigen	NT	Smith et al. (1984)
S. pneumoniae	m	Heat-killed whole cells	p (mice)	McDaniel et al. (1984)
S. pneumoniae	h	Vaccine	NT	Schwaber et al. (1984)
S. pneumoniae	h	Infection	NT	Steinitz et al. (1984)

Toxins

Organism	Species[a]	Immunogen	Action[b]	Ref.
Clostridium difficile toxin A	m	Toxoid A	non-n	Lyerly et al. (1985)

Organism	Species[a]	Immunogen	Action[b]	Ref.
C. botulinum toxin	m	Toxoid	n (in vitro)	Kamata et al. (1985)
Diptheria toxin	m	Toxoid	n (in vitro)	Hayakawa et al. (1983)
Diptheria toxin	h	Toxoid	n (rabbit)	Gigliotti et al. (1984)
Diptheria toxin	m	Toxoid	n (rabbit) n (in vitro)	Zucker and Murphy (1984)
E. coli enterotoxin	m	Toxin-BSA conjugate	n (mice)	Brandwein et al. (1985)
Pseudomonas exotoxin A	m	Toxoid or toxin	p (mice) n (in vitro)	Galloway et al. (1984)
Tetanus toxin	h	Toxoid	n (mice)	Gigliotti and Insel (1982)
Tetanus toxin	m	Toxoid or toxin + Ab	n (mice)	Ahnert-Hilger et al. (1983)
Tetanus toxin	h	Toxoid	n (mice)	Larrick et al.(1983)
Tetanus toxin	r	Toxoid	n (mice)	Sheppard et al. (1984)
Tetanus toxin	h	Toxoid	n (mice)	Tiebout et al. (1984)
Tetanus toxin	m	Toxoid	n (mice)	Volk et al. (1984)
Tetanus toxin	h	Toxoid	n (mice)	Ichimori et al. (1985)

Viruses

Organism	Species[a]	Immunogen	Action[b]	Ref.
Cytomegalovirus	h	Infection	non-p	Emanuel et al. (1984)
Cytomegalovirus	m	Whole virus	NT	Nowak et al.(1984)
Epstein-Barr virus	m	Whole virus	p (in vitro)	Hoffman et al. (1980)
Hepatitis A	m	Whole virus	p (in vitro)	Hughes et al.(1984)
Hepatitis B	h	Infection	NT	Ichimori et al. (1985)
Hepatitis B	h	Infection	NT	Stricker et al. (1985)

Organism	Species[a]	Immunogen	Action[b]	Ref.
Herpes simplex type 1	m	Whole virus	NT	Goldstein et al. (1983)
Herpes simplex type 2	h	Infection	non-p (in vitro)	Evans et al. (1984)
Herpes simplex types 1 and 2	h	Infection	p (in vitro)	Seigneurin et al. (1983)
Influenza	h	X31 (in vitro)	NT	Crawford et al. (1983b)
Influenza A and B	m	Infection	NT	McQuillin et al. (1985)
Measles	h	Infection	NT	Croce et al. (1980)
Mumps	m	Whole virus	p (in vitro) p (neonatal hamster)	Wolinsky et al. (1985)
Parainfluenza 3	m	Whole virus	NT	Waner et al. (1985)
Polio	m,r	Whole virus	p (in vitro)	Ferguson et al. (1984)
Polyoma virus	m	Whole virus	p (in vitro)	Marriott and Consigli (1985)
Respiratory syncitial virus	m	Infected cells	p (in vitro)	Routledge et al. (1985)
Rubella	h	Infection	NT	Ritts et al. (1983)
Vaccinia	m	UV-inactivated virus	p (in vitro)	Rodriguez et al. (1985)
Varicella zoster	h	Infection	p (in vitro)	Foung et al. (1985)
Vesicular stomatitis	m	Whole virus	p (mice) p (in vitro)	Lefrancois (1984)
Yellow fever	m	gp48	p (mice)	Schlesinger et al. (1985)

[a]m: murine, r: rat, h: human.
[b]NT: not tested, n: neutralizing, p: protective against infection.

REFERENCES

Abrams, P. G., Knost, J. A., Clarke, G., Wilburn, S., Oldham, R. K., and Foon, K. A. (1983). Determination of the optimal human cell lines for development of human hybridomas. *J. Immunol. 131*:1201-1204.

Ahnert-Hilger, G., Bizzini, B., Goretzki, K., Mühler, H., Völckers, C., and Habermann, E. (1983). Monoclonal antibodies against tetanus toxin and toxoid. *Med. Microbiol. Immunol. 172*:123-135.

Aman, P., Ehlin-Henriksson, B., and Klein, G. (1984). Epstein-Barr virus susceptibility of normal human B lymphocyte populations. *J. Exp. Med. 159*:208-220.

Apicella, M. A., Bennett, K. M., Hermerath, C. A., and Roberts, D. E. (1981). Monoclonal antibody analysis of lipopolysaccharide from *Neisseria gonorrhoeae* and *Neisseria meningitidis*. *Infect. Immun. 34*:751-756.

Astaldi, G. C. B. (1983). Use of human endothelial culture supernatant (HECS) as a growth factor for hybridomas. *Methods Enzymol. 92*:39-47.

Astaldi, G. C. B., Wright, E. P., Willems, C. H., Zeijlemaker, W. P., and Janssen, M. C. (1982). Increase of hybridoma formation by human lymphocytes after stimulation in vitro: Effect of antigen, endothelial cells and PWM. *J. Immunol. 128*:2539-2542.

Atlaw, T., Kozbor, D., and Roder, J. C. (1985). Human monoclonal antibodies against *Mycobacterium leprae*. *Infect. Immun. 49*:104-110.

Bankert, R. B., Dessoye, D., and Powers, L. (1980). Antigen-promoted cell fusion: Antigen-coated myeloma cells fuse with antigen-reactive spleen cells. *Trans. Proc. 12*:443-446.

Barski, G., Sorieul, S., and Cornefert, F. (1960). Production dans des cultures in vitro de deux souches cellulaires en association de cellules de caractere "hybride." *C.R. Acad. Sci. Paris 251*:1825-1827.

Baumal, R., Bloom, B., and Scharff, M. D. (1971). Induction of long-term lymphocyte lines from delayed hypersensitive human donors using specific antigen plus Epstein-Barr virus. *Nature 230*:20.

Bazin, H., Grych, J. M., Verwaerd, C., and Capron, A. (1980). A LOU rat nonsecreting myeloma cell-line suitable for the production of rat-rat hybridomas. *Ann. Immunol. D131*:359.

Berg, G. J. (1985). An integrated system for large scale cell culture. *Dev. Biol. Stand. 60*:297-303.

Birch, J. R., Boraston, R., and Wood, L. (1985). Bulk production of monoclonal antibodies in fermenters. *Trend Biotechnol. 3*:162-166.

Black, W. J., Schwalbe, R. S., Nachamkin, I., and Cannon, J. G. (1984). Characterization of *Neisseria gonorrhoeae* protein II phase variation by use of monoclonal antibodies. *Infect. Immun. 45*:453-457.

Bogard, Jr., W. C., Hornberger, E., and Kunk, P. C. (1985). Production and characterization of human monoclonal antibodies against gram-negative bacteria. In *Human Hybridomas and Monoclonal Antibodies* (E. G. Engleman, S. K. H. Foung, J. Larrick, and A. Raubitschek, eds.). Plenum Press, New York, pp. 95-112.

Borrebaeck, C. A. K. (1983). In vitro immunization for the production of antigen-specific lymphocyte hybridomas. *Scand. J. Immunol. 18*:9-12.

Boss, B. D. (1984). An improved in vitro immunization procedure for the production of monoclonal antibodies against neural and other antigens. *Brain Res. 291*:193-196.

Boumsell, L. and Bernard, A. (1980). High efficiency of Biozzi's high responder mouse strain in the generation of antibody secreting hybridomas. *J. Immunol. Methods 38*:225-229.

Brandwein, H., Deutsch, A., Thompson, M., and Giannella, R. (1985). Production of neutralising monoclonal antibodies to *Escherichia coli* heat-stable enterotoxin. *Infect. Immun. 47*:242-246.

Brennan, M., Davison, P. F., and Paulus, H. (1985). Preparation of bispecific antibodies by chemical recombination of monoclonal immunoglobulin G1 fragments. *Science 229*:81-83.

Brodeur, B. R., Larose, Y., Tsang, P., Hamel, J., Ashton, F., and Ryan, A. (1985). Protection against infection with *Neisseria menigitidis* group B serotype 2b by passive immunization with serotype-specific monoclonal antibody. *Infect. Immun. 50*:510-516.

Brodeur, B. R., Tsang, P., and Larose, Y. (1984). Parameters affecting ascites tumour formation in mice and monoclonal antibody production. *J. Immunol. Methods 71*:265-272.

Brodin, T., Olsson, L., and Sjögren, H. O. (1983). Cloning of human myeloma/ hybridoma and lymphoma cell lines by enriched human monocytes as feeder layer. *J. Immunol. Methods 61*:1-7.

Buck, D. W., Kennett, R. H., and McGarrity, G. (1982). Monoclonal antibodies specific for cell culture mycoplasmas. *In Vitro 18*:377-381.

Burnett, K. G., Leung, J. P., and Martinis, J. (1985). Human monoclonal antibodies to defined antigens. Toward clinical applications. In *Human Hybridomas and Monoclonal Antibodies* (E. G. Engleman, S. K. H. Foung, J. Larrick, and A. Raubitschek, eds.). Plenum Press, New York, pp. 113-133.

Bussard, A., Krichevsky, M. I., and Blaine, L. D. (1985). An International Hybridoma Data Bank: Aims, structure, function. In *Monoclonal Antibodies Against Bacteria*, Vol. 1 (A. J. L. Macario and E. C. de Macario, eds.). Academic Press, New York, pp. 288-311.

Butler, J. L., Ambrus, J. L., and Fauci, A. S. (1984). Characterization of monoclonal B cell growth factor (BCGF) produced by a human T-T hybridoma. *J. Immunol. 133*:251-255.

Butler, J. L., Lane, H. C., and Fauci, A. S. (1983). Delineation of optimal conditions for producing mouse-human heterohybridomas from human peripheral blood B cells of immunized subjects. *J. Immunol. 130*:165-168.

Byars, N. E. (1984). Two adjuvant-active muramyl dipeptide analogs induce differential production of lymphocyte-activating factor and a factor causing distress in guinea-pigs. *Infect. Immun. 44*:344-350.

Caldwell, H. D. and Hitchcock, P. J. (1984). Monoclonal antibody against a genus-specific antigen of *Chlamydia* species: Location of the epitope on chlamydia lipopolysaccharide. *Infect. Immun. 44*:306-314.

Callahan, L. T., Woodhour, A. F., Meeker, J. B., and Hilleman, M. R. (1979). Enzyme-linked immunosorbent assay for measurement of antibodies against pneumococcal polysaccharide antigens: Comparison with radio-immunoassay. *J. Clin. Microbiol. 10*:459-463.

Cannon, J. G., Black, W. J., Nachamkin, I., and Stewart, P. W. (1984). Monoclonal antibody that recognises an outer membrane antigen common to the pathogenic *Neisseria* species but not to most nonpathogenic *Neisseria* species. *Infect. Immun. 43*:994-999.

Carlsson, M., Hedin, A., Inganäs, M., Härfast, B., and Blomberg, F. (1985). Purification of in vitro produced mouse monoclonal antibodies. A two-step procedure utilizing cation exchange chromatography and gel filtration. *J. Immunol. Methods 79*:89-98.

Cavagnaro, J. and Osband, M. (1983). Successful in vitro primary immunization of human peripheral blood mononuclear cells and subsequent fusion with human myeloma cells to produce human-human hybridomas secreting specific monoclonal antibody. *Hybridoma 2*:128.

Celis, E., Chang, T. W., Stricker, L., Tiebout, R. F., and Zeijlemaker, W. P. (1985). Role for monoclonal hepatitis B antibody in hepatitis B immunization programmes. *Lancet 1*:1219.

Chiorazzi, N., Wasserman, R. L., and Kunkel, H. G. (1982). Use of Epstein-Barr virus-transformed B cell lines for the generation of immunoglobulin-producing human B cell hybridomas. *J. Exp. Med. 156*:930-935.

Cianfriglia, M., Armellini, D., Massone, A., and Mariani, M. (1983). Simple immunization protocol for high frequency production of soluble antigen-specific hybridomas. *Hybridoma 2*:451-457.

Clark, M., Cobold, S., Hale, G., and Waldman, H. (1983). Advantages of rat monoclonal antibodies. *Immunol. Today 4*:100-101.

Clark, M. R. and Milstein, C. (1981). Expression of spleen cell immunoglobulin phenotype in hybrids with myeloma cell lines. *Somatic Cell Genet. 7*:657-666.

Cleveland, W. L., Wood, I., and Erlanger, B. F. (1983). Routine large-scale production of monoclonal antibodies in a protein-free culture medium. *J. Immunol. Methods 56*:221-234.

Clezardin, P., McGregor, J. L., Manach, M., Boukerche, H., and Dechavanne, M. (1985). One-step procedure for the rapid isolation of mouse monoclonal antibodies and their protein liquid chromatography on a mono Q anion-exchange column. *J. Chromatog. 319*:67-77.

Cohn, M. (1967). Natural history of the myeloma. *Cold Spring Harbor Symp. Quant. Biol. 32*:211-221.

Cole, S. P. C., Vreeken, E. H., and Roder, J. C. (1985). Antibody production by human x human hybridomas in serum-free medium. *J. Immunol. Methods 78*:271-278.

Collier, A. M., Hu, P. C., and Clyde, Jr., W. A. (1983). Location of attachment moiety on *Mycoplasma pneumoniae. Yale J. Biol. Med. 56*:671-677.

Colwell, D. E., Gollahon, K. A., McGhee, J. R., and Michalek, S. M. (1982). IgA hybridomas: A method for generation in high numbers. *J. Immunol. Methods 54*:259-266.

Colwell, D. E., Michalek, S. M., Briles, D. E., Jirillo, E., and McGhee, J. R. (1984). Monoclonal antibodies to *Salmonella* lipopolysaccharide: anti-O-polysaccharide antibodies protect C3H mice against challenge with virulent *Salmonella typhimurium. J. Immunol. 133*:950-957.

Cote, R. J. and Houghton, A. N. (1985). The generation of human monoclonal antibodies and their use in the analysis of the humoral immune response to cancer. In *Human Hybridomas and Monoclonal Antibodies* (E. G. Engelman, S. K. H. Foung, J. Larrick, and A. Raubitschek, eds.). Plenum Press, New York, pp. 189-210.

Cote, R. J., Morrissey, D. M., Houghton, A. N., Beattie, E. J., Oettgen, H. F., and Old, L. J. (1983). Generation of human monoclonal antibodies reactive with cellular antigens. *Proc. Natl. Acad. Sci. USA 80*:2026-2030.

Cotton, R. G. H. and Milstein, C. (1973). Fusion of two immunoglobulin-producing myeloma cells. *Nature 244*:42-43.

Crawford, D. H., Barlow, M. J., Harrison, J. F., Winger, L., and Huehns, E. R. (1983a). Production of human monoclonal antibody to rhesus D antigen. *Lancet 1*:386-388.

Crawford, D. H., Callard, R. E., Muggeridge, M. I., Mitchell, D. M., Zanders, E. D., and Beverley, P. C. L. (1983b). Production of human monoclonal antibody to X31 influenza virus nucleoprotein. *J. Gen. Virol. 64*:697-700.

Crawford, D. H., Huehns, E. R., and Epstein, M. A. (1983c). Therapeutic use of human monoclonal antibodies. *Lancet 1*:1040.

Croce, C. M., Linnenbach, A., Hall, W., Steplewski, Z., and Koprowski, H. (1980). Production of human hybridomas secreting antibodies to measles virus. *Nature 288*:488-489.

Davidson, R. L. and Gerald, P. S. (1976). Improved techniques for induction of mammalian-cell hybridization by polyethylene glycol. *Somat. Cell Genet. 2*: 165-176.

Davis, J. M., Pennington, J. E., Kubler, A.-M., and Conscience, J.-F. (1982). A simple, single-step technique for selecting and cloning hybridomas for the production of monoclonal antibodies. *J. Immunol. Methods 50*:161-171.

Duff, R. G. (1985). Microencapsulation technology: A novel method for monoclonal antibody production. *Trends Biotechnol. 3*:167-170.

Edwards, M., McDade, R. L., Schoolnik, G., Rothbard, J. B., and Gotschlich, E. C. (1984). Antigenic analysis of gonococcal pili using monoclonal antibodies. *J. Exp. Med. 160*:1782-1791.

Edwards, P. A. W., Smith, C. M., Neville, A. M., and O'Hare, M. J. (1982). A human-human hybridoma system based on a fast-growing mutant of the ARH-77 plasma cell leukaemia-derived line. *Eur. J. Immunol. 12*:641-648.

Ehrlich, P. H., Moyle, W. R., and Moustafa, Z. A. (1983). Further characterization of co-operative interactions of monoclonal antibodies. *J. Immunol. 131*:1906-1912.

Ehrlich, P. H., Moyle, W. R., Moustafa, Z. A., and Canfield, R. E. (1982). Mixing two monoclonal antibodies yields enhanced affinity for antigen. *J. Immunol. 128*:2709-2715.

Emanuel, D., Gold, J., Colacino, J., Lopez, C., and Hammerling, U. (1984). A human monoclonal antibody to cytomegalovirus (CMV). *J. Immunol. 133*: 2202-2205.

Engvall, E. and Perlmann, P. (1972). Enzyme-linked immunosorbent assay, ELISA. III. Quantitation of specific antibodies by enzyme-labelled anti-immunoglobulin in antigen-coated tubes. *J. Immunol. 109*:129-135.

Evans, L., Maragos, C., and May, J. T. (1984). Human lymphoblastoid cell lines established from peripheral blood lymphocytes secreting immunoglobulins directed against herpes simplex virus. *Immunol. Lett. 8*:39-42.

Fazekas de St Groth, S. (1983). Automated production of monoclonal antibodies in a cytostat. *J. Immunol. Methods 57*:121-136.

Fazekas de St Groth, S. and Scheidegger, D. (1980). Production of monoclonal antibodies: Strategy and tactics. *J. Immunol. Methods 35*:1-21.

Feder, J. and Tolbert, W. R. (1983). The large-scale cultivation of mammalian cells. *Sci. Am. 248*:24-31.

Feit, C., Bartal, A. H., Tauber, G., Dymbort, G., and Hirshaut, Y. (1983). An enzyme-linked immunosorbent assay (ELISA) for the detection of monoclonal antibodies recognizing surface antigen expressed on viable cells. *J. Immunol. Methods 58*:301-308.

Feliu, E., Rozman, C., Berga, L. L., Vilella, R., Gallart, T., and Vives, J. (1983). Xenogeneic hybridoma cells contain and secrete virus particles. *Lancet 2*: 1255.

Ferguson, M., Minor, P. D., Magrath, D. I., Yi-Hua, Q., Spitz, M., and Schild, G. C. (1984). Neutralization epitopes on poliovirus type 3 particles: An analysis using monoclonal antibodies. *J. Gen. Virol. 65*:197-201.

Fong, S., Tsoukas, C. D., Pasquali, J.-L., Fox, R. I., Rose, J. E., Raiklen, D. A., Carson, D. A., and Vaughan, J. H. (1981). Fractionation of human lymphocyte subpopulations on Ig coated petri dishes. *J. Immunol. Methods 44*:171-182.

Foung, S. K. H., Perkins, S., Koropchak, C., Fishwild, D. M., Wittek, A. E., Engleman, E. G., Grumet, F. C., and Arvin, A. M. (1985). Human monoclonal antibodies neutralizing varicella-zoster virus. *J. Infect. Dis. 152*:280-285.

Foung, S. K. H., Perkins, S., Raubitschek, A., Larrick, J., Lizak, G., Fishwild, D., Engleman, E. G., and Grumet, F. C. (1984). Rescue of human monoclonal antibody production from an EBV-transformed B cell line by fusion to a human-mouse hybridoma. *J. Immunol. Methods 70*:83-90.

Fox, P. C., Berenstein, E. H., and Siraganian, R. P. (1981). Enhancing the frequency of antigen-specific hybridomas. *Eur. J. Immunol. 11*:431-434.

Frackelton, A. R. and Rotman, B. (1980). Functional diversity of antibodies elicited by bacterial β-D-galactosidase. *J. Biol. Chem. 255*:5286-5290.

Frade, R., Barel, M., Ehlin-Henriksson, B., and Klein, G. (1985). gp 140, the C3d receptor of human B lymphocytes is also the Epstein-Barr virus receptor. *Proc. Natl. Acad. Sci. USA 82*:1490-1493.

Franklin, R. M. (1982). Microcomputer inventory systems for stored cell lines. *J. Immunol. Methods 54*:141-157.

Gagnon, G. and Raymond, Y. (1985). Cloning of hybridomas by a single-cell transfer method. *J. Immunol. Methods 78*:267-269.

Galfre, G., Milstein, C., and Wright, B. (1979). Rat X rat hybrid myelomas and a monoclonal anti-Fd portion of mouse IgG. *Nature 277*:131-133.

Galfre, G. and Milstein, C. (1981). Preparation of monoclonal antibodies: Strategies and procedures. *Methods Enzymol. 73*:3-46.

Galloway, D. R., Hedstrom, R. C., and Pavlovski, O. R. (1984). Production and characterization of monoclonal antibodies to exotoxin A from *Pseudomonas aeruginosa. Infect. Immun. 44*:262-267.

Gefter, M. L., Marguilies, D. H., and Scharff, M. D. (1977). A simple method for polyethylene glycol-promoted hybridisation of mouse myeloma cells. *Somat. Cell Genet. 2*:231-236.

Gigliotti, F. and Insel, R. A. (1982). Protective human hybridoma antibody to tetanus toxin. *J. Clin. Invest. 70*:1306-1309.

Gigliotti, F., Smith, L., and Insel, R. A. (1984). Reproducible production of protective human monoclonal antibodies by fusion of peripheral blood lymphocytes with a mouse myeloma cell line. *J. Infect. Dis. 149*:43-47.

Gillis, T. P. and Buchanan, T. M. (1982). Production and partial characterization of monoclonal antibodies to *Mycobacterium leprae. Infect. Immun. 37*:172-178.

Glacken, M. W., Fleischaker, R. J., and Sinskey, A. J. (1983). Mammalian cell culture: Engineering principles and scale-up. *Trends Biotechnol. 1*:102-108.

Glassy, M. C., Handley, H. H., Hagiwara, H., and Royston, I. (1983). UC 729-6, a human lymphoblastoid B-cell line useful for generating antibody-secreting human-human hybridomas. *Proc. Natl. Acad. Sci. USA 80*:6327-6331.

Glassy, M. C. and Hofmann, G. (1985). Optimization of electrocell fusion parameters in generating human-human hybrids with UC 729-6. *Hybridoma 4*:61.

Goding, J. W. (1978). Use of staphylococcal protein A as an immunological reagent. *J. Immunol. Methods 20*:241-253.

Goding, J. W. (1980). Antibody production by hybridomas. *J. Immunol. Methods 39*:285-308.

Goding, J. W. (1983). *Monoclonal Antibodies: Principles and Practice.* Academic Press, New York.

Goldstein, L. C., Corey, L., McDougall, J. K., Tolentino, E., and Nowinski, R. C. (1983). Monoclonal antibodies to herpes simplex viruses: Use in antigenic typing and rapid diagnosis. *J. Infect. Dis. 147*:829-837.

Goodall, A. H., Miescher, G., Meek, F. L., Janossy, G., and Thomas, H. C. (1981). Monoclonal antibodies in a solid-phase radiometric assay for HBsAg. *Med. Lab. Sci. 38*:349-354.

Gordon, J., Ley, S. C., Melamed, M. D., English, L. S., and Hughes-Jones, N. C. (1984). Immortalized B lymphocytes produce B-cell growth factor. *Nature 310*:145-147.

Gravekamp, C., Bol, S. J. L., Hagemeijer, A., and Bolhuis, R. L. H. (1985). Production of human T-cell hybridomas by electrofusion. In *Human Hybridomas and Monoclonal Antibodies* (E. G. Engelman, S. K. H. Foung, J. Larrick, and A. Raubitschek, eds.). Plenum Press, New York, pp. 323-339.

Hanazawa, S., Saitoh, K., Ohmori, Y., Nishihara, H., Fujiwara, S., and Kitano, S. (1984). Production of monoclonal antibodies that recognise specific and cross-reactive antigens of *Bacteroides gingivalis. Infect. Immun. 46*:285-287.

Hansson, M., Falk, K., and Ernberg, I. (1983). Epstein-Barr virus transformation of human pre-B cells. *J. Exp. Med. 158*:616-622.

Harwell, L. W., Bolognino, M., Bidlack, J. M., Knapp, R. J., and Lord, E. M. (1984). A freezing method for cell fusions to distribute and reduce labor and permit more thorough early evaluation of hybridomas. *J. Immunol. Methods 66*:59-67.

Hayakawa, S., Uchida, I., Mekada, E., Moynihan, M. R., and Okada, Y. (1983). Monoclonal antibody against diptheria toxin. Effect on toxin binding and entry into cells. *J. Biol. Chem. 258*:4311-4317.

Hewitt, J., Coates, A. R. M., Mitchison, D. A., and Ivanyi, J. (1982). The use of murine monoclonal antibodies without purification of antigen in the sero-diagnosis of tuberculosis. *J. Immunol. Methods 55*:205-211.

Ho, M.-K., Rand, N., Murray, J., Kato, K., and Rabin, H. (1985). In vitro immunization of human lymphocytes. I. Production of human monoclonal antibodies against bombesin and tetanus toxoid. *J. Immunol. 135*:3831-3838.

Hoffman, G. J., Lazarowitz, S. G., and Hayward, S. D. (1980). Monoclonal antibody against a 250,000-dalton glycoprotein of Epstein-Barr virus identifies a membrane antigen and a neutralizing antigen. *Proc. Natl. Acad. Sci. USA 77*:2979-2983.

Hoogenraad, N., Heman, T., and Hoogenraad, J. (1983). The effect of pre-injection of mice with pristane on ascites tumour formation and monoclonal production. *J. Immunol. Methods 61*:317-320.

Hu, P. C., Collier, A. M., and Clyde, Jr., W. A. (1984). Serological comparison of virulent and avirulent *Mycoplasma pneumoniae* by monoclonal antibodies. *Isr. J. Med. Sci. 20*:870-873.

Hughes, J. V., Stanton, L. W., Tomassini, J. E., Long, W. J., and Scolnick, E. N. (1984). Neutralizing monoclonal antibodies to hepatitis A virus: Partial localization of a neutralizing antigenic site. *J. Virol. 52*:465-473.

Hunter, Jr., K. W. (1985). Human monoclonal antibodies for prophylaxis and therapy of bacterial infections. In *Monoclonal Antibodies Against Bacteria*, Vol I (A. J. L. Macario and E. C. de Macario, eds.). Academic Press, New York, pp. 207-231.

Hunter, K. W., Fischer, G. W., Hemming, V. G., Wilson, S. R., Hartzman, R. J., and Woody, J. N. (1982a). Antibacterial activity of a human monoclonal antibody to *Haemophilus influenzae* type b capsular polysaccharide. *Lancet 2*:798-799.

Hunter, W. M., Bennie, J. G., Budd, P. S., van Heyningen, V., James, K., Micklem, L., and Scott, A. (1982b). Immunoradiometric assays using monoclonal antibodies. In *Immunoassays for Clinical Chemistry* (W. M. Hunter and J. E. T. Corrie, eds.). Churchill Livingstone, Edinburgh, pp. 531-544.

Ichimori, Y., Sasano, K., Itoh, H., Hitotsumachi, S., Kimura, Y., Kaneko, K., Kida, M., and Tsukamoto, K. (1985). Establishment of hybridomas secreting human monoclonal antibodies against tetanus toxin and hepatitis B virus surface antigen. *Biochem. Biophys. Res. Comm. 129*:26-33.

Ivanyi, J., Sinha, S., Aston, R., Cussell, D., Keen, M., and Sengupta, U. (1983). Definition of species specific and cross-reactive antigenic determinants of *Mycobacterium leprae* using monoclonal antibodies. *Clin. Exp. Immunol. 52*:528-536.

James, K., Boyd, J. E., Micklem, L. R., Ritchie, A. W. S., Dawes, J., and McClelland, D. B. L. (1984). Monoclonal antibodies, their production and potential in clinical practice. *Scot. Med. J. 29*:67-83.

Jonak, Z. L., Braman, V., and Kennett, R. H. (1984). Production of continuous mouse plasma cell lines by transfection with human leukemia DNA. *Hybridoma 3*:107-118.

Jongkind, J. F., Verkerk, A., and Tanke, H. (1979). Isolation of human fibroblast hetero-karyons with two-color flow sorting (FACS II). *J. Exp. Res. 120*:444-448.

Kamata, Y., Kozaki, S., Nagai, T., and Sakaguchi, G. (1985). Production of monoclonal antibodies against *Clostridium botulinum* type E derivative toxin. *FEMS Microbiol. Lett. 26*:305-309.

Kaplan, M. E., Woodson, M., and Clark, A. (1976). Detection of human T lymphocytes by rosette formation with AET-treated sheep red cells. In *In Vitro Methods in Cell Mediated and Tumour Immunity* (B. R. Bloom and J. R. David, eds.). Academic Press, London, pp. 83-88.

Kawamoto, T., Sato, J. D., Le, A., McClure, D. B., and Sato, G. H. (1983). Development of a serum-free medium for growth of NS-1 mouse myeloma cells and its application to the isolation of NS-1 hybridomas. *Anal. Biochem. 130*:445-453.

Kearney, J. F., Radbruch, A., Liesegang, B., and Rajewsky, K. (1979). A new mouse myeloma cell line that has lost immunoglobulin expression but permits the construction of antibody-secreting hybrid cell lines. *J. Immunol. 123*:1548-1550.

Kennett, R. H. (1980). Enzyme-linked antibody assay with cells attached to polyvinyl chloride plates. In *Monoclonal Antibodies—Hybridomas: A New Dimension in Biological Analyses* (R. H. Kennett, T. J. McKearn, and K. B. Bechtel, eds.). Plenum Press, New York, pp. 376-377.

Kennett, R. H., McKearn, T. J., and Bechtel, K. B. (1980). *Monoclonal Antibodies—Hybridomas: A New Dimension in Biological Analyses.* Plenum Press, New York.

Kirkland, T. N. and Ziegler, E. J. (1984). An immunoprotective monoclonal antibody to lipopolysaccharide. *J. Immunol. 132*:2590-2592.

Köhler, G. (1985). Derivation and diversification of monoclonal antibodies. *Biosci. Rep. 5*:533-549.

Köhler, G., Howe, S. C., and Milstein, C. (1976). Fusion between immunoglobulin-secreting and nonsecreting myeloma cell lines. *Eur. J. Immunol. 6*:292-295.

Köhler, G. and Milstein, C. (1975). Continuous cultures of fused cells secreting antibody of predefined specificity. *Nature 256*:495-497.

Köhler, G. and Milstein, C. (1976). Derivation of specific antibody-producing tissue culture and tumour lines by cell fusion. *Eur. J. Immunol. 6*:511-519.

Kozbor, D., Abramow-Newerly, W., Tripputi, P., Cole, S. P. C., Weibel, J., Roder, J. C., and Croce, C. M. (1985). Specific immunoglobulin production and enhanced tumorigenicity following ascites growth of human hybridomas. *J. Immunol. Methods 81*:31-42.

Kozbor, D., Dexter, D., and Roder, J. C. (1983). A comparative analysis of the phenotypic characteristics of available fusion partners for the construction of human hybridomas. *Hybridoma 2*:7-16.

Kozbor, D., Lagarde, A. E., and Roder, J. C. (1982a). Human hybridomas constructed with antigen-specific, EBV-transformed cell lines. *Proc. Natl. Acad. Sci. USA 79*:6651-6655.

Kozbor, D. and Roder, J. C. (1984). In vitro stimulated lymphocytes as a source of human hybridomas. *Eur. J. Immunol. 14*:23-27.

Kozbor, D., Roder, J. C., Chang, T. H., Steplewski, Z., and Koprowski, H. (1982b). Human anti-tetanus toxoid monoclonal antibody secreted by EBV-transformed human B cells fused with a murine myeloma. *Hybridoma 1*:323-328.

Kozbor, D., Tripputi, P., Roder, J. C., and Croce, C. M. (1984). A human hybrid myeloma for production of human monoclonal antibodies. *J. Immunol. 133*: 3001-3005.

Lachmann, P. J., Oldroyd, R. G., Milstein, C., and Wright, B. W. (1980). Three rat monoclonal antibodies to human C3. *Immunology 41*:503.

Lamoyi, E. and Nisonoff, A. (1983). Preparation of F(ab')$_2$ fragments from mouse IgG of various subclasses. *J. Immunol. Methods 56*:235-243.

Lane, D. and Koprowski, H. (1982). Molecular recognition and the future of monoclonal antibodies. *Nature 296*:200-202.

Lane, R. D., Crissman, R. S., and Lachman, M. F. (1984). Comparison of polyethylene glycols as fusogens for producing lymphocyte-myeloma hybrids. *J. Immunol. Methods 72*:71-76.

Larrick, J. W., Truitt, K. E., Raubitschek, A., Senyk, G., and Wang, J. C. N. (1983). Characterization of human hybridomas secreting antibody to tetanus toxoid. *Proc. Natl. Acad. Sci. USA 80*:6376-6380.

Larsen, F. S., Selmer, J. C., and Hertz, J. B. (1984). Purification of *Bordetella pertusis* antigens using monoclonal antibodies. *Acta Pathol. Microbiol. Scand. Sect. C. Immunol. 92*:271-277.

Leaback, D. H. and Creme, S. (1980). A new experimental approach to fluorometric enzyme assays employing disposable microreaction chambers. *Anal. Biochem. 106*:314-321.

Lefrancois, L. (1984). Protection against lethal viral infection by neutralizing and nonneutralizing monoclonal antibodies: Distinct mechanisms of action in vivo. *J. Virol. 51*:208-214.

Levy, J. A., Lee, H. M., Kawahata, R. T., and Spitler, L. E. (1984). Purification of monoclonal antibodies from mouse ascites eliminates contaminating infectious mouse type C viruses and nucleic acids. *Clin. Exp. Immunol. 56*: 114-120.

Lindmark, R., Thoren-Tolling, K., and Sjöquist, J. (1983). Binding of immunoglobulins to protein A and immunoglobulin levels in mammalian sera. *J. Immunol. Methods 62*:1-13.

Linko-Kettunen, L., Arstila, P., Jalkanen, M., Jousimies-Somer, H., Lassila, O., Lehtonen, O.-P., Weintraub, A., and Vijanen, M. K. (1984). Monoclonal antibodies to *Bacteroides fragilis* lipopolysaccharide. *J. Clin. Microbiol. 20*:519-524.

Littlefield, J. W. (1964). Selection of hybrids from matings of fibroblasts in vitro and their presumed recombinants. *Science 145*:709-710.

Lo, M. M. S., Tsong, T. Y., Conrad, M. K., Strittmatter, S. M., Hester, L. D., and Snyder, S. H. (1984). Monoclonal antibody production by receptor-mediated electrically induced cell fusion. *Nature 310*:792-794.

Lucero, M. E. and Kuo, C.-C. (1985). Neutralization of *Chlamydia trachomatis* cell culture infection by serovar-specific monoclonal antibodies. *Infect. Immun. 50*:595-597.

Lyerly, D. M., Phelps, C. J., and Wilkins, T. D. (1985). Monoclonal and specific polyclonal antibodies for immunoassay of *Clostridium dificile* toxin a. *J. Clin. Microbiol. 21*:12-14.

Ma, M., Wu, S.-J., Howard, M., and Borkovec, A. B. (1984). Enhanced production of mouse hybridomas to picomoles of antigen using EL-4 conditioned media with an in vitro immunization protocol. *In Vitro 20*:739-742.

Macario, A. J. L. and Macario, E. C. de (1984). Antibacterial monoclonal antibodies and the dawn of a new era in the control of infection. *Surv. Synth. Pathol. Res. 3*:119-130.

Macario, A. J. L. and Macario, E. C. de (1985). *Monoclonal Antibodies against Bacteria*, Vol I, Academic Press, New York.

McClelland, D. B. L. and Yap, P. L. (1984). Clinical use of immunoglobulins. *Clin. Haematol. 13*:39-74.

McCullough, K. C. and Parkinson, D. (1984). The standardization of a "spot-test" ELISA for the rapid screening of sera and hybridoma cell products. *J. Biol. Stand. 12*:75-86.

McDaniel, L. S., Scott, G., Kearney, J. F., and Briles, D. E. (1984). Monoclonal antibodies against protease-sensitive pneumococcal antigens can protect mice from fatal infection with *Streptococcus pneumoniae. J. Exp. Med. 160*:386-397.

McDougal, J. S., Browning, S. W., Kennedy, S., and Moore, D. D. (1983). Immunodot assay for determining the isotype and light chain type of murine monoclonal antibodies in unconcentrated hybridoma culture supernates. *J. Immunol. Methods 63*:281-290.

McKearn, T. J. (1980). Fusion of cells in an adherent monolayer. In *Monoclonal Antibodies. Hybridomas: A New Dimension in Biological Analyses* (R. H. Kennett, T. J. McKearn, and K. B. Bechtol, eds.). Plenum Press, New York, pp. 368-369.

McQuillin, J., Madeley, C. R., and Kendal, A. P. (1985). Monoclonal antibodies for the rapid diagnosis of influenza A and B virus infections by immunofluorescence. *Lancet 2*:911-914.

Mao, S. J. T. and France, D. S. (1984). Enhancement of limiting dilution in cloning mouse myeloma-spleen hybridomas by human low density lipoproteins. *J. Immunol. Methods 75*:309-316.

Marciniak, R. A., Wands, J. R., Bruns, R. R., Malchesky, P. S., Nose, Y., and Haber, E. (1983). Quantitative removal of hepatitis B viral antigens from serum by a monoclonal IgM coupled to a biocompatable solid-phase support. *Proc. Natl. Acad. Sci. USA 80*:3821-3825.

Marguilies, D. H., Cieplinski, W., Dharmgrong-Artama, B., Gefter, M. L., Morrison, S. L., Kelly, T., and Scharff, M. D. (1976). Regulation of immunoglobulin expression in mouse myeloma cells. *Cold Spring Harbor Symp. Quant. Biol. 41*:781-791.

Marriott, S. J. and Consigli, R. A. (1985). Production and characterization of monoclonal antibodies to polyomavirus major capsid protein VP1. *J. Virol. 56*:365-372.

Massey, R. J. and Schochetman, G. (1985). Monoclonal antibodies to viruses. In *Immunochemistry of Viruses: The Basis for Serodiagnosis and Vaccines* (M. H. V. van Regenmortel and A. R. Neurath, eds.). Elsevier, Amsterdam, pp. 29-38.

Massicotte, H., Rauch, J., Schoenfeld, Y., and Tannenbaum, H. (1984). Influence of fusion cell ratio and cell plating density on production of human-human hybridomas secreting anti-DNA autoantibodies from patients with systemic lupus erthymatosus. *Hybridoma 3*:215-222.

Mattingly, J. A. (1984). An enzyme immunoassay for the detection of all *Salmonella* using a combination of a myeloma protein and a hybridoma antibody. *J. Immunol. Methods 73*:147-156.

Mierendorf, R. C., and Dimond, R. L. (1983). Functional heterogeneity of monoclonal antibodies obtained using different screening assays. *Anal. Biochem. 135*:221-229.

Miller, D. and Gilbride, K. J. (1985). The use of nephelometry for rapid detection of monoclonal antibody concentrations in cell suspensions and buffers. *Hybridoma 4*:69.

Miller, G. and Lipman, M. (1973). Comparison of the yield of infectious virus from clones of human and simian lymphoblastoid lines transformed by Epstein-Barr virus. *J. Exp. Med. 138*:1398-1412.

Milstein, C., Adetugbo, K., Cowan, N. J., Köhler, G., Secher, D. S., and Wilde, C. D. (1976). Somatic cell genetics of antibody-secreting cells: Studies of clonal diversification and analysis by cell fusion. *Cold Spring Harbor Symp. Quant. Biol. 41*:793-803.

Milstein, C. and Cuello, A. C. (1983). Hybrid hybridomas and their use in immunochemistry. *Nature 305*:537-540.

Milstein, C. and Köhler, G. (1977). Cell fusion and the derivation of cell lines producing specific antibody. In *Antibodies in Human Diagnosis and Therapy* (E. Haber and R. M. Krause, eds.). Raven Press, New York, pp. 271-286.

Miyazaki, T., Koga, H., Nakashima, M., Tomonaga, A., Hara, K., and Watanabe, T. (1985). Production of monoclonal antibodies against *Legionella pneumophila* serogroup 1. *Microbiol. Immunol. 29*:275-284.

Morrison-Plummer, J., Jones, D. H., and Baseman, J. B. (1983). An ELISA to detect monoclonal antibodies specific for lipid determinants of *Mycoplasma pneumoniae. J. Immunol. Methods 64*:165-178.

Morrow, D. L., Kline, J. B., Douglas, S. D., and Polin, R. A. (1984). Rapid detection of group B streptococcal antigen by monoclonal antibody sandwich enzyme assay. *J. Clin. Microbiol. 19*:457-459.

Murakami, H., Masui, H., Sato, G., and Raschke, W. C. (1981). Growth of mouse plasmacytoma cells in serum-free, hormone-supplemented medium: Procedure for the determination of hormone and growth factor requirements for cell growth. *Anal. Biochem. 114*:422-428.

Murakami, H., Masui, H., Sato, G. H., Sueoka, N., Chow, T. P., and Kano-Sueoka, T. (1982). Growth of hybridoma cells in serum-free medium: Ethanolamine is an essential component. *Proc. Natl. Acad. Sci. USA 79*:1158-1162.

Nachamkin, I., Cannon, J. G., and Mittler, R. S. (1981). Monoclonal antibodies against *Neisseria gonorrhoeae*: Production of antibodies directed against a strain-specific cell surface antigen. *Infect. Immun. 32*:641-648.

Ness, J., van, Laemmli, U. K., and Pettijohn, D. E. (1984). Immunization in vitro and production of monoclonal antibodies specific to insoluble and weakly immunogenic proteins. *Proc. Natl. Acad. Sci. USA 81*:7897-7901.

Neuberger, M. S. and Rajewsky, K. (1981). Activation of mouse complement by monoclonal mouse antibodies. *Eur. J. Immunol. 11*:1012-1016.

Nilsson, K., Scheirer, W., Merten, O. W., Ostberg, L., Liehl, E., Katinger, H. W. D., and Mosbach, K. (1983). Entrapment of animal cells for production of monoclonal antibodies and other bimolecules. *Nature 302*:629-630.

Nossal, G. J. V. and Lederberg, J. (1958). Antibody production by single cells. *Nature 181*:1419-1420.

Nowak, B., Sullivan, C., Sarnow, P., Thomas, R., Bricout, F., Nicolas, J. C., Fleckenstein, B., and Levine, A. J. (1984). Characterization of monoclonal antibodies and polyclonal immune sera directed against human cytomegalovirus virion proteins. *Virology 132*:325-338.

Nussbaum, S. R., Lin, C. S., Potts, Jr., J. T., Rosenthal, A. S., and Rosenblatt, M. (1985). Development of monoclonal antibodies against parathyroid hormone: Genetic control of the immune response to human PTH. *Methods Enzymol. 109*:625-638.

Ochi, A., Hawley, R. G., Hawley, T., Shirlman, M. J., Trauexker, A., Köhler, G., and Hozumi, N. (1983). Functional immunoglobulin M production after transfection of cloned immunoglobulin heavy and light chain genes into lymphoid cells. *Proc. Natl. Acad. Sci. USA 80*:6351-6355.

Oi, V. T. and Herzenberg, L. A. (1980). Immunoglobulin-producing hybrid cell lines. In *Selected Methods in Cellular Immunology* (B. B. Mishell and S. M. Shiigi, eds.). Freeman, San Francisco, pp. 351-372.

Okada, Y. and Tadokoro, J. (1962). Analysis of giant polynuclear cell formation caused by HVJ virus from Ehrlich's tumour cells. II. Quantitative analysis of giant polynuclear cell formation. *Exp. Cell Res. 26*:108-118.

Olsson, L. and Brams, P. (1985). Human-human hybridoma technology: Five years of technical improvements and its application in cancer biology. In *Human Hybridomas and Monoclonal Antibodies* (E. G. Engelman, S. K. H. Foung, J. Larrick, A. Raubitschek, eds.). Plenum Press, New York, pp. 227-244.

Olsson, L. and Kaplan, H. (1980). Human-human hybridomas producing monoclonal antibodies of predefined antigenic specificity. *Proc. Natl. Acad. Sci. USA 77*:5429-5431.

Olsson, L., Kronstrom, H., Cambon-de-Mouzon, A., Honsik, C., Brodin, T., and Jakobsen, B. (1983). Antibody producing human-human hybridomas. I. Technical aspects. *J. Immunol. Methods 61*:17-32.

Östberg, L. and Pursch, E. (1983). Human X (mouse X human) hybridomas stably producing human antibodies. *Hybridoma 2*:361-367.

Ouchterlony, O. (1958). Diffusion-in-gel methods for immunological analysis. *Progr. Allergy 5*:1-78.

Pardue, R. L., Brady, R. C., Perry, G. W., and Dedman, J. R. (1983). Production of monoclonal antibodies against calmodulin by in vitro immunization of spleen cells. *J. Cell Biol. 96*:1149-1154.

Parham, P. (1983). On the fragmentation of monoclonal IgG1, IgG2a and IgG2b from BALB/c mice. *J. Immunol. 131*:2895-2902.

Parks, D. R., Bryan, V. M., Oi, V. T., and Herzenberg, L. A. (1979). Antigen-specific identification and cloning of hybridomas with a fluorescence activated cell sorter. *Proc. Natl. Acad. Sci. USA 76*:1962-1966.

Peters, H., Jürs, M., Jann, B., Jann, K., Timmis, K. N., and Bitter-Suermann, D. (1985). Monoclonal antibodies to enterobacterial common antigen and to *Escherichia coli* lipopolysaccharide outer core: Demonstration of an antigenic determinant shared by enterobacterial common antigen and *E. coli* K5 capsular polysaccharide. *Infect. Immun. 50*:459-466.

Pizzocolo, G., Giammatteo, D., Barbiere, U., Boniolo, A., Callegaro, L., Palla, M., and Albertini, A. (1985). HBeAg/anti-HBe determination with a new monoclonal immunoradiometric assay. *Vox Sang. 48*:129-135.

Pluschke, G. and Achtman, M. (1985). Antibodies to O-antigen of lipopolysaccharide are protective against neonatal infection with *Escherichia coli* K1. *Infect. Immun. 49*:365-370.

Polin, R. A. (1984). Monoclonal antibodies against micro-organisms. *Eur. J. Clin. Microbiol. 3*:387-398.

Porterfield, J. S. and Tobin, J. O'H. (1984). Viral and bacterial infectious diseases. *Br. Med. Bull. 40*:283-290.

Posner, M. R., Schlossman, S. F., and Lazarus, H. (1983). Novel approach to construction of human "myeloma analogues" for production of human monoclonal antibodies. *Hybridoma 2*:369-381.

Potter, M. and Boyce, C. R. (1962). Induction of plasma neoplasms in strain BALB/c mice with mineral oil and mineral oil adjuvants. *Nature 193*:1086-1087.

Potter, M., Rudikoff, S., Radlan, E. A., and Vrana, M. (1977). Covalent structure of the antigen binding site: Antigen binding myeloma proteins of the BALB/c mouse. In *Human Diagnosis and Therapy* (E. Haber and R. M. Krause, eds.). Raven Press, New York, pp. 9-28.

Price, M. R. and Baldwin, R. W. (1984). A solid phase radioimmunoassay for the determination of immunoglobulin class and subclass of mouse monoclonal antibodies. *IRCS Med. Sci. 12*:1000-1001.

Raison, R. L., Walker, K. Z., Halnan, C. R. E., Briscoe, D., and Basten, A. (1982). Loss of secretion in mouse-human hybrids need not be due to the loss of a structural gene. *J. Exp. Med. 156*:1380-1389.

Rathjen, D. A. and Underwood, P. A. (1985). Optimization of conditions for in vitro antigenic stimulation of dissociated mouse spleen cells for the production of monoclonal antibodies against peptide hormones. *J. Immunol. Methods 78*:227-237.

Reading, C. L. (1982). Theory and methods for immunization in culture and monoclonal antibody production. *J. Immunol. Methods 53*:262-291.

Rickinson, A. B., Moss, D. J., and Pope, J. H. (1979). Long-term T-cell mediated immunity to Epstein-Barr virus in man. II. Components necessary for regression in virus infected leucocyte culture. *Int. J. Cancer 23*:610-617.

Ritts, R. E., Ruiz-Argüelles, A., Weyl, K. G., Bradley, A. L., Weihmeir, B., Jacobsen, D. J., and Strehlo, B. L. (1983). Establishment and characterization of a human non-secretory plasmacytoid cell line and its hybridization with human B cells. *Int. J. Cancer 31*:133-141.

Robertson, S. M., Frisch, C. F., Gulig, P. A., Kettman, J. R., Johnston, K. H., and Hansen, E. J. (1982). Monoclonal antibodies directed against a cell surface-exposed outer membrane protein of *Haemophilus influenzae* type b. *Infect. Immun. 36*:80-88.

Rodriguez, J. F., Janeczko, R., and Esteban, M. (1985). Isolation and characterization of neutralizing monoclonal antibodies to vaccinia virus. *J. Virol. 56*: 482-488.

Rosen, A., Persson, K., and Klein, G. (1983). Human monoclonal antibodies to a genus-specific chlamydial antigen, produced by EBV-transformed B cells. *J. Immunol. 130*:2899-2902.

Routledge, E. G., McQuillin, J., Samson, A. C. R., and Toms, G. L. (1985). The development of monoclonal antibodies to respiratory syncitial virus and their use in diagnosis by indirect immunofluorescence. *J. Med. Virol. 15*: 305-320.

Satoh, J., Prabhakar, B. S., Haspel, M. V., Ginsberg-Fellner, F., and Notkins, A. L. (1983). Human monoclonal auto-antibodies that react with multiple endocrine organs. *N. Engl. J. Med. 309*:217-220.

Sawada, S., Kawamura, T., Masuho, Y., and Tomibe, K. (1985). Characterization of a human monoclonal antibody to lipopolysaccharides of *Pseudomonas aeruginosa* serotype 5: A possible candidate as an immuno-therapeutic agent for infections with *P. aeruginosa. J. Infect. Dis. 152*:965-970.

Sawada, S., Suzuki, M., Kawamura, T., Fujinaga, S., Masuho, Y., and Tomibe, K. (1984). Protection against infection with *Pseudomonas aeruginosa* by passive transfer of monoclonal antibodies to lipopolysaccharides and outer membrane proteins. *J. Infect. Dis. 150*:570-576.

Scheinberg, D. A., Pan, X.-Q., Wilsnack, R., and Strand, M. (1983). Rapid screening of monoclonal antibodies: New "Microstick" radioimmunoassay. *J. Immunol. Methods 58*:285-292.

Schlesinger, J. J., Brandriss, M. W., and Walsh, E. E. (1985). Protection against 17D yellow fever encephalitis in mice by passive transfer of monoclonal antibodies to the nonstructural glycoprotein gp48 and by active immunization with gp48. *J. Immunol. 135*:2805-2809.

Schulman, M., Wilde, C. D., and Köhler, G. (1978). A better cell line for making hybridomas secreting specific antibodies. *Nature 276*:269-270.

Schwaber, J. and Cohen, E. P. (1973). Human/mouse somatic cell hybrid clone secreting immunoglobulin of both parental types. *Nature 244*:444-447.

Schwaber, J. F., Posner, M. R., Schlossman, S. F., and Lazarus, H. (1984). Human-human hybrids secreting pneumococcal antibodies. *Human Immunol. 9*:137-143.

Seigneurin, C., Desgranges, C., Seigneurin, D., Paire, J., Renversez, J. C., Jacquemont, B., and Micouin, C. (1983). Herpes simplex virus glycoprotein D: Human monoclonal antibody produced by bone marrow cell line. *Science 221*: 173-175.

Shay, J. W. (1985). The biology of cell fusion. In *Human Hybridomas and Monoclonal Antibodies* (E. G. Engelman, S. K. H. Foung, J. Larrick, and A. Raubitschek, eds.). Plenum Press, New York, pp. 5-20.

Sheppard, A. J., Cussell, D., and Hughes, M. (1984). Production and characterization of monoclonal antibodies to tetanus toxin. *Infect. Immun. 43*:710-714.

Shigeoka, A. O., Pincus, S. H., Rote, N. S., and Hill, H. R. (1984). Protective efficacy of hybridoma type-specific antibody against experimental infection with group B *Streptococcus*. *J. Infect. Dis. 149*:363-372.

Shoenfield, Y., Hsu Lin, S. C., Gabriels, J. E., Silberstein, L. E., Furie, B. C., Furie, B., Stollar, B. D., and Schwartz, R. S. (1982). Production of autoantibodies by human-human hybridomas. *J. Clin. Invest. 70*:205-208.

Siadak, A. W. and Lostrom, M. E. (1985). Cell-driven viral transformation. In *Human Hybridomas and Monoclonal Antibodies* (E. G. Engelman, S. K. H. Foung, J. Larrick, A. Raubitschek, eds.). Plenum Press, New York, pp. 167-185.

Smart, I. J. and Koh, L. Y. (1983). Competitive inhibition enzyme immunoassays for the measurement of human IgG, IgA and IgM. *J. Immunol. Methods 60*: 329-339.

Smith, R., Lehner, T., and Beverley, P. C. L. (1984). Characterization of monoclonal antibodies to *Streptococcus mutans* antigenic determinants I/II, I, II and III and their serotype specificities. *Infect. Immun. 46*:168-175.

Söderström, T., Stein, K., Brinton, Jr., C. C., Hosea, S., Burch, C., Hansson, H. A., Karpas, A., Schneerson, R., Sutton, A., Vann, W. I., and Hanson, L. A. (1983). Serological and functional properties of monoclonal antibodies to *Escherichia coli* type I pilus and capsular antigens. *Prog. Allergy 33*:259-274.

Spitz, M., Spitz, L., Thorpe, R., and Eugui, E. (1984). Intrasplenic primary immunization for the production of monoclonal antibodies. *J. Immunol. Methods 70*:39-43.

Springer, T. A. (1983). Quantitation of hybridoma immunoglobulins and selection of light-chain loss variants. *Methods Enzymol. 92*:147-160.

Stähli, C., Staehelin, T., Miggiano, V., Schmidt, J., and Häring, P. (1980). High frequencies of antigen-specific hybridomas: Dependence on immunization parameters and prediction by spleen cell analysis. *J. Immunol. Methods 32*: 297-304.

Stein, L. D. and Sigal, N. H. (1983). Limiting dilution analysis of Epstein-Barr virus-induced immunoglobulin production. *Cell. Immunol. 79*:309-319.

Steinitz, M., Izak, G., Cohen, S., Ehrenfeld, M., and Flechner, I. (1980). Continuous production of monoclonal rheumatoid factor by EBV-transformed lymphocytes. *Nature 287*:443-445.

Steinitz, M., Klein, G., Koskimies, S., and Mäkelä, O. (1977). EB virus-induced B lymphocyte cell lines producing specific antibody. *Nature 269*:420-422.

Steinitz, M., Koskimies, S., Klein, G., and Mäkelä, O. (1979). Establishment of specific antibody producing human lines by antigen preselection and Epstein-Barr virus (EBV)-transformation. *J. Clin. Lab. Immunol. 2*:1-7.

Steinitz, M., Tamir, S., and Goldfarb, A. (1984). Human antipneumococcal antibody produced by an Epstein-Barr virus (EBV)-immortalised cell line. *J. Immunol. 132*:877-882.

Stephenson, J. R., Lee, J. M., and Wilton-Smith, P. D. (1984). Production and purification of murine monoclonal antibodies: Aberrant elution from protein A-Sepharose 4B. *Anal. Biochem. 142*:189-195.

Stricker, E. A. M., Tiebout, R. F., Lelie, P. N., and Zeijlemaker, W. P. (1985). A human monoclonal IgG1 anti-hepatitis B surface antibody. *Scand. J. Immunol. 22*:337-343.

Strike, L. E., Devens, B. H., and Lundak, R. L. (1984). Production of human-human hybridomas secreting antibody to sheep erythrocytes after in vitro immunization. *J. Immunol. 132*:1798-1803.

Strosberg, A. D., Collins, J. J., Black, P. H., Malamud, D., Wilbert, S., Block, K. J., and Haber, E. (1974). Transformation by simian virus 40 of spleen cells from a hyperimmune rabbit: Demonstration of production of specific antibody to the immunizing antigen. *Proc. Natl. Acad. Sci. USA 71*:263-264.

Sugasawara, R. J., Prato, C., and Sippel, J. E. (1983). Monoclonal antibodies against *Neisseria meningitidis* lipopolysaccharide. *Infect. Immun. 42*:863-868.

Sugasawara, R. J., Prato, C. M., and Sippel, J. E. (1984). Enzyme-linked immunosorbent assay with a monoclonal antibody for detecting group A meningococcal antigens in cerebrospinal fluid. *J. Clin. Microbiol. 19*:230-234.

Sugasawara, R. J., Cahoon, B. E., and Karu, A. E. (1985). The influence of murine macrophage-conditioned medium on cloning efficiency, antibody synthesis and growth rate of hybridomas. *J. Immunol. Methods 79*:263-275.

Taggart, R. T. and Samloff, I. M. (1983). Stable antibody-producing murine hybridomas. *Science 219*:1228-1230.

Tam, M. R., Buchanan, T. M., Sandström, E. G., Holmes, K. K., Knapp J. S., Siadak, A. W., and Nowinski, R. C. (1982). Serological classification of *Neisseria gonorrhoeae* with monoclonal antibodies. *Infect. Immun. 36*:1042-1053.

Tanaka, T. and Kurth, R. (1984). A small scale indirect [125] iodine-labelled protein A binding assay for detection of monoclonal antibodies against avian oncoviral proteins. *J. Immunol. Methods 75*:217-226.

Teng, N. N. H., Kaplan, H. S., Hebert, J. M., Moore, C., Douglas, H., Wunderlich, A., and Braude, A. I. (1985a). Protection against gram-negative bacteremia and endotoxemia with human monoclonal IgM antibodies. *Proc. Natl. Acad. Sci. USA 82*:1790-1794.

Teng, N. N. H., Lam, K. S., Riera, F. C., and Kaplan, H. S. (1983). Construction and testing of mouse-human heteromyelomas for human monoclonal antibody production. *Proc. Natl. Acad. Sci. USA 80*:7308-7312.

Teng, N. N. H., Reyes, G. R., Birber, M., Fry, K. E., Lam, K. S., and Hebert, J. M. (1985b). Strategies for stable human monoclonal antibody production. In *Human Hybridomas and Monoclonal Antibodies* (E. G. Engelman, S. K. H. Foung, J. Larrick, A. Raubitschek, eds.). Plenum Press, New York, pp. 71-91.

Thirkill, C. E., Song, D. Y., and Gregerson, D. S. (1983). Application of monoclonal antibodies to detect intraocular *Mycoplasma* antigens in *Mycoplasma arthritidis*-infected Sprague-Dawley rats. *Infect. Immun. 40*:389-397.

Tiebout, R. F., Stricker, E. A. M., Hagenaars, R., and Zeijlemaker, W. P. (1984). Human lymphoblastoid cell line producing protective monoclonal IgG1,k anti-tetanus toxin. *Eur. J. Immunol. 14*:399-404.

Tosato, G., Blaese, R. M., and Yarchoan, R. (1985). Relationship between immunoglobulin production and immortalization by Epstein-Barr virus. *J. Immunol. 135*:959-964.

Truitt, K. E., Larrick, J. W., and Raubitschek, A. (1984a). Fusion of nonadherent human cell lines. In *Monoclonal Antibodies and Functional Cell Lines* (R. H. Kennett, K. B. Bechtol, and T. J. McKearn, eds.). Plenum Press, New York, pp. 371-373.

Truitt, K. E., Larrick, J. W., Raubitschek, A., Buck, D. W., and Jacobson, S. W. (1984b). Production of human monoclonal antibody in mouse ascites. *Hybridoma 3*:195-199.

Tsoi, M.-S., Aprile, J., Dobbs, S., Goehle, S., and Storb, R. (1982). Enrichment (and depletion) of human suppressor cells with monoclonal antibodies and immunoglobulin-coated plates. *J. Immunol. Methods 53*:293-305.

Underwood, P. A. and Bean, P. A. (1985). The influence of methods of production, purification and storage of monoclonal antibodies upon their observed specificities. *J. Immunol. Methods 80*:189-197.

Volk, W. A., Bizzini, B., Snyder, R. M., Bernhard, E., and Wagner, R. R. (1984). Neutralization of tetanus toxin by distinct monoclonal antibodies binding to multiple epitopes on the toxin molecule. *Infect. Immun. 45*:604-609.

Waner, J. L., Whitehurst, N. J., Downs, T., and Graves, D. G. (1985). Production of monoclonal antibodies against parainfluenza 3 virus and their use in diagnosis by immunofluorescence. *J. Clin. Microbiol. 22*:535-538.

Wang, S.-P., Kuo, E.-C., Barnes, R. C., Stephens, R. S., and Grayston, J. T. (1985). Immunotyping of *Chlamydia trachomatis* with monoclonal antibodies. *J. Infect. Dis. 152*:791-800.

Ware, C. F., Donato, N. J., and Dorshkind, K. (1985). Human, rat or mouse hybridomas secrete high levels of monoclonal antibodies following transplantation into mice with severe combined immunodeficiency disease (SCID). *J. Immunol. Methods 85*:353-361.

Weiss, R. A. (1982). Hybridomas produce viruses as well as antibodies. *Immunol. Today 3*:292-294.

Wells, D. E. and Price, P. J. (1983). Simple rapid methods for freezing hybridomas in 96-well microculture plates. *J. Immunol. Methods 59*:49-52.

Westerwoudt, R. J. (1985). Improved fusion methods. IV. Technical aspects. *J. Immunol. Methods 77*:181-196.

Westerwoudt, R. J., Blom, J., Naipal, A. M., and van Rood, J. J. (1983). Improved fusion technique. I. Human umbilical cord serum, a new and potent growth promoter, compared with other B cell and hybridoma activators. *J. Immunol. Methods 62*:59-67.

Winger, L., Winger, C., Shastry, P., Russell, A., and Longenecker, M. (1983). Efficient generation in vitro, from human peripheral blood cells, of monoclonal Epstein-Barr virus transformants producing specific antibody to a variety of antigens without prior deliberate immunization. *Proc. Natl. Acad. Sci. USA 80*:4484-4488.

Wolinsky, J. S., Waxham, M. N., and Server, A. C. (1985). Protective effects of glycoprotein-specific monoclonal antibodies on the course of experimental mumps virus meningo-encephalitis. *J. Virol. 53*:727-734.

Wong, V. C. W., Ip, H. M. H., Reesink, H. W., Lelie, P. N., Reerink-Brongers, E. E., Yeung, C. Y., and Ma, H. K. (1984). Prevention of the HBsAg carrier state in newborn infants of mothers who are chronic carriers of HBsAg by administration of hepatitis-B vaccine and hepatitis-B immunoglobulin: Double-blind randomised placebo-controlled study. *Lancet 1*:921-926.

Worobec, E. A., Shastry, P., Smart, W., Bradley, R., Singh, B., and Paranchych, W. (1983). Monoclonal antibodies against colonisation factor antigen I pili from enterotoxigenic *Escherichia coli*. *Infect. Immun. 41*:1296-1301.

Wright, J. F. and Hunter, W. M. (1982). The sucrose layering separation: A non-centrifugation system. In *Immunoassays for Clinical Chemistry* (W. M. Hunter and J. E. T. Corrie, eds.). Churchill Livingstone, Edinburgh, pp. 170-177.

Wright, W. E. (1978). The isolation of heterokaryons and hybrids by a selective system using irreversible biochemical inhibitors. *Exp. Cell Res. 112*:395-407.

Zimmermann, U. and Vienken, J. (1982). Electric field-induced cell-to-cell fusion. *J. Membr. Biol. 67*:165-182.

Zucker, D. R. and Murphy, J. R. (1984). Monoclonal antibody analysis of diptheria toxin I. Localisation of epitopes and neutralization of cytotoxicity. *Mol. Immunol. 21*:785-793.

TWO

Development of Monoclonal Antibodies Against *Neisseria gonorrhoeae*

Milton R. Tam
Genetic Systems Corporation
Seattle, Washington

Eric G. Sandström
Karolinska Institute
Stockholm, Sweden

I. INTRODUCTION

In the last decade an intense research effort has been directed toward characterization of gonococcal outer membrane components. Goals of this research have
included the development of a useful serotyping system, as well as an understanding of the pathogenesis and epidemiology of the disease. For these purposes the
pilus proteins, lipopolysaccharides (LPS), and outer membrane proteins have all
been isolated and examined to study their roles in bacterial virulence and pathogenesis, and to select possible antigens with which to study classification, serotyping, and immunoprophylaxis.

II. SURFACE ANTIGENS OF THE GONOCOCCUS

The surface layer of the gonococcus that interacts with the human mucosa consists of a complex mosaic of proteins, LPS, and phospholipids, that is tightly
bound together in the outer membrane structure. These surface molecules play
critical roles in establishing bacterial colonization and infection and in the resistance of the gonococcus to natural or induced host defenses. Recent studies have
given us a detailed picture of these surface antigens and their roles in pathogenesis.

A. Pili

Under an electron microscope, pili can be seen as hairlike filaments 1-4 μm long
and 7-9 nm in diameter protruding from the outer membrane. They are composed
of identical, repeating subunits of the protein pilin with apparent molecular
weights of 17,500-21,000 depending upon their type. In gram-negative bacteria
pili have been associated with transformation by DNA, and in gonococci they
have also been associated with virulence (Arko, 1972). When freshly isolated,
most strains express pili. They are, however, rapidly (but not irreversibly) lost
upon subculture in vitro. Presumably, the mode of action of pili is to mediate attachment of gonococci to epithelial or other cells, but the nature of these receptors has not been fully characterized. Not only have different gonococcal strains
been found that express antigenically diverse pili, but the antigenicity of pili expressed by a single strain has been found to undergo extensive variation over time
(Hagblom et al., 1985).

B. Lipopolysaccharides

Gonococci have been shown to produce only "rough" type LPS, which consists of lipid A and core polysaccharide, and lacks the repeating O antigen side chains characteristic of "smooth" LPS (Mintz et al., 1984). As with other gram-negative bacteria, gonococcal LPS is considered an endotoxin, with extracts demonstrated to be toxic for chick embryos (Bumgarner and Finkelstein, 1973) or explanted epithelial cells (Gregg et al., 1981). The LPS forms a stable association with outer membrane proteins, which resists denaturation by detergents and heat (Hitchcock, 1984). At least six types of serologically distinct gonococcal LPS have been identified (Apicella and Gagliardi, 1979). By differential testing of mutant strains varying in their LPS types, LPS has also been shown to mediate the resistance or sensitivity to bactericidal serum and complement (Rice and Kasper, 1977), pyocins (Connelly and Allen, 1983), or binding to lectins (Morse and Apicella, 1982).

C. Capsules

A number of investigators have reported the existence of gonococcal capsules (Hendley et al., 1977, 1981; James and Swenson, 1977; Richardson and Sadoff, 1977), the production of which was dependent upon on special media and fresh isolates. Currently, the existence of capsules is disputed because capsular material has not been isolated in pure form. Evidence against capsules in gonococci comes from the observation that wheat germ agglutinin, that can agglutinate noncapsulate meningococcal strains but not capsulate strains, could agglutinate all but a very small proportion of gonococcal strains (Rice et al., 1986). This suggested that gonococcal LPS was surface-exposed and lacked a protective capsular layer (Frasch, 1980). Because gonococci have been found to express high-molecular-weight polyphosphates on their surface, it is possible that these function as a capsular substance (Noegel and Gotschlich, 1983).

D. Outer Membrane Proteins

1. Protein I

Protein I (Pr I), also termed the principal or major outer membrane protein, accounts for about 60% of the total outer membrane protein and is present in all strains of gonococci. By polyacrylamide gel electrophoresis (PAGE), Pr I ranges from 32,000 to 39,000 in molecular weight (Johnston et al., 1976). Protein I is thought to occur in situ as a trimeric form (McDade and Johnston, 1980), serving as a porin which allows selective passage of hydrophilic molecules through the intrinsically hydrophobic outer membrane and into the cell (Douglas et al., 1981; Lynch et al., 1984). Protein I isolated from different strains of gonococci can be found as two "species," termed Pr IA and Pr IB, which distinctly differ from one another in their molecular weights, antigenic specificity, peptide maps, and susceptibility to proteolysis in situ (Sandstrom et al., 1982a). These two proteins contain multiple antigenic determinants that are stable in all strains studied. Almost all antigens identified on Pr I are species-specific (Tam et al., 1982).

2. Protein III

Protein III (Pr III), or associated protein, is thought to form a heteropolymer with Pr I in the outer membrane. Treatment of cells with cross-linking agents revealed several new types of protein complexes, suggesting that they exist, surface exposed, in close proximity with Pr I in the outer membrane (McDade and Johnston, 1980). Sarafian et al. (1983) have shown that antibodies to Pr I in normal human serum could block the binding of a monoclonal antibody (MAb) specific for Pr III, again demonstrating that Pr I and Pr III are closely associated within the outer membrane. The function of Pr III, common to all strains of gonococci, is unknown. Antigenically, Pr III shares determinants with all strains of meningococci and several species of commensal neisseriae (Tam, unpublished results).

3. Protein II

Protein(s) II (Pr II), or "opacity" proteins, comprise a group of related surface proteins that contribute to an "opaque" colony morphology but are generally absent from, or less well represented in, colonies with a "transparent" morphology (Swanson, 1978). Their apparent molecular weight when measured by PAGE or column chromatography depends upon the method and temperature with which they were isolated, but it is usually from 24 000 to 30,000. Every gonococcal strain has the potential to express several species of Pr II, although only one or two are usually expressed at any given time. The change, or "switch" rate of Pr II expression has been calculated at 10^{-3}/cell per generation in vitro, and therefore, variants can be produced even within the same colony (Mayer, 1982). Functionally, Pr IIs have been shown to differ in adherence to different types of cells (Watt and Ward, 1980), mediate serum sensitivity or resistance (Heckels and James, 1980), and resistance to antimicrobial agents (Heckels and James, 1980). Protein II expression also enables the gonococcus to aggregate or clump more readily. Variation of this protein may thus enable gonococci to adapt rapidly to a changing microenvironment within the host.

4. Other Proteins

Characterization of other proteins identified in the outer membrane include: (1) a 37,000 dalton iron-regulated protein that was found in higher amounts under iron-limiting conditions. Peptide mapping showed that this protein was distinct from Pr I and identical when isolated from Pr IA or Pr IB strains (Mietzner et al., 1984); and (2) a common gonococcal (and meningococcal) heat-modifiable outer membrane protein, H.8, with a molecular weight of 20,000 when extracted at 37°C, but 30,000 if extracted at 100°C (Cannon et al., 1984).

III. SELECTION OF REFERENCE STRAINS AND TARGET ANTIGENS FOR SEROLOGICAL CLASSIFICATION

A. Introduction

Serological classification or serogrouping of pathogenic bacteria has greatly aided the understanding of the clinical epidemiology of infections. For example, serogrouping of *N. meningitidis* on the basis of their capsular polysaccharides have shown that some serogroups, such as A, B, and C, are more virulent than others, which has led to the development of type-specific meningococcal vaccines. Before 1977 an equivalent serological classification system was lacking for gonococci. Early investigators were hampered by a lack of defined antigens and adequate technology, resulting in the failure to recognize the phenomenon of antigenic variation. The work of Wilson (1954) was never expanded, probably because the antigenic drift that he demonstrated within gonococcal strains was interpreted as a weakness in his classification scheme, rather than a novel property of the gonococci.

B. Serological Classification Using Lipopolysaccharides

One of the first attempts at serogrouping based on a single antigenic system was by Maeland (1969). Using only three strains, he identified six antigenic factors that were present in different combinations on all other gonococcal strains isolated. This line of investigation was continued by Apicella (1976) who showed unequivocally that gonococcal LPS carried distinct antigenic determinants. In searching for antigenically distinct strains of gonococci, he found four different types of LPS, termed GC1-4, which could be defined by specific antisera: all but 27 (16.5%) of 163 isolates could be grouped using the four antisera. Of the 136 typable strains, 85% possessed LPS in antigenically pure form, whereas the remaining 15% had an antigenic mosaic comprising two types of LPS. Apicella and Gagliardi (1979) found two more antigenic LPS determinants that were shared among the strains expressing LPS types 1-4, resulting in a total of six different LPS determinants.

C. Microimmunofluorescence with Whole Cell Antigen

Wang et al. (1977) also showed reproducible antigenic differences among another set of serotyping reference strains. By using the microimmunofluorescence method with mouse antisera raised against whole cells, they found that all but five of 180 gonococcal strains of diverse geographical origin could be grouped into three major and eight minor groups, A1-A3, B1-B3, and C1-C2. There were extensive cross-reactions among the gonococcal strains, and immunotyping was feasible only after absorption of antigen with an antigenically heterologous strain (NRL-5029) that showed little or no cross-reaction with the other gonococcal strains studied.

The need to absorb antisera may have contributed to the failure to type these five isolates.

D. Serological Classification Using Outer Membrane Proteins

Johnston et al. (1976) demonstrated that the outer membrane proteins could be used for gonococcal serogrouping. By use of strains isolated in New York and other parts of the world, they grouped all strains into 16 unique classes that correlated with the combined subunit molecular weight profiles of "major" and "minor" outer membrane proteins. Rabbit antisera raised against the outer membrane fragments of reference strains reacted specifically with the larger molecular weight proteins but cross-reacted with the smaller proteins. Once a strain was assigned to a serogroup, the antigens did not change with time, indicating that the defined antigens were stable.

1. Coagglutination Serogrouping

Sandström and Danielsson (1980) used a coagglutination (CoA) method for serogrouping of gonococci. With rabbit antisera generated against the 16 reference strains of Johnston et al. (1976), they found three antigenic classes of reactions, M, J, and W. Class M antigens were sensitive to periodate, resistant to pronase, and probably consisted of LPS. Six antigenic factors could be identified whose reaction patterns were analogous to those studied by Maeland (1969) and Apicella (1976). The patterns of reactivity were found to change spontaneously in serial isolates from the same patient but were stable on subculture in vitro. Class J antigens were less well defined and may, in part, have represented a number of reactivities to minor or variable Pr II outer membrane proteins. Class W antigens were pronase-sensitive but periodate-resistant. With CoA reagants to the W antigens, three serogroups, WI, WII, and WIII were identified using selectively absorbed polyclonal antisera. With minor exceptions, these three serogroups corresponded to the microimmunofluorescence groupings A, B, and C of Wang et al. (1977). These antigens were remarkably stable to various treatments, and were not modulated by the gonococci either in vivo or on subculture in vitro. Any given gonococcal strain possessed only one of the two different species of Pr I: Pr IA, which corresponded to serogroup WI, and Pr IB, which corresponded to serogroups WII/WIII. The W serogrouping system, further refined with use of MAbs, has been used extensively in epidemiological studies, and is reviewed in Chap. 4.

2. Enzyme-Linked Immunosorbent Assay Serotyping

Buchanan and Hildebrandt (1981) based their serotyping system exclusively upon Pr I. Using an enzyme-linked immunosorbent assay (ELISA) with a known amount of gonococci to inhibit typing sera, they could group 124 of 125 strains of gonococci, including the 16 reference strains of Johnston et al. (1976), into nine Pr I types. These types were organized such that types 1-3 corresponded to reactivity with serogroup WI, and types 4-9, in a spectrum based on assumptions of antigenic similarities, within serogroups WII and WIII. Types 3-9 were shown to be antigenically distinct, whereas types 1 and 2 were more closely related. Reactivity to LPS did not interfere with these reactions, as LPS contamination of the purified Pr I was minimal. More recently, Sandström et al. (1982b) found a close correlation between CoA serogrouping with W antigens and principal outer membrane protein serotypes: serogroup WI corresponded to Pr I serotypes 1-3, and WII/WIII corresponded to Pr I serotypes 4-9.

E. Summary

A meaningful serogrouping system should (1) define target gonococcal surface antigens that resist modulation with repeated subculture in vivo or in vitro over time, (2) define antigens that are neither too diverse nor too invariant, to produce a manageable number of subdivisions of strains, (3) be capable of grouping or classifying the overwhelming majority of strains isolated, including representative strains from geographically diverse origins, (4) preferably be based on antigens found only within the species to avoid misidentification of isolates, (5) allow standardization between different laboratories, and (6) have sufficient economy and ease of use to allow a wide dissemination. The advent of hybridoma technology has aided attempts to develop a system that fulfills these criteria.

IV. PRODUCTION AND CHARACTERIZATION OF MONOCLONAL ANTIBODIES AGAINST *NEISSERIA GONORRHOEAE*

In 1981 we applied hybridoma technology to the study of *N. gonorrhoeae*. Our goals were to prepare a panel of MAbs that were (1) broad in reactivity across a range of gonococcal strains and would possibly be valuable in the development of diagnostic reagents, and (2) that were of a more restricted specificity that would have applications in serotyping of strains in epidemiological studies and in mapping of individual antigenic determinants. On the basis of the studies outlined in the previous sections we selected gonococcal Pr I as the most suitable antigen for the production of MAbs with which to meet our goals.

A. Monoclonal Antibodies Against Outer Membrane Proteins

1. Protein I

Full details of the production and characterization of MAbs against Pr I are given by Tam et al. (1982), but the general approach was as follows:

a. Antibody Production. Strains representative of the W serogroups were chosen for immunization. BALB/c mice were immunized intraperitoneally (IP) on day 0 with 50-200 μg of purified Pr I (85% Pr I and less than 5% LPS) for fusions one to three and with Formalin-treated whole cells for fusion four. For some fusions, mice were immunized simultaneously with mixtures of Pr I and outer membrane extracts, whereas in others the mice were immunized with Pr I or outer membrane extracts from individual bacterial strains. Mice were boosted IP on days 14 and 21 with the same immunogen as they had received initially.

Lymphocytes from the spleen and lymphoid tissue were fused with NS-1 myeloma cells at a ratio of 4:1 in the presence of 40% polyethylene glycol (PEG). Cells were washed in RMPI 1640, mixed with an equal number of BALB/c thymocytes, and plated into a 96-well culture plate at a concentration of 10^6 cells per well in hypotanthine, aminopterin, thymidine (HAT) medium. After 5-6 days hybrid cells were routinely detected in every well of the plate. Because immunoglobulin production was unstable in most hybrid cells, low-density passage with thymocyte feeder cells (minicloning) was used to rescue immunoglobulin-positive hybrids before cloning by endpoint dilution.

b. Antibody Selection. For the selection of MAbs it was advantageous to obtain maximum information regarding their specificity in early screening. Although purified Pr I was used for immunization, the mice could have responded to the small amounts of other gonococcal antigens or contaminants present. Also, we usually generated many more hybrids secreting gonococcus-specific antibodies than could be conveniently handled. For example, assays with culture fluids from 2400 wells, representing four different fusions, showed that 254 wells (10.6%) contained antibodies that reacted with outer membrane preparations from one or more gonococcal strains. This necessitated a quick and accurate assessment of those antibodies produced to select and stabilize those of desired specificity. The culture fluids from a 96-well culture plate were tested by replica plating onto Pr I preparations of three or more strains of gonococci. The plates were then developed with ^{125}I-labeled protein A and autoradiography. The strains for assay were chosen with reference to the previous studies of Buchanan and Hildebrandt (1981) who showed that strains could be grouped on the basis of their Pr I heterogeneity. We thus assayed our fusions on two or more closely related strains and at least one other strain which was not closely related. In this manner we could accurately assess and select a number of antibodies, each exhibiting different patterns of reactions, for further cloning and study. Figure 1 illustrates the replicate-plate method used. Strains 7122 and 7929 are closely related, and are both within the WI serogroup bearing Pr IA, whereas strain 8035 is of WII serogroup or Pr IB origin. Several antibodies with differing specificities can be seen, D3 and A11, which are serotype-specific; F10, which reacts with both members of the WI group; and H7, which defines a genus or species-specific antigen. With multiple immunizations of mice using representative

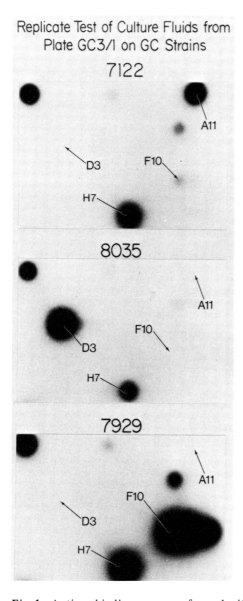

Replicate Test of Culture Fluids from
Plate GC3/1 on GC Strains

Fig. 1 Antigen-binding assays performed with MAbs using culture fluid of a primary plate. Culture fluids from the primary plate were replicate-plated into microtest plates into which three·different gonococcal protein I extracts were adsorbed. Immune binding was detected by addition of ^{125}I-labeled protein A and subsequent autoradiography. A positive control (polyvalent rabbit antiserum 1:50) was included on the top left corner of each plate.

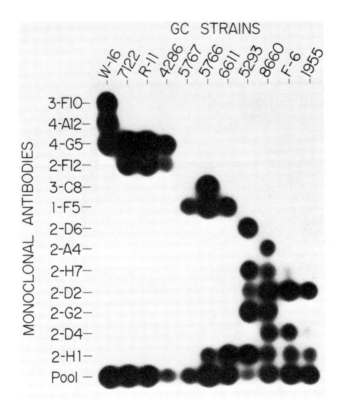

Fig. 2   Antigen-binding assays of monoclonal antibodies with a panel of protein I or outer membrane preparations from gonococcal serotyping reference strains. Culture fluids from 13 prototype hybrid cell lines were tested against outer membrane extracts from 11 strains of gonococci. Immune reactions were detected by the addition of ^{125}I-labeled protein A and subsequent autoradiography. Also included in the last row of this assay is a test using a pool of four culture fluids (3F10, 2F12, 1F5, and 2D2).

gonococcal reference strains and similar assay protocols, we were able to generate a spectrum of *N. gonorrhoeae*-specific MAbs, primarily those with narrow to moderate serotype-specific reactivity (Fig. 2). Those MAbs with broad species reactivity invariably reacted with other species of pathogenic or commensal *Neisseria*.

Cells from 79 of the 254 antibody-producing wells from the first four fusions were selected according to the serological specificity of their antibodies and continually propagated. From these, 56 phenotypically stable, independently cloned cell lines were obtained. Cells from each of these lines were inoculated into pristane-primed syngeneic mice to produce ascites fluids containing high-titer MAbs. These 56 MAbs selected from our first four fusions were examined by antigen-binding assays for reactivity with 34 gonococcal reference strains. On this basis, 16 MAbs were initially chosen for further study (Tam et al., 1982). Each of the 16 MAbs reacted with a discrete subpopulation of the reference strains, did not react with any of the 17 other species of *Neisseria* or with *Branhamella catarrhalis*, and was confirmed as specific for Pr I by radioimmune precipitation assays in PAGE. Three of the patterns of antibody reactivities approximated those identified previously in CoA assays using polyvalent antisera, i.e., reacting only within the previously defined CoA WI, WII, or WIII serogroups. A fourth pattern of reactivity was revealed when certain MAbs reacted with strains in both the WII and WIII serogroups. This was interpreted as a serological relatedness between groups WII and WIII, which is consistent with peptide-mapping studies revealing two distinctively different Pr I molecules, Pr IA for group WI and Pr IB for groups WII/WIII (Sandstrom et al., 1982a). More recently, we have generated additional Pr IA-specific MAbs and have selected 12 MAbs, six specific to Pr IA and six specific to Pr IB for use in serological classification studies (Knapp et al., 1984). These results are summarized in Sect. V and discussed in detail in Chap. 4.

2. Protein II

Nachamkin et al. (1981) were the first to report successful production of an MAb to a gonococcal-specific surface antigen. This antibody, termed 10.1, was described as highly strain-specific and reacted only with a subset of clones of strain FA1090 selected for variations in opacity. This MAb was later shown to be directed against a variable Pr II (Sugasawara et al., 1983).

The MAb 10.1 and an additional antibody (H138.2) to a different Pr II were used to directly identify the expression of antigenic epitopes in certain forms of Pr II proteins. Monoclonal antibody 10.1, bound to both Pr IIb and Pr IId but was bactericidal for only those variants expressing Pr IIb. The MAb H138.2 reacted with, and was bactericidal for, only the Pr IIa variant (Black et al., 1984). Newhall et al. (1985) have also prepared MAbs each specific for three Pr II variants of strain F62. No cross-reactions of these antibodies were observed for heterologous Pr IIs in six other gonococcal strains tested. These studies point to the considerable antigenic variation found within Pr II molecules in the gonococcus.

3. Protein III

An MAb specific for gonococcal Pr III has been used to study some properties of Pr III in the outer membrane (Swanson et al., 1982). Western blot transfer indicates that MAb 2E6 reacted with a single Pr III band at 30,000-31,000 daltons. This antibody recognized a common, surface-exposed epitope present on three gonococcal strains of different origins, suggesting that the Pr III antigenic epitopes are conserved. Further studies with MAb 2E6 showed that it reacted in CoA assays with all 34 serotyping reference strains, supporting the view that the Pr III epitopes are conserved in most if not all strains of gonococci (Tam, unpublished results).

4. Other Proteins

By using MAb H.8 Cannon et al. (1984) have defined an additional antigen common to all strains of *N. gonorrhoeae* and *N. meningitidis*, as well as *N. lactamica* and *N. cinerea*. This antigen was described as surface-exposed, heat-modifiable, and banding at an apparent molecular weight of 20,000 if extracted at 37°C. This heat-modifiable property distinguishes the antigen defined by H.8 as distinct from Pr I and Pr III.

B. Monoclonal Antibodies Against Lipopolysaccharides

Apicella et al. (1981) reported production of a MAb reactive with a determinant common to the LPS found on all strains of gonococci and partially shared by some strains of meningococci. Similar preparations of LPS from representative strains of *Escherichia coli* and *Salmonella* failed to inhibit antibody binding. This MAb was completely inhibited from binding to gonococcal LPS by D-galactosamine, and was partially inhibited by a a-lactose and β-lactose, findings that led to the conclusion that the determinant recognized was D-galactosamine-O-D-galactopyranosyl-(1-4)-D-glucopyranose.

C. Monoclonal Antibodies Against Pili

Monoclonal antibodies were used by Virji et al. (1983) as a means of probing the distribution of antigens and demonstrating the antigenic heterogeneity in the pilus protein (pilin). They produced type-specific as well as broadly cross-reactive MAbs that were used in competition assays to determine the number of distinct epitopes present. They concluded that two distinct regions exist on pilin: a common region shared by all types and a highly variable type-specific region. Both regions were found to contain multiple antigenic epitopes. In functional assays, the type-specific MAbs, but not the cross-reactive antibodies, could inhibit the adhesion of pili to human buccal epithelial cells, and could also protect Chang epithelial cells growing in culture from damage from virulent gonococci (Virji and Heckels, 1985).

Edwards et al. (1984) were also able to define both cross-reactive and type-specific pilin epitopes using MAbs and could separate their type-specific antibodies into those that did or that did not react with the cyanogen bromide-generated pilin fragment CB-3 (the carboxy-terminal part of the molecule containing the type-specific antigenic determinants). Cross-reactive antibodies were not reactive with CB-3. Certain pilin epitopes as defined by MAbs were shown to be linear protein structures, because antibodies would bind to the synthetic peptides generated. Other MAbs were shown to be specific for intact pili, but did not bind to synthetic peptides or peptide fragments. These latter antibodies probably reacted with secondary or tertiary structural determinants which were lost with confirmational changes in the protein.

V. USES OF MONOCLONAL ANTIBODIES

A. Intraspecies Serotyping for Epidemiological Studies

Following our initial work describing 16 MAbs specific for Pr I (Tam et al., 1982), we generated additional Pr IA-specific MAbs, from which we have selected a definitive panel of six MAbs specific for gonococcal Pr IA and another six to Pr IB for use in serological classification studies. By CoA studies we were able to classify 1433 strains, collected in a worldwide survey, into 19 Pr IA and 28 Pr IB serovars. Because gonococcal strains can be also classified by auxotyping, a stable biochemical characteristic, the combination of serovar/auxotype categorization served to further separate the strains which were otherwise identical by serotyping. We were now able to classify the isolates into 107 unique, stable classes (Knapp et al., 1984). As discussed in Chap. 4, this dual, fine-point classification method can be used to: (1) identify patterns of gonococcal transmission; (2) identify related gonococcal strains to test focused measures of control; (3) analyze patterns of antibiotic resistance; (4) monitor the migration and establishment of strains between different geographic areas; (5) identify the association of auxotypes/serovars with various types of complicated infection; and (6) identify temporal changes in gonococcal populations within a community. Once strains are classified in this manner, the effectiveness of public health intervention upon disease incidence can be directly assessed.

B. Identification of Structures Responsible for Pathogenesis

Attachment functions of proteins associated with pathogenesis of gonococci have been studied with specific MAbs. For example, Sugasawara et al. (1983) reported that the Pr II-specific MAb 10.1 interfered with attachment to HeLa cells of gonococcal strain FA1090 bearing the homologous species of Pr II but did not interfere with the variant of the same strain not expressing the Pr II molecule. A nonspecific MAb used as a control also had no effect on binding of FA1090 to HeLa cells.

Similar studies to determine the effect of antipilin MAbs on the binding of pili to epithelial cells were reported by Heckels and Virji (1985). They found that MAbs reactive with the variable domains of pilin (type-specific antibodies) inhibited the attachment of purified preparations of pili to human buccal epithelial cells, whereas MAbs reactive with conserved regions (cross-reactive antibodies) did not. To further investigate these interactions using live organisms, the authors noted that the type-specific antipilin MAbs prevented attachment and subsequent damage of Chang epithelial cells by piliated gonococci, whereas the cross-reactive MAbs were ineffective. They concluded that the variable region, but not the conserved region of pilin contains the epithelial cell receptor sequence, which is sterically hindered by attachment of the MAb. It is possible that receptor sites may also reside in the constant region of pilin, but MAbs were not produced to define those epitopes.

These findings are relevant to the development of a vaccine for control of gonorrhea and highlight problems likely to be encountered using vaccines that incorporate pili or other highly variable proteins as immunogens. Whereas antibodies to the common regions are seemingly ineffective for protection against the pathogenic effects of gonococci, antibodies to the variable regions are likely to produce a selective pressure on the organism to shift the antigenic specificity of the protein. Even if more stable proteins, such as Pr I, are chosen, care must be taken to select the precise antigenic sequences of the immunogens to ensure the production of bactericidal antibodies. For example, Joiner et al. (1985) investigated the bactericidal effects of MAbs directed against Pr I. Their results indicated that if a first anti-Pr I MAb was reacted with viable gonococci, it could block the bactericidal activity of a second MAb specific for a similar or identical Pr I epitope. Thus, for Pr I or other vaccines, efforts should be made to exclude those amino acid sequences responsible for production of "blocking" antibodies.

C. Interspecies Classification for Phylogenetic Studies

Monoclonal antibodies directed to gonococcal antigens may be used to determine phylogenetic relationships between the members of the genus *Neisseria*. For example, MAb H.8 produced by Cannon et al. (1984) from a mouse inoculated with gonococcal outer membrane proteins reacted with all gonococci and meningococci tested. Monoclonal antibody H.8 also bound to four of five strains of *N. lactamica*, and the one strain of *N. cinerea* tested, but bound to only one of 34 other strains of commensal neisseriae and *B. catarrhalis* tested (the one positive was an "atypical" strain of *N. sicca*). These results are consistent with other investigations such as DNA hybridization studies which indicate that the two commensal *Neisseria* species, *N. lactamica* and *N. cinerea*, are most closely related to the pathogens *N. gonorrhoeae* and *N. meningitidis*. The role or function of this conserved H.8 antigen among the related species of *Neisseria* is not known.

Other antigens may be used to investigate phylogenetic relationships within the *Neisseria*. Monoclonal antibodies against LPS (Apicella et al., 1981) and pilus antigens (Heckels and Virji, 1985) react with both gonococci and meningococci. Although the MAbs described as reactive with LPS or pili do not react with *Sal-*

monella spp. or *E. coli*, there are no reports of testing for such antibodies with a complete panel of commensal *Neisseria* spp.

D. Diagnosis of Gonococcal Infection

Monoclonal antibody technology has the potential to produce highly sensitive and specific immunological reagents, which can be made widely available for the diagnosis of infectious diseases (Nowinski et al., 1983; Tam et al., 1985). For example, Nowinski et al. (1983), reported that a CoA reagent agent using a mixture of three broadly reactive anti-Pr I MAbs identified 99.6% (716/719) of gonococcal isolates without cross-reacting with 17 other closely related *Neisseria* spp. The use of MAbs in the diagnosis of gonorrhea is reviewed in Chap. 3.

VI. CONCLUSIONS

In a few short years the application of hybridoma technology has made a major impact on our understanding of the gonococcus. The precise specificity of MAbs has made possible the definition of common, unique, and previously unrecognized gonococcal antigenic determinants on membrane proteins, pilus proteins, and LPS. The dissection and analysis of the immune response to gonococcal antigens with MAbs has resulted in the definition of epitopes or regions on molecules that contribute to pathogenicity. Using this knowledge, more effective vaccines or methods of therapy may be produced. To establish more effective serotyping methods, panels of MAbs have been generated that react with different epitopes on a single stable membrane protein. Measures for control of gonococcal infection by public health intervention may be more effectively tested and implemented with these improved typing and epidemiological tracing methods. Initial formulations of MAbs for diagnosis of gonococcal infection have been reported. Improved diagnostic reagents should result from the generation of more complete libraries of MAbs and will undoubtedly lead to more sensitive, specific, and rapid methods for diagnosis than are currently available. In summary the utilization of MAbs in gonococcal research and diagnosis of disease has just begun. Monoclonal antibodies will find further applications in vaccine development, as an aid to molecular cloning of gonococcal-specific antigens, and in purification of antigens from complex mixtures.

REFERENCES

Arko, R. J. (1972). *Neisseria gonorrhoeae*: Experimental infection of experimental animals. *Science 177*:1200-1203.

Apicella, M. A. (1976). Serogrouping of *Neisseria gonorrhoeae*: Identification of four immunologically distinct acidic polysaccharides. *J. Infect. Dis. 134*: 377-383.

Apicella, M. A., Bennett, K. M., Hermerath, C. A., and Roberts, D. E. (1981). Monoclonal antibody analysis of lipopolysaccharide from *Neisseria gonorrhoeae* and *Neisseria meningitidis*. *Infect. Immun. 34*:751-756.

Apicella, M. and Gagliardi, N. C. (1979). Antigenic heterogeneity of the non-serogroup antigen structure of *Neisseria gonorrhoeae* lipopolysaccharides. *Infect. Immun. 26*:870-874.

Black, W. J., Schwalbe, R. S., Nachamkin, I., and Cannon, J. G. (1984). Characterization of *Neisseria gonorrhoeae* protein II phase variation by use of monoclonal antibodies. *Infect. Immun. 45*:453-457.

Buchanan, T. M. and Hildebrandt, J. F. (1981). Antigen-specific serotyping of *Neisseria gonorrhoeae*: Characterization based upon principal outer membrane protein. *Infect. Immun. 32*:985-993.

Bumgarner, L. R. and Finkelstein, R. A. (1973). Pathogenesis and immunology of experimental gonococcal infection: Virulence of colony type of *Neisseria gonorrhoeae* for chicken embryos. *Infect. Immun. 8*:919-924.

Cannon, J. G., Black, W. J., Nachamkin, I., and Stewart, P. W. (1984). A monoclonal antibody that recognizes an outer membrane antigen common to the pathogenic *Neisseria* species, but not to most nonpathogenic *Neisseria* species. *Infect. Immun. 43*:994-999.

Connelly, M. D. and Allen, P. Z. (1983). Antigenic specificity and heterogeneity of lipopolysaccharides from pyocin-sensitive and resistant strains of *Neisseria gonorrhoeae*. *Infect. Immun. 41*:1046-1055.

Dillon, J. R., Bygdeman, S., and Sandström, E. (1987). Serovar, anxotype, plasmid profile, and antibiotic susceptibility of 113 gonococcal isolates from Canada. *Genitourin. Med.* (In press).

Douglas, J. T., Lee, M. D., Nikaido, H. (1981). Protein I of *Neisseria gonorrhoeae* outer membrane is a porin. *FEMS Microbiol. Lett. 12*:305-309.

Edwards, M., McDade, R. L., Schoolnik, G., Rothbard, J. B., and Gotschlich, E. C. (1984). Antigenic analysis of gonococcal pili using monoclonal antibodies. *J. Exp. Med. 160*:1782-1791.

Frasch, C. E. (1980). Role of lipopolysaccharide in wheat germ agglutinin-mediated agglutination of *Neisseria meningitidis* and *Neisseria gonorrhoeae*. *J. Clin. Microbiol. 12*:498-501.

Gregg, C. R., Melly, M. A., Hellerqvist, C. G., Coniglio, J. G., and McGee, Z. A. (1981). Toxic activity of purified lipopolysaccharide of *Neisseria gonorrhoeae* for human fallopian tube mucosa. *J. Infect. Dis. 150*:49-56.

Hagblom, P., Segal, E., Billyard, E., and So, M. (1985). Intragenic recombination leads to pilus antigenic variation in *Neisseria gonorrhoeae*. *Nature 315*:156-158.

Heckels, J. E. (1981). Structural comparison of *Neisseria gonorrhoeae* outer membrane proteins. *J. Bacteriol. 145*:736-742.

Heckels, J. E. and James, L. T. (1980). The structural organization of the gono-coccal cell envelope and its influence on pathogenesis. In *Genetics and Immunobiology of Pathogenic Neisseria* (D. Danielsson and S. Normark, eds.). University of Umea, Sweden, p. 75.

Heckels, J. E. and Virji, M. (1985). Monoclonal antibodies against gonococcal pili: Uses in the analysis of gonococcal immunochemistry and virulence. In *Monoclonal Antibodies Against Bacteria* (A. J. L. Macario and E. C. de Macario, eds.). Academic Press, New York, pp. 2-35.

Hendley, J. O., Powell, K. R., Rodewall, R., Holzgrefe, H. H., and Lyles, R. (1977). Demonstration of a capsule on *Neisseria gonorrhoeae*. *N. Engl. J. Med. 296*:608-611.

Hendley, J. O., Powell, K. R., Salomonsky, N. L., and Rodewald, R. R. (1981). Electron microscopy of the gonococcal capsule. *J. Infect. Dis. 143*:796-802.

Hitchcock, P. J. (1984). Analyses of gonococcal lipopolysaccharide in whole cell lysates by sodium dodecyl sulfate and polyacrylamide gel electrophoresis: Stable association of lipopolysaccharide with the major outer membrane protein (protein I) of *Neisseria gonorrhoeae*. *Infect. Immun. 46*:202-212.

James, J. F. and Swanson, J. (1977). The capsule of the gonococcus. *J. Exp. Med. 145*:1082-1086.

James, J. F., Zurlinden, E., Lammel, C. J., and Brooks, G. F. (1982). Relation of protein I and colony opacity to serum killing of *Neisseria gonorrhoeae*. *J. Infect. Dis. 145*:37-43.

Johnston, K. H., Holmes, K. K., and Gotschlich, E. C. (1976). The serological classification of *Neisseria gonorrhoeae*. I. Isolation of the outer membrane complex responsible for serotypic specificity. *J. Exp. Med. 143*:741-758.

Joiner, K. A., Warren, K. A., Tam, M. R., and Frank, M. M. (1985). Monoclonal antibodies directed against gonococcal protein I vary in bactericidal activity. *J. Immunol. 134*:3411-3419.

Knapp, J. S., Tam, M. R., Nowinski, R. C., Holmes, K. K., and Sandström, E. G. (1984). Serological classification of *Neisseria gonorrhoeae* with use of monoclonal antibodies to gonococcal outer membrane protein I. *J. Infect. Dis. 150*:44-48.

Lynch, E. C., Blake, M. S., Gotschlich, E. C., and Mauro, A. (1984). Studies of porins: Spontaneously transferred from whole cells and reconstituted from purified proteins of *Neisseria gonorrhoeae* and *Neisseria meningitidis*. *Biophys. J. 45*:104-107.

McDade, Jr., R. and Johnston, K. H. (1980). Characterization of serologically dominant outer membrane proteins of *Neisseria gonorrhoeae*. *J. Bacteriol. 141*:1183-1191.

Maeland, J. A. (1969). Serological cross-reactivity of aqueous ether extracted endotoxin from *Neisseria gonorrhoeae* strains. *Acta Pathol. Microbiol. Scand. 77*:505-517.

Mayer, L. W. (1982). Rates of in vitro changes of gonococcal colony opacity phenotypes. *Infect. Immun. 37*:481-485.

Mietzner, T. A., Luginbuhl, G. H., Sandström, E., and Morse, S. A. (1984). Identification of an iron-regulated 37,000 dalton protein in the cell envelope of *Neisseria gonorrhoeae. Infect. Immun. 45*:410-416.

Mintz, C. S., Apicella, M. A., and Morse, S. A. (1984). Electrophoretic and serological characterization of the lipopolysaccharide produced by *Neisseria gonorrhoeae. J. Infect. Dis. 149*:544-551.

Morse, S. A. and Apicella, M. A. (1982). Isolation of a lipopolysaccharide mutant of *Neisseria gonorrhoeae*: An analysis of the antigenic and biologic differences. *J. Infect. Dis. 145*:206-216.

Nachamkin, I., Cannon, J. C., and Mittler, R. S. (1981). Monoclonal antibodies against *Neisseria gonorrhoeae*: Production of antibodies directed against a strain-specific cell surface antigen. *Infect. Immun. 32*:641-648.

Newhall V, W. J., Sawyer, W. D., and Haak, R. A. (1980). Cross-binding analysis of the outer membrane proteins of *Neisseria gonorrhoeae. Infect. Immun. 28*:785-791.

Newhall V, W. J., Mail, L. B., Wilde III, C. E., and Jones, R. B. (1985). Purification and antigenic relatedness of proteins II of *Neisseria gonorrhoeae. Infect. Immun. 49*:576-580.

Noegel, A. and Gotschlich, E. C. (1983). Isolation of a high molecular weight polyphosphate from *Neisseria gonorrhoeae. J. Exp. Med. 157*:2049-2060.

Nowinski, R. C., Tam, M. R., Goldstein, L. C., Stong, L., Kuo, C. C., Corey, L., Stamm, W. E., Handsfield, H. H., Knapp, J. S., and Holmes, K. K. (1983). Monoclonal antibodies for diagnosis of infectious diseases in humans. *Science 219*:637-644.

Rice, P. A. and Kasper, D. L. (1977). Characterization of gonococcal antigens responsible for induction of bacterial antibody in disseminated infection: The role of gonococcal endotoxins. *J. Clin. Invest. 60*:1149-1158.

Rice, R. J., Schalla, W. O., Whittington, W. L., JeanLouis, Y., Biddle, J., Goldberg, M., DeWitt, W., Pasquariello, C. A., Arbrutyn, E., and Swenson, R. (1986). Phenotypic characterization of *Neisseria gonorrhoeae* isolated from three cases of meningitis. *J. Infect. Dis. 153*:362-365.

Richardson, W. P. and Sadoff, J. C. (1977). Production of a capsule by *Neisseria gonorrhoeae. Infect. Immun. 15*:663-664.

Sandström, E. G., Chen, K. C. S., and Buchanan, T. M. (1982a). Serology of *Neisseria gonorrhoeae*: Coagglutination serogroups WI and WII/WIII correspond to different outer membrane protein I molecules. *Infect. Immun. 38*:462-470.

Sandström, E. G. and Danielsson, D. (1980). Serology of *Neisseria gonorrhoeae*: Classification by coagglutination. *Acta Pathol. Microbiol. Scand. Sect. B. 88*:27-29.

Sandström, E. G., Knapp, J. S., and Buchanan, T. B. (1982b). Serology of *Neisseria gonorrhoeae*: W-antigen serogrouping by coagglutination and protein I serotyping by enzyme-linked immunosorbent assay both detect protein I antigens. *Infect. Immun. 35*:229-239.

Sarafian, S. K., Tam, M. R., and Morse, S. A. (1983). Gonococcal protein I-specific opsonic IgG in normal serum. *J. Infect. Dis. 148*:1025-1032.

Sugasawara, R. J., Cannon, J. C., Black, W. J., Nachamkin, I., Sweet, R. L., and Brooks, G. F. (1983). Inhibition of *Neisseria gonorrhoeae* attachment to HeLa cells with monoclonal antibody directed against a protein II. *Infect. Immun. 42*:980-985.

Swanson, J. (1978). Studies on gonococcus infection: XIV. Cell wall protein differences among color/opacity colony variants of *Neisseria gonorrhoea*. *Infect. Immun. 21*:292-296.

Swanson, J., Mayer, L. W., and Tam, M. R. (1982). Antigenicity of *Neisseria gonorrhoeae* outer membrane protein(s) III detected by immunoprecipitation and Western blot transfer with a monoclonal antibody. *Infect. Immun. 38*:668-672.

Tam, M. R., Buchanan, T. M., Sandström, E. G., Holmes, K. K., Knapp, J. S., Siadak, A. W., and Nowinski, R. C. (1982). Serological classification of *Neisseria gonorrhoeae* with monoclonal antibodies. *Infect. Immun. 36*: 1042-1053.

Tam, M. R., Goldstein, L. C., and Yelton, D. E. (1985). Monoclonal antibodies in clinical microbiology. In *Manual of Clinical Microbiology*, 4th Ed. (E. H. Lenette, A. Balows, W. J. Hausler, and H. J. Shadomy, eds.). American Society for Microbiology, Washington, DC, pp. 905-909.

Virji, M. and Heckels, J. E. (1985). Role of anti-pilus antibodies in host defense against gonococcal infection studied with monoclonal anti-pilus antibodies. *Infect. Immun. 49*:621-628.

Virji, M., Heckels, J. E., and Watt, P. J. (1983). Monoclonal antibodies to gonococcal pili: Studies on antigenic determinants on pili from variants of strain P9. *J. Gen. Microbiol. 129*:1965-1973.

Wang, S. P., Holmes, K. K., Knapp, J. S., Ott, S., and Kyzer, D. D. (1977). Immunologic classification of *Neisseria gonorrhoeae* with microimmunofluorescence. *J. Immunol. 119*:795-803.

Watt, P. J. and Ward, M. E. (1980). Adherence of *Neisseria gonorrhoeae* and other *Neisseria* species to mammalian cells. In *Bacterial Adherence* (E. Beachey, ed.). Chapman and Hall, New York, pp. 253-288.

Wilson, J. F. (1954). A serological study of *Neisseria gonorrhoeae*. *J. Pathol. 68*: 495-510.

THREE

Immunological Diagnosis of Gonococcal Infection

Hugh Young
Edinburgh University
Medical School
Edinburgh, Scotland

Katherine G. Reid
Protein Fractionation Centre
Scottish Blood Transfusion Service
Edinburgh, Scotland

I. INTRODUCTION

Gonorrhea, an infection of the mucosal surfaces of the genitourinary tract, is transmitted mainly by sexual intercourse and is common in developed as well as in developing countries. The global incidence of approximately 200 million cases a year clearly indicates the need for improved control. Prompt and accurate diagnosis followed by effective treatment is an important component of any gonorrhea control program. This chapter first outlines the nature of the infection and discusses this in relation to diagnostic strategies before dealing with the immunological diagnosis.

A. Disease Entities

1. Genital Infection

Acute anterior urethritis is the most common manifestation of gonococcal infection in men and results in a purulent discharge. The incubation period is, on average, 3-4 days with a range of 2-14 days. Before effective antimicrobial agents were available most patients had symptomatic resolution within 8 weeks and 95% were free of symptoms within 6 months (Holmes, 1974).

The columnar epithelium of the endocervix is the primary site of infection in women. The cervix is involved in 85-90% and the urethra in 65-75% of the patients (Robertson et al., 1988). The most common symptoms among women infected with *Neisseria gonorrhoeae* are abnormal or increased vaginal discharge, abnormal uterine bleeding, dysuria, and urinary frequency and urgency (Handsfield, 1977). Most women with endocervical gonococcal infections, however, develop very slight or nonspecific symptoms and do not seek medical attention.

Asymptomatic urethral infections are also found in men. Overall, 10% of men acquire infections in which few or no symptoms develop (Handsfield et al., 1980), although a figure of 40% was reported for men who were known contacts of women with gonorrhea. John and Donald (1978) found that 17% of 203 cases of urethral gonorrhea were asymptomatic and a further 7% of cases had symptoms so mild that they failed to seek medical attention. All of these cases were brought to attention by contact tracing.

a. Complications of Local Genital Infection. Local spread of urethral gonococcal infections in men may result in prostatitis, seminal vesiculitis, epididymitis, inflammation, and abscess formation in the urethral glands (Robertson et al., 1988). Urethral strictures and fistulae, once common in the preantibiotic era are now rare in the Western world. In West Africa, and probably also in other developing countries where medical facilities are inadequate and improper self-treatment with antibiotics occurs, all of the mentioned complications are frequently seen (Osoba and Alausa, 1976).

Local complications in women include involvement of the paraurethral and greater vestibular (Bartholin's) glands. Pelvic inflammatory disease (PID) occurs in up to 10% of untreated patients, with 20% of such women developing impaired fertility (Eschenbach and Holmes, 1975). It has been estimated that the cost of PID in the United States is 700 million dollars per year (U.S. Department of Health and Human Services, 1981), thus there is a strong economic incentive to control gonorrhea. The World Health Organization (WHO, 1978) considers that gonorrhea is a major cause for the high prevalence of infertility in parts of Africa.

2. Rectal Infection

Rectal infections occur in both men and women. Anorectal infections in men result from receptive anal intercourse. In 1977, 10.9% of men with gonorrhea had acquired their infection as a result of homosexual contact (British Cooperative Clinical Group, 1980). The majority of male patients with rectal gonorrhea produce no symptoms (Bygdeman, 1981; McMillan and Young, 1978), and the proctoscopic appearance of the rectal mucosa is normal in 84% of these men (McMillan et al., 1983).

The rectum is involved in approximately 25-50% of women with gonorrhea (Handsfield et al., 1980; Willcox, 1981). Rectal infection is mainly due to contamination of the anus by infected vaginal discharge (Willcox, 1981) but may also result from rectal coitus (Cornthwaite et al., 1974; Kinghorn and Rashid, 1979).

3. Pharyngeal Infection

Lack of correlation between pharyngeal colonization and symptoms of pharyngitis (Wiesner, 1975; Young and Bain, 1983), combined with the reluctance of many patients to admit to orogenital contact (fellatio and, less commonly, cunnilingus), make it difficult for the clinician to use these criteria in selecting patients from whom to take throat cultures. Although the prevalence of pharyngeal infection is highest in homosexual men, there has been a marked increase in heterosexually acquired pharyngeal infection in Edinburgh in recent years (Robertson et al., 1988): during 1985, 9% of heterosexual men, 14.6% of women, and 27.8% of homosexual men with gonorrhea had pharyngeal infection. Pharyngeal transfer of gonococci by kissing is very rare (Tice and Rodriguez, 1981). Oral-to-genital transmission is rare, although it has been reported in relation to subsets of prostitutes in Southeast Asia who specialize in oral sex (Soendjojo, 1983).

4. Disseminated Infection

In a small percentage of untreated cases of mucosal gonorrhea, systemic spread gives rise to the entity termed disseminated gonococcal infection (DGI), often referred to as the arthritis-dermatitis syndrome. Clinically, DGI can be divided into two stages: an initial bacteremic stage associated with fever, leukocytosis, and skin lesions, closely followed by a second stage associated with tenosynovitis or septic arthritis (Brooks, 1985). Occasionally the two stages overlap (Brogadir et al., 1979), and rarely, DGI may be followed by the more severe manifestations of endocarditis or meningitis (Masi and Eisenstein, 1981).

Disseminated infection is more likely to occur in women than in men, possibly because a greater proportion of women are symptomless (Holmes et al., 1971). Barr and Danielsson (1971) found that the overall prevalence of septic gonococcal dermatitis was 1.9%, 3% for women and 0.7% for men. The incubation period for DGI ranges from seven to 30 days, but it is difficult to determine accurately as most cases result from asymptomatic infection. The disseminated form occurs most commonly in women at the time of menstruation when the incubation period may represent the time between the acquisition of infection and the onset of menstruation.

5. Infection in Infants and Children

Gonococcal conjunctivitis of the newborn (ophthalmia neonatorum) was the single largest cause of blindness during the preantibiotic era. Nowadays this condition is uncommon in developed countries owing to general improvements in antenatal care and the detection and treatment of gonococcal infection. Gonococcal conjunctivitis in older children and in adults is usually acquired by contact with fingers and/or moist towels contaminated with fresh pus. Although genital and rectal infection in young children under the age of puberty may result from accidental contamination of the child with discharge when sleeping with an infected parent, sexual contact and abuse probably occur much more frequently than is generally supposed (Alexander et al., 1984; Sgroi, 1982).

B. Epidemiology

1. Prevalence of Gonorrhea

Differences and inadequacies in reporting systems make absolute comparison of data between countries difficult. The available data, however, give a useful guide about trends. In many countries, as illustrated by data from the United Kingdom (Fig. 1), there was a sharp rise in the incidence of gonorrhea in the late 1950s and throughout the 1960s, reaching a peak of 65,997 recorded cases in 1973. Numbers stabilized and declined thereafter with 53,802 cases recorded in 1984. Most infections occur in the 20- to 25-year-old group

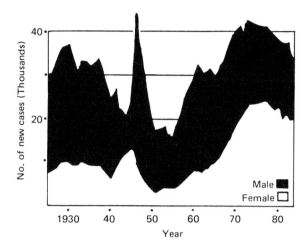

Fig. 1 Clinic returns for gonorrhea in the United Kingdom 1925-1984. Data not available for Northern Ireland before 1958 (*Source*: reproduced from *Communicable Diseases Scotland Weekly Report* 86/31 by permission of Dr. J. Emslie, Medical Editor and Dr. N. S. Galbraith, Director PHLS Communicable Disease Surveillance Centre, Colindale, London).

In England in 1982, the reported incidence rate was 111.4/100,000 population and the male/female ratio was 1.7:1 (Extract from the report of the Chief Medical Officer, 1985). In the United States in 1981 990,864 cases were reported (435/100,000 population): 92% of cases occurred in those under the age of 35. The male/female ratio decreased from 2.4:1 in 1960 to 1.4:1 in 1981 (U.S. Department of Health and Human Services, 1982). The decrease in the male/female ratio is in part due to public health service programs of more culture screening to detect infected women who are often symptomless.

In developing countries in Asia, Africa, Central and South America the prevalence of gonorrhea is not known because of inadequacies in the reporting systems. Data from several studies from Africa suggest that there are very high levels of infection. In Nairobi 17.5% of women attending a family planning clinic had gonorrhea (Hopcraft et al., 1973); in rural Uganda infection was found in 9% of men and 18% of women randomly selected for testing (Arya et al., 1973); and in Salisbury, Zimbabwe, 35% of women attending an STD clinic were infected (Latif, 1981).

2. Properties of the Organism

Apart from behavioral factors of the host, the spread of gonorrhea is to some extent dependent upon properties of the organism. Gonococcal typing and the association of certain strains with specific clinical and epidemiological situations is considered in detail in Chap. 4. Certain of these organismal factors, may, however, affect diagnosis and hence the spread of infection.

Strains that require arginine, hypoxanthine, and uracil for growth (the AHU⁻ auxotype) are associated with asymptomatic infection in men (Crawford et al., 1975), thus allowing these strains a greater opportunity to disseminate within the community. In addition, difficulty may be experienced in detecting these strains by culture as a result of their antibiotic hypersensitivity: there is a significant correlation between the AHU⁻ auxotype and sensitivity to vancomycin, one of the antibiotics used in certain gonococcal selective media (Mirrett et al., 1981).

Provided that virulence is not adversely affected, antibiotic-resistant gonococci that are associated with treatment failure have a greater opportunity to spread. Currently recommended dosages of penicillin and ampicillin/amoxycillin tend to be ineffective in the treatment of infections with isolates with a minimum inhibitory concentration (MIC) $\geqslant 1$ mg/L.

Strains showing chromosomal antibiotic resistance that is mediated through changes in the cell envelope and resistance that is mediated through plasmid-encoded β-lactamase (penicillinase) enzymes are now prevalent in many areas. There is considerable geographical variation in the proportion of strains showing significant levels of resistance to penicillin. Strains from Southeast Asia tend to be most resistant. In Singapore 64% of the strains have MICs $\geqslant 0.5$ mg/L resulting from chromosomally mediated resistance (Sng et al., 1984). Similar levels of resistance are common in parts of Africa (Sparling, 1977).

In one large London clinic the prevalence of strains with a penicillin MIC of $\geqslant 1$ mg/L was 8.5% (Easmon, 1985). In the United States chromosomally mediated resistant gonococci have been reported in 23 states (Rice et al., 1986). As prevalence data were not given, it is impossible to gauge the size of the problem.

Penicillinase-producing *N. gonorrhoeae* (PPNG) were first reported simultaneously in the United Kingdom (Phillips, 1976) and the United States (Ashford et al., 1976); the respective isolates were linked epidemiologically with West Africa and Southeast Asia. The PPNG now occur throughout the world and have become endemic in many countries, albeit at a low level. The prevalence of PPNG decreased in the United States during 1983 and in some parts of the United Kingdom during 1984 (Easmon, 1985). Early diagnosis, effective therapy and intensive contact tracing have undoubtedly contributed to the decrease in PPNG. Certain serogroups and serovars of gonococci are correlated with antibiotic resistance (Chap. 4).

II. DIAGNOSTIC STRATEGIES

The main aim of diagnosis is to determine whether or not *N. gonorrhoeae* is present in a specimen and, if present, whether or not the strain produces β-lactamase.

The greater the number of sites examined, the better will be the chance of detecting gonococcal infection.

A. Multiple-Specimen Versus Single-Specimen Screening

In women seen at genitourinary medicine clinics, specimens for culture should be taken from the urethra, endocervix, rectum, and if the contact of a man with gonorrhea, from the pharynx. Smears should be taken from the endocervix for examination after Gram staining. In studies involving repeated examinations of multiple sites, the proportion of infected women detected at their first clinic attendance has been reported as 91% (Chipperfield and Catterall, 1976), 97% (Barlow et al., 1976), and 98% (Young et al., 1979).

The effectiveness of screening by a single endocervical culture varies widely with reported values as disparate as 40% (Norins, 1974) and 90% (Young et al., 1979). In terms of a screening schedule, more infections are detected by testing additional sites than by rescreening by endocervical culture: 97.6% of 451 infections were detected by testing multiple sites compared with only 92.4% by three endocervical cultures. One in three infected women is likely to be missed if a high vaginal swab is the only specimen taken (Bhattacharyya et al., 1973).

Multiple infections are also common in homosexual men. In a study of 278 cases of homosexually acquired infection, the urethra, rectum, and throat were infected in 60.8%, 41.0%, and 8.3% of the patients, respectively (McMillan and Young, 1978). If only one set of tests had been relied upon, 7% of patients with rectal and 26% of patients with pharyngeal gonorrhea would not have been identified. Detection of rectal infection in homosexual men is particularly important because the biological properties of gonococci associated with homosexually acquired infection tend to make them more refractory to treatment. Rectal infection in women is also linked with treatment failure, although to a lesser extent.

Pharyngeal gonorrhea in both sexes requires a higher penicillin dosage than does uncomplicated infection. There is, however, little risk associated with pharyngeal gonorrhea, either to the individual, or to their sexual partner(s). Consequently, the detection of pharyngeal gonorrhea will have little impact on the overall control of infection and has low priority compared with the detection of endocervical infection, anorectal infection in homosexual men, and urethral gonorrhea in males. Anogenital examination is also important in diagnosing DGI because most patients, including those without genital symptoms, are likely to yield gonococci from an anogenital site (Barr and Danielsson, 1971).

Although repeated examination of multiple sites should be the goal within genitourinary medical clinics, there is also an important role for widespread screening based on the examination of a single specimen. Screening with a single endocervical specimen has the potential to detect up to 90% of infected women, many of whom would be symptomless. Provided that "target groups" are properly selected, even a low positivity rate would have an amplified effect in decreasing the level of infection within the community at large. Whereas examination of a single urethral specimen is highly effective in heterosexually acquired urethral gonorrhea, single-specimen screening is unsuitable for rectal infection in homosexual men and for pharyngeal infection in both men and women.

B. Spectrum of Neisserial Colonization

As the spectrum of colonization with neisseriae other than the gonococcus varies markedly between different anatomical sites, this also has an important bearing on the utility of identification methods. Genital sites that form the mainstay of single-specimen noncultural immunological diagnosis are least subject to interference by related neisseriae such as *N. meningitidis* and *N. lactamica* (Sect. III.C.1.a).

III. NONIMMUNOLOGICAL DIAGNOSIS

This section provides an overview of conventional diagnostic methods as a background with which to compare the advantages and disadvantages of immunological diagnosis.

A. Immediate Diagnosis

Gram staining of genital secretions remains the only widely accepted routine procedure for making an immediate diagnosis of gonorrhea. In men, Gram-stained smears of urethral discharge provided an immediate differential diagnosis between gonococcal and nongonococcal urethritis in 85% of patients (Jacobs and Kraus, 1975). The sensitivity and specificity in relation to urethral smears from symptomatic men ranges from 83 to 96% and 95 to 99%, respectively (Goodhart et al., 1982). Although Gram staining is a simple method, the experience of the observer is of paramount importance. The probability of gonorrhea in men whose smears were reported as containing typical intracellular gram-negative diplococci (GNDC) dropped from 94.8 to 53.9% when an inexperienced technician interpreted smears from men with urethritis (Goodhart et al., 1982). The Gram stain method is unsuitable for men without clinical features of urethritis. In a symptomless population in which the prevalence of gonorrhea was 2%, the probability of infection in patients whose smears were reported positive by an experienced observer was only 34.9% (Goodhart et al., 1982).

The sensitivity and specificity of the Gram stain for cervical smears ranges from 23 to 65% and 88 to 100%, respectively (Goodhart et al., 1982). The poorer performance in women is related to the asymptomatic nature of the infection as well as the difficulty of differentiating GNDC within the normal vaginal flora. The experience of the observer is even more important than in the male.

The quality of the culture system used as a standard influences the observed sensitivity and specificity of microscopy. A poor culture system that fails to detect infections with low numbers of gonococci, i.e., those most likely to be missed by microscopy, will result in a Gram stain that gives falsely high sensitivity. Conversely, specificity will be falsely poor if vancomycin-sensitive gonococci are missed with a culture medium containing vancomycin. Patients who have taken antibiotics before examination are also likely to yield positive smears and negative cultures.

Because of the complexity of the gut flora, rectal smears are not routinely taken. Rectal smears may be of value in homosexual men with proctitis if pus or mucopus can be collected by proctoscopy (William et al., 1981). A Gram stain has no place in the diagnosis of pharyngeal infection.

1. Simplified Staining Procedures

Single stains, such as methylene blue or safranin, or a single reagent, such as methyl-green pyronin, have been investigated as a means of shortening the time required to stain smears. The rapid exclusion of gram-positive organisms, however, saves more technician time than does shortening of the staining procedure (Oxtoby et al., 1982).

B. Culture

With over 70% of the laboratories in England and Wales using some form of selective medium (Adler et al., 1978), its importance is firmly established. A combination of a selective and a nonselective medium has been recommended by some workers. While this may be theoretically desirable, it is too time-consuming and technically demanding, and it is not cost-effective in areas where the prevalence of antibiotic-sensitive strains is low (Bonin et al., 1984). Most selective media contain a rich nutrient base supplemented with blood, partially lysed by heat (chocolate agar) or completely lysed by saponin; an antimicrobial cocktail is added to inhibit microorganisms other than pathogenic neisseriae. The following are the most widely used selective media.

1. Thayer-Martin Medium and Its Modifications

The original selective medium of Thayer and Martin (1966) contains the antimicrobials vancomycin, colistin, and nystatin. Although widely used in many laboratories Thayer-Martin (TM) medium has been criticized because a proportion of gonococcal strains are inhibited by vancomycin; growth is slow and colonies are small on TM medium; *Proteus* spp. and yeasts are not suppressed effectively. These problems were overcome to some extent with the introduction of modified TM medium (Martin et al., 1974). Modified TM medium contained double the concentration of agar, glucose (0.25%) was added to promote more rapid growth, and trimethoprim added to inhibit *Proteus* spp. Unfortunately, modified TM medium does not overcome the problem of vancomycin sensitivity. As vancomycin sensitivity varies geographically and has been reported to be as high as 30% (Windall et al., 1980), this is more important in some areas than in others.

2. Martin-Lewis Medium

Martin-Lewis medium is similar to modified TM medium but contains anisomycin in place of nystatin to inhibit yeasts (Martin and Lewis, 1977). Anisomycin is more stable than nystatin and is useful in providing commercially prepared selective media with longer shelf-lives. Smeltzer et al. (1979) found the enhanced inhibition of yeasts on Martin-Lewis medium made screening plates for gonococcal colonies much easier.

3. New York City Medium and Its Modification

New York City (NYC) medium was devised originally by Faur et al. (1973) to provide a luxuriant growth of pathogenic neisseriae after incubation for 24 hr. The NYC medium essentially consists of a proteose peptone-corn starch agar-buffered base to which is added a hemoglobin solution prepared from fresh horse erythrocytes, horse plasma, yeast dialysate, glucose, and vancomycin, colistin, amphotericin B, and trimethoprim lactate. This medium is inconvenient for many service laboratories to prepare, and the modified NYC (MNYC) medium described by Young (1978a) may be more suitable for routine use. The MNYC medium uses a commercially prepared gonococcal base, completely lysed whole blood in place of plasma and hemoglobin solution made from fresh horse erythrocytes, and lincomycin in place of vancomycin.

   In comparison with TM medium, MNYC medium improved the overall isolation rate and enabled a larger percentage of isolates to be identified after 24 hr. Svarva and Maeland (1979) and Hookham (1981) also noted an improvement in culture results with MNYC medium and adopted it for routine use. It is, however, important to examine cultures after 24 hr of incubation. Because lincomycin is less inhibitory than vancomycin, if rectal cultures are not examined until after 48 hr of incubation, contaminants may mask small numbers of gonococcal colonies. Lawton and Koch (1982) compared commercially available NYC and Martin-Lewis media and found the NYC medium to be much superior.

   Comparing smear and culture results is an essential part of the quality control of gonorrhea diagnosis. If the proportion of patients giving positive smears but negative cultures is high, or increases, the culture procedures should be investigated. In Atlanta, Georgia, the proportion of cervical specimens yielding typical positive smears but negative cultures on selective media containing vancomycin varied from 2.6% (Oxtoby et al., 1982) to 5.6% (Goodhart et al., 1982). Young et al. (1979), by using MNYC medium containing lincomycin, showed that only 1% of infections in women gave typical positive smears that were not confirmed by culture.

C. Identification

1. Introduction

The use of a selective medium aids in the identification of *N. gonorrhoeae* because commensal neisseriae are inhibited. *Neisseria meningitidis* and *Branhamella catarrhalis*, however, are two organisms most often confused with *N. gonorrhoeae* (Arko et al., 1982). As *N. meningitidis* grows well on selective media it is important to know its prevalence in the population of GNDC isolated from anatomical sites examined for gonococcal infection. Because the spectrum of nongonococcal neisseriae (including *B. catarrhalis*) (NGN) varies markedly with anatomical site, identification methods that are of acceptable sensitivity and specificity for one site may be unsuitable for another site.

a. Spectrum of Neisserial Colonization. The prevalence of NGN isolated by routine culture of various anatomical sites on MNYC medium from patients attending the Department of Genito-Urinary Medicine, Edinburgh between 1978 and 1985 is shown in Tables 1 to 4.

The results shown in Table 1 for pharyngeal cultures illustrates the effectiveness of selective media in inhibiting nonpathogenic neisseriae. The mucosal membranes of the oropharynx are the natural habitat of commensal neisseriae, yet such organisms accounted for only 6.2% of all GNDC, or 2.4% if *N. lactamica* is excluded. Although *N. lactamica* is regarded as a commensal organism, it grows well on selective media with a colonial morphology similar to *N. meningitidis*. It is obviously important to have reliable methods for differentiating the gonococcus from the meningococcus when examining pharyngeal cultures, as almost 70% of the GNDC isolated are meningococci. As GNDC isolated from anogenital sites in heterosexual patients have a high probability of being gonococci, less accurate

Table 1 Identity of 2553 Oxidase-Positive Gram-Negative Diplococci (GNDC) Isolated from 6443 Pharyngeal Cultures from Patients with Gonorrhea (Edinburgh 1978-1985)

Organism	Number of isolates	% of total pharyngeal cultures	% of oxidase positive GNDC
N. gonorrhoeae	632	9.8	24.7
N. meningitidis	1763	27.4	69.1
N. lactamica	97	1.5	3.8
N. flava	3	<0.1	0.1
N. perflava	32	0.5	1.3
B. catarrhalis	23	0.4	0.9
Unidentified	3	<0.1	0.1
Total	2553	39.6	100.0

Table 2   Anogenital Isolation of Nongonococcal Neisseriae[a] (NGN) in Women (Edinburgh 1978-1985)

Year	Number of patients with anogenital GNDC	Number of isolates of NGN from following sites			
		Urethra	Cervix	Rectum	Total
1978	456	0	0	3[b]	3
1979	424	0	0	0	0
1980	404	1[c]	1[c]	0	2
1981	333	0	1	1	2
1982	336	1[d]	1[d]	2	4
1983	325	0	1	5[e]	6
1984	266	2[f]	0	0	2
1985	332	0	0	0	0
Total	2876	4	4	11	19
	(100%)	(0.14%)	(0.14%)	(0.38%)	(0.66%)

[a]*N. meningitidis* unless denoted otherwise.
[b]Includes one *B. catarrhalis*.
[c]Same patient.
[d]Same patient.
[e]Includes two *B. catarrhalis*.
[f]Both *B. catarrhalis*.

Table 3   Heterosexually Acquired Genital Nongonococcal Neisseriae[a] (NGN) in Men (Edinburgh 1978-1985)

Year	Number of urethral GNDC	Number (%) shown to be NGN
1978	614	3 (0.49)
1979	544	1 (0.18)
1980	519	2 (0.39)
1981	477	0
1982	458	1 (0.22)
1983	420	3 (0.71)
1984	419	1 (0.24)
1985	451	4[b] (0.89)
Total	3902	15 (0.38)

[a]*N. meningitidis* unless denoted otherwise.
[b]Includes one *B. catarrhalis*.

Table 4   Homosexually Acquired Anogenital Nongonococcal Neisseriae[a] (NGN) (Edinburgh 1978-1985)

Year	Number of patients with urethral GNDC	Number (%) shown to be NGN	Number of patients with rectal GNDC	Number (%) shown to be NGN
1978	50	0	46	4 (8.7)
1979	25	1 (4.0)	31	1[b] (3.2)
1980	32	0	35	3 (8.6)
1981	32	0	41	4 (9.8)
1982	42	1[c] (2.4)	75	9[c,d] (12.0)
1983	46	1 (2.2)	65	8 (12.3)
1984	38	3 (7.9)	54	9[e] (16.7)
1985	27	0	38	6 (15.8)
Total	292	6 (2.1)	385	44 (11.4)

[a]*N. meningitidis* unless denoted otherwise.
[b]*N. perflava.*
[c]Same patient with *B. catarrhalis.*
[d]One *N. perflava.*
[e]Two *B. catarrhalis*, one *N. lactamica.*

methods may be sufficient. The NGN accounted for only 0.7% of anogenital GNDC from women (Table 2) and 0.4% of GNDC from urethral cultures from heterosexual men (Table 3). Depending upon the sexual orientation of the patient, the same site may have a different spectrum of colonization. For example, in homosexual men NGN are much more common, accounting for 2.1% of urethral isolates and 11.4% of rectal isolates of GNDC (Table 4). *Neisseria meningitidis* and *B. catarrhalis* accounted for 84.5 and 11.9%, respectively, of the 84 NGN isolated from anogenital sites (see Tables 2-4).

2. Presumptive Identification

The data presented in Table 2 show that in a female population in whom the prevalence of gonorrhea is around 10%, a presumptive identification of *N. gonorrhoeae* made on the basis of oxidase-positive GNDC growing on selective medium is approximately 99.8% accurate for genital cultures and 99.4% accurate for rectal cultures. Smeltzer et al. (1980) evaluated a low-prevalence population (1.4%) and showed that 98.5% of the presumptive positive cervical isolates available for confirmation were identified as *N. gonorrhoeae*. Presumptive identification is 99.6 and 98% accurate for urethral GNDC from heterosexual men (see Table 3) and homosexual men (see Table 4), respectively. Accuracy of presumptive identification is poor (89%) for male rectal cultures and is totally unsuitable for throat culture because most GNDC isolated are meningococci (see Table 1).

3. Carbohydrate Utilization Tests

A definitive diagnosis has traditionally been made on the basis of carbohydrate utilization tests.

a. Conventional Tests. In conventional tests for carbohydrate utilization a solid medium containing the appropriate carbohydrate and pH indicator is inoculated with the test organism. Although widely used, these tests are unsuitable because a positive reaction is dependent upon adequate growth of the test organism, which may take up to 72 hr (Pollock, 1976).

Failure to support gonococcal growth is a major problem with the commercially available cystine-trypticase agar (CTA) system widely used in the United States. Inconclusive results and other problems with CTA medium accounted for 44% of 141 gonococcal cultures sent to the Centers for Disease Control (CDC), Atlanta, for confirmation (Arko et al., 1982). The poor performance of CTA medium has led to the acceptance of "glucose-negative" gonococci, a concept that may cause diagnostic problems. Knapp et al. (1984) described an asaccharolytic diplococcus that had been isolated from the cervix of a patient with arthritis. The isolate was presumptively identified as a glucose-negative gonococcus but later identified as *N. cinerea*.

Certain meningococci fail to give a positive reaction with maltose in the CTA system owing to deficiencies in maltose permease or phosphorylase (Saez-Nieto et al., 1982). Colonization with "maltose-negative" meningococci has been misdiagnosed as pharyngeal gonorrhea (Noble and Cooper, 1979).

The excellent growth-supporting capacity of MNYC medium has been utilized in the commercially available MNYC carbohydrate medium, which was shown to provide more accurate and reliable results than CTA medium (Simms and Lue, 1982). Knapp and Holmes (1983) developed a semisolid medium which they termed modified oxidation-fermentation (MOF) medium. This medium proved much more reliable than CTA medium. Up to 24 hr of incubation may be required to obtain results.

b. Rapid Carbohydrate Utilization Test. In the rapid carbohydrate utilization test (RCUT) preformed enzyme is measured by adding a suspension of the overnight growth of the suspect organism to a buffered, nonnutrient solution containing the sugar to be tested and a pH indicator (Young et al., 1976). Apart from rapidity, the ability to identify other neisseriae and confirm *N. gonorrhoeae* within 24-72 hr of seeing the patient, the RCUT, in measuring preformed enzyme, has the advantage of being independent of growth. Results of the RCUT are usually available after 1-3 hr incubation at 37°C.

If the test reagents are properly quality controlled and suspensions are prepared with young 18 to 24-hr cultures grown on medium containing glucose, RCUT methods are more accurate than conventional tests (Tapsall and Cheng, 1981). It is important to use extra pure maltose. Many batches of maltose are contaminated with glucose, which may result in gonococci giving false-positive reactions. In our experience, glucose-negative gonococci are not encountered, and meningococci found to be maltose-negative in the CTA test utilize maltose in the RCUT (Wood and Young, 1986).

The RCUT methods have the additional advantage that isolates can be characterized, including penicillinase testing, from the primary isolation plate (Young, 1978b). Considerable saving in time and reagents can be made by performing the test in microtiter plates. Plates containing reagents can be prepared in batches and stored at −20°C for several months.

Commercially available adaptations of the RCUT method include the Minitek system (BBL Microbiology Systems) and Oxoid *Neisseria* Identification Discs. Recently a 1-hr test was developed by incorporating chloroform in the incubation mixture (Lairscey and Kelly, 1985), presumably to increase bacterial permeability.

c. Other Carbohydrate Utilization Methods.   Yong and Prytula (1978) described a modified RCUT that used both preformed enzymes and enzymes formed as a result of growth in a superenriched medium. The combined action of the two sources of enzyme make this method suitable for very small inocula. Because of possible contamination by other bacteria, the method cannot be used to characterize isolates directly from primary isolation cultures.

The BACTEC *Neisseria* differentiation kits are available commercially. They are designed to identify *N. gonorrhoeae, N. meningitidis,* and *N. lactamica* in 3 hr by detecting $[^{14}C]CO_2$ resulting from the metabolism of $[^{14}C]$ sugars by a bacterial suspension in a closed bottle. Apart from the disadvantages of working with radiolabeled material and the expense of monitoring equipment, the system is oversensitive and gives positive results with *N. cinerea* (Boyce et al., 1985). This resulted in proctitis associated with *N. cinerea* being misdiagnosed as a gonococcal infection in an 8-year-old boy (Dossett et al., 1985).

4. Biochemical Identification Systems

A number of neisserial identification systems such as the RapID NH System (Innovative Diagnostics Systems Inc.) and Gonocheck (E-Y Laboratories) are now available commercially (Philip and Garton, 1985).

a. RapID NH System.   The RapID NH system is a 4-hr test designed to differentiate *Neisseria* spp., *Branhamella, Moraxella,* and *Haemophilus* spp. and is based on both sugar utilization tests and single-substrate chromogenic biochemical tests. A suspension of the test organism is added to reconstituted dehydrated reagents in the appropriate wells of a plastic tray. In addition to sugar utilization, tests such as β-D-galactosidase, aminopeptidase, indole production, urea hydrolysis, and phosphate and nitrate degradation, are included. Robinson and Oberhofer (1983) found that there were considerable problems associated with the use of this system. *Branhamella catarrhalis* could not be distinguished from species of the gram-negative coccobacilli *Moraxella* and *Kingella*; 44% of gonococcal isolates tested did not utilize glucose, and the other tests had to be relied upon to give definitive identification. Similar problems were found with isolates of *N. meningitidis*. This system also failed to differentiate accurately between *N. gonorrhoeae* and *N. cinerea* (Boyce and Mitchell, 1985).

b. Gonocheck. Gonocheck is a single-tube, multiple chromogenic substrate test designed to identify *N. gonorrhoeae, N. meningitidis, N. lactamica,* and *B. catarrhalis.* The enzymes produced by *N. gonorrhoeae, N. meningitidis,* and *N. lactamica* are proline aminopeptidase, γ-glutamyl aminopeptidase, and β-galactosidase, respectively; *B. catarrhalis* does not produce these enzymes.

Oxidase-positive GNDC are added to the reconstituted tubes which are then incubated at 35°C for 30 min. A blue coloration designates *N. lactamica*; yellow designates *N. meningitidis*. If there is no color development a diazonium salt derivative (EY 20) is added. If the tube subsequently turns red, the isolate is a gonococcus. If no color develops after the addition of EY 20, then the isolate is *B. catarrhalis.*

Welborn et al. (1984), comparing the Gonocheck with RapID NH and the RCUT system of Young et al. (1976), found that Gonocheck compared well with the RCUT provided that the tubes were read carefully for color production before the addition of the EY 20 reagents. The addition of EY 20 to tubes that had developed a slight blue would produce false-positive red, resulting in *N. lactamica* being falsely identified as a gonococcus. The RapID NH performed poorly and was not recommended.

Wood and Young (1986) found that some meningococci produced very low levels of γ-glutamyl aminopeptidase and very little or no yellow developed. This resulted in the misidentification of three strains, two as *N. gonorrhoeae* and one as *B. catarrhalis* on first testing from primary culture plates. After 24-hr subculture these strains were identified correctly. Gonocheck persistently misidentified one gonococcal strain as *B. catarrhalis.* Boyce and Mitchell (1985) reported that Gonocheck could not differentiate between *N. gonorrhoeae* and *N. cinerea.*

These newer test systems have been evaluated with only small numbers of isolates. The evaluation of the RapID NH System by Robinson and Oberhofer (1983) included 28 meningococci, while the Gonocheck evaluations of Welborn et al. (1984) and Wood and Young (1986) included only six and 65 meningococci, respectively. The reliability of differentiating gonococci and meningococci on the basis of enzyme profiles remains to be established in large scale "in-use" evaluations. Throat meningococci form a more heterogeneous group and have lower mean γ-glutamyl aminopeptidase levels and higher mean hydroxyproline activity than systemic strains (Ison et al., 1982). Unlike systemic strains that are almost always groupable, a large proportion (36.5%) of meningococci isolated from the throat of patients with gonorrhea are nongroupable (Young et al., 1983a).

c. Miscellaneous Identification Methods. These include identification using lectins and the superoxol test. Lectins are plant proteins that react with carbohydrates: certain lectins agglutinate gonococci and can be used in a slide test. Curtis and Slack (1981) tested 168 gonococci and 96 meningococci with wheat germ lectin and found a sensitivity of 94.6% and a specificity of 78.1%. The poor specificity is caused by lectin agglutination of nongroupable meningococci. Lectins fail to agglutinate groupable meningococci because the capsular polysaccharide blocks the *N*-acetylglucosamine receptor. Lectin agglutination has also been used in conjunction with chromogenic peptidase assays (Yajko et al., 1984).

The superoxol test (Saginur et al., 1982) is essentially a catalase test performed with 20-30% hydrogen peroxide in place of 3%. A positive superoxol test reaction is of limited diagnostic value because a considerable number of meningococci and some commensal neisseriae give a positive reaction (Young et al., 1984). In contrast, an isolate is almost certainly not a gonococcus if it gives a negative superoxol test result, as all but one of 596 gonococcal isolates tested gave positive results. Odugbemi and Arko (1983) found a negative superoxol test result valuable in differentiating *N. gonorrhoeae* from *Kingella denitrifcians*. The latter has a colonial morphology similar to the gonococcus, and on Gram staining may appear as coccoid or short rod-shaped.

D. Antibiotic Susceptibility Tests

Detection of PPNG is the most important aspect of sensitivity testing, and all isolates should be screened immediately. Because most patients with gonococcal infection who attend genitourinary medical clinics will have been treated on the basis of a positive Gram-stained smear, susceptibility tests, other than those to detect PPNG, are of little help in the initial management of the patient. Routine testing of at least a proportion of isolates is worthwhile, however, as it provides epidemiological data on which to plan rational therapy.

1. Penicillinase-Producing Neisseria gonorrhoeae

Screening for PPNG can be performed very simply by inoculating several colonies from the primary isolation plate onto a suitable nonselective medium and placing a 6 μg disk on the well. After overnight incubation, any isolate showing a zone of inhibition of < 20 mm is likely to be a PPNG and should be confirmed by one of the specific penicillinase detection methods (World Health Organization, 1978).

One of the most sensitive and convenient methods uses commercially available paper strips impregnated with a chromogenic cephalosporin.

If all isolates are not screened routinely for penicillinase production, it is most important to test all strains isolated after treatment. All strains with decreased susceptibility to penicillin (MIC $\geqslant 0.125$ mg/L) should also be tested.

Recently Taylor et al. (1985) described the detection of PPNG in urethral exudates by measuring the fluorescent end products of β-lactamase activity on an ampicillin substrate. Although the sensitivity and specificity of this method were 91 and 96%, respectively, there were occasional unresolved technical difficulties with the test.

2. Minimum Inhibitory Concentration

A proportion of strains may show chromosomally mediated resistance to penicillin at a level ($\geqslant 1$ mg/L), which makes failure likely with current penicillin treatment regimens.

These strains that have been common in Southeast Asia for some years (Sng et al., 1984) are now becoming more common in the United Kingdom (Easmon, 1985) and the United States (Rice et al., 1986). Such strains tend to be more resistant to tetracycline and erythromycin.

Although standardization of MIC testing is desirable, most laboratories use disk or agar dilution methods with media and inocula to suit their individual needs and preferences. Disk susceptibility testing has been widely used because it is simple and can give a rapid guide to the sensitivity or resistance of an isolate. Although more accurate results are obtained with an agar dilution method, this can be tedious and time-consuming for small numbers of isolates. Large numbers of isolates can be conveniently tested in batches using multipoint inoculation technology. Much useful information is accumulating on the correlation between gonococcal serovar, as determined with monoclonal antibodies (MAbs) and antibiotic susceptibility (Chap. 4). It may be that in the future, serovar analysis will provide a rapid guide to the antibiotic susceptibility pattern of an isolate.

E. Transport and Culture Systems

The most suitable transport and culture system must be related to local constraints imposed on individual geographical areas. Direct plating should be used whenever possible as it produces the best results for specimens from all sites. In comparison with specimens cultured following transport, cultures plated directly yield larger colonies at 18-24 hr. This is important in providing rapid identification, as many of the newer identification methods can be used directly with the growth from primary cultures.

When direct plating and immediate incubation are impractical a conventional nonnutrient transport medium such as Amies' modification of Stuart's medium

(Amies, 1967) or a nutrient transport and culture system based on a selective medium contained in a biological environment chamber (JEMBEC) (Martin and Jackson, 1975) should be used.

Nutrient transport and culture systems are expensive and would seem to offer little advantage over a nonnutrient medium when the transit time is about 3 hr. A significant loss of viability occurs when specimens are in transit for longer than 3 hr (Ebright et al., 1982; Sng et al., 1982; Spence et al., 1983). Amies' medium is more effective than Stuart's in maintaining gonococcal viability (Human and Jones, 1986). When transit times longer than 3 hr are anticipated, it is best to use a transport/culture system and to incubate the container overnight before forwarding to the laboratory. Faur et al. (1977) found that NYC medium in a biological environment chamber was an effective method for the handling, transport, and culture of *N. gonorrhoeae*, provided the delay in transport did not exceed 24 hr: a delay of 48 hr resulted in 17.5% fewer positive cultures than direct plating and immediate incubation.

Because of the problems associated with maintaining the viability of gonococci during transit, particularly when the inoculum is low, several noncultural methods have been developed. These include both immunological (Sect. IV.C) and nonimmunological methods (Sect. V).

IV. IMMUNOLOGICAL DIAGNOSIS

In detecting gonococcal antigen, immunological diagnosis obviates problems associated with the transport and culture of the gonococcus. Immunological diagnosis is also adaptable and has the potential for immediate diagnosis, the identification of *N. gonorrhoeae* following culture, and detection of antigen in exudates transported to a central laboratory.

A. Immediate Diagnosis

1. *Polyclonal Antibodies*

The limitations of the Gram-stained smear (Sect. III.A), particularly in female patients, led to the development of immediate diagnosis based on direct fluorescent antibody (FA) staining of urogenital smears. Although FA staining of smears can provide results in less than 1 hr, there were inconsistencies in test performance when results from several published trials were compared (Hare, 1974). In spite of FA staining being superior to Gram staining in many of the trials, Hare (1974) considered that the direct FA test was unsuitable for routine work but could be useful in the investigation of special cases and in research. A similar conclusion was reached by Danielsson and Forsum (1975) in a detailed discussion of the methodology of FA staining.

Subsequent laboratory procedures have not included routine FA staining thus endorsing these early recommendations. Apart from the need for a highly experienced staff and a fluorescence microscope on site, the reading of FA tests was difficult owing to various degrees of cross-reaction with other organisms. Although reagents were absorbed to remove cross-reacting antibodies, this also tended to decrease the specific staining with gonococci. In addition, the pool of polyclonal antibodies used in preparing the FA reagents were chosen without the benefit of the serogrouping and serotyping system described in Chap. 4.

2. Monoclonal Antibodies

The advent of MAbs reactive with epitopes on protein I of *N. gonorrhoeae* (Chap. 2) has revitalized interest in FA staining. Monoclonal antibody reagents for direct FA staining have been developed jointly by Syva and Genetic Systems Inc. As yet, these reagents are not available for routine use. A preliminary evaluation, however, showed that they were superior to Gram staining for specimens from women but not from men (Ison et al., 1985).

Urethral specimens from 105 men and urethral and cervical specimens from 60 women were examined. For the 45 positive cultures from men, the FA test had a sensitivity of 85% and a specificity of 100%: Gram stains gave values of 94 and 100%, respectively. For the 17 positive cultures from women, the FA test had a sensitivity of 65% and a specificity of 98% for urethral samples; the corresponding values for cervical samples were 72 and 94%, respectively. The sensitivity of Gram stains was 40% for both sites.

The FA staining had no advantage over Gram staining for detecting gonorrhea in men, but the superior sensitivity was a marked advantage when dealing with female patients. Testing duplicate smears increased the sensitivity from 85 to 89% in men and from 72 to 88% for cervical samples. This indicates that the failure of the FA test to detect infected patients was most likely due to specimen collection (sample variation) rather than a failure of the MAbs to recognize epitopes on certain strains of gonococci. Direct FA staining with MAbs awaits wide-scale evaluation. If sufficiently sensitive and specific, it could be of great value in the rapid diagnosis of rectal gonorrhea in men.

B. Identification of *Neisseria gonorrhoeae*

Advantages of confirming the identity of *N. gonorrhoeae* by immunological methods include rapidity and the use of very small amounts of bacterial growth. These factors, combined with the early difficulties with culture and carbohydrate utilization, stimulated the development of immunological methods.

1. Polyclonal Antibodies

Methods such as direct FA staining and coagglutination (CoA) have been used widely in identifying gonococci. Experience with other systems such as agglutination with antigonococcal lipopolysaccharide hen serum is extremely limited (Maly-sheff et al., 1978; Wallace et al., 1978).

Although FA staining was the first method to be used, CoA is simpler to perform, easier to interpret, and does not require expensive immunofluorescence equipment (Young and McMillan, 1982). Coagglutination is a rapid slide test that uses protein A-containing staphylococci with rabbit antigonococcal antibodies bound by their Fc portion to the protein A (Danielsson and Kronvall, 1974). When this reagent is mixed with gonococci, a readily visible agglutination is pro-duced. This reaction is compared with a control in which the staphylococci have not been coated with specific antibodies.

The sensitivity and specificity obtained with commercial reagents for CoA (Phadebact Gonococcus Test, Pharmacia) and direct FA staining (Difco Labora-tories) are comparable (Shanker et al., 1981; Young and McMillan, 1982). These and other groups (Carlson et al., 1982; Lim and Wall, 1980) reported CoA sensi-tivities and specificities in the range of 92.6-97.8% and 93.0-96.8%, respectively. Insofar as they fail to detect a small proportion of gonococcal isolates and fail to give clear-cut negative reactions with a similar proportion of NGN, both FA staining and CoA suffer from the same disadvantages. Although CoA testing ef-fectively replaced the FA method in most laboratories, it was particularly prone to cross-reaction with *N. lactamica.* This made the test unsuitable for confirming the identity of pharyngeal isolates.

2. Monoclonal Antibodies

Immunological identification of *N. gonorrhoeae* with MAb CoA reagents has super-seded both FA and CoA polyclonal antibody tests. Two commercial test systems are available.

a. Gono Gen. The Gono Gen CoA test (New Horizons Diagnostic Company, Columbia, MD) consists of a single test reagent prepared from a pool of murine MAbs reactive with protein I (Tam et al., 1982; see also Chap. 2) and a control reagent (nonimmune rabbit IgG bound to staphylococci). The test is performed with growth from the primary isolation plate. A light suspension of organisms is made in distilled water and boiled for 5 min before mixing with test and control reagents. A positive reaction is indicated within 1 min by substantially stronger agglutination with test reagent than with control reagent.

The sensitivity of the Gono Gen test was 99.1% for 110 isolates (Lawton and Battaglioli, 1983) and 96.6% in evaluations involving 56 (Philip et al., 1984) and 205 gonococcal isolates (Young and Reid, 1984). Lawton and Battaglioli (1983) tested 57 meningococcal isolates and reported a specificity of 100% as did Philip et al. (1984) who tested 24 meningococci and three isolates of *N. lactamica.* Young and Reid (1984) reported one of 52 meningococci reactive when tested from the primary isolates plate but negative after two subcultures. One of three clinical isolates of *N. lactamica* reacted with control reagent as well as the test reagent.

Thirteen stock cultures of *N. lactamica* were negative with Gono Gen, whereas seven were positive with the Phadebact Gonococcus Test which used polyclonal reagents. If the absolute specificity of the Gono Gen MAb reagent is confirmed in larger surveys, it would mean that a positive reaction with an isolated from any anatomical site, including the pharynx, could be regarded as a gonococcus without recourse to further testing: a specificity of 100% yields no false-positive reactions, hence the positive predictive value is also 100%.

Unfortunately, the sensitivity of Gono Gen was only 96 6% in the two evaluations reported from the United Kingdom (Philip et al., 1984; Young and Reid, 1984). The 99.1% sensitivity reported by Lawton and Battaglioli (1983) in New York may suggest differences in the antigenic profile of gonococci circulating in these different geographical areas. Knapp (1985) reporting on unpublished observations from the United States noted that a panel of 10 MAb reagents detected 100% of 839 strains and a panel of three of these reagents detected 99.5% (835) of the strains. It may be that MAb pools will have to be "tailored" to suit broad geographical areas. Each time a pool is changed by the addition of a new reagent, however, it is important to ensure that this does not have an adverse effect on the overall performance of the new composite reagent. A sensitivity marginally less than 100% has a very marked effect on the negative predictive value, particularly when testing anogenital isolates from heterosexual patients. The low prevalence of NGN in anogenital sites means that a negative Gono Gen result is more likely to be due to a nonreactive gonococcus than to NGN: this is reflected in the poor negative predictive value (10.68%) indicating the need to confirm Gono Gen-negative anogenital isolates by biochemical tests (Young and Reid, 1984). Conversely, because of the preponderance of NGN, mainly meningococci among pharnygeal isolates, a negative Gono Gen result has a high predictive value (99.13%) for NGN.

b. Phadebact Monoclonal GC Test. The Phadebact Monoclonal GC test contains two separate reagents, WI and WII/III, prepared with different pools of MAbs reactive with protein IA and protein IB, respectively (Sandström et al., 1985). The pools of MAbs are selected from the Ph-antibodies used in serovar determination (Chap. 4).

The test is performed on suspect gonococci (oxidase-positive GNDC) from primary isolation cultures. It is important to follow the manufacturer's instructions to make a light suspension in 0.9% saline and boil for 5 min. When the boiled antigen is cooled it is tested against both the WI and WII/III reagents: a substantially stronger reaction in either the WI or WII/III reagent constitutes a positive result and provides instant serogrouping. Positive results tend to be stronger and appear more quickly than with those with polyclonal reagents.

The Phadebact Monoclonal GC test was shown to be 100% sensitive and specific when tested against 550 gonococcal and 197 nongonococcal GNDC including

N. meningitidis, N. lactamica, N. cinerea, and *B. catarrhalis* (Blomqvist et al., 1985).

A prolonged "in-use" evaluation (Young, unpublished results) has confirmed the absolute specificity and extremely high sensitivity. All 861 NGN (784 *N. meningitidis,* 46 *N. lactamica,* 18 *N. perflava,* 8 *N. flava,* and 5 *B. catarrhalis*) identified by the rapid carbohydrate utilization test gave unequivocal negative reactions. Of 1017 gonococci tested 1014 were unequivocally positive, giving an overall sensitivity of 99.7%. An analysis of the results with the individual reagents showed that all 480 serogroup WI strains were reactive, whereas three of the 537 serogroup WII strains were nonreactive, giving a sensitivity of 99.4%. All three nonreactive WII/III strains were of the extremely rare serovar Bj/Bro (see Chap. 4) and were isolated over a restricted period.

Because of the occurrence, albeit very rarely, of nonreactive gonococci, it is advisable to confirm the identity of any nonreactive anogenital isolate but particularly those from heterosexual patients.

Using the formula of Vecchio (1960) the spectrum of neisserial colonization given in Tables 1 to 4 can be used to calculate predictive values for results on isolates from various anatomical sites. As shown in Table 5 a small decrease in sensitivity is translated into a marked decrease in the predictive value of a negative test.

Table 5 Effect of Decreasing Sensitivity on Negative Predictive Value (NPV) for GNDC Isolated From Various Anatomical Sites

	NPV based on proportion of gonococcal GNDC from the following sites				
			Homosexual male		
Sensitivity	Heterosexual male urethra[a]	Female anogenital[b]	Urethra[c]	Rectum[d]	Throat (all groups)[e]
100.00	100.00	100.00	100.00	100.00	100.00
99.90	80.06	87.58	95.55	99.23	99.97
99.70	57.24	70.12	87.73	97.72	99.90
99.50	44.54	58.50	81.10	95.94	99.84
99.30	36.46	50.18	75.40	94.84	99.77
99.10	30.85	43.92	70.44	93.46	99.71
98.00	16.72	26.06	51.75	86.55	99.35

Specificity 100%: Positive Predictive Value 100% for all groups.
[a]Proportion of gonococcal GNDC = 0.996 (Table 3).
[b]Proportion of gonococcal GNDC = 0.993 (Table 2).
[c]Proportion of gonococcal GNDC = 0.979 (Table 4).
[d]Proportion of gonococcal GNDC = 0.886 (Table 4).
[e]Proportion of gonococcal GNDC = 0.247 (Table 1).

This is most noticeable for sites, such as the male urethra, where NGN are rarely isolated. For example, at a sensitivity between 99.5 and 99.7% the negative predictive value is around 50%, indicating that a negative test result is as likely to be due to a nonreactive gonococcus as the NGN. Even at a sensitivity of 99.9% two of 10 negative test results from male urethral isolates will be false-negative. Because NGN are isolated more frequently from homosexual patients, negative predictive values are higher. When dealing with isolates from the throat, the negative predictive value remains high, even at a sensitivity of 98%.

The absolute specificity of the test makes it suitable for confirming the identity of throat isolates. In our experience this is particularly useful when characterizing isolates from primary cultures. Cultures with apparently characteristic meningococcal growth have, on several occasions, given a positive Phadebact Monoclonal GC test. On careful investigation, these cultures were shown to be a mixed infection with gonococci and meningococci. Likewise the test is useful in the rapid identification of gonococci in rectal cultures that may be contaminated with organisms other than neisseriae.

An omnireagent combining protein IA and IB MAb pools is also available in certain areas. As agglutination of the test reagent must be compared with a control reagent, the test is not any simpler to perform. In addition, an omnireagent is less flexible, and it would be more difficult to "modify" the MAb pool to cover nonreactive strains should the proportion of such strains increase.

C. Detection of Antigen in Exudates

A reliable method for the detection of gonococcal antigen in patient exudates would remove the need to maintain the viability of the gonococcus during transport, as well as overcoming problems associated with biochemical identification methods. Although a few groups have attempted to develop antigen detection systems based on enzyme-linked immunoadsorbent assay (ELISA) methods (Sarafian and Young, 1982; Young et al., 1983b) most published studies have evaluated the commercially available Gonozyme test (Abbott Diagnostics).

1. Gonozyme Test

The Gonozyme test is performed with urethral or cervical exudate collected on a swab and transported to the laboratory in a special transport tube containing a preservative. The swab should be processed to extract antigen within 5 days. Polystyrene beads (pretreated in an unspecified manner) are used as the solid phase to capture antigen, which is detected by polyclonal antibodies. Initially, the test was based on 15-min incubation periods and results could be obtained in 90 min. The test was later modified by extending the incubations to 45 min which increased the time taken to obtain results to over 3 hr.

a. Diagnosis from Urethral Swabs from Men. As shown in Table 6, the sensitivity, specificity, positive, and negative values are high in the case of symptomatic

Table 6 Detection of Gonococcal Antigen in Male Urethral Specimens by Gonozyme

Author	Study population	Prevalence of gonorrhea by culture (%)	Culture system	Sensitivity (%)	Specificity (%)	PVP[a]	PVN[b]	Comment
Aardoom et al. (1982)	Symptomatic ($n = 52$)	67	Direct plating: TM and chocolate agar	100 (90-100)[c]	100 (81-100)[c]	—	—	Same swab; plate inoculated first
Demetriou et al. (1984)	Symptomatic ($n = 57$)	42	Direct plating: JEMBEC with Martin-Lewis medium	100	100	100	100	Same swab; plate inoculated first
Papasian et al. (1984)	Symptomatic ($n = 208$)	54	Direct plating: Martin-Lewis or MTM medium	97.3	95.8	96.5	96.8	Two swabs; plate inoculated with first
Stamm et al. (1984)	Symptomatic ($n = 465$)	36	Direct plating: TM and chocolate agar biplate	95	98	97	97	Same swab used in order: Gram stain, biplate, Gonozyme
	Asymptomatic ($n = 664$)	2	Direct plating: TM and chocolate agar biplate	67	98	30	99	Same swab used in order: Gram stain, biplate, Gonozyme
Granato and Roefaro (1985)	Symptomatic ($n = 217$)	33	Direct plating: JEMBEC with Martin-Lewis medium	95.3	99.4	97.6	98.8	Culture and Gonozyme performed with eluate from a single swab

[a]PVP, predictive value for a positive test.
[b]PVN, predictive value for a negative test.
[c]95% confidence intervals given as probability percentages.

Table 7 Detection of Gonococcal Antigen in Cervical Specimens by Gonozyme

Author	Study population	Prevalence of gonorrhea by culture (%)	Culture system	Sensitivity (%)	Specificity (%)	PVP[a]	PVN[b]	Comment
Aardoom et al. (1982)	Contacts of suspected gonorrhea (n = 54)	24	Direct plating: TM and chocolate agar	86.7 (60-98)[c]	89.7 (76-97)[c]	—	—	Same swab; plate inoculated first
	Prostitutes STD control screen (n = 102)	12	Direct plating: TM and chocolate agar	91.7 (62-100)[c]	96.7 (91-99)[c]	—	—	Same swab; plate inoculated first
Demetriou et al. (1984)	Symptomatic, asymptomatic, high and low risk (n = 782)	12	Direct plating: JEMBEC with Martin-Lewis medium	87.5	98.0	85.7	98.2	Same swab; plate inoculated first
Papsian et al. (1984)	Symptomatic and asymptomatic (n = 252)	29	Direct plating: Martin-Lewis MTM medium	79.2	87.2	71.3	91.3	Two swabs; plate inoculated with first
Stamm et al. (1984)	STD clinic attenders (n = 723)	15	Direct plating: TM and chocolate agar biplate	78 76[d]	98 99[d]	85 88[d]	96 96[d]	Same swab used in order: Gram stain, biplate, Gonozyme
Granato and Roefaro (1985)	STD clinic attenders (n = 158)	28	Direct plating: JEMBEC with Martin-Lewis medium	100 100[e]	70.7 92.3[e]	49.3 85.4[e]	100 100[e]	Culture and Gonozyme performed with eluate from a single swab

[a]PVP, predictive value for a positive test.
[b]PVN, predictive value for a negative test.
[c]95% confidence intervals given as probability percentages.
[d]Results after retesting equivocal specimens.
[e]Excluding 30 specimens from contacts of infected men and test-of-cure specimens.

patients. The test is not reliable, however, for diagnosing infection in men without urethral discharge (Stamm et al., 1984); although the specificity was the same for both symptomatic and asymptomatic patients, the reduction in sensitivity from 95 to 67% was significant ($p < .001$) as was the reduction in positive predictive value from 97 to 30%. In symptomatic patients Gram staining, which is both inexpensive and simple to perform, correlated well with Gonozyme (Demetriou et al., 1984; Granato and Roefaro, 1985; Stamm et al., 1984). Consequently, when examining male urethral specimens there would seem to be little need for the more expensive Gonozyme assay.

b.   Diagnosis from Cervical Swabs.   In comparison with the results from men, antigen detection from cervical swabs (Table 7) is generally less sensitive and less specific. Demetriou et al. (1984) found the difference in sensitivity was significant ($p = .03$). There was no significant difference in sensitivity among the various subgroups of female patients (Demetriou et al., 1984). The lowest values for sensitivity were obtained by Stamm et al. (1984) who used the same specimen to make a Gram-stained smear and to inoculate a biplate before testing for antigen. It is likely that progressive loss of antigen during these procedures contributed to the lower sensitivity found in this study. Nevertheless, the sensitivity of Gonozyme (78%) was significantly greater than that of the Gram stain (48%). Unfortunately, as the test takes about 3-4 hr to perform, a result cannot be obtained when the patient is at the clinic.

The poorer sensitivity in women compared with men most probably results from less antigen in certain specimens. On the basis of semiquantitative counts, Demetriou et al. (1984) were able to show that cultures from six of 12 women with false-negative antigen assays had fewer than 100 colony-forming units (CFU) compared with 9 (10.8%) of 83 for whom quantitation was available in the true positive group ($p = .006$). The number of gonococci recovered from cervical aspirates varies widely. Young et al. (1983b) reported a range of 5.0×10^3 to 8.0×10^6 CFU/ml (mean 1.0×10^6 CFU/ml) in 37 infected women. The numbers in combined cervicovaginal washings from 52 women ranged from 4.0×10^2 to 1.8×10^7 (mean 1.45×10^5) (Lowe and Kraus, 1976).

Papasian et al. (1984) considered the poorer sensitivity in women may also be related to the more complex microbial flora of the female genital tract. If nongonococcal antigens adsorb onto the bead they could compete with gonococcal antigen for binding sites. Adsorption of nongonococcal antigens combined with cross-reactivity of the polyclonal detection antiserum may also account for the poorer specificity in women. Demetriou et al. (1984) found the difference in positive predictive value between male and female patients was statistically significant ($p = .02$). Because the detection antiserum may cross-react with other neisseriae, such as *N. meningitidis* and *N. lactamica*, the Gonozyme test is not recommended for pharyngeal or rectal specimens.

Unless a test exhibits absolute specificity, its positive predictive value will decline rapidly as the prevalence of the disease in the population decreases. Using the sensitivity and specificity values shown in Table 7 Demetriou et al. (1984) calculated that in a population with a 2% prevalence rate, as typically found in many family-planning clinics, the positive and negative predictive values would be 47.2 and 99.7%, respectively. Under such circumstances, the Gonozyme test could be used only for screening: as over one-half of the positives would be false-positive, culture confirmation under optimum conditions is essential. The high negative predictive value, however, means that screening with Gonozyme is likely to be more reliable for excluding gonococcal infection than culture techniques after prolonged transport. Martin et al. (1984) evaluated 510 patients (282 women and 140 men) with Gonozyme and Transgrow, containing Martin-Lewis medium, shipped to the laboratory after overnight incubation. The prevalence of gonorrhea by culture was approximately 15%. When specificity and sensitivity were calculated on the basis of clinical, epidemiological, and on-site laboratory data, Gonozyme had a sensitivity of 95% and a specificity of 99%. Transgrow had a sensitivity of only 69% but was 100% specific. More extensive evaluation of Gonozyme is required, however, for low-prevalence populations.

c. *Diagnosis from First-Voided Urine.*   Schachter et al. (1986) compared the Gonozyme test, performed on centrifuged urinary sediment, with conventional urethral culture in 196 men attending an STD clinic. The men were either asymptomatic, requesting routine investigation, or were named contacts. The prevalence of infection was 14% by culture. The sensitivity and specificity of Gonozyme were 93% (25 of 27) and 99% (167 of 169), respectively, and the negative and positive predictive values were 99 and 93%, respectively. The ability to detect gonococcal antigen in urinary sediment may provide the basis for a noninvasive method of screening for male infection. Again, evaluation of the test in the low-prevalence populations is required.

Detection of antigen in urine is ultimately to provide the optimum screen for infected women as urethral infection occurs in only around 75% (Young et al., 1979). In a direct comparison, Chapel and Smeltzer (1975) found that culture of urinary sediment was only 80% as productive as cervical culture.

d. *Detection of Antigen in Treated Patients.*   Granato and Roefaro (1985) considered that almost all of their false-positive Gonozyme test results occurred in either test-of-cure samples or specimens from women who were recent contacts of infected men. Because of the possible persistence of antigen in endocervical secretions, the Gonozyme test was not recommended for evaluating test-of-cure specimens. In a more detailed evaluation Stamm et al. (1984) tested 10 men and 10 women daily until both culture and immunoassay results became negative. On the first day after treatment all 10 men were culture-negative and specimens from seven of the men were also antigen test-negative. Two men did not become immunoassay-negative until the second day after treatment, while one man yielded persistent positive immunoassays, despite negative cultures, for 5 days after treatment. All 10 women yielded negative cultures on the first day after treatment and were immunoassay-negative by the second day.

D. Detection of Antibody

1. Humoral Antibody

The gonococcal complement fixation test (GCFT) is the only test that has been used to any extent in routine diagnosis. The test has fallen into disrepute over the years and it should not be relied upon either to detect or exclude uncomplicated infection. The GCFT has been withdrawn from most laboratories. As genital examination does not lend itself to large-scale-screening programs there is a real need for a sensitive and specific serological test to screen large groups of individuals, particularly asymptomatic women. Modern approaches using radioimmunoassay (RIA) and ELISA techniques with highly purified antigens, such as gonococcal pilus protein or outer membrane protein, have failed to provide a suitable test. The main problem is that antibody levels in infected and noninfected individuals overlap to such an extent that it is impossible to define an antibody level that gives a reliable indication of infection. Monoclonal antibodies by defining antigens specific for gonococcal infection, may aid the development of a suitable serological test(s). The serological diagnosis of gonococcal infection is reviewed in detail by Donegan (1985).

2. Local Antibody

The production of secretory IgA can be detected in cervical secretions by an indirect immunofluorescent (IF) method (McMillan et al., 1980). The use of exudates collected on swabs detected antigonococcal IgA in 72% of 78 infected women, but it was detected in only 5% of 490 noninfected women. Although this test could be developed further, it suffers from the disadvantage of requiring a genital specimen and must therefore be considered in relation to other noncultural methods.

V. NONCULTURAL, NONIMMUNOLOGICAL DIAGNOSIS

The following nonimmunological methods are available for detecting gonococcal components. These methods, however, have not been evaluated, or exploited commercially, to the same extent as immunological methods.

A. Endotoxin

The limulus amebocyte lysate (LAL) assay is a test to detect endotoxin. It can be used to detect gonococcal endotoxin in urethral and cervical exudates. The assay is not specific for gonococcal endotoxin but depends upon the absence of other bacteria producing endotoxin in amounts that would give a positive result. Because of the qualitative and quantitative differences in the genital tract flora of men and women the LAL assay performs best with male urethral exudates. Results with cervical exudates vary widely depending upon the dilution of exudate used in the test (Spagna et al., 1982).

Prior and Spagna (1985) evaluated the LAL assay on 200 men with varying quantities of urethral discharge. Pyrogen-free Dacron swabs were used for sample collection and a chromogenic substrate was used for visible endpoint determination after incubation for 10 min. The prevalence of gonorrhea by culture was 40% and the sensitivity and specificity of the LAL assay were 95 and 97%, respectively. There was no statistical difference between these results and those of Gram-stained smears read by an experienced microscopist. Five of 80 men with culture-proven gonorrhea and 52 of 120 men with nongonococcal urethritis had a minimal amount of urethral discharge and could not be evaluated by the LAL assay. Although the test is described as a simple, fast, and accurate method for the evaluation of exudative urethritis in an office setting, great care is required to ensure that all materials are pyrogen-free. The LAL assay is not suitable for populations with a low prevalence of gonorrhea (Judson et al., 1985).

B. Genetic Transformation

Gonococcal DNA can be detected in clinical specimens by transforming auxotrophic indicator gonococci to protrophy (Janik et al., 1976). This assay is extremely sensitive and can detect as few as 50 CFU of donor gonococci. One of the main limitations of this method is that clinical isolates of *N. gonorrhoeae* may themselves be auxotrophic for the same marker as the indicator strain and thus unable to transform it. The proportion of such auxotrophs will vary geographically. Although it may be possible to overcome these problems by using a temperature-sensitive mutant as indicator (Zubrzycki and Weinberger, 1980), the test remains difficult to perform and interpret.

C. DNA Hybridization

Gonococcal DNA has been detected in urethral exudates by hybridization with the 2.6 megadalton (Md) gonococcal cryptic plasmid as a radiolabeled [^{32}P] probe (Totten et al., 1983). Again, this test is very sensitive, detecting about 100 CFU of gonococci or 0.1 pg of gonococcal cryptic plasmid DNA. Unfortunately, certain strains of gonococci such as the PCU$^-$ auxotroph that are common in certain geographical areas, especially Canada (Chap. 4), lack the 2.6 Md cryptic plasmid and would not be identified by this assay.

Perine et al. (1985) used both the 2.6 Md plasmid and the 4.4 Md β-lactamase-encoding plasmid as probes for the detection of African and Asian strains of *N.*

gonorrhoeae in men with urethritis. With use of the 2.6 Md plasmid, the sensitivity and specificity of the hybridization method were 96% (180 of 187) and 93% (27 of 29), respectively. The 4.4 Md probe also detected infection with strains carrying the 3.2 Md plasmid and gave an overall sensitivity of 91% (59 of 65) and a specificity of 98% (136 of 139) compared with the chromogenic cephalosporin assay on cultured gonococci. Because organisms such as *Haemophilus influenzae* and *Escherichia coli* may contain β-lactamase-encoding plasmids that would react with the gonococcal plasmid probe, the hybridization method could not be used for specimens from the cervix, rectum, and throat. As the test takes at least 3 days to perform, it is useful only for epidemiological purposes. The use of biotin-labeled probes coupled with an avidin detection system provides the potential for results within 1 hr making the test useful in diagnosis.

VI. CONCLUSIONS

The accurate diagnosis of gonorrhea is particularly challenging because infection may involve a variety of anatomical sites with marked quantitative and qualitative differences in normal flora. Because of the medicolegal and social aspects of the disease, however, the level of accuracy required of tests to identify *N. gonorrhoeae* is greater than that accepted for many other organisms. Unless tests have a specificity in the region of 99% and a sensitivity greater than 99.9% they cannot be used reliably for confirming and excluding *N. gonorrhoeae* from all anatomical sites.

Monoclonal antibodies have an important role in the simple and reliable identification of gonococci. The new coagglutination identification reagents employing pools of MAbs offer 100% specificity and by careful selection and monitoring of MAb pools, approach a sensitivity of 99.9%. Serovar determination with MAbs as outlined in Chap. 4 is important in monitoring the antigenic profile of circulating gonococci and in constructing appropriate pools of MAb reagents.

Much smaller numbers of isolates have been evaluated using the newer biochemical identification methods, and their ability to give comparable levels of accuracy remains to be established. Biochemical methods do have the advantage, however, of identifying NGN to species level rather than simply differentiating between gonococci and NGN.

The use of MAbs in the direct detection of gonococci in genital exudates remains to be evaluated as an "on-the-spot" test for use in the clinic setting. It also remains to be shown that MAbs are useful for detecting gonococcal antigen in transported genital exudates. Gonozyme, the only immunological antigen detection method currently available commercially, uses a mixture of polyclonal antibodies. The levels of sensitivity and specificity of the Gonozyme test make it more suitable for excluding, rather than confirming, gonococcal infection. By combining polyclonal antibodies for antigen capture with MAbs for specific antigen recognition it should be possible to develop more specific, and possibly more sensitive, tests.

Because of the variety of diagnostic problems, some of which have been outlined in this chapter, there is an impetus for the increased use of immunological detection for the large-scale screening of genital specimens. Before this happens a more comprehensive evaluation of the performance of antigen detection tests in populations with a low prevalence of gonorrhea is required. Provided that such tests perform well in low-prevalence populations, and provided that screening programs are effective in reaching women with asymptomatic infection, they should have a marked effect on gonorrhea control. Although screening will be expensive, cost/benefit analysis must take into account the enormous cost of hospitalization because of PID resulting from untreated infection. Immunological detection is now best regarded as screening rather than diagnostic. Whenever possible, patients with positive antigen tests should be fully investigated by culture of the appropriate sites. Apart from confirming the diagnosis, culture will identify antibiotic-resistant strains.

REFERENCES

Aardoom, H. A., De Hoop, D., Iserief, C. O. A., Michel, M. F., and Stolz, E. (1982). Detection of *Neisseria gonorrhoeae* antigen by a solid-phase enzyme immunoassay. *Br. J. Vener. Dis. 58*:359-362.

Adler, M. W., Belsey, E. M., O'Conner, B. H., Catterall, R. D., and Miller, D. L. (1978). Facilities and diagnostic criteria in sexually transmitted disease clinics in England and Wales. *Br. J. Vener. Dis. 54*:2-9.

Alexander, W. J., Griffith, H., Housch, G., and Holmes, J. R. (1984). Infections in sexual contacts and associates of children with gonorrhea. *Sex. Transm. Dis. 11*:156-158.

Amies, C. R. (1967). A modified formula for the preparation of Stuart's transport medium. *Can. J. Public Health 58*:296-300.

Anand, C. M. and Kadis, E. M. (1980). Evaluation of the Phadebact Gonococcus test for confirmation of *Neisseria gonorrhoeae*. *J. Clin. Microbiol. 12*:15-17.

Arko, R. J., Finley-Price, K. G., Wong, K.-H., Johnson, S. R., and Reising, G. (1982). Identification of problem *Neisseria gonorrhoeae* cultures by standard and experimental tests. *J. Clin. Microbiol. 15*:435-438.

Arya, O. P., Nsanzumuhire, M., and Taber, S. R. (1973). Clinical, cultural, and demographic aspects of gonorrhoea in a rural community in Uganda. *Bull. WHO 49*:587-595.

Ashford, W. A., Golash, R. G., and Hemming, V. A. (1976). Penicillinase-producing *Neisseria gonorrhoeae*. *Lancet 2*:657-658.

Barlow, D., Nayyar, K., Phillips, I., and Barrow, J. (1976). Diagnosis of gonorrhoea in women. *Br. J. Vener. Dis. 52*:326-328.

Barr, J. and Danielsson, D. (1971). Septic gonococcal dermatitis. *Br. Med. J. 1*: 482-485.

Bhattacharyya, M. N., Jephcott, A. E., and Morton, R. S. (1973). Diagnosis of gonorrhoea in women: Comparison of sampling sites. *Br. Med. J. 2*:748-750.

Blomqvist, C., Ryden, A.-C., Amuso, P., Frankel, J., Lewis, J., and Young, H. (1985). Evaluation of the new Padebact Monoclonal GC test. 6th International Meeting of the International Society for STD Research, Brighton, England, p. 148.

Bonin, P., Tanino, T. T., and Handsfield, H. H. (1984). Isolation of *Neisseria gonorrhoeae* on selective and non-selective media in a sexually transmitted disease clinic. *J. Clin. Microbiol. 19*:218-220.

Boyce, J. M. and Mitchell, E. B. (1985). Difficulties in differentiating *Neisseria cinerea* from *Neisseria gonorrhoeae* in rapid systems used for identifying pathogenic *Neisseria* species. *J. Clin. Microbiol. 22*:731-734.

Boyce, J. M., Mitchell, E. B., Knapp, J. S., and Buttke, T. M. (1985). Production of ^{14}C-labeled gas in BACTEC *Neisseria* Differentiation Kits by *Neisseria cinerea*. *J. Clin. Microbiol. 22*:416-418.

British Co-operative Clinical Group (1980). Homosexuality and venereal disease in the United Kingdom: A second study. *Br. J. Vener. Dis. 56*:6-11.

Brogadir, S. P., Schimmer, B. M., and Meyers, A. R. (1979). Spectrum of the gonococcal arthritis-dermatitis syndrome. *Semin. Arthritis Rheum. 8*:177-183.

Brooks, G. F. (1985). Disseminated gonococcal infection. In *Gonococcal Infection* (G. F. Brooks and E. A. Donegan, eds.). Edward Arnold, London, pp. 121-131.

Bygdeman, S. (1981). Gonorrhoea in men with homosexual contacts. Serogroups of isolated gonococcal strains related to antibiotic susceptibility, site of infection and symptoms. *Br. J. Vener. Dis. 57*:320-324.

Carlson, B. L., Haley, M. S., Kelly, J. R., and McCormack, W. M. (1982). Evaluation of the Phadebact test for the identification of *Neisseria gonorrhoeae*. *J. Clin. Microbiol. 15*:231-234.

Chapel, T. A. and Smeltzer, M. (1975). Culture of urinary sediment for the diagnosis of gonorrhoea in women. *Br. J. Vener. Dis. 51*:25-27.

Chipperfield, E. J. and Catterall, R. D. (1976). Reappraisal of Gram-staining and cultural techniques for the diagnosis of gonorrhoea in women. *Br. J. Vener. Dis. 52*:36-39.

Communicable Diseases Scotland (1986). *Sexually Transmitted Disease Surveillance, United Kingdom, 1984.* Communicable Diseases Scotland Unit, 86/31, Glasgow, pp. 5-11.

Cornthwaite, S. A., Savage, W. D., and Willcox, R. R. (1974). Oral and rectal coitus amongst female gonorrhoea contacts in London. *Br. J. Clin. Pract. 28*:305-306.

Crawford, G., Knapp, J. S., Hale, J., and Holmes, K. K. (1975). Asymptomatic gonorrhoea in men: Caused by gonococci with unique nutritional requirements. *Science 196*:1352-1353.

Curtis, G. D. W. and Slack, M. P. E. (1981). Wheat-germ agglutination of *Neisseria gonorrhoeae*: A laboratory investigation. *Br. J. Vener. Dis. 57*:253-255.

Danielsson, D. and Forsum, U. (1975). Diagnosis of *Neisseria* infections by defined immunofluorescence. Methodologic aspects and applications. *Ann. N.Y. Acad. Sci. 254*:334-349.

Danielsson, D. and Kronvall, G. (1974). Slide agglutination method for the serological identification of *Neisseria gonorrhoeae* with anti-gonococcal antibodies adsorbed to protein A-containing staphylococci. *Appl. Microbiol. 27*: 368-374.

Demetriou, E., Sackett, E., Welch, D. F., and Kaplan, D. W. (1984). Evaluation of an enzyme immunoassay for detection of *Neisseria gonorrhoeae* in an adolescent population. *J. Am. Med. Assoc. 252*:247-250.

Donegan, E. A. (1985). Serological tests to diagnose gonococcal infections. In *Gonococcal Infection* (G. F. Brooks and E. A. Donegan, eds.). Edward Arnold, London, pp. 168-177.

Dossett, J. H., Appelbaum, P. C., Knapp, J. S., and Totten, P. A. (1985). Proctitis associated with *Neisseria cinerea* misidentified as *Neisseria gonorrhoeae* in a child. *J. Clin. Microbiol. 21*:575-577.

Easmon, C. S. F. (1985). Gonococcal resistance to antibiotics. *J. Antimicrob. Chemother. 16*:409-417.

Ebright, J. R., Smith, K. E., Drexler, L., Ivsin, R., Krogstad, S., and Farmer, S. G. (1982). Evaluation of modified Stuart's medium in culturettes for transport of *Neisseria gonorrhoeae*. *Sex. Transm. Dis. 9*:44-47.

Eschenbach, D. A. and Holmes, K. K. (1975). Acute pelvic inflammatory disease: Current concepts of pathogenesis, etiology and management. *Clin. Obstet. Gynecol. 18*:35-56.

Extract from the report of the Chief Medical Officer (1985). Sexually transmitted diseases: Extract from the annual report of the Chief Medical Officer of the Department of Health and Social Security for the year 1983. *Genitourin. Med. 61*:204-207.

Faur, Y. C., Weisburd, M. H., Wilson, M. E., and May, P. S. (1973). A new medium for the isolation of pathogenic *Neisseria* (NYC medium). I. Formulation and comparisons with standard media. *Health Lab. Sci. 10*:44-54

Faur, Y. C., Weisburd, M. H., Wilson, M. E., and May, P. S. (1977). Field evaluation of New York City medium in the biological environment—CO_2 chamber in recovery of *Neisseria gonorrhoeae* and urogenital mycoplasmas. *J. Clin. Microbiol. 5*:137-141.

Goodhart, M. E., Ogden, J., Zaidi, A. A., and Kraus, S. J. (1982). Factors affecting the performance of smear and culture tests for the detection of *Neisseria gonorrhoeae*. *Sex. Transm. Dis. 9*:63-69.

Granato, P. A. and Roefaro, M. (1985). Comparative evaluation of enzyme immunoassay and culture for the laboratory diagnosis of gonorrhoea. *Am. J. Clin. Pathol. 83*:613-618.

Handsfield, H. H. (1977). Clinical aspects of gonococcal infections. In *The Gonococcus* (R. B. Roberts, ed.). John Wiley & Sons, New York, pp. 68-69.

Handsfield, H. H., Knapp, J. S., Diehr, P. K., and Holmes, K. K. (1980). Correlation of auxotype and penicillin susceptibility of *Neisseria gonorrhoeae* with sexual preference and clinical manifestations of gonorrhea. *Sex. Transm. Dis.* 7:1-5.

Handsfield, H. H., Lipman, T. O., Harnisch, J. P., Tronca, E., and Holmes, K. K. (1974). Asymptomatic gonorrhea in men: Diagnosis, natural course, prevalence and significance. *N. Engl. J. Med. 290*:117-123

Hare, M. J. (1974). Comparative assessment of microbiological methods for the diagnosis of gonorrhoea in women. *Br. J. Vener. Dis. 50*:437-441.

Holmes, K. K. (1974). Gonococcal infection. *Adv. Intern. Med. 19*:259-285.

Holmes, K. K., Counts, G. W., and Beaty, H. N. (1971). Disseminated gonococcal infection. *Ann. Intern. Med. 74*:979-993.

Hopcraft, M., Verhagen, A. R., Ngigi, S., and Haga, A. C. A. (1973). Genital infections in developing countries: Experience in a family planning clinic. *Bull. WHO 48*:581-586.

Hookham, A. B. (1981). Thayer-Martin medium and modified New York City medium for the cultural diagnosis of gonorrhoea. *Br. J. Vener. Dis. 57*: 213.

Human, R. P. and Jones, G. A. (1986). Survival of bacteria in swab transport packs. *Med. Lab. Sci. 43*:14-18.

Ison, C., Glynn, A. A., and Bascomb, S. (1982). Acquisition of new genes by oral *Neisseria. J. Clin. Pathol. 35*:1153-1157.

Ison, C. A., McLean, K., Gedney, J., Munday, P. E., Coghill, D., Smith, R., Harris, J. R. W., and Easmon, C. S. F. (1985). Immunofluorescence for the rapid diagnosis of gonorrhoea. 6th International Meeting of the International Society for STD Research, Brighton, England, Abstract 95.

Jacobs, N. F. Jr. and Kraus, S. J. (1975). Gonococcal and nongonococcal urethritis in men. Clinical and laboratory differentiation. *Ann. Intern. Med. 82*:7-12.

Janik, A., Juni, E., and Heyn, G. A. (1976). Genetic transformation as a tool for detection of *Neisseria gonorrhoeae. J. Clin. Microbiol. 4*:71-81.

John, J. and Donald, W. H. (1978). Asymptomatic urethral gonorrhoea in men. *Br. J. Vener. Dis. 54*:322-323.

Judson, F. N., Werners, B. A., and Shahan, M. R. (1985). Lack of utility of a *Limulus* amoebocyte lysate assay in the diagnosis of urethral discharge in men. *J. Clin. Microbiol. 21*:152-154.

Kinghorn, G. R. and Rashid, S. (1979). Prevalence of rectal and pharyngeal infection in women with gonorrhoea in Sheffield. *Br. J. Vener. Dis. 55*:408-410.

Knapp, J. S. (1985). Typing of gonococci. In *Gonococcal Infection* (G. F. Brooks and E. A. Donegan, eds.). Edward Arnold, London, pp. 159-167.

Knapp, J. S. and Holmes, K. K. (1983). Modified oxidation-fermentation medium for detection of acid production from carbohydrates by *Neisseria* spp. and *Branhamella catarrhalis. J. Clin. Microbiol. 18*:56-62.

Knapp, J. S., Totten, P. A., Mulks, M. H., and Minshen, B. H. (1984). Characterization of *Neisseria cinerea*, a nonpathogenic species isolated on Martin-Lewis medium selective for pathogenic *Neisseria* spp. *J. Clin. Microbiol. 19*:63-67.

Lairscey, R. C. and Kelly, M. T. (1985). Evaluation of a one-hour test for the identification of neisseriae species. *J. Clin. Microbiol.* 22:238-240.

Latif, A. S. (1981). Sexually transmitted disease in clinic patients in Salisbury, Zimbabwe. *Br. J. Vener. Dis.* 57:181-183

Lawton, W. D. and Battaglioli, G. J. (1983). Gono Gen coagglutination test for confirmation of *Neisseria gonorrhoeae*. *J. Clin. Microbiol.* 18:1264-1265.

Lawton, W. D. and Koch, L. W. (1982). Comparison of commercially available New York City and Martin-Lewis medium for recovery of *Neisseria gonorrhoeae* from clinical specimens. *J. Clin. Microbiol.* 18:1264-1265.

Lim, D. V. and Wall, T. (1980). Confirmatory identification of *Neisseria gonorrhoeae* by slide agglutination. *Can. J. Microbiol.* 26:218-222.

Lowe, T. L. and Kraus, S. J. (1976). Quantitation of *Neisseria gonorrhoeae* from women with gonorrhea. *J. Infect. Dis.* 133:621-626.

McMillan, A., McNeillage, G., Gilmour, H. M., and Lee, F. D. (1983). Histology of rectal gonorrhoea in men, with a note on anorectal infection with *Neisseria meningitidis*. *J. Clin. Pathol.* 36:511-514.

McMillan, A., McNeillage, G., Young, H., and Bain, S. S. R. (1980). Detection of anti-gonococcal IgA in cervical secretions by indirect immunofluorescence: An evaluation as a diagnostic test. *Br. J. Vener. Dis.* 56:223-226.

McMillan, A. and Young, H. (1978). Gonorrhea in the homosexual man: Frequency of infection by culture site. *Sex. Transm. Dis.* 5:146-150.

Malysheff, C., Wallace, R., Ashton, F. E., Diena, B. B., and Perry, M. B. (1978). Identification of *Neisseria gonorrhoeae* from primary cultures by a slide agglutination test. *J. Clin. Microbiol.* 8:260-261.

Martin, J. E., Armstrong, J. H., and Smith, P. B. (1974). New system for cultivation of *Neisseria gonorrhoeae*. *Appl. Microbiol.* 27:802-805.

Martin, J. E. and Jackson, R. L. (1975). Biological environmental chamber for the culture of *Neisseria gonorrhoeae*. *J. Am. Vener. Dis. Assoc.* 2:28-30.

Martin, J. E. and Lewis, J. S. (1977). Anisomycin: Improved anti-mycotic activity in modified Thayer-Martin medium. *Public Health. Lab.* 35:53-60.

Martin, R., Wentworth, B. B., Coopes, S., and Larson, E. H. (1984). Comparison of Transgrow and Gonozyme for the detection of *Neisseria gonorrhoeae* in mailed specimens. *J. Clin. Microbiol.* 19:893-895.

Masi, A. T. and Eisenstein, B. I. (1981). Disseminated gonococcal infection (DGI) and gonococcal arthritis (GCA). II. Clinical manifestations, diagnosis, complications, treatment, and prevention. *Semin. Arthritis Rheum.* 10:173-197.

Mirrett, S., Reller, L. B., and Knapp, J. S. (1981). *Neisseria gonorrhoeae* strains inhibited by vancomycin in selective media and correlation with auxotype. *J. Clin. Microbiol.* 14:94-99.

Noble, R. C. and Cooper, R. M. (1979). Meningococcal colonisation misdiagnosed as gonococcal pharyngeal infection. *Br. J. Vener. Dis.* 55:336-339.

Norins, L. C. (1974). The case for gonococcal serology. *J. Infect. Dis.* 130:677-679.

Odugbemi, T. and Arko, R. J. (1983). Differentiation of *Kingella denitrificans* from *Neisseria gonorrhoeae* by growth on a semisolid medium and sensitivity to amylase. *J. Clin. Microbiol.* 17:389-391.

Osoba, A. O. and Alausa, O. (1976). Gonococcal urethral stricture and watering-can perineum. *Br. J. Vener. Dis. 52*:387-393.

Oxtoby, M. J., Arnold, A. J., Zaidi, A. A., Kleris, G. S., and Kraus, S. J. (1982). Potential shortcuts in the laboratory diagnosis of gonorrhea: A single stain for smears and nonremoval of cervical secretions before obtaining test specimens. *Sex. Transm. Dis. 9*:59-62.

Papasian, C. J., Bartholomew, W. R., and Amsterdam, D. (1984). Validity of an enzyme immunoassay for detection of *Neisseria gonorrhoeae* antigens. *J. Clin. Microbiol. 19*:347-350.

Perine, P. L., Totten, P. A., Holmes, K. K., Sng, E. H., Ratnam, A. V., Widy-Wersky, R., Nsanze, H., Habte-Gabr, E., and Westbrook, W. G. (1985). Evaluation of a DNA-hybridization method for detection of African and Asian strains of *Neisseria gonorrhoeae* in men with urethritis. *J. Infect. Dis. 152*: 59-63.

Philip, A. and Garton, G. C. (1985). Comparative evaluation of five commercial systems for the rapid identification of pathogenic *Neisseria* species. *J. Clin. Microbiol. 22*:101-104.

Philip, S. K., Ison, C. A., and Easmon, C. S. F. (1984). Coagglutination identification of *Neisseria gonorrhoeae*. *Br. J. Vener. Dis. 60*:66

Phillips, I. (1976). β-Lactamase-producing penicillin resistant gonococcus. *Lancet 2*:656-657.

Pollock, H. M. (1976). Evaluation of methods for the rapid identification of *Neisseria gonorrhoeae* in a routine clinical laboratory. *J. Clin. Microbiol. 4*: 19-21.

Prior, R. B. and Spagna, V. A. (1985). Improved utility of Gonoscreen a *Limulus* amoebocyte lysate assay in the evaluation of urethral discharges in men. *J. Clin. Microbiol. 22*:141-144.

Rice, R. J., Biddle, J. W., Jean Louis, Y. A., De Witt, W. E., Blount, J. H., and Morse, S. A. (1986). Chromosomally mediated resistance in *Neisseria gonorrhoeae* in the United States: Results of surveillance and reporting, 1983-1984. *J. Infect. Dis. 153*:340-345.

Robertson, D. H. H., McMillan, A., and Young, H. (1988). Diagnosis of gonorrhoea: Laboratory and clinical procedures. In *Clinical Practice in Sexually Transmissible Diseases*. Churchill Livingstone, Edinburgh.

Robinson, M. J. and Oberhofer, T. R. (1983). Identification of pathogenic *Neisseria* species with the RapID NH system. *J. Clin. Microbiol. 17*:400-404.

Saez-Nieto, J. A., Fenoll, A., Vazquez, J., and Casal, J. (1982). Prevalence of maltose-negative *Neisseria meningitidis* variants during an epidemic period in Spain. *J. Clin. Microbiol. 15*:78-81.

Saginur, R., Clecner, B., Portnoy, J., and Mendelson, J. (1982). Superoxol (catalase) test for identification of *Neisseria gonorrhoeae*. *J. Clin. Microbiol. 15*: 475-476.

Sandström, E., Lindell, P., Harfast, B., Blomberg, F., Ryden, A.-C., and Bygdeman, S. (1985). Evaluation of a new set of *Neisseria gonorrhoeae* serogroup W-specific monoclonal antibodies for serovar determination. In *The Patho-*

genic Neisseriae (G. K. Schoolnick, G. F. Brooks, S. Falkow, C. E. Frasch, J. S. Knapp, J. A. McCutchan, and S. A. Morse, eds.). American Society for Microbiology, Washington, DC, pp. 26-30.

Sarafian, S. K. and Young, H. (1982). Detection of gonococcal antigens by an indirect sandwich enzyme-linked immunosorbent assay, *J. Med. Microbiol. 15*: 541-550.

Schachter, J., Pang, F., Parks, R. M., Smith, R. F., and Armstrong, A. S. (1986). Use of Gonozyme on urine sediment for diagnosis of gonorrhea in males. *J. Clin. Microbiol. 23*:124-125.

Sgroi, S. M. (1982). Pediatric gonorrhea and child sexual abuse: The venereal disease connection. *Sex. Transm. Dis. 9*:154-156.

Shanker, S., Daley, D. A., and Sorrell, T. C. (1981). A rapid slide coagglutination test—an alternative to the fluorescent antibody test for the identification of *Neisseria gonorrhoeae. J. Clin. Pathol. 34*:420-423.

Simms, D. H. and Lue, Y. A. (1982). Evaluation of modified New York City carbohydrate medium for speciation of *Neisseria. Sex. Transm. Dis. 9*:34-36.

Smeltzer, M. P., Curran, J. W., Brown, S. T., and Pass, J. (1980). Accuracy of presumptive criteria for culture diagnosis of *Neisseria gonorrhoeae* in low-prevalence populations of women. *J. Clin. Microbiol. 11*:485-487.

Smeltzer, M. P., Curran, J. W., and Lossick, J. A. (1979). A comparative evaluation of media used to culture *N. gonorrhoeae. Public Health Lab. 37*:43-56.

Sng, E. H., Lim, A. L., and Yeo, K. L. (1984). Susceptibility to antimicrobials of *Neisseria gonorrhoeae* isolated in Singapore: Implications on the need for more effective treatment regimens and control strategies. *Br. J. Vener. Dis. 60*:374-379.

Sng, E. H., Rajan, V. S., Yeo, K. L., and Goh, A. J. (1982). The recovery of *Neisseria gonorrhoeae* from clinical specimens: Effects of different temperatures, transport times and media. *Sex. Transm. Dis. 9*:74-78.

Soendjojo, A. (1983). Gonococcal urethritis due to fellatio. *Sex. Transm. Dis. 10*:41-42.

Spagna, V. A., Prior, R. B., and Sawaya, G. A. (1982). Sensitivity, specificity, and predictive values of the *Limulus* lysate assay for detection or exclusion of gonococcal cervicitis. *J. Clin. Microbiol. 16*:77-81.

Sparling, P. F. (1977). Antibiotic resistance in the gonococcus. In *The Gonococcus* (R. B. Roberts, eds.). John Wiley & Sons, New York, pp. 111-135.

Spence, M. R., Guzick, D. S., and Katta, L. R. (1983). The isolation of *Neisseria gonorrhoeae*: A comparison of three culture transport systems. *Sex. Transm. Dis. 10*:138-140.

Stamm, W. E., Cole, B., Fennell, C., Bonin, P., Armstrong, A. S., Herrmann, J. E., and Holmes, K. K. (1984). Antigen detection for the diagnosis of gonorrhea. *J. Clin. Microbiol. 19*:399-403.

Svarva, P. L. and Maeland, J. A. (1979). Comparison of two selective media in the cultural diagnosis of gonorrhoea. *Acta Pathol. Microbiol. Scand. Sect. B 87*:391-392.

Tam, M. R., Buchanan, T. M., Sandstrom, E. G., Holmes, K. K., Knapp, J. S., Siadak, A. W., and Nowinski, R. C. (1982). Serological classification of *Neisseria gonorrhoeae* with monoclonal antibodies. *Infect. Immun. 36*:1042-1053.

Tapsall, J. W. and Cheng, J. (1981). Rapid identification of pathogenic species of *Neisseria* by carbohydrate degradation tests: Importance of glucose in media for preparation of inocula. *Br. J. Vener. Dis. 57*:249-252.

Taylor, D. N., Chen, K. C. S., Panikabutra, K., Wangba, C., Chitwarakern, A., Echeverria, P., and Holmes, K. K. (1985). Rapid identification of penicillinase-producing *Neisseria gonorrhoeae* by detection of beta-lactamase in urethral exudates. *Lancet 2*:625-626.

Thayer, J. D. and Martin, J. E. (1966). Improved medium selective for cultivation of *N. gonorrhoeae* and *N. meningitidis. Public Health Rep. 81*:559-562.

Tice, A. W. and Rodriguez, V. L. (1981). Pharyngeal gonorrhea. *J. Am. Med. Assoc. 246*:2717-2719.

Totten, P. A., Holmes, K. K., Handsfield, H. H., Knapp, J. S., Perine, P. L., and Falkow, S. (1983). DNA hybridization technique for the detection of *Neisseria gonorrhoeae* in men with urethritis. *J. Infect. Dis. 148*:462-471.

U.S. Department of Health and Human Services (1981). *STD Fact Sheet 35. Basic Statistics on the Sexually Transmitted Disease Problem in the United States.* Public Health Service, Centers for Disease Control, VD Control Division, Atlanta, Georgia, HHS Publication (CDC): 81-8195, pp. 1-35.

U.S. Department of Health and Human Services (1982). *Sexually Transmitted Diseases (STD) Statistical Letter* (formerly *VD Statistical Letter*), Calendar Year 1981. Public Health Service, Center for Disease Control, VD Control Division, Atlanta, Georgia, pp. 1-55.

Vecchio, T. J. (1960). Predictive value of a single diagnostic test in unselected populations. *N. Engl. J. Med. 274*:1171-1173.

Wallace, R., Ashton, F. E., Ryan, A., Diena, B. B., Malysheff, C., and Perry, M. B. (1978). The lipopolysaccharide (R type) as a common antigen of *Neisseria gonorrhoeae.* II. Use of less antiserum to gonococcal lipopolysaccharide in a rapid slide test for the identification of *N. gonorrhoeae* from primary isolates and secondary cultures. *Can. J. Microbiol. 24*:124-128.

Welborn, P. P., Uyeda, C. T., and Ellison-Birang, N. (1984). Evaluation of Gonocheck-II as a rapid identification system for pathogenic *Neisseria* species. *J. Clin. Microbiol. 20*:680-683.

Wiesner, P. J. (1975). Gonococcal pharyngeal infection. *Clin. Obstet. Gynecol. 18*:121-129.

Willcox, R. R. (1981). The rectum as viewed by the venerologist. *Br. J. Vener. Dis. 57*:1-6.

William, D. C., Felman, Y. M., and Riccardi, N. B. (1981). The utility of anoscopy in the rapid diagnosis of symptomatic anorectal gonorrhea in men. *Sex. Transm. Dis. 8*:16-17.

Windall, J. J., Hall, M. M., Washington, J. A., Douglass, T. J., and Weed, L. A. (1980). Inhibitory effects of vancomycin on *Neisseria gonorrhoeae* in Thayer-Martin medium. *J. Infect. Dis. 142*:775.

Wood, I. A. and Young, H. (1986). Identification of pathogenic *Neisseria* by enzyme profiles determined with chromogenic substrates. *Med. Lab. Sci. 43*: 24-27.

World Health Organization (1978). *Neisseria gonorrhoeae and Gonococcal Infections.* Technical Report Series 616. WHO, Geneva.

Yajko, D. M., Chu, A., and Hadley, W. K. (1984). Rapid laboratory identification of *Neisseria gonorrhoeae* with lectins and chromogenic substrates. *J. Clin. Microbiol. 19*:380-382.

Yong, D. C. T. and Prytula, A. (1978). Rapid micro-carbohydrate test for confirmation of *Neisseria gonorrhoeae. J. Clin. Microbiol. 8*:643-647.

Young, H. (1978a). Cultural diagnosis of gonorrhoea with modified New York City (MNYC) medium. *Br. J. Vener. Dis. 54*:36-40.

Young, H. (1978b). Identification and penicillinase testing of *Neisseria gonorrhoeae* from primary isolation cultures on New York City medium. *J. Clin. Microbiol. 7*:247-250.

Young, H. and Bain, S. S. R. (1983). Neisserial colonisation of the pharynx. *Br. J. Vener. Dis. 59*:228-231.

Young, H., Harris, A. B., Robertson, D. H. H., and Fallon, R. J. (1983a). Anogenital gonorrhoea and pharngeal colonisation with meningococci: A serogroup analysis. *J. Infect. 6*:49-54.

Young, H., Harris, A. B., and Tapsall, J. W. (1984). Differentiation of gonococcal and non-gonococcal neisseriae by the superoxol test. *Br. J. Vener. Dis. 60*:87-89.

Young, H., Harris, A. B., Urquhart, D., and Robertson, D. H. H. (1979). Screening by culture for the detection of gonorrhoea in women. *Scot. Med. J. 24*: 302-306.

Young, H. and McMillan, A. (1982). Rapidity and reliability of gonococcal identification by coagglutination after culture on modified New York City medium. *Br. J. Vener. Dis. 58*:109-112.

Young, H., Paterson, I. C., and McDonald, D. R. (1976). Rapid carbohydrate utilisation test for the identification of *Neisseria gonorrhoeae. Br. J. Vener. Dis. 52*:172-175.

Young, H. and Reid, K. G. (1984). Immunological identification of *Neisseria gonorrhoeae* with monoclonal and polyclonal antibody coagglutination reagents. *J. Clin. Pathol. 37*:1276-1281.

Young, H., Sarafian, S. K., Harris, A. B., and McMillan, A. (1983b). Non-cultural detection of *Neisseria gonorrhoeae* in cervical and vaginal washings. *J. Med. Microbiol. 16*:183-191.

Zubrzycki, L. and Weinberger, S. S. (1980). Laboratory diagnosis of gonorrhoea by a simple transformation test with a temperature-sensitive mutant of *Neisseria gonorrhoeae. Sex. Transm. Dis. 7*:183-187.

FOUR

Polyclonal and Monoclonal Antibodies Applied to the Epidemiology of Gonococcal Infection

Solgun M. Bygdeman
Karolinska Institute
Huddinge University Hospital
Huddinge, Stockholm, Sweden

I. INTRODUCTION

It is well known that different types or groups of microorganisms within the same species may differ in pathogenicity and virulence and in their resistance to different drugs. In epidemiological work it is of great importance to be able to divide the causal agents into groups and subgroups to follow the routes of transmission of these infections. In this chapter the different methods of strain differentiation of *Neisseria gonorrhoeae* will be reviewed and special reference to the application of serological classification, alone or in combination with other methods, in the epidemiology of gonococcal infection will be made.

II. METHODS OF STRAIN DIFFERENTIATION

A. Antibiotic Susceptibility Testing

After the advent of chemotherapeutic agents and antibiotics the gonococcus demonstrated its ability to acquire decreased susceptibility or resistance of chromosomal origin to these drugs. Resistance to streptomycin and spectinomycin have been used as markers. The appearance of penicillinase (β-lactamase)-producing *N. gonorrhoeae* (PPNG) strains, first reported in 1976 (Ashford et al., 1976; Phillips, 1976), created a new situation concerning treatment and epidemiology. Surveillance of antibiotic susceptibility patterns has demonstrated different epidemiological situations in various parts of the world and in different subpopulations.

B. Auxotyping

In 1973 Catlin described a defined nutritional medium for investigation of the growth requirements of *N. gonorrhoeae*. By the exclusion of single or multiple components such a medium can be used for the so-called auxotyping of gonococci. Because the medium described by Catlin was rather complex for routine use, Hendry and Stewart (1979) described a defined medium from which several constituents were deleted or changed compared with the Catlin medium. Several other modifications of the nutritional medium used for auxotyping gonococci have been published (see Ansink-Schipper, 1985).

The auxotypes are often distinguished according to the requirements of the tested strains for proline (Pro$^-$), arginine (Arg$^-$), hypoxanthine (Hyx$^-$), uracil (Ura$^-$), and methionine (Met$^-$). Citrulline (Cit$^-$) and ornithine (Orn$^-$), as well as a mixture of vitamins have sometimes been added to the components of the medium. Strains without specific requirements for these substances are called prototrophic (Proto) or wild type.

Auxotyping is a valuable tool for clinical and epidemiological investigations. Because the method is complicated and needs a well-equipped laboratory, it has been used mainly for research purposes.

C. Determination of the Plasmid Profile

Most gonococcal strains contain a small cryptic 2.6-megadalton (Md) plasmid (Maness and Sparling, 1972). Isolates lacking this plasmid have, however, been described by Dillon and Pauzé (1981a). Many isolates have also been found to harbor a so-called transfer plasmid of 24.5 Md.

The PPNG strains have been shown to contain either a β-lactamase-encoding plasmid of 4.4 Md (the Asian type) or a smaller β-lactamase-encoding plasmid of 3.2 Md (the African type) (Eisenstein et al., 1977; Elwell et al., 1977; Perine et al., 1977; Kirven and Thornsberry, 1977). Many of the PPNG strains of the Asian type contain, in addition to the 4.4-Md plasmid, the 24.5-Md transfer plasmid, which was not found in the PPNG strains of the African type during the first years (Ashford et al., 1976). The ability of a coexisting 24.5-Md plasmid to mobilize by conjugation the 4.4-Md plasmid into a penicillin-sensitive recipient has been described by Roberts and Falkow (1977). More recently, the 24.5-Md plasmid has also been found for the first time in strains carrying the β-lactamase-encoding 3.2 Md plasmid (Ansink-Schipper et al., 1982; Dillon and Pauzé, 1981b; van Embden et al., 1981; Johnston and Kolator, 1982).

The analysis of the plasmid profile of gonococcal isolates is a valuable contribution to the methods of strain differentiation of gonococci. It is particularly suited to research purposes.

D. Restriction Endonuclease Digestion and DNA Mapping

Restriction endonucleases are enzymes that cleave both strands of DNA at internal sites containing specific nucleotide sequences. Several methods have been used to construct restriction endonuclease maps of bacterial DNA (Dillon et al., 1985). The technique chosen for DNA mapping is determined by the level of detail required. To describe the methods for detailed maps of the gonococcal genome is beyond the purpose of this chapter. The different patterns of bands (fingerprints) in the gel after digestion of the gonococcal DNA by a single restriction endonuclease (Hind III) and subsequent separation of the fragments by electrophoresis have, however, been useful for the characterization of individual isolates (Falk et al., 1984; Falk et al., 1985).

E. Serological Classification

The selection of reference strains and target antigens for serological classification are reviewed in Chap. 2, Sect. III. Of the various classification schemes described, only the coagglutination (CoA) system based on W antigens (Sandström, 1979; Sandström and Danielsson, 1980) is suitable for extensive epidemiological studies. The value of this system in clinical and epidemiological studies was established by Bygdeman (1981a). Copley et al. (1983) showed that W antigens detected by CoA were stable during natural transmission, thus confirming their usefulness in epidemiological studies. The correlations found between the different serogroups with respect to antibiotic susceptibility and auxotype, and the epidemiological applications of the system, are described in the following section.

III. W SEROGROUPING SYSTEM USING POLYCLONAL ANTIBODIES

A. Geographical Distribution of Serogroups

Differences in the distribution of the three serogroups WI, WII, and WIII are found between different geographical regions and between PPNG and non-PPNG strains from the same geographical area (Fig. 1). The WI strains predominate in smaller Swedish cities (Bygdeman et al., 1981a; Danielsson et al., 1983). WI is also the most common serogroup among PPNG isolates from Hong Kong, the Philippines, and Africa. Serogroup WII, however, predominates among non-PPNG strains from these regions. Isolates in all other areas studied, both PPNG and non-PPNG, were most frequently serogroup WII with a maximum of 100% of the PPNG strains from Korea (Bygdeman et al., 1981b; Bygdeman et al., 1983; Handsfield et al., 1982; Odugbemi et al., 1983a,b). Southeast Asia seemed to be the focus of infection for WIII strains (Bygdeman et al., 1981b; Handsfield et al., 1982).

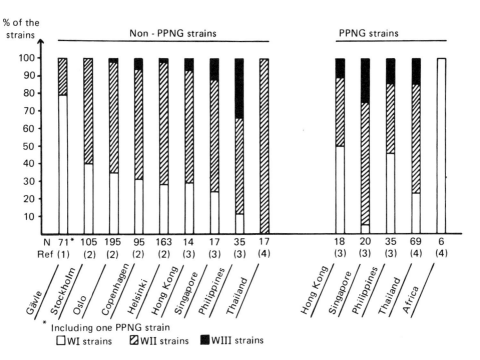

Fig. 1 Distribution into W serogroups of gonococcal isolates from patients in Scandinavia, Hong Kong, Singapore, the Philippines, Thailand, and Africa. (*Source*: from (1) Danielsson et al., 1983; (2) Bygdeman et al., 1983; (3) Handsfield et al., 1982; (4) Bygdeman et al., 1981.)

B. Serogroups in Relation to Sex and Sexual Preference

Differences in serogroup patterns have been shown between women and men. Although Danielsson et al. (1983) isolated WI strains more frequently from women than from men in Swedish cities, the opposite was found by Reid and Young (1984) in Edinburgh, Scotland. The predominant serogroup infecting homosexual men is WII, accounting for up to 90% of isolates from these men (Bygdeman, 1981a,b; Morse et al., 1982; Reid and Young, 1984). The difference in the prevalence of WII strains between homosexual men and other groups of patients is highly significant.

C. Serogroups in Relation to Auxotypes

Among non-PPNG strains isolated in Sweden, a great variety of auxotypes were seen. Four of them, Pro⁻Arg⁻, Hyx⁻Ura⁻, Met⁻Arg⁻Hyx⁻Ura⁻ (Met⁻AHU⁻), and Pro⁻AHU⁻, were seen only among WI strains (Danielsson et al., 1983). There

Table 1 Predominant Serogroup/Auxotype Combination Among Gonococcal
Strains from Different Geographical Regions

Region	PPNG or non-PPNG	Serogroup	Auxotype
The Philippines	PPNG	WI	Pro⁻
Hong Kong	PPNG	WI	Pro⁻
Africa	PPNG	WI	Proto
Thailand	PPNG	WII	Pro⁻
Singapore	PPNG	WII	Proto
Singapore	non-PPNG	WII	Pro⁻
Korea	PPNG and non-PPNG	WII	Proto

was also a strong correlation between AHU⁻ strains and serogroup WI (Danielsson et al., 1983; Sandström, 1979; Sandström et al., 1984). Apart from AHU⁻,
three other auxotypes, Proto, Pro⁻, and Pro⁻ Arg⁻ Ura⁻, were frequent (Danielsson et al., 1983). They were identified among strains of all three serogroups.

A more restricted number of auxotypes were represented among PPNG
strains isolated in Sweden, with Proto and Pro⁻ strains predominating (Bygdeman
et al., 1981b). Table 1 shows the preponderant serogroup/auxotype combination
in isolates from different geographical areas (Bygdeman et al., 1981b; Handsfield
et al., 1982; Odugbemi et al., 1983a,b). These data lend support to epidemiological observations concerning PPNG outbreaks in the United States (Handsfield et
al., 1982). The majority of isolates from patients with PPNG infections in Washington State were WI/Pro⁻ supporting the finding that the Philippines were mentioned as the site of foreign contact for many of these patients. A PPNG outbreak
in Shreveport, Louisiana, associated with WII/Pro⁻ strains was most likely due to
strains imported from Thailand.

Although the patterns of strains, as judged by serogrouping, were apparently
similar in different geographical regions (see Fig. 1), these patterns could be different when auxotyping was added as a method of strain differentiation (see
Table 1).

D. Serogroups in Relation to Plasmid Profiles and Auxotypes

The PPNG strains from Korea were WII/Proto and harbored the 4.4-Md plasmid,
usually in association with the 24.5-Md transfer plasmid (Odugbemi et al., 1983b).
The serovar/auxotype combination WI/Proto that was preponderant among African PPNG strains (see Table 1) was found only among strains carrying the 3.2-
Md plasmid: only one WII/Proto strain was seen among 39 PPNG isolates. This

strain was one of the seven strains harboring the 4.4-Md plasmid, and it was also one of the two strains carrying the transfer plasmid. Four of the 4.4-Md plasmid strains that originated from West Africa were WI/Pro⁻; the remaining 4.4-Md plasmid strains were WII/Pro⁻ (Odugbemi et al., 1983a).

E. Serogroups in Relation to Antibiotic Susceptibility

During the first decade after penicillin was introduced for the treatment of gonorrhea, the minimum inhibitory concentrations (MICs) of benzylpenicillin rarely exceeded 0.06 mg/L (Love and Finland, 1955; Martin et al., 1970; Reyn et al., 1958; Reyn, 1961) and the distribution of the MICs showed one single peak (Reyn et al., 1958; Reyn, 1961). After 1956 the frequency of gonococci from different parts of the world that show decreased susceptibility to penicillin has increased, and the MICs have shown a bimodal distribution with two peaks at about 0.01 and 0.2 mg/L, respectively (Reyn et al., 1958; Reyn, 1961). In some parts of the world, e.g., Africa and Southeast Asia, gonococcal isolates with MICs of > 0.5 mg/L are prevalent, even among non-PPNG strains (Araya and Phillips, 1970; Willcox, 1970). A parallel increase in the frequency of decreased susceptibility or resistance to other drugs used for the treatment of gonorrhea has occurred.

Because regional and other variations in antibiotic susceptibility had been noticed, it seemed interesting to investigate if they were correlated to differences in serogroup patterns.

1. Penicillins

Significant differences in susceptibility to benzylpenicillin (Fig. 2) and ampicillin among non-PPNG strains of the three serogroups have been demonstrated with WI strains as the most sensitive and WIII strains as the least susceptible (Bygdeman, 1981c). Thus, 94% of 46 WI strains isolated in Sweden were inhibited by ≤ 0.06 mg/L of benzylpenicillin and by ≤ 0.125 mg/L of ampicillin, whereas all nine WIII strains had MICs of ≥ 0.25 mg/L for these antibiotics. Among the 66 WII strains, isolated in Sweden and without known foreign origin, 45% were sensitive (MIC ≤ 0.06 mg/L) to benzylpenicillin and 47% were sensitive (MIC ≤ 0.125 mg/L) to ampicillin, whereas among the 17 non-PPNG strains imported from Thailand, none was sensitive to benzylpenicillin (see Fig. 2) or ampicillin.

2. Cefuroxime and Doxycycline

Significant differences in susceptibility to cefuroxime (Fig. 3) were found between WI, WII, and WIII non-PPNG strains. Differences in the susceptibility of WI and WIII and WII and WIII non-PPNG strains to doxycycline were also noted. There were no significant differences in susceptibility to these antibiotics between WII PPNG strains and WII non-PPNG strains imported from Thailand nor between

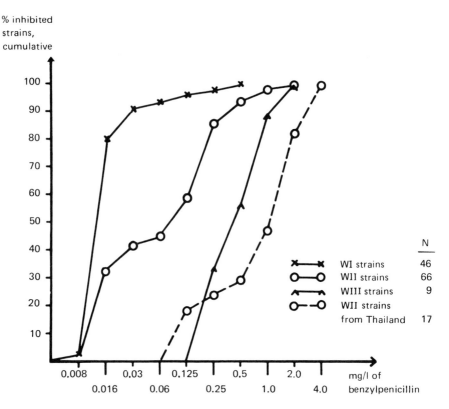

Fig. 2   In vitro susceptibility of non-PPNG strains to benzylpenicillin in relation to serogroup.

WIII PPNG strains and WIII non-PPNG strains. WI non-PPNG strains, however, were more sensitive to cefuroxime and doxycycline than the WI PPNG strains, which were more sensitive to these antibiotics than the WII PPNG strains.

Differences in susceptibility to other antibiotics also correlated to serogroup.

3. Geographical Differences

In another study (Danielsson et al., 1983), 726 gonococcal isolates from 10 different cities in Sweden were tested for susceptibility to ampicillin, cefuroxime, and doxycycline. In this study the correlation between susceptibility to ampicillin and cefuroxime, on the one hand, and serogroup, on the other hand, was confirmed. It was also shown that WI strains were more sensitive to doxycycline than WII strains. As expected, in the cities with a high prevalence of WI strains, the frequency of gonococcal isolates sensitive to ampicillin and cefuroxime was higher than in those cities where WII/WIII strains dominated.

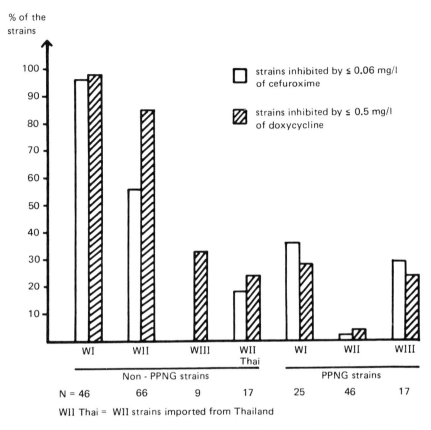

Fig. 3   Distribution of cefuroxime and doxycycline susceptibility in relation to W serogroup of strains isolated in Sweden.

4. Sex and Sexual Preference: Multiresistant Strains

The significantly higher prevalence of WII strains among men than among women is paralleled by a significantly higher frequency of gonococcal isolates with decreased susceptibility to ampicillin and doxycycline among the men (Bygdeman, 1981a).

The few WI strains isolated from homosexual men were significantly less susceptible to penicillin, ampicillin, cefuroxime, and doxycycline than WI strains from unselected patients in the same city (Bygdeman, 1981b). Gonococcal isolates from homosexual men, from whom WII strains were isolated more frequently than from heterosexual men, were significantly less susceptible to ampicillin, cefuroxime, and doxycycline than were those isolates from unselected men (Bygdeman, 1981a).

In transformation assays a genetic linkage between WII specificity and resistance to several antibiotics, detergents, and dyes has been shown (Bygdeman et al., 1982). This is in agreement with the decreased antibiotic susceptibility of WII strains.

Another genetic locus, *mtr*, also confers resistance to antibiotics, detergents, and hydrophobic dyes (Sparling et al., 1975; Sparling et al., 1976). Consequently, the *mtr* strains might predominate in environments, such as the rectum, that are rich in hydrophobic molecules. The *mtr* strains were significantly more prevalent among isolates from 43 homosexual men than among those from matched heterosexual controls (Morse et al., 1982). These strains also belonged to serogroup WII significantly more often than non-*mtr* strains. Data in another study by McFarland et al. (1983) suggested that the host environments could select for increased resistance to hydrophobic molecules by an *mtr*-independent mechanism. Reid and Young (1984) compared the relative distribution of WI and WII strains isolated from different sites of male and female heterosexual patients and suggested that selective pressures might be exerted at sites of infection other than the hydrophobic rectal environment.

F. Serogroups in Relation to Clinical Findings

Disseminated gonococcal infection (DGI) has been associated with WI strains (Sandström et al., 1984). Although earlier studies reported an association between DGI and the AHU⁻ auxotype (Knapp and Holmes, 1975), there is a better correlation between DGI and serogroup WI.

WIII strains have been reported to be relatively more common than WI and WII strains in patients from whom repeated gonococcal isolates have been obtained on different occasions. This indicates that WIII strains might be important for treatment failures (Danielsson et al., 1983) and is in keeping with their higher MICs.

G. Subgrouping of the Serogroups

During the studies with polyclonal antibodies, different reference strains were used for immunization of rabbits and also for absorption of the antisera (Bygdeman, 1981a). The CoA reagents finally chosen for the serological classification with polyclonal antibodies are listed in Table 2.

Using properly absorbed antibodies for the serological classification of *N. gonorrhoeae*, the same results were obtained when isolates were tested at different laboratories. Gonococcal strains that were serogrouped, stored, and retested some months later were referred to the same serogroup on each occasion. This indicated that the antigens involved were stable and the method was reproducible (Bygdeman, 1981a).

Table 2 Immunization and Absorption Scheme for the Preparation of Polyclonal Coagglutination Reagents for the Identification of Serogroups WI, WII, and WIII

Serogroup	Immunizing strain	Absorption strain	WI			WII				WIII
			Combinations of CoA patterns[a]							
WI	NRL[b] 7122	MOMP[c] A-1	+	+	–	–	–	–	–	–
WI	MOMP D-4	MOMP C-3 & F-6	–	+	+	–	–	–	–	–
WII	MOMP N-10	MOMP B-2 & F-6	–	–	–	+	+	–	–	–
WII	MOMP A-1	MOMP F-6 & NRL 7122	–	–	–	–	+	+	–	–
WII	MOMP H-8	MOMP B-2 & F-6	–	–	–	–	–	+	+	–
WIII	MOMP F-6	MOMP R-11 & A-1	–	–	–	–	–	–	–	+
No. of strains			27	456	8	243	45	65	14	21

[a]Patterns obtained on analyzing 879 gonococcal strains from Sweden (Danielsson et al., 1983).
[b]Obtained from the *Neisseria* Reference Laboratory, USPHS Hospital, Seattle, Washington.
[c]Major outer membrane protein reference strains (Johnston et al., 1976).

Unabsorbed antisera cross-reacted with *N. lactamica* and *N. meningitidis*. The selectively absorbed CoA reagents, however, cross-reacted neither with these species nor with the other oxidase-positive bacteria tested (Bygdeman, 1981a; Sandström, 1979). These findings indicated a species specificity for the W antigens, namely, protein I (Pr I).

If the polyclonal antisera were absorbed in the same way, the different CoA patterns (see Table 2) obtained within each serogroup were identical for each strain when the CoA was repeated and when multiple isolates from the same patient and isolates from their sexual partners were tested. If, however, the sera were absorbed with different strains, the CoA patterns within each serogroup might be different. Serogroup WI strains, which reacted only with the reagent anti-D-4, did, however, react only with anti-D-4 independently of the strains and methods used for the absorption. Furthermore, they belonged to different auxotypes compared with other WI strains and they were preponderantly isolated from homosexual men or were contracted abroad. It was obvious that these strains, WI-D-4, constituted a distinct subgroup within serogroup WI. Similarly, some WII subgroups could be distinguished (Bygdeman, 1981a).

Because WIII strains were found to have a Pr I molecule similar to that of WII strains (Pr IB) (Sandström et al., 1982) it was obvious that strains with different WII CoA patterns and those of serogroup WIII should be regarded as subgroups of the same serogroup, which was subsequently named WII/III.

H. Conclusions

During the studies with polyclonal antibodies it was evident that a system with better resolution was needed. As judged by the different patterns obtained with the polyclonal CoA reagents, it was apparent that strains of the same serogroup, in different parts of the world or in different subpopulations in the same area, were not identical. Among WII strains, some were sensitive to antibiotics and others had decreased susceptibility, suggesting that they might belong to different subgroups. WII strains from Thailand belonged, for instance, to those with decreased antibiotic susceptibility. WI strains, isolated from homosexual men were more resistant to antibiotics than those isolated from unselected patients. Did these findings indicate that WI strains from homosexual men belonged to different WI subgroups than those isolated from heterosexual patients?

With improved resolution of the serogroups into subgroups a better understanding of the macro- and microepidemiology of gonococcal infection might be achieved. With polyclonal antibodies it was impossible to resolve isolates into subgroups with reproducible results.

IV. SELECTION OF MONOCLONAL ANTIBODIES FOR USE IN THE SUBGROUPING OF W SEROGROUPS INTO SEROVARS

A. Selection of Monoclonal Antibodies for Subgrouping into Serovars

1. Development of Monoclonal Antibodies

In the efforts to circumvent the problems encountered in the serological classifica-tion of gonococci with polyclonal antibodies, especially those concerning subgroup-ing of the serogroups, monoclonal antibodies (MAbs) directed against epitopes on the Pr I, were produced in Seattle (Tam et al., 1982). For further information about the development of these Genetic Systems (GS) antibodies see Chap. 2.

2. Selection of Monoclonal Antibodies

About 30 different Pr I-specific MAbs from nine fusions performed in Seattle were selected for further analysis on clinical gonococcal isolates (Bygdeman and Sandström, unpublished data). The aim of this further selection of antibodies was to obtain a panel of monoclonal CoA reagents that identified epitopes on Pr I of all existing variants of *N. gonorrhoeae* but did not react with other bac-terial species. Furthermore, this panel should provide a maximum of resolution into subgroups with a limited number of reagents. It was also desirable to choose MAbs that could define subgroups of strains with clinically or epidemiologically important characteristics. The CoA reactions should be clear-cut and reproducible, resulting in identical CoA reactions on repeated testing of the same strain.

On the basis of these criteria, 11 Pr IA- and nine Pr IB-specific antibodies (Table 3) were selected for evaluation in more extended clinical studies (Bäckman et al.,1985; Bygdeman et al.,1983; Bygdeman et al.,1985; Ramstedt et al.,1985). Although all 20 MAbs (see Table 3) have been used for the analysis of the iso-lates in these studies, the results of the reactions with some of the antibodies have not been reported, and are discussed in Sect. IV.A.4.

3. Designation of Monoclonal Antibodies and Serovar Nomenclature

In Table 3 the original names of the MAbs are listed together with a more practi-cal designation with lower-case letters after a capital *A* for antibodies identifying WI strains and after a capital *B* for those detecting epitopes on WII/III strains. A serovar is defined as the pattern of reactivity of each strain with the monoclonal reagents. For example, the serovar of a WI strain reacting with the reagents Ae and Ad would be named Aed and a WII/III strain reacting with the reagents Ba, Bc, and Bk would be designated Back. This nomenclature for the gonococcal sero-vars has subsequently been used by our research group (Bygdeman et al., 1985).

Table 3 Monoclonal Antibodies (GS-Antibodies) Used for the Serological Classification of *N. gonorrhoeae* into W Serogroups and into Serovars

Serogroup WI protein IA-specific MAbs

Original name:	6G9	4A12	4G5	2F12	6D9	5C2	5G9	5D1	9D2	9G1	9F11
Designation:	Af	Ab	Ae	Ad	Ag	Ak	Ai	Ah	An	Al	Am
Standard panel according to Bygdeman and Sandström[a]	x		x	x	x	x	x	x			
Standard panel according to Knapp et al.[b]		x	x	x	x		x	x			

Serogroup WII/III protein IB-specific MAbs

Original name:	3C8	1F5	2D6	2H7	2G2	2D4	3C1	3B10	2H1
Designation:	Ba	Bb	Bc	Be	Bg	Bh	Bi	Bj	Bk
Standard panel according to Bygdeman and Sandström[a]	x		x	x	x	x		x	x
Standard panel according to Knapp et al.[b]	x	x	x		x	x			x

[a]From Bygdeman, S. and Sandström, E. (unpublished data) and Bygdeman et al., 1985.
[b]From Knapp et al., 1984.

Knapp and coworkers (Knapp et al., 1984) use a different serovar nomenclature. This is based on the use of the prefix IA or IB to indicate whether a strain is reactive with Pr IA- or Pr IB-specific reagents. The prefix is followed by a numerical designation according to the frequency with which strains of this serovar were encountered in a survey of gonococcal isolates from several countries (Knapp et al., 1984) using a fixed panel of 12 MAbs (see Table 3). The MAbs used by Knapp and coworkers were selected independently by them from the pool of MAbs obtained from the same nine fusions in Seattle. (For further information about the two systems of nomenclature for the gonococcal serovars see Knapp et al., 1985).

4. Notes on Special Monoclonal Antibodies

Three of the MAbs, listed in Table 3, have been excluded from our standard panel, i.e., Ab, Bb, and Bi, because in some of our studies, they have been found to give nonreproducible reactions. The three antibodies, An, Al, and Am, are not included in our standard panel but are always used by us. The antibody An is of value because it is reactive with almost all WI strains, whereas Al and Am are valuable because they usually react only with strains of the serovar Ae (corresponding to the polyclonal subgroup WI-D-4): reactions with the Ae reagent are often weak, making such isolates difficult to identify. The antibody Af may sometimes give weak reactions, but it is an essential member of the panel because some isolates from Singapore and also more recently from Canada (Dillon et al., 1986) have been shown to be reactive only with this monoclonal reagent. Ideally Bj should be excluded from the panel because it has been shown to cross-react with strains of some other *Neisseria* spp. However, as some gonococcal isolates from Singapore and one from Helsinki have been detected that react only with this reagent, it should be included in the panel until another MAb is found that identifies the Bj serovar strains. Bh is a stable antibody and, because it detects the strains formerly called WIII, it is of interest. Better resolution of the system is obtained by including Be in the panel.

5. Conclusions

Worldwide evaluation of the serovar patterns of gonococcal isolates may yield strains that are nonreactive with the present panel of antibodies. Even if the present panel covered all existing variants of the gonococcus, this might not be so in the future, as genetic changes in the gonococcus may occur. New antibodies that identify clinically or epidemiologically important strains may also be found.

Therefore, as new reagents may have to be added to the panel, a system for serovar nomenclature that is not based on a fixed set of antibodies is preferable.

B. Development of a Second Panel of Monoclonal Antibodies for the Serological Classification into Serovars

In an attempt to obtain better resolution of serovars than that obtained with our standard GS-panel, a new panel of MAbs (the Ph-panel) was developed (Sandström

Table 4 Monoclonal Antibodies (Ph-Antibodies) Used for the Serological Classification of *N. gonorrhoeae* into W Serogroups and into Ph-serovars

	Serogroup WI-specific MAbs								
Original name:	A13.3	A30.1	B18.1	B6.3	266B				
Designation:	Ar	Ao	As	At	Av				

	Serogroup WII/III-specific MAbs								
Original name:	D14.3	D12.2	D1.3	A15.2	A41.2	A29.1	A57.3	C6.2	254B
Designation:	Br	Bo	Bp	By	Bv	Bu	Bs	Bt	Bx

et al., 1985a). Five antibodies that detected WI strains and nine antibodies that identified WII/III strains were selected for the Ph-panel (Table 4), according to the criteria described earlier. Corresponding to the system for the GS-antibodies, the new antibodies, included in the Ph-panel, were named by means of lower-case letters from the second half of the alphabet after an *A* or a *B* for antibodies detecting WI and WII/III strains, respectively. None of these antibodies identified a previously recognized epitope on the Pr I.

C. Comparison Between the Two Panels of Monoclonal Antibodies

A comparison of the two different sets of MAbs was made on 253 PPNG strains isolated in Sweden during 1982 and 1983 (Bygdeman et al., 1985). The two sets of reagents showed good correlation. The resolution into serovars obtained by the two systems was equal and would, for either of the two systems, be greater if additional monoclonal reagents were added to each panel. The reactions with the Ph-reagents were clear-cut and reproducible.

A total of 165 WI strains isolated from patients in Australia, New Zealand, Bangkok, and Singapore (Bygdeman and others, unpublished data) and in the Republic of Korea (Bygdeman and others, unpublished data) and 395 WII/III strains isolated from patients in Bangkok, Singapore, and Korea were classified into GS- and Ph-serovars (Figs. 4 and 5).

Only seven WI serovars were identified with either of the two panels, and a total of eight GS-/Ph- serovar combinations were seen. With few exceptions, each WI serovar of one system corresponded to one specific serovar of the other system.

For WII/III serovars a diversity of GS-/Ph-serovar combinations was seen. Thus, each serovar of either system usually corresponded to one to three serovars

Fig. 4 table:

GS-serovars	\multicolumn{7}{c	}{Ph- serovars}	Total no.
	Arost	Aros	Arst	At	Ars	Ar	Av	
Aedgkih	54							54
Aedgki		1						1
Aedih			50					50
Aed			4	1				5
Af					3			3
Afe						2		2
Ae							50	50
Total no.	54	1	54	1	3	2	50	165

Fig. 4 Correlation between GS- and Ph-serovars for 165 serogroup WI isolates from Australia, New Zealand, Thailand, Singapore, and Korea.

Fig. 5 table — Ph - serovars:

GS-serovars	Brpyus	Brpyust	Brpyut	Bpyust	Byust	Bpyus	Bpyvust	Bpyvut	Bpyvu	Bopyvt	Bopyvst	Bopyst	Bopst	Bops	Bopys	Bys	Bropyst	Bropyt	Bopyt	Bopt	Bropt	Brpt	Bropst	Brops	Bo	Total no.
Bacejk	1	4	1																							6
Bcegk				3																						3
Bcegjk				47	1	1																				49
Bceghjk							1	11																		12
Beghjk								60	1																	61
Beghk							1	5																		6
Bcghk										1																1
Bhk										2																2
Bgjk												1														1
Bcgjk												1	13	5												19
Bcgk											1	50			17											68
Bacgk												1														1
Bck															14	3										17
Back																	7	2	14							23
Bak																		1	6							7
Bajk																				19	11	1				31
Bacjk																		2	4	19	52		7	1		85
Bachjk																							1			1
Bj																									2	2
Total no.	1	4	1	50	1	1	2	76	1	3	1	53	13	5	31	3	7	5	24	38	63	1	8	1	2	395

Fig. 5 Correlation between GS- and Ph-serovars for 395 serogroup WII/III isolates from Thailand, Singapore, and Korea.

of the other system. Among strains of the GS-serovar Bacjk, however, six different Ph-serovars were recognized. A total of 19 WII/III GS-serovars and 25 Ph-
serovars were seen and 41 GS-/Ph-serovar combinations. The resolution into
WII/III serovars consequently is much greater using the two systems or a combination of monoclonal reagents from the two systems.

V. EPIDEMIOLOGICAL DATA IN RELATION TO SEROVARS CURRENTLY RECOGNIZED BY MONOCLONAL ANTIBODIES

A. Geographical Distribution of Serovars

1. WI Serovars

a. General. In Fig. 6 the distribution into the three most frequently encountered WI serovars, Aedgkih, Ae, and Aedih, is presented for a total of 533 WI isolates from different geographical areas: these three serovars represented 490 (92%)
of the isolates.

The distribution into serogroups of the gonococcal isolates from the Scandinavian cities, except Trondheim, was described in Fig. 1 in relation to the classification using polyclonal antibodies. The results obtained by a serogrouping of
the isolates were the same with both polyclonal and monoclonal reagents. As in
the Scandinavian capitals, a preponderance of WII/III strains was seen in Trondheim (62% of all strains), among strains imported to Helsinki from Russia (85%),
in Sydney (82%), Perth (79%), Adelaide (67%), Darwin (60%), and Auckland
(73%), as well as among PPNG and non-PPNG strains from Bangkok (82 and
74%, respectively), Singapore (76 and 86%) and Korea (100 and 94%, respectively). Among PPNG strains isolated from patients in Sweden, 55% belonged
to serogroup WII/III, and among gonococcal isolates from Gabon the proportion
of WII/III strains was 51%.

b. Aedgkih. The serovar Aedgkih dominated among WI strains in all Scandinavian cities and in Perth and Adelaide (71-92% of the WI strains in each city); and
it was also the most common WI serovar in Sydney (43% of the WI strains). (In
the Scandinavian study Ah was not reported but all of the reported Aedgki strains
also reacted with the reagent Ah.) Aedgkih was also the most common WI serovar among gonococcal strains isolated in Canada [65 (82%) of 79 WI strains]
(Dillon et al., 1987). This serovar was not identified in Bangkok and Singapore
and rarely encountered in Gabon. In Korea a few Aedgkih strains were seen, all
non-PPNG strains, constituting 29% of the WI strains but only 1% of all strains.
Among 117 WI PPNG and 141 WII/III PPNG strains isolated in Sweden during
1982 and 1983, 162 of which were introduced from at least 35 different countries, only nine belonged to the serovar Aedgkih, of which seven had been introduced from Europe, Saudi Arabia, or African countries but not from Asia (Fig. 7).

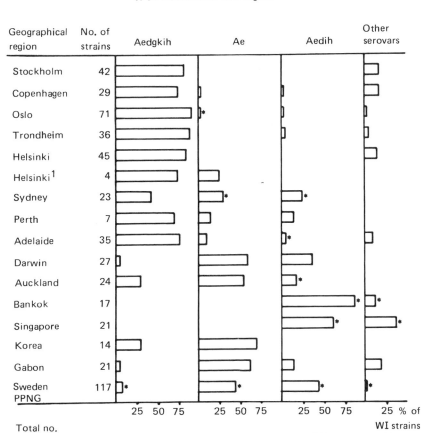

Fig. 6 Distribution into serovars of gonococcal strains of serogroup WI isolated from patients in Scandinavia, Australia, New Zealand, Bangkok, Singapore, the Republic of Korea, and Gabon. (*Source*: data from Bygdeman et al., 1983; Bygdeman and others,* unpublished data.) *Sandström, E. (Stockholm), Lassus, A. (Helsinki). Philpot, R., Tapsall, J., Handke, G., Blums, M., and Dyrting, A. (Australia), Say, P. J. (New Zealand), Panikabutra, K. (Bangkok), Sng, E. H. (Singapore), McChesney, D., Boslego, J. and Tramont, E. (Washington-Korea) and Frost, E. (Gabon).

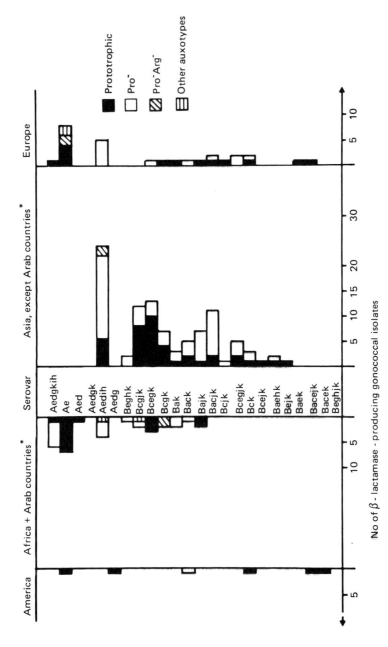

Fig. 7 Serovar and auxotype of 162 PPNG strains imported to Sweden during 1982 and 1983 in relation to probable geographical origin. The serovars Aedgk and Beghjk were represented only among indigenous isolates. *One isolate each from Kuwait and Saudi Arabia.

Among 142 WI strains isolated in the United States, 101 (71%) belonged to the serovars IA-1 and IA-2, corresponding to the serovar Aedgkih (Knapp et al., 1984).

Important foci for the Aedgkih serovar strains seem to be Europe, North America, and some parts of Australia, but not Southeast Asia.

c. Ae. The serovar Ae dominated among WI strains from Darwin, Auckland, and Gabon. In Korea gonococcal strains of this serovar constituted 71% of the WI strains but only 4% of all strains; there were no PPNG strains. Ae strains were also fairly common among WI strains from Sydney, and one of the four WI strains introduced to Helsinki from Russia belonged to this serovar. In Scandinavia, Ae strains were rarely seen among non-PPNG strains but accounted for 45% of the WI PPNG strains in Sweden. The Ae PPNG strains in Sweden, acquired abroad, were either introduced from other European countries, from Africa, or from the United States (one strain) but never from Asia (see Fig. 7). No Ae strain was identified in Bangkok or Singapore.

There are grounds to suggest that the geographical origin of the Ae strains is Africa. Other foci for Ae strains might be some parts of the Western Pacific such as New Zealand and the northern parts of Australia.

d. Aedih. The serovar Aedih dominated among WI strains in Bangkok (86% of the WI PPNG strains and 90% of the WI non-PPNG strains) and accounted for 80% of the WI PPNG strains in Singapore. Aedih was also common among non-PPNG strains in Singapore (45%). More than one-third of the WI strains in Darwin and one-fourth of those in Sydney were of this serovar, but they were rarely encountered among non-PPNG strains in Scandinavia or in Gabon (14%) and not at all in isolates from Korea. Among PPNG strains in Sweden, Aedih strains represented 45% of the WI strains. The majority (76%) of the 33 Aedih PPNG strains, imported to Sweden, had been acquired in Asia (see Fig. 7), 85% in Thailand or in the Philippines. Six of the seven WI PPNG strains seen in Australia and New Zealand belonged to the serovar Aedih and one was Ae.

Southeast Asia seems to be an important focus for Aedih serovar strains.

e. Other WI Serovars. Only 43 (8%) WI strains of serovars other than Aedgkih, Ae, and Aedih were seen, (see Fig. 6). Six of these WI strains of unusual serovars were PPNG, corresponding to 4% of the 143 WI PPNG strains. In Scandinavia nine other serovars were identified among non-PPNG strains, representing 10% of all 221 WI non-PPNG strains. In each Scandinavian city, between four and six different WI serovars were seen. In Sydney, Perth, Darwin, Auckland, and Korea, WI serovars other than two or all three of the serovars Aedgkih, Ae, and Aedih were not identified. Singapore seemed to be a source of gonococcal strains of unusual WI serovars, such as Aed, Ad, Afe, and Af, together accounting for 38% of the WI strains. Aed and Afe strains were also seen in Bangkok. Gonococcal strains of the serovar Af have hitherto only been identified in Singapore and Canada (Dillon et al., 1986). The six PPNG strains of more unusual serovars were classified as Aed, Afe, Aedg, or Aedgk.

In a survey of the serovars of 430 gonococcal isolates of serogroup WI from different parts of the world (Knapp et al., 1984) 13 different WI serovars were recognized and 59% of the isolates belonged to the serovars IA-1, IA-2, IA-4, and IA-6, corresponding to the serovars Aedgkih, Ae, and Aedih. In this study the serovar IA-3, corresponding to Aedi or Aedki, was the second most common serovar, accounting for 23% of the isolates. The geographical origin of these strains was not reported.

2. WII/III Serovars

a. General. Figures 8 and 9 show the serovars identified among WII/III gonococcal isolates from the same studies as the serogroup WI data presented in Fig. 6 (except those from Gabon). A wide variety of WII/III serovars were seen among both PPNG and non-PPNG strains. Of 1333 WII/III strains 36 serovars were identified. The 10 most commonly represented serovars are shown in Fig. 8 in relation to the geographical regions from which they originated; 89% (1192) of all WII/III strains belonged to these 10 serovars. The prevalence of each of the remaining 26 serovars (Fig. 9) ranged from 2.5% (32 isolates of serovar Bck) to 0.1% (representing a single isolate) of all WII/III strains.

Although there were great differences in the WII/III serovar patterns between the different geographical regions, the serovar Bajk was identified in all. Also, the three most common serovars in each region belonged to the 10 most common WII/III serovars. There were, however, differences in the serovar patterns between different cities in Australia and in Scandinavia; strains of the more unusual serovars were not seen in Perth or Darwin. Thirteen of the 26 serovars seen in Fig. 9 were found in only one of the geographical areas where they were usually represented by only one or two isolates. The more unusual serovars, however, accounted for 26% of the PPNG strains isolated in Sweden. As the Swedish PPNG strains were imported from at least 35 different countries, some of the "more unusual" serovars might predominate in other regions.

b. Serovars of the Former WIII Strains. In the Scandinavian study (Bygdeman et al., 1983), 14 WIII strains were identified with the polyclonal CoA reagents. With the monoclonal reagents, nine of the WIII strains were shown to belong to the serovar Beghjk and five to Beghk. In another study, comparing the results of the serological classification of gonococci with polyclonal and MAb reagents, 31, 13, and 1 of 44 WIII strains isolated in the United States, were found to belong to the serovars IB-4, IB-12, and IB-15, respectively (Knapp et al., 1984). The serovar IB-4 corresponds to the serovars Bghk, Bghjk, Beghk, and Beghjk, IB-12 to

Serovar	No. of strains	% of all WII/III strains	% of the WII/III gonococcal strains isolated in each area														
			Stockholm	Copenhagen	Oslo	Trondheim	Helsinki	Helsinki (Russia)	Sydney	Perth	Adelaide	Darwin	Auckland	Bangkok	Singapore	Korea	PPNG in Sweden
Bajk	309	23	35	37	38	28	34	26	34	59	30	2.	30	7*	14*	8*	12*
Bacejk	119	9	29	20	7		22	17	30	4	4		6	3*	1	1	2*
Bak	104	8	13	4	5	10	24	26	11			15	20*	2	7*	1	4*
Bacek	93	7	6	3	32	50	10					2					2*
Bacjk	176	13	11	1	2			4	7	11	37	30	8	23*	19*	21*	16*
Bcgjk	62	5	2	4	1		2	4	1*	7	7*	22	4	7*	8*	3*	11*
Back	75	6	2	9	3		2		8*		17	15	4	20*	7*	2	6*
Beghjk	87	6		9			2	4	3	11	1	10		21*	8*	16	2*
Bcegjk	76	6	2	6					3	7	1		8*	10*	10*	14*	7*
Bcgk	91	7				2				7		2	3	5	10*	22*	11*
Subtotal no.	1192		61	65	112	52	115	19	99	27	70	40	55	59	84	230	104
Total no.	1333		63	70	128	58	120	23	103	27	71	40	66	61	100	262	141
% of WII/III		89	97	93	88	90	96	83	96	100	99	100	83	97	84	88	76

Fig. 8 Proportion of WII/III gonococcal strains isolated in Scandinavia, Australia, Auckland, Bangkok, Singapore, and Korea belonging to the 10 most common WII/III serovars. *PPNG strains of this serovar were found. In addition, PPNG strains isolated in the Scandinavian cities belonged to the serovars Bacejk, Bcgik, Bcegjk, and Bcgk. Helsinki (Russia) strains isolated in Helsinki but introduced from Russia.

No. of gonococcal strains isolated in each area

Serovar	No. of strains	Stockholm	Copenhagen	Oslo	Trondheim	Helsinki	Helsinki (Russia)	Sydney	Perth	Adelaide	Darwin	Auckland	Bangkok	Singapore	Korea	PPNG in Sweden
Bcghjk	1						1									
Bceghjk	12														12*	
Bgjk	1														1	
Bachjk	1														1	
Bcghk	1												1*			
Bhk	2													2		
Bghjk	3						2							1		
Bj	3					1								2*		
Bk	6			1	4	1										
Baehk	2											2*				2*
Bejk	1															1*
Bcegk	24			3									1*	4*	12	17*
Bck	32						1							6*	6	10*
Beghk	14			4	1							1				3*
Bcjk	3	1														2*
Bcejk	5		2	2	1											1*
Baek	10		2	2		1						4				1
Baejk	3			1		1										
Bgk	3			1		1										
Bcek	1		1	1												
Bacej	1		1													
Ba	2			1						1						
Bahj	6	1		1				1				4				
Bagk	1							1								
Bacj	2							2								
Total no. 141		2	5	16	6	5	4	4	0	1	0	11	2	16	32	37

Fig. 9 Number of gonococcal strains isolated in Scandinavia, Australia, Auckland, Bangkok, Singapore, and Korea belonging to the more unusual WII/III serovars. *PPNG strains of this serovar found. In addition, PPNG strains isolated in the Scandinavian cities belonged to the serovars Bcegk and Bgk. Helsinki (Russia) strains isolated in Helsinki but introduced from Russia.

Bcghk, Bcghjk, Bceghk, and Bceghjk, and IB-15 corresponds to Bhk, Bhjk, Behk, and Behjk (Knapp et al., 1985).

In both the above studies all gonococcal strains identified as WI or WII/WIII with the polyclonal antibody reagents were referred to the same serogroup with the MAb reagents.

Gonococcal strains of the serovars that corresponded to the former serogroup WIII were most commonly seen in Bangkok and Korea, representing 23% of the WII/III strains in each area. In Bangkok all but one of the strains belonged to the serovar Beghjk, whereas in Korea, 30% belonged to either of the two serovars Beghk or Bceghjk; the remaining strains were of the more common serovar Beghjk. Beghk strains were also identified in Norway and among PPNG strains isolated in Sweden. The serovar Bcghjk was represented by only one strain, which originated from Russia.

c. *Serovars of Penicillinase-Producing* Neisseria gonorrhoeae *Strains.* Eighteen different serovars were seen among the WII/III PPNG strains in Sweden. In Bangkok, Singapore, and Korea, PPNG strains of 9, 11, and 6 different serovars, respectively, were identified with a total of 14 different serovars. Only three of them were not encountered among PPNG strains in Sweden. Eleven WII/III PPNG strains that belonged to serovars that were also seen in Bangkok, Singapore, or both, were isolated in Australia and Auckland. Nine WII/III PPNG strains were isolated in the Scandinavian countries (apart from the PPNG material from Sweden). Only one of them belonged to a serovar, Bgk, that was not identified among PPNG strains from the other areas. Thus, 22 different serovars were seen among PPNG strains in the entire material. With the exception of Bcghk, each serovar was also found among non-PPNG strains.

3. WII/III Serovars Compared with WI Serovars

Successive changes have been noted during the last few years with an increasing proportion of isolates in Sweden belonging to WII/III serovars (Danielsson et al., 1985).

A greater diversity of serovars is found among WII/III strains than among WI strains. The serovar patterns in different geographical regions are much more complex for WII/III strains than for WI strains, with greater differences even in adjacent geographical areas. The spread of β-lactamase-encoding plasmids to strains of new serovars with the capacity to survive seems also to be more developed among strains of serogroup WII/III than among those of serogroup WI.

In reported studies only 10 WII/III serovars were represented by up to 89% of all WII/III strains. Are gonococcal strains of the same serovar antigenically identical, as judged by the Pr I epitopes, in different geographical regions? Looking at Fig. 5, where the GS-/Ph-serovar combinations of the WII/III gonococcal strains from Bangkok, Singapore, and Korea are listed, it is obvious that strains of the same GS-serovar may have other epitopes on their Pr I that distinguish them from each other. The GS-serovar Bacjk corresponds to six different Ph-serovars, the GS-serovars Bacejk, Bcegjk, Bcgjk, Bcgk, Back, and Bajk, each correspond to three different Ph-serovars, and Beghjk and Bak each correspond to two Ph-serovars. The serovar Bacek was not identified in these areas. Nine of the "10 most common" WI/III serovars may, consequently, be resolved into 28 antigenically different serovars, as judged by this material from a comparatively restricted geographical area. By using an expanded panel of monoclonal reagents for the identification of WII/III serovars, it might be discovered that no serovar is, in fact, seen in all geographical regions.

As judged by the results presented in Fig. 4, corresponding resolution of WI serovars into a larger number of different serovar combinations is not possible; one serovar obtained with either panel of reagents, almost exclusively corresponds to one serovar obtained with the other panel of monoclonal reagents.

Similar results for WI and WII/III strains were obtained in another study by Bygdeman et al. (1985).

This means that the epidemiological differences are even more pronounced than they may appear between WI and WII/III strains.

B. Serovars in Relation to Sex and Sexual Preference

A correlation between gonococcal serovar and individual sexual preferences was found in a study in Stockholm of 378 gonococcal strains isolated from 330 women, 318 heterosexual men, and 83 homosexual men, including 21 bisexual men (Bäckman et al., 1985). Gonococcal isolates from women and heterosexual men belonged significantly more often to the WI serovar Aedgih (corresponding also to Aedgkih) and to the WII/III serovar Baik (corresponding to Bak and Bajk) than those isolated from homosexual men. The serovars Ae and Bacek (corresponding to Bacek and Bacejk), on the other hand, were more frequently identified in isolates from homosexual men. The serovar Ae corresponds to the subgroup WI-D-4, identified with polyclonal CoA reagents, which was seen preponderantly among homosexual men or which was acquired abroad (Bygdeman, 1981a).

Among gonococcal isolates from 221 women and heterosexual men and from 35 homosexual men in Sydney, Adelaide, and Auckland (female prostitutes excluded), those isolated from homosexual men belong to the serovar Bacejk significantly more often than those isolated from heterosexual patients. Only one strain of the serovar Bacek was found, and it was isolated from a homosexual man (Bygdeman and others, unpublished data). Three of the five WI strains isolated from the 35 homosexual men in Sydney, Adelaide, and Auckland belonged to the serovar Ae in contrast to 15 (25%) of the 61 WI strains isolated from women (prostitutes excluded) and heterosexual men.

C. Serovars in Relation to Auxotypes

1. General

A correlation between auxotype and serovar was found in a study of 1433 gonococcal strains from different parts of the world (Knapp et al., 1984). The serovars IA-1 and IA-2, corresponding to Aedgkih, accounted for 143 (98%) of 146 AHU⁻ strains and for only 32 (11%) of 287 WI strains belonging to other auxotypes. Among the other auxotypes no correlation with serovars was apparent. Proto strains were found among all serovars, except two, and Pro⁻ strains among all serovars, except four. The 13 WI and the 25 WII/III serovars could be resolved into 107 serovar/auxotype combinations.

Correlation between the serovar Aedgih (corresponding also to Aedgkih) and AHU⁻ was also found in a study of 731 gonococcal strains from patients in Stockholm (Bäckman and others, unpublished data). Correlation between several other serovars and auxotypes was also noticed, but this was interpreted as the effect of a local spread of strains of these serovar/auxotype combinations.

2. Penicillinase-Producing Neisseria gonorrhoeae Strains

Among 258 PPNG strains isolated in Sweden, the auxotypes Proto and Pro⁻ accounted for 53% and 42% of the strains. This corresponds well to the earlier finding that 93% of 98 PPNG strains were either Proto or Pro⁻ (Bygdeman et al., 1981b). Only four other auxotypes, Pro⁻ Arg⁻, Arg⁻, Met⁻, and Pro⁻ Met⁻, were represented. All six WI serovars and all 18 WII/III serovars (see Fig. 7), except Beghk, were represented among the Proto strains and 14 of the serovars were seen among Pro⁻ strains.

The Aedgkih PPNG strains, isolated in Sweden, were either Proto or Pro⁻, but none was AHU⁻. The majority, 91%, of the 53 Ae strains was Proto, and none was Pro⁻. The preponderant auxotype among the 52 Aedih strains was Pro⁻ (77%) and 15% were Proto. The auxotype Pro⁻ Arg⁻ was represented by strains of the serovars Ae, Aedih, and Bcgk.

The 258 PPNG strains could be resolved into 24 different serovars and only six auxotypes but as many as 43 different serovar/auxotype combinations.

a. Geographical Origin of WI Penicillinase-Producing Neisseria gonorrhoeae Strains.

Among the WI PPNG strains introduced to Sweden from other European countries, from Africa, or from Asia (see Fig. 7), Aedgkih and Ae strains were acquired in Africa or Europe and Aedih strains were acquired from all three continents.

Of the 10 serovar/auxotype combinations, represented by these, only Aedih/Pro⁻ strains were seen in all three geographical regions (Fig. 10). Ae/Proto and Aedgkih/Proto strains were acquired in Africa or Europe and strains of seven different serovar auxotype combinations were found to be introduced from any of

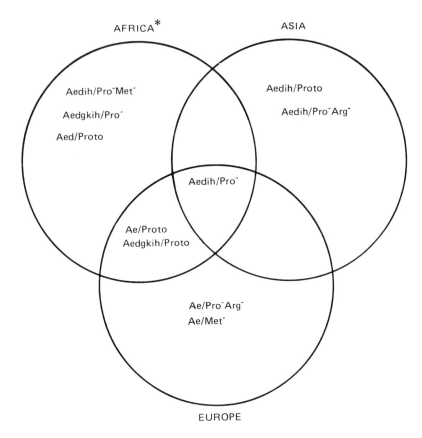

Fig. 10   The probable geographical origin of 56 PPNG strains of serogroup WI, isolated from patients in Sweden who had acquired their infection in other European countries, in Africa, or in Asia, related to serovar and auxotype of the isolates. *One Aedgkih/Pro⁻ strain from Saudi Arabia included.

the three continents. The Ae/Proto strains, brought into Sweden from Europe might, like strains of other serovar/auxotype combinations, initially have been imported to Europe. Ae/Pro⁻Arg⁻ and Ae/Met⁻ strains were acquired only in Europe and Aedih/Proto and Aedih/Pro⁻Arg⁻ strains only in Asia.

The earlier suggestion that the geographical origin of the Ae strains might be Africa may be valid for Ae/Proto strains. This is in accordance with the findings by Odugbemi et al. (1983a) that most of WI PPNG strains in Africa were Proto.

b.   Geographical Origin of WII/III Penicillinase-Producing Neisseria gonorrhoeae *Strains.*   Correspondingly, it was shown that the 11 serovars seen among WII/III gonococcal strains, imported from two or from all three continents (see Fig. 7), could be resolved into 23 serovar/auxotype combinations, nine of which were found among strains introduced from only one of these regions. In all, 10 serovar/auxotype combinations were seen only among strains originating from Asia, and two, Bcgjk/Arg⁻ and Bcgk/Pro⁻Arg⁻, only among those from Africa. This may indicate that Asia is a major source of WII/III PPNG strains of new serovar/auxotype combinations. The finding that Bcgjk/Arg⁻ strains were imported from Africa is in accordance with the report about WII PPNG strains in Africa belonging to the auxotype Arg⁻ (Odugbemi et al., 1983a). Strains of only two serovar/auxotype combinations, Bacejk/Proto and Baek/Proto, were acquired only in Europe, both in Spain (Bacejk/Proto also in Barbados) and six were acquired in Asia and Africa.

D. Serogroups and Serovars in Relation to Auxotypes and Plasmid Profiles

1. Non-Penicillinase-Producing Neisseria gonorrhoeae *Strains*

In a study comprising 113 non-PPNG strains isolated in Canada and selected to reflect geographical and auxotype diversities (Dillon et al., 1987), it was found that 16 (89%) of 18 isolates carrying the cryptic 2.6-Md palsmid in conjunction with the 24.5-Md transfer plasmid belonged to serogroup WII/III. The Pro⁻Cit⁻Ura⁻ auxotype, which was the most prevalent auxotype in Canada and distinguished by its absence of all plasmids, including the cryptic plasmid, was represented by 45 isolates belonging to either of four WII/III serovars, with Bacejk representing 93% of these strains.

2. Penicillinase-Producing Neisseria gonorrhoeae *Strains*

a. General. The changing patterns among PPNG strains—from the originally described African type of the auxotype Arg⁻ containing a 3.2-Md plasmid and the Asian type of the auxotypes Proto and Pro⁻ containing a 4.4-Md plasmid, mostly in conjunction with a 24.5-Md transfer plasmid (Perine et al., 1977)—have become clear. The PPNG strains of a diversity of auxotypes and serovars have emerged, representing the spread of the β-lactamase-encoding plasmids between strains of different serovar/auxotype combinations.

The PPNG strains harboring the 3.2-Md plasmid are represented by strains of auxotypes other than Arg⁻, i.e., Proto and Pro⁻, and although most of them belonged to serogroup WI, a few WII strains have also been seen (Odugbemi et al., 1983a). By using commercially available reagents for the detection of WI and WII strains, Yvert et al. (1985) found that all groupable PPNG strains isolated from patients in Gabon, belonged to serogroup WI and to the auxotypes Proto, Pro⁻, or Arg⁻.

b. Strains Carrying the 3.2-Md Plus the 24.5-Md Plasmid. The emergence of the 24.5-Md plasmid in strains carrying the 3.2-Md plasmid (Ansink-Schipper et

Table 5   Serovar, Auxotype, and Plasmid Profile Identified Among β-Lactamase-Producing Gonococcal Strains of Serogroup WI

Serovar	Auxotype	Plasmid profile[a]	Isolated in	Imported from	No. of strains	Ref.
Aedgkih	Pro⁻	3.2 Md	Sweden	Africa	1	1
Aedgkih	Pro⁻	3.2 Md + 24.5 Md	Sweden	Africa	1	1
Aedgkih	Pro⁻	4.4 Md + 24.5 Md	Sweden	Africa	2	1
Aedgkih	Proto	3.2 Md	Sweden	Canary I.	1	1
Aedgkih	Pro⁻Orn⁻	3.2 Md	Canada			3
Ae	Pro⁻	4.5 Md + 24.5 Md	Amsterdam		2	2
Ae	Proto	3.2 Md	Sweden	Africa	6	1
Ae	Proto	3.2 Md	Amsterdam		4	2
Ae	Proto	3.2 Md + 24.5 Md	Amsterdam		198	2
Ae	Pro⁻Orn⁻[b]	4.5 Md + 24.5 Md	Canada		51	3
Ae	Pro⁻Hyx⁻Ura⁻	4.5 Md + 24.5 Md	Amsterdam		5	2
Aedih	Pro⁻	4.5 Md	Amsterdam		17	2
Aedih	Pro⁻	4.5 Md + 24.5 Md	Amsterdam		1	2
Aedih	Pro⁻	4.4 Md + 24.5 Md	Sweden	Africa	3	1
Aedih	Proto	3.2 Md	Amsterdam		15	2
Aedih	Proto	3.2 Md + 24.5 Md	Amsterdam		11	2
Aedih	Pro⁻Met⁻	3.2 Md	Sweden	Africa	1	1
Aed	Pro⁻	4.5 Md	Amsterdam		1	2
Aed	Proto	3.2 Md	Amsterdam		1	2
Aed	Proto	3.2 Md	Sweden	Africa	1	1
Aedg	Pro⁻	4.5 Md	Amsterdam		2	2
Af	Pro⁻Orn⁻	4.5 Md	Canada	Philippines or Malaysia	4	3
Afe	Pro⁻	4.5 Md + 24.5 Md	Amsterdam		1	2

[a]The cryptic 2.6 Md plasmid not listed.
[b]Corresponding to Pro⁻Arg⁻.
Sources: Ref. 1. Falk and others (unpublished data). 2. Ansink-Schipper et al. (1987). 3. Dillon et al. (1987).

al., 1982; Dillon and Pauzé, 1981b; van Embden et al., 1981; Johnston and Kolator, 1982) has further changed our concept about African versus Asian PPNG strains.

Among 14 PPNG strains introduced into Sweden from Africa that carried the 3.2-Md plasmid, three were serogroup WII/III of serovar/auxotype combination Bcgjk/Arg⁻ or Bcgk/Pro⁻Arg⁻. The 11 serogroup WI PPNG strains are shown in Table 5. Six of these strains belonged to the combination Ae/Proto, two to Aedgkih/Pro⁻ and one to each of Aedgkih/Proto, Aedih/Pro⁻Met⁻, and Aed/Proto. Only one of the 14 3.2-Md plasmid strains (Aedgkih/Pro⁻) had a coexisting 24.5-Md transfer plasmid (Falk and others, unpublished data).

Aedgkih PPNG strains have not been reported from Asia and they were not among those brought into Sweden from Asia (see Fig. 10), indicating that the Aedgkih/Pro⁻ strains carrying both the 3.2-Md and the transfer plasmid are not the result of deletion of the 4.4-Md plasmid in Asian-type PPNG strains, but rather the result of a genetic exchange between existing local strains. Both the Aedgkih/Pro⁻ strains, with and without the 24.5-Md plasmid, originated from Nigeria.

In Amsterdam, the first PPNG strains harboring the 3.2-Md plasmid in conjunction with the transfer plasmid, were found in October 1980 (Ansink-Schipper et al., 1982). Between 1976 and 1978 almost all PPNG strains isolated in Amsterdam contained the 4.4-Md plasmid, most of them in conjunction with the 24.5-Md plasmid, and only sporadic cases of infection with 3.2-Md plasmid PPNG strains were seen, most of them imported from Africa.

During 1980 the number of PPNG infections in Amsterdam began increasing and peaked in January 1981. Among 54 PPNG strains isolated in October 1980 and Februrary to March 1981, 38 carried a 3.3-Md and a 24-Md plasmid (van Embden et al., 1981). Of 729 PPNG strains isolated in Amsterdam between March 1981 and September 1982 (Ansink-Schipper et al., 1987) 367 (50%) harbored both the 3.2-Md plasmid and the transfer plasmid (Afr⁺ strains) and were Proto (most were also inhibited by phenylalanine). Only nine Afr⁺ strains belonged to other auxotypes. Another 106 (15%) PPNG strains carried the 3.2-Md plasmid but not the transfer plasmid (Afr⁻ strains) and all but two were Proto (and inhibited by phenylalanine). Thus, the 1981-1982 PPNG outbreak in Amsterdam was caused mainly by Proto strains harboring the 3.2-Md plasmid, with or without the transfer plasmid (65% of the strains).

Serovar analysis of 234 Afr⁺Proto strains and 99 Afr⁻Proto strains showed marked differences. Serovar Ae accounted for 85% of Afr⁺ strains and 4% of Afr⁻ strains. The serovars Aedih and Bacejk accounted for 5 and 9%, respectively, of the Afr⁺ strains and 15 and 79%, respectively, of Afr⁻ strains. Only 2% each of the Afr⁺Proto strains and the Afr⁻Proto strains belonged to other serovars. These findings suggest that Proto strains of serovar Ae have a great capacity to survive and spread, a capacity that is more pronounced for Afr⁺ strains.

Ae/Proto strains were neither identified among PPNG strains in Amsterdam, carrying the 4.4-Md plasmid (see Table 5), nor among PPNG strains imported to Sweden from Asia (see Figs. 7 and 10). Furthermore, the serovar Ae has not been identified among PPNG strains in Southeast Asia (see Fig. 6). Thus, it is reasonable to suggest that the Ae/Proto strains, harboring both the 3.2- and the 24.5-Md plasmids, involved in the PPNG outbreak in Amsterdam, are not the result of a deletion of the 4.4-Md plasmid in Asian-type PPNG strains of the same serovar/ auxotype combination.

c. 4.4-Md Plasmid Strains in Africa. Some PPNG strains isolated in African countries have been found to carry the 4.4-Md plasmid, with or without the transfer plasmid (Anderson et al., 1982). Odugbemi et al. (1983a) reported that four PPNG strains, carrying the 4.4-Md plasmid, were isolated in West Africa. They all belonged to serogroup WI and were Pro⁻, while three 4.4-Md plasmid strains from other African countries belonged to serogroup WII and were either Proto or Pro⁻. They concluded that the 4.4-Md plasmid strains of serogroup WI were indigenous to West Africa, whereas those of serogroup WII had been imported.

Perine et al. (1983) noted that two PPNG strains with a 4.4-Md plasmid, isolated in Ghana, belonged to serogroup WI and were Pro⁻: similar serovars were common among PPNG strains isolated in Asia but these are usually Proto.

Twelve of 26 PPNG strains introduced into Sweden from Africa carried the 4.4-Md plasmid. All 12 strains also carried the 24.5-Md plasmid (Falk and others, unpublished data). Five of the isolates were serogroup WI and seven WII/III. The WI strains, which were all Pro⁻, included three isolates from Gambia, two of serovar Aedih and one Aedgkih. One strain from Sudan was also Aedih and one of unknown African origin Aedgkih (see Table 5). The PPNG strains of the serovar Aedgkih have not been identified in Southeast Asia (see Fig. 6). The Aedgkih/ Pro⁻ strains, carrying the 4.4 Md-plasmid and the transfer plasmid are, consequently, probably indigenous to Africa.

The Aedih PPNG strains are, on the other hand, currently isolated in Southeast Asia (see Fig. 6) and Aedih/Pro⁻ PPNG strains are often imported from this part of the world (see Figs. 7 and 10). None of the PPNG strains introduced from Africa and carrying the 3.2-Md plasmid were Aedih/Pro⁻. The PPNG strains of this serovar/auxotype combination, harboring the 4.4-Md plasmid, are then likely to have been brought into Africa.

Seven of the 12 4.4 Md-plasmid strains from Africa belonged to five different WII/III serovars and were either Proto or Pro⁻. No PPNG strain carrying the 3.2 Md plasmid was found to belong to the same serovar/auxotype combinations. The PPNG strains of four of these five serovars, i.e., Bcegk, Back, Bak, and Bcgjk, have been isolated in Thailand and/or Singapore (see Figs. 8 and 9), and PPNG strains belonging to the same serovar/auxotype combinations as the African WII/ III PPNG strains have been introduced into Sweden from Thailand (see Fig. 7).

The WII/III PPNG strains, carrying the 4.4-Md plasmid and brought into Sweden from Africa might, as with the Aedih/Pro⁻ PPNG strains, not have been originally indigenous to Africa.

d. Ae Strains with Asian-Type Plasmid. During a PPNG outbreak in Canada, 51 cases of infection with strains of the serovar/auxotype combination Ae/Pro⁻Orn⁻ (corresponding to Ae/Pro⁻Arg⁻) were identified: they were all Asia⁺. This is the first report of PPNG strains of the Asia⁺/Ae/Pro⁻Arg⁻ phenotype (Dillon et al., 1986). Ae/Pro⁻Arg⁻ strains are rarely seen among PPNG or non-PPNG strains in Canada, although seven cases of infection with non-PPNG strains of the same type were identified in connection with the PPNG outbreak. Ae/Pro⁻Arg⁻ PPNG strains have been introduced into Sweden from Hungary (see Figs. 7 and 10). Asia⁺Ae strains of auxotypes other than Pro⁻Arg⁻ have been isolated in Amsterdam (see Table 5).

e. Conclusion. It may be concluded that a combination of the three genetically independent methods of strain differentiation, namely, serological classification into serovars, auxotyping, and the determination of the plasmid profile, is very useful for the analysis of the epidemiology of gonococcal infection. A basic knowledge of the serovar/auxotype patterns of gonococcal isolates from different parts of the world is, however, a prerequisite for the interpretation of the results. It has been possible to present epidemiological circumstantial evidence for the origin of PPNG strains of new plasmid combinations.

E. Serovars in Relation to Antibiotic Susceptibility

1. WII/III Serovars

The earlier findings of a correlation between decreased susceptibility to different antibiotics and gonococcal strains of serogroups WII and WIII (see Figs. 2 and 3), prompted the question of whether or not antibiotic resistance was correlated to certain WII/III serovars.

The susceptibility of 85 gonococcal strains, including 28 PPNG strains, to thiamphenicol and rifampin was related to the serovars of these strains (Bygdeman et al., 1984). It was found that decreased susceptibility to thiamphenicol (MIC ≥ 1.0 mg/L) and rifampin (MIC ≥ 0.5 mg/L) was associated with WII strains. Both WI and WIII strains were significantly more sensitive than were the WII strains. Among the WII strains, decreased susceptibility to both drugs was also characterized by a reaction with Bg. Because Bh is a marker for WIII strains and because WII/III serovars are grouped together, this correlation is valid only for WII/III strains reacting with Bg but not with Bh.

Among 289 WII/III non-PPNG strains isolated in Australia and Auckland (Bygdeman and others, unpublished data) the MIC_{50} of benzylpenicillin for the 28 strains of the serovars Bcgjk, Bcegjk, Bcgk, and Bagk was 0.5 mg/L and that

for the 10 Beghjk strains was 0.125 mg/L. None of these 38 strains had a MIC of
< 0.06 mg/L. For the 251 strains of the remaining 12 serovars not characterized
by a reaction with Bg (see Figs. 8 and 9), the MIC_{50} was 0.06 mg/L with a range
from 0.004 to 2.0 mg/L. In this material all serovars, characterized by a reaction
with Bg were found to be associated with decreased susceptibility to benzylpenicillin (MIC ≥ 0.125 mg/L)..Forty-one (14%) of the 296 WII/III non-PPNG strains
from Australia and Auckland belonged to serovars characterized by a reaction
with Bg, compared with 40 (41%) of the 98 WII/III non-PPNG strains from
Bangkok and Singapore. Although the MIC_{50} for strains not reacting with Bg
was comparatively low, some did have high MIC values.

In a clinical trial of rosoxacin, Rudén et al. (1985) found that 92% of 24
gonococcal isolates of serogroup WI had a MIC of ≤ 0.03 mg/L of rosoxacin
compared with 59% of 17 WII isolates. Among the WII serovars Bacek was found
to correlate with decreased susceptibility to this drug. This is interesting because
gonococcal strains of the serovar Bacek have been isolated significantly more often from homosexual men than from heterosexual patients (p. 142) (Bäckman et
al., 1985).

2. WI Serovars

Gonococcal strains of the serovar Ae have been correlated to homosexual preference among men (p. 142) (Bäckman et al., 1985) and WI strains isolated from
homosexual men have been shown to be significantly more resistant to benzylpenicillin and other antibiotics than those isolated from unselected patients (p.
125) (Bygdeman, 1981b).

Among 108 WI non-PPNG strains isolated from patients in Australia and
Auckland (Bygdeman and others, unpublished data) the MIC_{50} of benzylpenicillin was 0.03 mg/L. The MIC_{50} for the 39 Ae strains and for the 16 Aedih strains
was, however, 0.06 mg/L compared with 0.016 mg/L for the 50 Aedgkih strains.
Gonococcal strains (WII/III strains included), isolated from women (prostitutes
excluded) and heterosexual men in Sydney, Adelaide, and Auckland were inhibited significantly more often by ≤ 0.016 mg/L than those isolated from homosexual men. Isolates from women and heterosexual men belonged significantly
more often to serovars with MIC_{50} of ≤ 0.016 mg/L than those from homosexual men.

3. Spectinomycin-Resistant Strains

A number of spectinomycin-resistant gonococcal strains were isolated in London
during 1983. Microbiological evidence suggested that they all belonged to a single clone, but no epidemiological evidence could support this hypothesis, which
was supported further by the fact that all strains belonged to the serovar Bacjk
(Easmon et al., 1984). A single spectinomycin-resistant gonococcal strain has, so
far, been isolated in Sweden. It belonged to the same serovar as the strains from

London, indicating an epidemiological link (Bygdeman and Sandström, unpublished data).

4. Conclusions

Multiresistance to antibiotics has been shown to be linked to serogroup WII. In transformation assays with DNA from a multiresistant WII strain as donor and an antibiotic-sensitive WI strain as recipient, the multiresistant transformants showed an increase in Pr I molecular weight compared with the recipient (Bygdeman et al., 1982). Because the MAbs used for serological classification react with epitopes on Pr I, which functions as a porin in the gonococcus (Blake and Gotschlich, 1983), a certain correlation between antibiotic susceptibility and gonococcal serovars could be expected. Because decreased susceptibility to penicillin, for example, is controlled by several genetic loci that are not linked to the Pr I gene, differences in antibiotic susceptibility between strains of the same serovar are likely.

F. Serovars in the Microepidemiology of Gonococcal Infection

Serological classification of gonococci should aid the control of gonorrhea in high-risk populations. The detailed information provided by serotyping, in conjunction with contact tracing has proved useful in the recognition and control of microepidemics, the recognition of double infections, the differentiation of reinfection and therapeutic failure, and in medicolegal cases.

1. Sexual Partners and Double Infections

When nonidentity of the strains isolated from two sexual partners occurs, both of them must have had additional sexual contact, unless one of them had been infected with two different strains, only one of which was identified.

In Stockholm, data from 731 patients (330 women, 318 heterosexual men, and 83 homosexual men) with gonorrhea were examined to assess the occurrence of double infections and to correlate the serovars of isolates from known contact pairs (Bäckman et al., 1985).

Homosexual men were infected significantly more often with two different strains than were women and heterosexual men. Two strains of gonococci with different serovars were isolated from two (1%) of 218 women, two (7%) of 28 heterosexual men, and three (25%) of 12 homosexual men who had two or more gonococcal isolates on the same occasion. Only two of these seven patients were found to have two different strains at the same site. They were infected with strains of different serogroups. The remaining five patients were infected with two strains of the same serogroup but with different serovars that were isolated from different sites. This reflects the problem of recognizing double infections deriving from one site when the different strains belong to the same serogroup but different serovars. With the knowledge of the currently existing serovars in a geographical region, finding an unusual coagglutination pattern should suggest a double infection and lead to a number of single colonies being subcultured and classified separately.

Gonococcal strains, isolated from 80 (95%) of 84 known contact pairs, belonged to the same serovar within each couple. The strains from the remaining four pairs of sexual partners belonged to different serovars. Nine contact chains with three persons involved were also included in the study. In one of these chains, two of the three patients were infected with identical strains, but the third patient, who had had additional sexual partners, was infected with a strain of a different serovar. Strains of different serovars were isolated significantly more often from homosexual couples than from heterosexual partners.

Infections with multiple strains are common in other areas. In Adelaide, among 106 patients with gonorrhea, one of 13 "known" pairs of sexual partners had gonococcal isolates of nonidentical serovars (Bygdeman and others, unpublished data). This couple was homosexual.

During a treatment trial of gonococcal ophthalmia neonatorum in Nairobi, gonococcal isolates were obtained from the eyes of 41 newborns and from the nasopharynx of seven and from the cervix of 18 of the mothers (Brunham et al., 1985). Four of the 18 maternal-neonatal strain pairs belonged to different serovar/auxotypes. These results suggested that maternal infection with multiple strains had occurred. This hypothesis agreed with the finding that two of seven eye-nasopharyngeal strain pairs from the neonates also were discordant in their serovar/auxotype patterns.

Infections with multiple strains are more likely to occur in individuals who are members of a core group of high-frequency transmitters of gonococcal infection (Yorke et al., 1978) such as prostitutes and certain sexually active homosexual men.

2. *Control and Analysis of Penicillinase-Producing* Neisseria gonorrhoeae *Outbreaks*

Isolates from 253 patients with PPNG infection in Sweden were classified serologically into GS- and Ph-serovars (Bygdeman et al., 1985). Serovar analysis identified 25 known or suspected contact pairs or chains accounting for 77 isolates. The index patient in 16 of these 25 cases of indigenous spread was known to have acquired the infection abroad. Of the remaining 61 patients involved in the pairs or chains of PPNG infection, 31 (51%) belonged to the serovar/auxotype Ae/Proto. Eleven of the 61 strains belonged to the serovar Aedih, one to Aedgkih, and the remaining 18 strains to 11 different WII/III serovar/auxotype combinations. This also suggests, as found in the PPNG outbreak in Amsterdam (Sect. V.D.2.b), that the capacity to survive and spread may be more developed for Ae/Proto strains than for PPNG strains of other serovar/auxotype combinations.

Ae/Proto strains were responsible for an outbreak of PPNG infection in Gothenburg during 1983. Knowledge of the serovars of the PPNG strains enabled the outbreak to be recognized early and contact-tracing efforts to be concentrated on those persons infected with the epidemic strain. During June to August 1983 43 PPNG strains were isolated from 42 patients in Gothenburg (Ramstedt et al., 1985). The first eight patients, who were seen before the end of March, had acquired their infection abroad and the isolates belonged to various WII/III serovars. At the end of March and during the first week in April, five men infected with Ae/Proto PPNG strains reported local prostitutes as the source of their infections. When the outbreak was stopped in July 1983, 27 patients including six prostitutes had been infected with the Ae/Proto PPNG strain. Five of seven patients who could not be epidemiologically linked to the outbreak, apart from their isolates being Ae/Proto, were treated at clinics with inadequate contact-tracing facilities. Serovar analysis was able to link another four patients in different parts of Sweden with the Gothenburg outbreak and to determine when the outbreak had ended.

The PPNG strains may lose the β-lactamase-encoding plasmid (Bygdeman, 1981a). It is important to take this into account when contact tracing is undertaken during a PPNG outbreak and also when an infection with two different strains is suspected. For example, during a study in Adelaide, isolates from a husband and wife belonged to the serovar combination Bcgjk/Bopst (Bygdeman and others, unpublished data). The isolate from the man was a PPNG, but that from the wife did not produce β-lactamase. The subsequent isolate obtained from his wife was a PPNG of the same serovar as her first isolate. Only those three strains of the serovar combination Bcgjk/Bopst were seen in Adelaide during the study period, indicating that the non-PPNG isolate from the woman had lost its β-lactamase-encoding plasmid.

3. Medicolegal Cases

Serological classification into serovars may also be useful in medicolegal cases, such as sexual abuse of children or rape. In some the establishment of the identity or nonidentity of gonococcal strains isolated from small girls and adult men accused of child abuse has helped clarify the situation (Bygdeman and Sandström, unpublished data). In these circumstances, it is important to be able to relate the serovar of the tested strains to their frequency in the geographical region in question.

For example, gonococcal isolates were obtained from a 2-year-old girl in New Zealand and from two adult men who were accused of having sexually interfered with her (Say and Bygdeman, unpublished data). The strain from the girl belonged to the GS-/Ph-serovar combination Bcgjk/Bopys. The same serovar was seen in the isolate from one of the two men, whereas, the other man was infected with an Aedgkih/Arost strain. The serovar Bopys was seen in nine (10%) of 90 gonococcal strains isolated in the same city. The serovar combination Bcgjk/Bopys was, however, seen in only two (2%) of these strains. Thus, the probability that the girl had acquired her infection from the man with an identical strain was considered high.

4. Reinfection Versus Therapeutic Failure

The classification of a patient with a positive test-of-cure culture after treatment as a therapeutic failure or a case of reinfection often must be made on the basis of epidemiological evidence that may be difficult to interpret. A proper classification of the treatment results is of great importance for the individual patient and his or her sexual partner(s) as, for example, in the evaluation of the effect of new drugs for the treatment of gonorrhea.

In a clinical trial of rosoxacin in Stockholm (Rudén et al., 1985), eight of the 48 patients included in the study were found to have positive test-of-cure cultures, either on day 2 or on day 7 after treatment. For four of these patients, who were initially considered as therapeutic failures on clinical evaluation, this classification was supported by the finding of identical serovars before and after treatment. For one of the patients, initially considered to have been reinfected, this classification had to be reconsidered because the two isolates belonged to the same serovar, which was unusual in Stockholm ($<1\%$ of the strains). This patients only admitted to have had different anonymous homosexual partners. The probability was considered as low that this man had been reinfected by another anonymous partner who was infected with a strain of the same serovar. On the other hand, the different serovars of the pre- and posttreatment isolates from another man confirmed that he had been reinfected.

In the study of 731 patients in Stockholm (Sect. V.F.1), 31 of them were infected twice during the study period. Twenty-one (68%) of these 31 patients were infected with strains of different serovars on the two occasions. Ten patients were infected more than once with strains of the same serovar. For patients infected with the same serovar, it is difficult to differentiate between reinfection and therapeutic failure because many cases of reinfection result from further contact with the original untreated partner.

In such circumstances, however, the use of additional methods of strain differentiation may be helpful.

G. Serogroups in Relation to Objective Symptoms and *Chlamydia trachomatis* Infection

A correlation between absence of clinical signs and serogroup WI has been found in a study consisting of 292 heterosexual men with urethral gonorrhea in Stockholm (Rudén et al., 1986a). Men infected with WI strains had fewer signs of urethritis, as judged by the number of leukocytes per high-power field, than those infected with WII/III strains ($p < .05$). Discharge from the urethra was also less common among patients infected with WI strains (60%) than among those from whom WII/III strains were isolated (79%) ($p < .01$). There was, however, no difference between the two groups of patients in the number attending the clinic for urethral symptoms.

In the same study, 20% of the patients with gonorrhea had a coexisting *C. trachomatis* infection. Corresponding frequencies for patients with WI and WII/III strains were 30% and 16%, respectively ($p < .01$).

A correlation between chlamydial infection and infection with WI gonococcal strains was also found in a study of patients with gonorrhea in three Swedish counties (Rudén et al., 1986a). Chlamydial infection was more common in all three regions, among both heterosexual men and women infected with WI strains than among those infected with WII/III strains, but the differences were significant only in two regions. The differences were most pronounced in the Halmstad region where 85 and 68% of the women and the men infected with WI strains had a coexisting chlamydial infection compared with 48 and 30% for those infected with WII/III strains ($p < .01$).

H. Conclusions

Many of the questions prompted by the results of the studies with polyclonal antibodies have been answered during the first years using Mabs for the serological classification of gonococci. We have learned that the epidemiology of WI strains is essentially different from that of WII/III strains, that WI strains from one part of the world are different from those in other parts of the world, and that the pattern of WII/III serovars may differ even in adjacent geographical regions. A greater diversity of serovars has been found among non-PPNG, as well as among PPNG strains of serogroup WII/III, than among those of serogroup WI. The potential for a better resolution of the WII/III serogroup has raised the possibility of the use of an expanded panel of MAb reagents for the classification of WII/III strains into serovars.

Serological classification in combination with auxotyping and plasmid profile analysis has been useful for the understanding of the epidemiology of PPNG infections. The probable geographical origin of strains of certain serovar/auxotype combinations has been proposed. Certain serovars have been correlated to sexual preference. Decreased susceptibility to antibiotics has been found to be correlated with some WII/III serovars. Even among the comparatively antibiotic-sensitive WI strains, differences in antibiotic susceptibility between strains of different serovars have been noticed.

Gonococcal infection is a global problem, but it is, in fact, composed of a multitude of local microepidemics. The understanding of the transmission between individuals is a prerequisite for the development of meaningful strategies to reduce the global problem. For this reason serological classification of gonococci applied to the microepidemiology of gonococcal infection is important. We have learned that gonococcal isolates from sexual partners mostly belonged to identical serovars. Discordance between serovars of strains from presumed sexual partners indicates that additional sexual partners have to be traced, unless there is double infection. Correspondingly, discordance between the serovars of gonococcal isolates from mother-neonate, indicates an infection with more than one strain, at least in the mother. Multiple infections, as with differences in serovar between isolates from sexual partners, were more common among homosexual men than among heterosexual patients. The identity of or differences between pre- and posttreatment isolates, as judged by the serovars, facilitated the classification into therapeutic failure or reinfection.

Serological classification into serovars using the CoA method is technically easy to perform, even in poorly equipped laboratories. With the use of the same panel of MAbs in the different laboratories, the system will be standardized, so that results obtained in studies from different parts of the world will be comparable. Serological classification into serovars, alone or in combination with other methods of strain differentiation based on different genetic mechanisms, will continue to help us to achieve a better understanding of the epidemiology of gonococcal infection.

VI. PROSPECTS

Many questions remain to be answered. For example, why is infection with WI strains more prevalent in women and associated with lack of clinical signs but more likely to be associated with *C. trachomatis* infection?

Although we have acquired knowledge of the gonococcal serogroup and serovar patterns in different parts of the world, we have little understanding of the many different factors that bring about epidemiological change in a particular region or area. We need to know the properties that appear to endow certain strains (e.g., Ae/Proto PPNG) with a greater capacity to survive and spread than others have.

In a given area, the pattern of gonococcal strains of different types may be transformed either by importation of new strains (Rudén et al., 1986b) or by genetic changes of locally existing strains. Both mechanisms are likely to operate most effectively when strains are introduced into a subpopulation of high-frequency transmitters. Infection with multiple strains of gonococci may be particularly important in the overall ecology of gonococci because exchange of plasmids and chromosomal DNA may occur in vivo and allow the development of phenotypic change (Brunham et al., 1985).

Studies involving serovar analysis should also prove useful in the development and assessment of gonococcal vaccines. Because repeated gonococcal infections are not unusual, if protective antibodies are produced against epitopes on the Pr I, gonococcal strains of new serovars might have an advantage over those that are more common in a given area. The possibility of being reexposed to a strain of the same serogroup but antigenically different from that of an earlier infection is greater for WII/III strains than for WI strains because in each region a greater diversity of serovars has been found within the WII/III serogroup than within the WI serogroup (Bygdeman et al., 1983). This hypothesis might explain why WII/III strains are more common among homosexual than among heterosexual men and more frequent among heterosexual men than among women, because repeated gonococcal infections are seen more often among homosexual than among heterosexual men and also more often among heterosexual men than among women (Bäckman et al., 1985). If this hypothesis is valid, women prostitutes would be infected with WI strains less frequently than other women. This was found among patients from Sydney and Adelaide (Fig. 11) (Bygdeman and others, unpublished data). The number of patients, however, was too small to obtain statistical significance. In Bangkok and Singapore the proportion of WI strains among women was not higher than among men, which might be

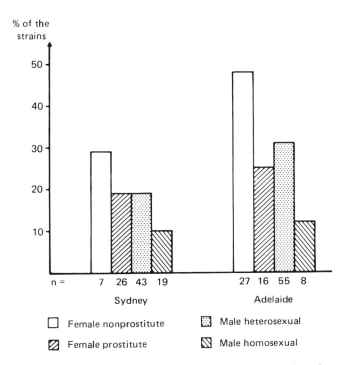

Fig. 11   Proportion of WI strains related to sex, sexual preference, and prostitution.

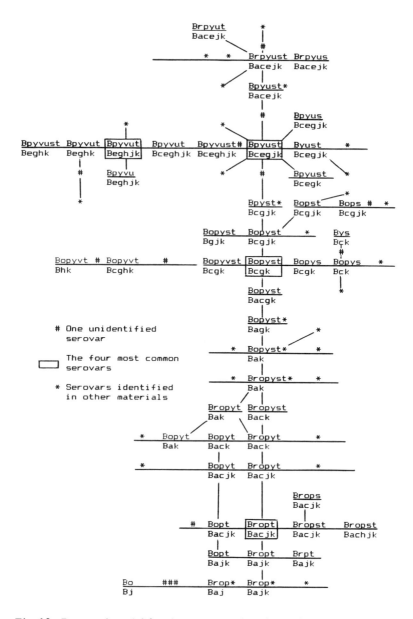

Fig. 12 Proposed model for the gonococcal evolution by antigenic drift. Gonococcal Ph-/GS-serovar combinations, identified among strains isolated in Bangkok, Singapore, Korea, and some other countries and arranged according to a stepwise random loss or acquisition of one protein I epitope.

explained by the fact that almost all women included in the study were prostitutes. Further studies to clarify this hypothesis seem essential for the discussion and development of a gonococcal vaccine.

Finally, the two panels of MAbs can be used for the phylogenetic classification of gonococci at the subspecies level. Gonococcal strains, 27 WI and 93 WII/III GS-/Ph-serovar combinations, served as a model to demonstrate the temporal accumulation of mutational changes (antigenic drift) in Pr I (Sandström et al., 1985b). When these serovars were analyzed for a proposed random loss of one antigenic epitope, it was found that they could be interconnected in two different "evolutionary" trees.

The WI serovars were clustered around a frequently isolated serovar (Aedgkih/Arost), from which three different major branches seem to have evolved. The situation with regard to WII/III serovars is more complex. Because multiple intermediary serovars were missing among the currently isolated WII/III serovars, these had to be postulated as having once existed or as not yet having been identified. Four very divergent branches, however, could best demonstrate the proposed hypothesis. It was striking that, in spite of the multitude of possible pathways of epitope variation, only a few "branches" seem to have been successful.

In Fig. 12 the GS-/Ph-serovar combinations, identified among WII/III strains from Bangkok, Singapore, and Korea (see Fig. 5) are arranged according to the proposed evolution. With the addition of a few serovar combinations that have been identified among gonococcal isolates from other countries, a maximum of one intermediary type was missing to connect the various serovars (with the exception of Bo/Bj) to branches of the same tree. The four most common serovar combinations occupy a central position in different branches of the tree. In any given area a few serovars dominate (see Figs. 6 and 8). Gonococcal strains of these preponderant serovars may serve as the basis for future evolution because of their proven superior adaptability.

The pronounced differences found between WI and WII/III strains in epidemiology as well as in clinical findings have sometimes provoked the question of whether or not they belong to "the same species." Lately a few very special gonococcal strains have, however, been identified that seem to have both WI and WII/III characteristics. Table 6 lists the serovars and the geographical origin of these strains. Two main types have been recognized, i.e., those of the Ph-serovar Av/Bx, identified in Gabon and Europe and those of the Ph-serovar Ar/Bo, isolated in Singapore and Europe. Further studies of these strains, which may be the missing link between the two serogroups, may contribute to our understanding of gonococcal infection.

Serological classification of other bacterial species, such as salmonellae and streptococci, is accepted as of great importance for epidemiological and clinical reasons. Similarly, the serological classification of gonococci should be included

Table 6 Serovars and Geographical Origin of Gonococcal Strains with Both Serogroup WI and WII/III Characteristics

GS-serovar	Ph-serovar	No. of isolates	Isolated in	Year of isolation
Al/Bej	Av/Bx	7	Rotterdam[a]	1977
Al/Be	Av/Bx	2	Gabon[b]	1983 (?)
Al/Be	ND	9	Gabon[b]	1983 (?)
Al/Bej	Av/Bx	2	Halmstad, Sweden[c]	1985
Al/Be	Av/Bx	1	London[d]	1985
Al/Beh	Av/Bx	3	Norge[a]	1984
Al/Beh	Av/Bx	3	Stockholm, Sweden	1985
Al/Beh	Av/Bx	4	Sweden (PPNG)[f]	1985
Al/Bacejk	Av/Bx	1	London[d]	1985
Anlm/Baejk	Av/Bx	1	Sundsvall, Sweden[g]	1985
Al/Behj	Av/Bx	6	Edinburgh[h]	1985
Al/Behj	Av/Bx	11	Edinburgh[h]	1986
An/Bj	Ar/Bo	2	Singapore[i]	1983
An/Bjk	Ar/Bo	1	Sweden (PPNG)	1985

The strains or the antigens kindly provided by [a]Prof. E. Stoltz; [b]Dr. E. Frost; [c]Dr. T. Ripa; [d]Dr. C. Ison; [e]Dr. J. Fuglesang; [f]one of the strains imported from North Africa; [g]Dr. K. Dornbusch; [h]classified by Dr. H. Young and D. C. Coghill; [i]Dr. E. H. Sng. [h]Reactions with A1 were weak. ND = not done.

in the national and local surveillance programs for the control of infectious diseases.

REFERENCES

Anderson, B., Odugbemi, T., and Johnson, S. (1982). Penicillinase producing *Neisseria gonorrhoeae* from Nigeria with Far Eastern type plasmid. *Lancet 1*:676.

Ansink-Schipper, M. C. (1985). Auxanographic typing of *Neisseria gonorrhoeae*. Ph.D. Thesis, Amsterdam, The Netherlands.

Ansink-Schipper, M. C., Embden, J. D. A. van, Klingeren, B. van, and Woudstra, R. (1982). Further spread of plasmids among different auxotypes of penicillinase-producing gonococci. *Lancet 1*:445.

Ansink-Schipper, M. C., Bygdeman, S. M., Klingeren, B. van, and Sandström, E. G. (1987). Serological classification, auxanographic typing and plasmid profile determination in the analysis of a PPNG outbreak in Amsterdam. *Genitourin. Med.* (In press).

Araya, O. P. and Phillips, I. (1970). Antibiotic sensitivity of gonococci and treatment of gonorrhoea in Uganda. *Br. J. Vener. Dis. 46*:149-152.

Ashford, W. A., Golash, R. G., and Hemming, V. G. (1976). Penicillinase-producing *Neisseria gonorrhoeae*. *Lancet 2*:657-658.

Bäckman, M., Rudén, A.-K. M., Bygdeman, S. M., Jonson, A., Rigertz, O., and Sandström, E. G. (1985). Gonococcal serovar distribution in Stockholm with special reference to multiple infections and infected partners. *Acta Pathol. Microbiol. Immunol. Scand. Sect. B 93*:225-232.

Blake, M. S. and Gotschlich, E. C. (1983). Gonococcal membrane proteins: Speculation on their role in pathogenesis. *Prog. Allergy 33*:298-313.

Brunham, R., Franzén, L., Plummer, F., Piot, P., Slaney, L., Bygdeman, S., and Nsanze, H. (1985). Antimicrobial sensitivity testing and phenotyping of *Neisseria gonorrhoeae* isolated from cases of ophthalmia neonatorum in Nairobi, Kenya. *Antimicrob. Agents Chemother. 28*:393-396.

Bygdeman, S. (1981a). Serological classification of *Neisseria gonorrhoeae*. Relation to antibiotic susceptibility and auxotypes. Epidemiological applications. Ph.D. Thesis, Stockholm, Karolinska Institute, Stockholm, Sweden.

Bygdeman, S. (1981b). Gonorrhoea in men with homosexual contacts. Serogroups of isolated gonococcal strains related to antibiotic susceptibility, site of infection and symptoms. *Br. J. Vener. Dis. 57*:320-324.

Bygdeman, S. (1981c). Antibiotic susceptibility of *Neisseria gonorrhoeae* in relation to serogroups. *Acta Pathol. Microbiol. Scand. Sect. B 89*:227-237.

Bygdeman, S., Bäckman, M., Danielsson, D., and Norgren, M. (1982). Genetic linkage between serogroup specificity and antibiotic resistance in *Neisseria gonorrhoeae*. *Acta Pathol. Microbiol. Immunol. Scand. Sect. B 90*:243-250.

Bygdeman, S., Danielsson, D., and Sandström, E. (1981a). Classification of *Neisseria gonorrhoeae* by coagglutination. A study of serological patterns in two geographical areas of Sweden. *Acta Dermato-Venereol. 61*:423-427.

Bygdeman, S., Danielsson, D., and Sandström, E. (1983). Gonococcal W serogroups in Scandinavia. A study with polyclonal and monoclonal antibodies. *Acta Pathol. Microbiol. Immunol. Scand. Sect. B 91*:293-305.

Bygdeman, S. M., Gillenius, E.-C., and Sandström, E. G. (1985). A comparison between two different sets of monoclonal antibodies for the serological classification of *Neisseria gonorrhoeae*. In *The Pathogenic Neisseriae* (G. K. Schoolnik, G. Brooks, S. Falkow, J. S. Knapp, A. McCutchan, and S. Morse, eds.). American Society for Microbiology, Washington, DC, pp. 31-36.

Bygdeman, S., Kallings, I., and Danielsson, D. (1981b). Serogrouping and auxotyping for epidemiological study of beta-lactamase producing *Neisseria gonorrhoeae* strains isolated in Sweden. *Acta Dermato-Venereol. 61*:329-334.

Bygdeman, S., Mardh, P.-A., and Sandström, E. (1984). Susceptibility of *Neisseria gonorrhoeae* to rifampicin and thiamphenicol. Correlation to protein I antigenic determinants. *Sex. Transm. Dis. 11*:366-370.

Catlin, B. W. (1973). Nutritional profiles of *Neisseria gonorrhoeae*, *Neisseria meningitidis* and *Neisseria lactamica* in chemically defined media and the use of growth requirements for gonococcal typing. *J. Infect. Dis. 128*:178-194.

Copley, C. G., Chiswell, C. P., and Egglestone, S. I. (1983). *Neisseria gonorrhoeae*: Stability of typing markers after natural transmission. *Br. J. Vener. Dis. 59*: 237-241.

Danielsson, D., Bygdeman, S., and Kallings, I. (1983). Epidemiology of gonorrhoeae. Serogroup, antibiotic susceptibility and auxotype patterns of consecutive gonococcal isolates from ten different areas of Sweden. *Scand. J. Infect. Dis. 15*:33-42.

Danielsson, D., Sandström, E., Bygdeman, S., Bäckman, M., and Gnarpe, H. (1985). W-serogroup (protein I) and serovar patterns of gonococci isolated during two different periods in urban and rural districts of Sweden. In *The Pathogenic Neisseriae* (G. K. Schoolnik, G. Brooks, S. Falkow, J. S. Knapp, A. McCutchan, and S. Morse, eds.). American Society for Microbiology, Washington, DC, pp. 71-77.

Dillon, J.-A. R., Bezanson, G. S., and Yeung, K.-H. (1985). Basic techniques. In *Recombinant DNA Methodology* (J.-A. R. Dillon, A. Nasim, and E. R. Nestmann, eds.). John Wiley & Sons, New York, pp. 1-126.

Dillon, J.-A. and Pauzé, M. (1981a). Relationship between plasmid content and auxotype in *Neisseria gonorrhoeae* isolates. *Infect. Immun. 33*:625-628.

Dillon, J.-A. and Pauzé, M. (1981b). Appearance in Canada of *Neisseria gonorrhoeae* strains with a 3.2 megadalton penicillinase-producing plasmid and a 24.5 megadalton transfer plasmid. *Lancet 2*:700.

Dillon, J. R., Pauzé, M., Gould, R., Sutherland, R., and Romanowski, B. (1986). Penicillinase-producing *Neisseria gonorrhoeae* with Pro Orn, WI, Asia phenotype. *Lancet 1*:103-104.

Dillon, J. R., Bygdeman, S. M., and Sandström, E. G. (1987). Serological ecology of *Neisseria gonorrhoeae* (PPNG and nonPPNG): A Canadian perspective. *Genitourin. Med.* (In press).

Easmon, C. S. S., Forster, G. E., Walker, G. D., Ison, C. A., Harris, J. R. W., and Munday, P. E. (1984). Spectinomycin as initial treatment for gonorrhoea. *Br. Med. J. 289*:1032-1034.

Eisenstein, B. I., Sox, T., Biswas, G., Blackman, E., and Sparling, P. F. (1977). Conjugal transfer of the gonococcal penicillinase plasmid. *Science 195*: 998-1000.

Elwell, L. P., Roberts, M., Mayer, L. W., and Falkow, S. (1977). Plasmid-mediated beta-lactamase production by *Neisseria gonorrhoeae*. *Antimicrob. Agents Chemother. 11*:528-533.

Embden, J. D. A. van, Klingeren, B. van, Dessens-Kroon, M., and Wijngaarden, L. J. van (1981). Emergence in the Netherlands of penicillinase-producing gonococci carrying "Africa" plasmid in combination with transfer plasmid. *Lancet 1*:938.

Falk, E. S., Bjorvatn, G., Danielsson, D., Kristiansen, B.-E., Melby, K., and Sörensen, B. (1984). Restriction endonuclease fingerprinting of chromosomal DNA of *Neisseria gonorrhoeae*. *Acta Pathol. Microbiol. Immunol. Sect. B 92*:271-278.

Falk, E. S., Danielsson, D., Bjorvatn, B., Melby, K., Sörensen, B., and Kristiansen, B.-E. (1985). Genomic fingerprinting in the epidemiology of gonorrhoea. *Acta Dermatol-Venereol. 65*:235-239.

Handsfield, H. H., Sandström, E. G., Knapp, J. S., Perine, P. L., Whittington, W. L., Sayers, B. S., and Holmes, K. K. (1982). Epidemiology of penicillinase-producing *Neisseria gonorrhoeae* infections. Analysis by auxotyping and serogrouping. *N. Engl. J. Med. 306*:950-954.

Hendry, A. T. and Stewart, I. O. (1979). Auxanographic grouping and typing of *Neisseria gonorrhoeae. Can. J. Microbiol. 25*:512-521.

Johnston, K. H., Holmes, K. K., and Gotschlich, E. C. (1976). The serological classification of *Neisseria gonorrhoeae*. I. Isolation of the outer membrane complex responsible for serotypic specificity. *J. Exp. Med. 143*:741-758.

Johnston, N. A. and Kolator, B. (1982). Emergence in Britain of beta-lactamase-producing gonococci with new plasmid combinations. *Lancet 1*:445-446.

Kirven, L. A. and Thornsberry, C. (1977). Transfer of beta-lactamase genes of *Neisseria gonorrhoeae* by conjugation. *Antimicrob. Agents Chemother. 5*: 1004-1006.

Knapp, J. S., Bygdeman, S., Sandström, E., and Holmes, K. K. (1985). A note on the nomenclature for the serological classification of *Neisseria gonorrhoeae*. In *The Pathogenic Neisseriae* (G. K. Schoolnik, G. Brooks, S. Falkow, J. S. Knapp, A. McCuthan, and S. Morse, eds.). American Society for Microbiology, Washington, DC, pp. 4-5.

Knapp, J. S. and Holmes, K. K. (1975). Disseminated gonococcal infection caused by *Neisseria gonorrhoeae* with unique nutritional requirements. *J. Infect. Dis. 132*:204-208.

Knapp, J. S., Tam, M. R., Novinski, R. C., Holmes, K. K., and Sandström, E. G. (1984). Serological classification of *Neisseria gonorrhoeae* with use of monoclonal antibodies to gonococcal outer membrane protein I. *J. Infect. Dis. 150*:44-48.

Love, B. D. and Finland, M. (1955). Susceptibility of *Neisseria gonorrhoeae* to eleven antibiotics and sulfadiazine. *Arch. Intern. Med. 95*:66-73.

McFarland, L., Mietzner, T. A., Knapp, J. S., Sandström, E., Holmes, K. K., and Morse, S. A. (1983). Gonococcal sensitivity to faecal lipids can be mediated by an *mtr* independent mechanism. *J. Clin. Microbiol. 18*:121-127.

Maness, M. J. and Sparling, P. F. (1972). Antibiotic resistance in *Neisseria gonorrhoeae. Clin. Res. 20*:52-53.

Martin, J. E. Jr., Lester, A., Price, E. V., and Schmale, J. D. (1970). Comparative study of gonococcal susceptibility to penicillin in the United States 1955-1969. *J. Infect. Dis. 122*:459-461.

Morse, S. A., Lysko, P. G., McFarland, L., Knapp, J. S., Sandström, E., Critchlow, C., and Holmes, K. K. (1982). Gonococcal strains from homosexual men have outer membranes with reduced permeability to hydrophobic molecules. *Infect. Immun. 37*:432-438.

Odugbemi, T. O., Brown, S. T., Biddle, J., Johnson, S., Perkins, G., DeWitt, W., and Albritton, W. L. (1983a). Plasmid profile, serogrouping and auxotyping of *Neisseria gonorrhoeae* isolates from Africa. *Br. J. Vener. Dis. 59*:41-43.

Odugbemi, T. O., Whittington, W. L., DeWitt, W., Perkins, G., Johnson, S., Biddle, J., Piziak, M., and Albritton, W. L. (1983b). Epidemiological characterisation of *Neisseria gonorrhoeae* isolated from the Far East. *Br. J. Vener. Dis.* *59*:285-288.

Perine, P. L., Thornsberry, C., Schalla, W., Biddle, J., Siegel, M. S., Wong, H. K., and Thompson, S. E. (1977). Evidence for two distinct types of penicillinase producing *Neisseria gonorrhoeae*. *Lancet 2*:993-995.

Perine, P. L., Totten, P. A., Knapp, J. S., Holmes, K. K., Bentsi, C., and Klufio, C. A. (1983). Diversity of gonococcal plasmids, auxotypes and serotypes in Ghana. *Lancet 1*:1051-1052.

Phillips, I. (1976). β-Lactamase-producing penicillin-resistant gonococcus. *Lancet 2*:656-657.

Ramstedt, K., Hallhagen, G., Bygdeman, S., Lincoln, K., Kallings, I., Gillenius, T., and Sandström, E. (1985). Serological classification and contact-tracing in the control of microepidemics with β-lactamase producing *Neisseria gonorrhoeae*. *Sex. Transm. Dis. 12*:209-214.

Reid, K. G. and Young, H. (1984). Serogrouping of *Neisseria gonorrhoeae*: Correlation of coagglutination serogroup WII with homosexually acquired infection. *Br. J. Vener. Dis. 60*:302-305.

Reyn, A. (1961). Sensitivity of *N. gonorrhoeae* to antibiotics. *Br. J. Vener. Dis. 37*:145-157.

Reyn, A., Korner, B., and Benzon, M. W. (1958). Effects of penicillin, streptomycin and tetracycline on *N. gonorrhoeae* isolated in 1944 and in 1957. *Br. J. Vener. Dis. 34*:227-239.

Roberts, M. and Falkow, S. (1977). Conjugal transfer of R-plasmids in *Neisseria gonorrhoeae*. *Nature 266*:630-631.

Rudén, A.-K., Bäckman, M., Bygdeman, S., Jonsson, A., Ringertz, O., and Sandström, E. (1986a). Gonorrhoea in heterosexual men. Correlation between gonococcal W serogroup, *Chlamydia trachomatis* infection and objective symptoms. *Acta Dermato-Venereol. 66*:453-456.

Rudén, A.-K., Bäckman, M., Bygdeman, S., Jonsson, A., Ringertz, O., and Sandström, E. (1986b). Analysis of serovar distribution as a tool in epidemiological studies in gonorrhoea. *Acta Dermato-Venereol. 66*:325-333.

Rudén, A.-K., Werner, Y. K., Ringertz, O., Bygdeman, S. M., Bäckman, M., and Sandström, E. G. (1985). Use of gonococcal W serogrouping in the evaluation of a clinical trial of rosoxacine. *Sex. Transm. Dis. 12*:19-24.

Sandström, E. (1979). Studies on the serology of *Neisseria gonorrhoeae*. Ph.D. Thesis, Stockholm. Karolinska Institute, Stockholm, Sweden.

Sandström, E., Chen, K. C. S., and Buchanan, T. M. (1982). Serology of *Neisseria gonorrhoeae*. Coagglutination serogroups WI and WII/III correspond to different outer membrane protein I molecules. *Infect. Immun. 38*:462-470.

Sandström, E. and Danielsson, D. (1980). Serology of *Neisseria gonorrhoeae*: Classification with coagglutionation. *Acta Pathol. Microbiol. Scand. Sect. B 88*:27-38.

Sandström, E., Knapp, J. S., Reller, B., Thompson, S., Hook, E. W., and Holmes, K. K. (1984). Serogrouping of *Neisseria gonorrhoeae*: Correlation of serogroup with disseminated gonococcal infection. *Sex. Transm. Dis. 11*:77-80.

Sandström, E., Lindell, P., Harfest, B., Blomberg, F., Rydén, A.-C., and Bygdeman, S. (1985a). Evaluation of a new set of *Neisseria gonorrhoeae* serogroup W-specific monoclonal antibodies for serovar determination. In *The Pathogenic Neisseriae* (G. K. Schoolnik, G. Brooks, S. Falkow, J. S. Knapp, A. McCuthan, and S. Morse, eds.). American Society for Microbiology, Washington, DC, pp. 26-30.

Sandström, E., Tam, M., and Bygdeman, S. (1985b). Antigenic drift of gonococcal protein I as judged by serovar determination. In *The Pathogenic Neisseriae* (G. K. Schoolnik, G. Brooks, S. Falkow, J. S. Knapp, A. McCutchan, and S. Morse, eds.). American Society for Microbiology, Washington, DC, pp. 13-19.

Sparling, P. F., Guymon, I., and Biswas, G. (1976). Antibiotic resistance in the gonococcus. In *Microbiology* (D. Schlesinger, ed.). American Society for Microbiology, Washington, DC, pp. 494-500.

Sparling, P. F., Sarubbi, F. A., Jr., and Blackman, E. (1975). Inheritance of low-level resistance to penicillin, tetracycline and chloramphenicol in *Neisseria gonorrhoeae*. *J. Bacteriol. 124*:740-749.

Tam, M. R., Buchanan, T. M., Sandström, E. G., Holmes, K. K., Knapp, J. S., Siadak, A. W., and Novinski, R. C. (1982). Serological classification of *Neisseria gonorrhoeae* with monoclonal antibodies. *Infect. Immun. 36*: 1042-1053.

Willcox, R. R. (1970). A survey of problems in the antibiotic treatment with gonorrhoea. With special reference to South-East Asia. *Br. J. Vener. Dis. 46*:217-242.

Yorke, J., Hethcote, H., and Nold, A. (1978). Dynamics and control of the transmission of gonorrhea. *Sex. Transm. Dis. 5*:51-56.

Yvert, F., Frost, E., Guibourdenche, M., Riou, J. Y., and Ivanoff, B. (1985). Auxotypes and serogroups of penicillinase producing and non-producing strains of *Neisseria gonorrhoeae* isolated in Franceville, Gabon. *Genitourin. Med. 61*:99-102.

FIVE

Development of Monoclonal Antibodies Against *Chlamydia trachomatis*

Richard S. Stephens*
School of Public Health
University of California
Berkeley, California

*Current affiliation: University of California, San Francisco, California.

I. INTRODUCTION

Chlamydia trachomatis is an obligate intracellular bacterium that is responsible
for a variety of diseases in humans. Since the development in the 1950s of tissue culture systems capable of isolating *C. trachomatis*, chlamydial infection is
now recognized as the most prevalent sexually transmitted disease in the United
States, Britain, and other developed countries (Thompson and Washington, 1983).
Sexually transmitted chlamydial infections are usually limited to mucosal surfaces, but chlamydiae are capable of causing systemic diseases. Strains of *C. trachomatis* that infect humans consist of two biovars, lymphogranuloma venereum
(LGV) and trachoma. The LGV biovar strains are more invasive than the trachoma biovar strains and typically proliferate in lymphatic tissues causing lymphogranuloma venereum. The trachoma biovar strains are usually limited to the mucosal surfaces of the eye and the respiratory and the genitourinary tracts. However, trachoma strains are often responsible for diseases such as epididymitis
(Berger et al., 1978), salpingitis (Sweet et al., 1983), and maternal and infant
infections following delivery (Alexander and Harrison, 1983). Additional complications that have been associated with infections of trachoma strains include
endometritis (Mardh et al., 1981), perihepatitis (Wolner-Hanse et al., 1980), and
Reiter's syndrome (Martin et al., 1982). Interest is also increasing in the potential
role of *C. trachomatis* infections in cervical dysplasia (Schachter et al., 1975).

Chlamydia trachomatis infections are readily treatable if the diagnosis can
be made. Unfortunately, the clinical presentations of these infections are nonspecific and, indeed, asymptomatic infections are common (Stamm and Holmes,
1984). Historically, the laboratory diagnosis of chlamydial infections has relied
upon difficult, time-consuming, and expensive tissue culture isolation. Culture of
chlamydiae requires a minimum of 3 days for each passage, and one blind passage
should be performed (Schachter and Dawson, 1978). Despite improvement and
standardization of culture techniques, culture facilities are not readily available
in many areas. Even where tissue culture isolation of chlamydiae is available, the
sensitivity of isolation is estimated to be only 80% (Schachter, 1984).

The development and use of monoclonal antibodies (MAbs) for improved
diagnostic assays for *C. trachomatis* has led the way for major improvements in
diagnostic capabilities for culture techniques as well as for laboratories without
culture facilities. Although the currently available test formats are relatively unsophisticated, the activity of various groups and commercial operations in this
field offer the potential for considerable, and needed, improvements in chlamydial detection systems. The details of the available assays and their performance
are covered in Chap. 6. This chapter addresses the molecular considerations and
the technical issues of MAb development that are unique to *C. trachomatis*. This
will be prefaced by an introduction to the essential microbiological components

of these organisms. Complete microbiological reviews are available for the interested reader (Becker, 1978; Schachter, 1984; Schachter and Caldwell, 1980).

II. MICROBIOLOGY OF *CHLAMYDIA TRACHOMATIS*

Chlamydiae grow only within eukaryotic cells. Although these organisms have considerable biosynthetic capabilities, they lack metabolic pathways that are essential for the production of energy (Becker, 1978). Chlamydiae rely upon the host cell's ATP for their own use (Hatch, 1975) and have been termed energy parasites (Moulder, 1966). The genus *Chlamydia* is composed of two species, *C. trachomatis* and *C. psittaci*. Although the two species have similar morphological and developmental properties, they are readily separable based upon essential differences in these properties (Moulder et al., 1984). Furthermore, the natural host range for each species differs, such that *C. trachomatis* is primarily a pathogen of humans and *C. psittaci* is primarily a pathogen of birds and feral animals. Interestingly, DNA homology studies performed to assess the genetic relatedness between these two species reveal less than 10% DNA homology (Kingsbury and Weiss, 1968). Nevertheless, these species share at least one common antigen (Barwell, 1952; Kuo et al., 1971), their protein profiles by polyacrylamide gel electrophoresis (PAGE) are very similar (Hatch et al., 1981), and they have similar developmental cycle characteristics (Schachter and Caldwell, 1980).

A. Developmental Cycle

Chlamydiae have a unique biphasic growth cycle that facilitates survival in two discontinuous habitats. The elementary body (EB) is a small (200-300 nm), extracellular infectious form. The EBs are metabolically inactive and their attachment to host cells triggers endocytic mechanisms that mediate the uptake of the organisms into a host cell endosome or phagosome (Byrne and Moulder, 1978). The growth of *C. trachomatis* takes place within this membrane-bound vesicle and, significantly, the natural response of lysosomes to fuse with phagosomes is specifically inhibited only in those phagosomes that harbor chlamydiae (Eissenberg and Wyrick, 1981). The properties of attachment, uptake, and inhibition of phagolysosomal fusion do not require metabolic activity from chlamydiae; the same properties can be observed for EB cell wall preparations (Eissenberg et al., 1983). Furthermore, these activities can be inhibited with specific polyvalent antibody (Todd and Storz, 1975). It appears, then, that EBs display some preformed structures on their surfaces that mediate these important biological functions.

Once an EB has entered a cell it begins a transformation into the noninfectious, metabolically active, and replicative reticulate body (RB) form. Several notable changes have been defined for the transition from the EB to RB form. Aside from metabolic activity, the most notable changes affect the properties of the chlamydial outer membrane. Whereas the EB is resistant to osmotic stress, the RB membrane, although plastic, is very fragile. The RB membrane is more permeable to solutes and increases in size, such that the mature RB form measures 500-1000 nm in diameter. The current model for these membrane changes attributes these differences to highly cross-linked membrane proteins in the EB that are not cross-linked in the RB (Hatch et al., 1984).

Approximately 20 hr after infection, an initiating EB can produce about 1000 RBs which then begin the transition back to the infectious EB form. This is not a totally synchronous event; thus, by the end of the growth cycle the phagosome contains predominantly EB forms but also contains substantial populations of RBs and intermediate-staged forms. During this RB-EB transition, *C. trachomatis* often produces large quantities of glycogen which is deposited in the phagosome matrix. Approximately 36-48 hr after infection, the mature phagosome occupies nearly the entire host cell cytoplasmic volume and is visualized as a large vacuolar intracellular inclusion (Fig. 1). The identification of this intracellular inclusion in tissue culture has been the morphological hallmark for the presence of chlamydiae. Ultimately infectious EB are released to initiate new rounds of infection, but how chlamydiae are released from the host cell is unclear.

B. Antigenic Structure

The progress of MAb development for *C. trachomatis* is dependent upon an understanding of the antigenic structure and composition of these organisms. Although the two chlamydial species share a common lipopolysaccharide (LPS) antigen and their surface protein components are analogous, the surface proteins are not antigenically cross-reactive. Within *C. trachomatis*, serological reactivities define antigens that display species-, subspecies-, and type-specific protein antigens.

1. Lipopolysaccharide

One of the first antigenic reactivities recognized for chlamydiae was a heat-stable, periodate-sensitive, genus-specific antigen. This component was soluble in ether and formed the basis for the complement fixation test for psittacosis (Hillman and Nigg, 1946). When glycolipid extracts were saponified, the immunologic activity was identified with a high-molecular-weight acidic polysaccharide and the antigenic moiety was similar to the 2-keto-3-deoxyoctanoic acid (KDO) of salmonella LPS (Dhir et al., 1972).

The genus reactivity of the chlamydial LPS has been confirmed by the development of genus-specific MAb to *Chlamydia* that react with a protease-resistant, periodate-sensitive, and heat-stable component that displays a molecular weight of less than 10,000 in immunoblots of PAGE gels (Stephens et al., 1982c). We

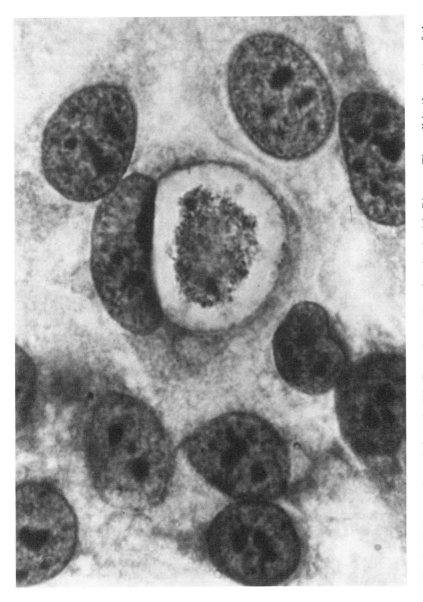

Fig. 1 Cell monolayer infected with *C. trachomatis* and stained with Giemsa. The cell in the center of the field shows a large vacular inclusion which has apparently deformed the nucleus (top).

observed that some genus-specific MAbs bound LPS after mild periodate oxidation, whereas others did not, suggesting that more than one antigenic determinant
was present on chlamydial LPS (Stephens et al., 1982c). Recently, more detailed
analyses have been completed on the chlamydial LPS. Chemical characterization
of chlamydial LPS has shown it to be similar to enterobacterial LPS (Nurminen
et al., 1984). They share a common lipid A and terminal KDO that is similar to
the immunodominant KDO for salmonella Re-type LPS (Nurminen et al., 1983).
At least two antigenic determinants for chlamydial LPS have been described; one
that cross-reacts with enterobacterial Re LPS and one that is chlamydia-specific
(Caldwell and Hitchcock, 1984; Brade et al., 1985; Thornley et al., 1985).

2. Protein

The principal protein antigens that are associated with the outer membrane include proteins that display approximate molecular weights of 155,000, 62,000,
60,000, 40,000, and 30,000. The 155,000 molecular weight protein was characterized from nonionic detergent extraction as a highly immunogenic species-
specific antigen that is quantitatively a minor protein constituent (Caldwell and
Kuo, 1977). The 62,000 and 60,000 molecular weight proteins are very antigenic;
however, little, if any, of the reactivity can be attributed to the exposed surface
of the organism (Newhall et al., 1982). The 60,000 molecular weight protein can
be isolated from cell wall preparations and appears to form oligomeric complexes
in the EB cell wall (Newhall and Jones, 1983). The 30,000 molecular weight protein has been defined as a type-specific antigen that can be isolated by mild extraction with nonionic detergents (Sacks and MacDonald, 1979; Hourihan et al.,
1980) or isolated from tissue culture supernatants (MacDonald et al., 1985). This
protein can be labeled with ^{125}I by surface labeling procedures and is characterized as a heat-labile antigen. This antigen seems to be loosely associated with the
surface of the organism and is quantitatively a minor constituent.

The quantitatively preponderant protein is the 40,000 molecular weight major
outer membrane protein (MOMP). This protein constitutes over 60% of the cell
outer membrane, is exposed on the surface (Caldwell et al., 1981), is essential
for the structural integrity of the EB (Newhall and Jones, 1983), and is involved
in the conversion of the EB to the fragile RB (Hatch et al., 1984). The MOMP
also has pore-forming properties that regulate the exchange of solutes for the
metabolically active RB (Bavoil et al., 1984). The structural and porin functions
of the MOMP are both controlled by disulfide bond interactions which appear to
play a central role in mediating the developmental cycle of chlamydiae. The MOMP
is not only an important functional protein but is also a complex antigen that displays determinants with multiple specificities (Caldwell and Schachter, 1982;
Stephens et al., 1982c).

Because the MOMP of chlamydiae is prominently exposed on the surface and
is a critical element involved with the stability and conversion of EB during the

growth cycle, much of the effort to investigate the antigenic components of these organisms has centered upon the MOMP. The MOMP and LPS account for the bulk of the surface immunogenic responses and are also the quantitatively preponderant antigens, consequently most of the MAbs produced to *C. trachomatis* are specific to one of these antigens.

C. Serological Relationships

The development of the microimmunofluorescence test by Wang and Grayston (1973) facilitated their extensive evaluations of the serological diversity of *C. trachomatis* isolates. Wang and Grayston's elegant studies used polyvalent antisera raised to each new isolate, then these antibodies were reacted with 15 different prototype strains. Comparisons were evaluated by testing serial dilutions of antisera against each prototype strain (one-way test). Similarly, antisera raised to the prototype strains were tested against the isolate (two-way test). The endpoint reactivity of each of these antisera to the isolate and to the prototype strains, provides the ability to identify over 15 serotypes or serovars of *C. trachomatis*. The contribution of this advance to serodiagnosis, epidemiology, and an understanding of pathogenesis cannot be overestimated; nevertheless, this test is difficult to perform and requires considerable experience and skill.

Wang and Grayston (1982) have shown a hierarchy of relationships among serovars that can be broadly classified into two groups (C-complex and B-complex) depending upon the extent of serological cross-reactivity. Within each group the serovars can be ordered in a hierarchy of antigenic complexity based upon the evaluation of predominantly one-way serological cross-reactions (Fig. 2). For example, serovars C and A are serologically related in the C-complex, and antiserum derived to serovar A reacts with A antigen, but no reactivity is observed with C antigen. Conversely, antiserum to serovar C reacts with C antigen and serovar A antigen.

Caldwell and his colleagues have made considerable advances in our understanding of the antigenic composition of *C. trachomatis* using polyvalent antisera. Over 18 antigens can be identified by crossed-immunoelectrophoresis (Caldwell et al., 1975). Particularly challenging for polyvalent antisera are characterizations of molecular components that are antigenically complex such as the chlamydial MOMP. This protein displays multiple antigenic specificities that are not apparent using antisera derived from chlamydial organisms and was only appreciated after the development of MAbs (Stephens et al., 1982c) and monospecific antibodies (Caldwell and Schachter, 1982) to MOMP. By using MAbs it was shown that each MOMP displayed common, multiple, and unique antigenic specificities (Stephens et al., 1982c).

Antibodies elicited using purified MOMP from different serovars display the same endpoint reactivity patterns as those observed in the microimmunofluorescence test (Caldwell and Schachter, 1982). Furthermore, MAbs specific to the

Immunotypes of Chlamydia trachomatis

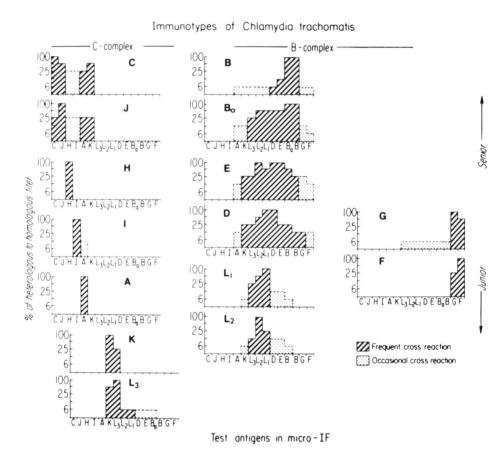

Test antigens in micro-IF

Fig. 2 Serological relationships between 15 *C. trachomatis* serovars utilizing polyvalent antisera (Y axis). The extent of cross-reactions delineate C-complex and B-complex serogroups and the senior-junior relationships within serogroups (*Source*: from Wang and Grayston, 1982).

MOMP also reflect the serological relationships defined by the micro-IF test (Stephens et al., 1982c). This data attributes these important determinants to the chlamydial MOMP.

Conventional polyvalent antisera have been used for antigenic analysis, serotyping, and detection of inclusions for *C. trachomatis* isolates. The use of such reagents has been very valuable; however, there are inherent limitations for polyvalent sera in these applications. The lack of specificity of antichlamydial polyvalent antisera is clearly the paramount limitation. This has been particularly problematic for *C. trachomatis*, primarily because of the limited, and obligate intracellular growth of these organisms. Consequently, it is difficult to obtain chlamydiae sufficiently free of host cell contaminants that these contaminants do not represent a substantial immunogenic component.

III. MONOCLONAL ANTIBODIES TO *CHLAMYDIA TRACHOMATIS*

There are two factors that greatly influence the outcome of MAb development. These are the components used for immunization and the components used for screening culture fluids.

The experience with *C. trachomatis* illustrates a common theme when intact organism preparations are used for either immunization or screening. Intact organisms represent a large repertoire of antigens; however, each antigen will be represented by its relative abundance and availability on the surface of the organism. Because selection is biased toward monoclones that produce the strongest signals, the antibodies are almost always specific to quantitatively preponderant components of the organism. This is probably advantageous when developing probes for immunodiagnostic assays.

The technical procedures employed for the production of MAbs to chlamydiae represent standard procedures, and usually cell lines such as NS-1 or NS-0 have been employed. In spite of the fact that purified *C. trachomatis* organisms contain considerable host immunogenic components, MAbs specific to *C. trachomatis* can be readily selected.

A. Specificities

Four classes of specificity can be recognized for MAbs to *C. trachomatis* using a variety of detection techniques (i.e., ELISA, immunofluorescence, or immunoblot). Examples of the various reactivity patterns observed with MAbs to chlamydiae are shown in Fig. 3.

1. Genus-Specific Antibodies

The genus-specific antibodies represented by 1G6 react to all strains of *Chlamydia*, which includes *C. trachomatis* and *C. psittaci*. By immunofluorescence, antibodies to the genus-specific LPS react well with inclusions in cell culture and RB forms, yet these antibodies react relatively poorly to the EB forms (Stephens et al., 1982c). This suggests that these antigens are not readily accessible on the cell surface of the condensed EB form. Recently, Fuentes et al. (1985) reported the production of MAbs to *C. psittaci*, and several of these antibodies displayed genus-specific reactivity patterns. Interestingly, some of the antibodies reacted to the

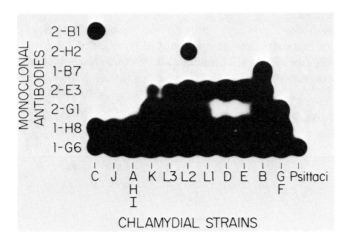

Fig. 3   Autoradiograph of antibody-binding assays performed with culture fluids and EB of various chlamydial strains. *Chlamydia trachomatis* immunotypes A-K and *C. psittaci* strains Mn were adsorbed to wells of a microtest plate and reacted with MAb. Immune reactions were detected with ^{125}I-labeled protein A. Immunotypes A, H, and I, as well as immunotypes G and F, were pooled before adsorption. Representative MAb reaction patterns were: type-specific, 2-B1, 2-H2, and 1-B7; subspecies-specific, 2-E3 and 2-G1; species-specific, 1-H8; genus-specific, 1-G6 (*Source*: from Stephens et al., 1982c).

MOMP in immunoblots of MOMP from *C. trachomatis*; however, it is not known whether or not these determinants are exposed on the surface of the organisms.

2. Species-Specific Reactivities

The species-specific reactivities represented in 1H8 are characterized by roughly equivalent reactivities with all *C. trachomatis* serovars and these determinants are not represented in *C. psittaci* strains (Stephens et al., 1982c).

3. Subspecies-Specific Determinants

Subspecies-specific determinants can be recognized by reactivities to specific groups of two or more serovars but not with all serovars (i.e., 2E3 and 2G1). Numerous multitype specificities have been represented by MAbs that recognize unique groupings of two to 10 serovars.

4. Type-Specific Determinants

Type-specific determinants are exemplified by MAbs that react with only one serovar such as antibodies 2B1, 2H2, and 1B7 (Stephens et al., 1982c). Monoclonal antibodies are particularly valuable for discriminating fine differences between serovars. The best example may be represented by a Mab that can differentiate between serovars B and Ba, although the only difference previously demonstrated with polyvalent antisera is that Ba antisera cross-react more extensively with other serovars.

B. Antigens and Immunization Schedules

The use of chlamydial organisms (EBs) has been effective for the development of immunodiagnostic probes. The immunization schedule can also influence the definition of the desired specificities. For example, when interest is primarily directed toward the development of broadly reacting MAbs for *C. trachomatis*, multiple serovars can either be mixed before immunization or different serovars can be used sequentially for immunizations. Furthermore, relatively long-term immunization schedules have been employed. When our interests changed toward serovar-specific MAbs, it was found that two IV immunizations within 1-2 weeks increased by 40-fold the frequency of MAbs that recognized type-specific antigens (Stephens et al., 1982b).

C. Screening Methods and Strategies

Two approaches have been used to select MAbs specific to *C. trachomatis*. One is to screen hybrid cell culture fluids on replicate-plated chlamydial preparations and noninfected host cell material. This approach showed that most cell culture fluids were specific for host cell components (Stephens et al., 1982c). The second approach utilizes two different host cell systems, which simplifies the selection process. Here, yolk sac-grown chlamydiae were used for immunizing mice, and antibody assays were performed using HeLa cell-grown organisms (Stephens et al., 1982b).

Because of the antigenic complexities, the success of the MAb endeavor depends upon the types or forms of antigen employed and the spectrum of antigens screened. While enzyme-linked immunosorbent assay (ELISA) reactivities are often employed as the first screening assay, it is also clear that it is especially useful to employ multiple assay formats in the initial screening phase. Other assay systems, such as immunoblot and immunofluorescence, have been employed with success. The initial screenings should generate information that will permit selection of the most useful antibody-producing cells. This is particularly true given the large expense and labor-intensive commitments necessary for MAb development. A successful approach for chlamydiae has encompassed a preliminary ELISA assay against usually four different antigen preparations. These antigens are selected based upon the desired MAbs specificities and knowledge of the antigenic relationships among strains. For example, to identify type-specific MAbs to serovar D, culture fluids can be tested with serovar D, serovar E, serovar L_1, and a host cell control. Serovars E and L_1 are the closest relatives to serovar D, thus this step focuses activity to putative type D-specific culture fluids. These culture fluids are next assessed against all 15 serovars using the micro-IF procedure. This is also the time to make any physicochemical assessments of interest such as heat sensitivity or lability. All the information is gathered before cloning, and it is at this point that cell lines are most unstable. Consequently, rational decisions can now be made concerning the extent of effort to be applied for each cell line depending upon the level of interest. For potentially very important cell lines, much larger efforts may be made to ensure the outcome of a stable phenotype. It can be difficult to produce an MAb to a quantitatively minor outer membrane constituent of chlamydiae. We have used the 155,000-molecular-weight protein purified by Caldwell and Kuo (1977) for immunization and assayed the resulting culture fluids against intact organisms. Two levels of reactivities were observed; one strong and one relatively weak. The strong-reacting clones represented antibodies to the predominant MOMP, whereas the weak-reacting clones were either phenotypically unstable and no longer producing antibody, or they were clones that were specific to the minor protein constituent. The latter reactivity can usually be differentiated by serial titration of culture fluids because weak binding caused by antigen limitations will nevertheless show high titers. An MAb developed by this approach identified the 155,000-molecular-weight component in immunoblots of Triton-X100 extracts from all *C. trachomatis* serovars.

D. Characterization

Characterization of antichlamydial MAbs involves sequential tiers of evaluation including immunological, morphological, physicochemical, biological, and format suitability.

1. Immunological Specificity

Because of the antigenic diversity among chlamydiae, the first evaluation is of the spectrum of serovars identified. The classic evaluation is made by titrations of each antibody against all serovars of *C. trachomatis* using the micro-IF test. Even at low dilutions of high-titered ascites fluids, the reactivities are usually consistent with those observed within two dilutions of the endpoint. The ELISA assay sometimes demonstrates a bit broader reactivity profile at low dilutions because of its increased sensitivity over immunofluorescence, but ELISA assays provide essentially the same information (Stephens et al., 1982c). The one exception is the reactivity of MAbs to chlamydial LPS. With such antibodies, reactivities by ELISA are strong when EB antigen preparations are used; however, they react aberrantly to EBs by immunofluorescence (Stephens et al., 1982c). This differential reactivity is probably because of limited access to LPS antigens on the surface of EBs, whereas there is considerable LPS antigen that is not cell associated that is available for binding in ELISA assays.

2. Morphological

Morphological evaluation is also important. Differential morphological staining of EB and RB forms with genus-specific antibodies is an example. This is clearly an issue for immunodiagnostic assay formats that include morphological criteria for evaluation (i.e., culture-independent immunofluorescent assays). The poor staining of EBs with MAbs to the genus-specific LPS makes these antibodies unsuitable for use in culture-independent immunofluorescent assays. Species and subspecies MAbs to the MOMP of *C. trachomatis* are most suitable for the direct staining of individual EBs in clinical specimens. Highly sensitive and specific reagents are of paramount importance in immunofluorescent assays. Because of the very small size of these organisms, which are just above the resolving power of the light microscope, they could easily be confused with the nonspecific staining that is evident using polyclonal antibodies. From another viewpoint, immune electron microscopy of MAbs by Clark et al. (1982) demonstrated unique differences in surface-binding patterns that were correlated with differences in biological activities. Determination of surface binding could be important for some assay formats such as coagglutination.

3. Physicochemical

Physicochemical evaluations have included identification of macromolecular components recognized by MAbs as well as evaluation of antibody reactivities following physical and chemical treatments of antigens. Because of various technical limitations to using immunoprecipitation assays for chlamydiae, the immunoblot has served as the method of choice for the identification of specific macromolecular components. The immunoblot assay simply involves the electrophoretic separation of molecular components by PAGE and the transfer of these separated components to nitrocellulose sheets. The nitrocellulose sheets can then be probed with antibodies and the specific components can be visualized. Using this assay we demonstrated strong binding of genus-specific MAbs to the low-molecular-weight LPS as well as strong binding of species- and subspecies-specific MAbs to the chlamydial MOMP (Fig. 4) (Stephens et al., 1982c). In contrast, type-specific MAbs reacted weakly to MOMP. The immunoblot characterization of type-specific antibodies by Terho et al. (1982) showed similar weak binding, and these observations probably reflect some conformational loss of activity to SDS-denatured protein. Immunoblots of MAbs do not always demonstrate the same pattern of reactivity as observed by assays on intact organisms (Stephens and Kuo, 1984). Presumably the denatured protein can expose epitopes that are structurally hindered in native protein conformations.

Physical and chemical treatments of antigens have provided a rapid, albeit crude, evaluation of whether MAbs recognize protein or carbohydrate moieties (Stephens et al., 1982c). The differential reactivities of genus-specific MAbs to

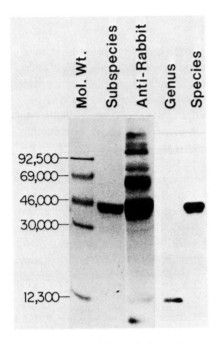

Fig. 4 Immunoblots of *C. trachomatis* probed with subspecies-, genus-, and species-specific MAbs and polyvalent rabbit serum. Subspecies- and species-specific monoclonal antibodies identify the MOMP, and the genus-specific antibody identifies LPS (*Source*: Stephens et al., 1982c).

LPS and MAbs to MOMP after periodate and proteinase treatments of antigens or organisms, indicated that the former was recognizing a carbohydrate determinant sensitive to periodate, whereas the latter group of antibodies recognized protease-sensitive determinants. All reactivities, however, were very resistant to heat treatments (Fig. 5).

4. Biological

Biological activity of a variety of MAbs has been assessed. Several investigators have used MAbs for in vitro neutralization of chlamydiae in cell culture systems. Peeling et al. (1984) demonstrated complement-independent neutralization of infectivity with a species-specific MAb. Lucero and Kuo (1985) used the same species-specific MAb as Peeling et al. (1984) and this antibody did not neutralize in a complement-dependent system. Clark et al. (1982) and Lucero and Kuo (1985) demonstrated complement-dependent neutralization of chlamydiae by type-specific MAbs. Interestingly, not all type-specific MAbs were capable of neutralization. Clark et al. (1982) reported on one type-specific MAb that did

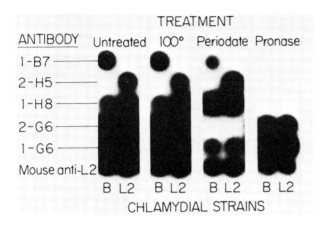

TREATMENT

ANTIBODY   Untreated   100°   Periodate   Pronase

1-B7
2-H5
1-H8
2-G6
1-G6
Mouse anti-L2

B L2   B L2   B L2   B L2

CHLAMYDIAL STRAINS

Fig. 5   Autoradiograph of antibody-binding assays comparing MAb reactivities after heat treatment, periodate oxidation, or pronase digestion of *C. trachomatis* immunotypes B and L_2. As determined by the micro-IF test, MAbs 1-B7 and 2-H5 identified type-specific antigens B and L_2, respectively. Monoclonal antibody 1-H8 identified a species-specific antigen. Monoclonal antibodies 2-G6 and 1-G6 identified genus-specific antigens. Conventional antisera from mice that had been immunized with *C. trachomatis* immunotype L_2 were used as positive controls (*Source*: Stephens et al., 1982c).

not neutralize infectivity, and this antibody displayed different surface binding patterns by immune electron microscopy than type-specific antibodies that did neutralize. Lucero and Kuo (1985) showed that the differential neutralizing capabilities of MAbs was not an artifact of immunoglobulin isotype.

Depending upon the test format to be utilized, some of the characterizations discussed previously are of more or less relevance. Decisions concerning whether an assay will be designed to detect protein or carbohydrate antigens, or whether the assay should be limited to species or genus level detection will influence the approach for maximum efficiency. The development of more sophisticated formats may require more than one antibody to different determinants on a particular antigen or require a specific immunoglobulin isotype. However the criteria of the test format may be defined, these factors should be considered before a MAb development effort because of the high costs in time and materials.

IV. MONOCLONAL ANTIBODY APPLICATIONS TO *CHLAMYDIA TRACHOMATIS*

The defined specificity of MAbs make them unique reagents for many applications that conventional polyvalent sera cannot duplicate. For *C. trachomatis* research,

MAbs have now been utilized primarily for immunodiagnostic probes, for immunotyping isolates, and as probes of molecular structure.

The details of the immunodiagnostic applications of MAbs for *C. trachomatis* are covered in Chap. 6 of this book. This section will cover the development of immunotyping schemes using MAbs.

A. Immunotyping with Serovar-Specific Probes

The development of the micro-IF test has enabled the definition of 15 distinct serovars for *C. trachomatis*. The exhaustive quantitative analysis of the cross-reactions between antibody derived from prototype strains to an isolate and between antibody derived from the isolate to the prototype antigens encompasses the two-way test (Wang and Grayston, 1982). Few laboratories are typing new isolates, and those that are typing some isolates usually employ the simplified one-way test (Wang et al., 1973). However, the one-way test fails to provide unequivocal classification of closely related serovars. Because the initial findings that type-specific and subspecies-specific MAbs provided the same serotyping data that was obtained by the conventional micro-IF test, it was proposed that MAbs could be applied to these evaluations without rigorous isolation procedures and concomitant immunizations to produce antibody for the micro-IF test (Stephens, 1983). A test of the efficacy of this approach encompassed the proposition that closely related serovars could be differentiated and, more importantly, that a type-specific antibody detected on the prototype strains was a determinant shared by other strains of the same serovar (i.e., serovar-specificity). Type-specific MAbs to serovars F, B, D, and E were used to test the reactivity to over 60 isolates that had been previously typed by the micro-IF test. The results from this study demonstrated the breadth of reactivity required for typing strains and that MAbs readily accomplish rapid immunoclassification of chlamydial isolates (Stephens, 1983). This approach has recently been extended to all serovars. Utilizing a diverse panel of MAbs, over 300 strains were serotyped that previously had been classified by the micro-IF test (Wang et al., 1985). These results showed that the serotyping determinations provided by MAbs were similar to the results obtained by the micro-IF test and that serotyping with MAbs was very rapid, used less antigen, and most importantly, was much more precise. For these evaluations we used a two-step test in which the first analysis grouped the isolate into one of three classes, which then defined the antibodies to be used in the second analysis (Table 1). This allowed typing of isolates using six to eight separate MAbs instead of 15 different antibody assays representative of each serovar. As confidence grows concerning the suitability of each serovar-specific antibody, it should be possible to pool sets of antibodies. The use of combinatorial pooling will facilitate the definitive serotyping of chlamydial isolates by the pattern of reactions obtained from as few as four single tests in one assay (Table 2).

Table 1 Serological Classification of 313 *C. trachomatis* Isolates Using a Two-Step Microimmunofluorescence Test with Monoclonal Antibodies

Serovar or subtype (no. of strains)

MA (ascites)	C group					Intermediate group					B group							
	C	J	H	A	I	I'	G	L3	F	K	B	Ba	L2	L2'	E	L1	D	D'
	(15)	(23)	(19)	(12)	(5)	(17)	(18)	(4)	(29)	(19)	(31)	(23)	(13)	(3)	(55)	(3)	(19)	(5)
First step																		
LE-4	+	+	+	+	+	−	−	−	−	−	−	−	−	−	−	−	−	−
G/F/K	−	−	−	−	−	+	+	+	+	+	−	−	−	−	−	−	−	−
BB-11	−	−	−	−	−	−	−	−	−	−	+	+	+	+	+	+	+	+
BB-3	−	−	−	−	−	−	−	−	−	−	+	+	+	+	−	−	−	−
Second step																		
CC-1	+	+																
LA-10			+															
AC-11				+	+													
PE-5					+													
PE-5						+		+										
GG-11						+	+	+										
FC-2									+									
KK-1										+								
DD-1											+							
2F-1													+	+				
155-35													+					
KB-8															+	+	−	−
JG-9															−		+	−

Note: + = positive fluorescence; − = negative fluorescence; MA = monoclonal antibodies; G/F/K = pooled GG-11, FC-2, and KK-1 ascites, with equal antibody titer; I', D', and L2' indicate subtypes of I, D, and L2, respectively.
Source: Wang, Kuo, Barnes, Stephens, and Grayston, 1985.

Table 2   Combinatorial Evaluation of 15 Serovar-Specific Monoclonal Antibodies

Pool	Monoclonal antibody number														
	1	2	3	4	5	6	7	8	9	10	11	12	13	14	15
A	1	2	3	4					9	10				14	15
B		2	3	4	5	6					11		13		15
C			3	4		6	7	8	9		11			14	
D				4		6	7			10		12	13	14	15

Fifteen monoclonal antibodies are distributed into four separate pools (A-D). The reactivity pattern observed, following the testing of an isolate with pools A through D, identifies a reaction by one unique monoclonal antibody. For example, if pools A and B were positive and pools C and D were negative, then only antibody 2 reacted.

The rapidity and ease of use of such MAb reagents will provide the opportunity for expanded epidemiological assessments of chlamydial infections. A recent study has demonstrated an additional advantage of this assay (Barnes et al., 1985) in that isolates from patients that were coinfected with multiple serovars were easily identified. The classic approach of growing these isolates to sufficient titers for immunization of mice and subsequent evaluation of their serotypic response with polyvalent antisera would result in either the selection of serovars that grow more efficiently in cell culture or in the production of polyvalent antibody that provides equivocal reactivities.

V. CONCLUSIONS

The development of MAbs reactive with *C. trachomatis* have already made a considerable impact on the diagnosis of chlamydial infection (Chap. 6). The commercial immunodiagnostic assays currently available for *C. trachomatis* encompass culture confirmation assays and culture-independent assays. The rapidly growing prevalence of sexually transmitted chlamydial infections and the concomitant damaging sequelae are related to the chronic asymptomatic and latent characteristics of chlamydial infections. Thus, there is an appreciation of the market and of the need for diagnostic capabilities that are effective for the detection of chlamydiae in low-prevalence and asymptomatic populations (*Morbidity and Mortality Weekly Report Supplement*, 1985). Clearly this requires assays with greater sensitivities than are now available and in formats that are rapid and preferably automated.

Potential directions for the development of these assays are homogeneous or competitive assay formats. Such applications require readily available defined antigens. The development of monoclonal antigens (i.e., peptides of predefined immunological specificity) for use in conjunction with MAbs provides the essential and standardized components for the development of a sensitive homogeneous or competitive assay system. Using recombinant DNA-cloning techniques, portions of the chlamydial MOMP have been expressed in *Escherichia coli* and these recombinant products are specifically recognized by many of the MAbs developed to *C. trachomatis* (Stephens et al., 1985). The use of both antigens and antibodies of predefined specificity may not only provide a novel and sensitive assay format but would also eliminate problems of nonimmune binding of antibodies by organisms or components with protein A-like receptors for immunoglobulin. The demonstrated efficacy of employing MAbs for culture-independent immunodiagnostic evaluations for *C. trachomatis* infection offers a model system with defined variables and challenges. This system is an excellent candidate for use in the development of new immunodiagnostic methods because they must produce sensitive and specific results from complex clinical material, and ultimately there is a medical need and a sufficient market to warrant these efforts. Finally, the direct immunotyping of clinical isolates with MAbs should provide the opportunity for expanding epidemiological studies of chlamydial infections and aid in the development and application of effective control programs.

REFERENCES

Alexander, E. R. and Harrison, H. R. (1983). Role of *Chlamydia trachomatis* in perinatal infections. *Rev. Infect. Dis. 5*:713-719.

Barnes, R. C., Suchland, J. R., Wang, S.-P., Kuo, C.-C., and Stamm, W. E. (1985). Detection of multiple serovars of *Chlamydia trachomatis* in genital infections. *J. Infect. Dis. 152*:985-989.

Barwell, C. F. (1952). Some observations on the antigenic structure of psittacosis and lymphogranuloma venereum viruses. *Br. J. Exp. Pathol. 33*:258-261.

Bavoil, P., Ohlin, A., and Schachter, J. (1984). Role of disulfide bonding in outer membrane structure and permeability in *Chlamydia trachomatis. Infect. Immun. 44*:479-485.

Becker, Y. (1978). The chlamydia: Molecular biology of procaryotic obligate parasites of *eukaryotes. Microbiol. Rev. 42*:274-306.

Berger, R. E., Alexander, E. R., Monda, G. O., Ansell, J., McCormick, G., and Holmes, K. K. (1978). *Chlamydia trachomatis* as a cause of acute "idiopathic" epididymitis. *N. Engl. J. Med. 298*:301-303.

Brade, L., Nurminen, M., Makela, P. H., and Brade, H. (1985). Antigenic properties of *Chlamydia trachomatis* lipopolysaccharide. *Infect. Immun. 48*:569-572.

Byrne, G. I. and Moulder, J. W. (1978). Parasite-specified phagocytosis of *Chlamydia psittaci* and *Chlamydia trachomatis* by L and HeLa cells. *Infect. Immun. 19*:598-606.

Caldwell, H. D. and Hitchcock, P. J. (1984). Monoclonal antibody against a genus-specific antigen of *Chlamydia* species: Location of the epitope on chlamydial lipopolysaccharide. *Infect. Immun. 44*:306-314.

Caldwell, H. D., Kromhout, J., and Schachter, J. (1981). Purification and partial characterization of the major outer membrane protein of *Chlamydia trachomatis*. *Infect. Immun.* *31*:1161-1176.

Caldwell, H. D. and Kuo, C.-C. (1977). Purification of a *Chlamydia trachomatis*-specific antigen by immunoadsorption with monospecific antibody. *J. Immunol.* *118*:437-441.

Caldwell, H. D., Kuo, C.-C., and Kenny, G. E. (1975). Antigenic analysis of chlamydiae by two-dimensional immunoelectrophoresis. I. Antigenic heterogeneity between *C. trachomatis* and *C. psittaci*. *J. Immunol.* *115*:963-975.

Caldwell, H. D. and Schachter, J. (1982). Antigenic analysis of the major outer membrane protein of *Chlamydia* spp. *Infect. Immun.* *35*:1024-1031.

Clark, R. B., Nachamkin, I., Schatzki, P. F., and Dalton, H. P. (1982). Localization of distinct surface antigens on *Chlamydia trachomatis* HAR-13 by immune electron microscopy with monoclonal antibodies. *Infect. Immun. 38*: 1273-1278.

Dhir, S. P., Hakomori, S., Kenny, G. E., and Grayston, J. T. (1972). Immunochemical studies on chlamydial group antigen (presence of a 2-keto-3-deoxycarbohydrate as immunodominant group). *J. Immunol. 109*:116-121.

Eissenberg, L. G. and Wyrick, P. B. (1981). Inhibition of phagolysosome fusion is localized to *Chlamydia psittaci*-laden vacuoles. *Infect. Immun. 32*:889-896.

Eissenberg, L. G., Wyrick, P. B., Davis, C. H., and Rumpp, J. W. (1983). *Chlamydia psittaci* elementary body envelopes: Ingestion and inhibition of phagolysosome fusion. *Infect. Immun. 40*:741-751.

Fuentes, V., Lefebvre, J. F., Lema, F., Bissac, E., and Orfila, J. (1985). Establishment of hybridomas secreting monoclonal antibodies to *Chlamydia psittaci*. *Immunol. Lett. 10*:325-327.

Hanna, L., Okumoto, M., Thygeson, P., Rose, L., and Dawson, C. R. (1965). TRIC agents isolated in the United States. X. Immunofluorescence in the diagnosis of TRIC agent infection in man. *Proc. Soc. Exp. Biol. Med. 119*: 722-728.

Hatch, T. P. (1975). Utilization of L-cell nucleoside triphosphates by *Chlamydia psittaci* for ribonucleic acid synthesis. *J. Bacteriol. 122*:393.

Hatch, T. P., Allan, I., and Pearce, J. H. (1984). Structural and polypeptide differences between envelopes of infective and reproductive life cycle forms of *Chlamydia* spp. *J. Bacteriol. 157*:13-20.

Hatch, T. P., Vance, D. W., and Al-Hossainy, E. (1981). Identification of a major envelope protein in *Chlamydia* spp. *J. Bacteriol. 146*:426-429.

Hillman, R. M. and Nigg, C. (1946). Studies of lymphogranuloma venereum complement-fixing antigens. *J. Immunol. 59*:349-364.

Hourihan, J. T., Rota, T. R., and MacDonald, A. B. (1980). Isolation and purification of a type-specific antigen from *Chlamydia trachomatis* propagated in cell culture utilizing molecular shift chromatography. *J. Immunol. 124*:2399-2404.

Kingsbury, D. T. and Weiss, E. (1968). Lack of deoxyribonucleic acid homology between species of the genus *Chlamydia*. *J. Bacteriol. 96*:1421-1423.

Kuo, C.-C., Kenny, G. E., and Wang, S.-P. (1971). Trachoma and psittacosis antigens in agar gel double immunodiffusion. In *Trachoma and Related Disorders Caused by Chlamydial Agents* (R. L. Nichols, eds.). Experpta Medica, Amsterdam, pp. 113-123.

Lucero, M. E. and Kuo, C.-C. (1985). Neutralization of *Chlamydia trachomatis* cell culture infection by serovar-specific monoclonal antibodies. *Infect. Immun. 50*:595-597.

MacDonald, A. B., Stuart, E. S., Reddish, M. A., Tirrell, S., and De Toma, F. J. (1985). Isolation of genus and serotype specific antigens from supernatants of *Chlamydia trachomatis* infected tissue culture. (Abstract), International Society for Sexually Transmitted Diseases Research, Brighton, England.

Mardh, P. A., Moller, B. R., Ingerslev, H. J., Nussler, E., Westrom, L., and Wolner-Hansen, P. (1981). Endometritis caused by *Chlamydia trachomatis. Br. J. Vener. Dis. 57*:191-193.

Martin, D. H., Pollack, S., Kuo, C.-C., Wang, S.-P., Brunham, R. C., and Holmes, K. K. (1982). Urethral chlamydial infections in men with Reiter's syndrome. In *Chlamydial Infections* (P.-A. Mardh, K. K. Holmes, J. D. Oriel, P. Piot, and J. Schachter, eds.). Elsevier Biomedical Press, New York, pp. 107-110.

Morbidity and Mortality Weekly Report Supplement (1985). *Chlamydia trachomatis* infections. Policy guidelines for prevention and control. Centers for Disease Control, *34*:53S-74S.

Moulder, J. W. (1966). The relation of the psittacosis group (chlamydiae) to bacteria and viruses. *Ann. Rev. Microbiol. 20*:107-130.

Moulder, J. W., Hatch, T. P., Kuo, C.-C., Schachter, J., and Storz, J. (1984). Genus I. *Chlamydia*. In *Bergey's Manual of Systemic Bacteriology*, Vol. 1 (N. Kreig, ed.). Williams & Williams, Baltimore, pp. 729-739.

Newhall, W. J., Batteiger, V. B., and Jones, R. B. (1982). Analysis of the human serological response to proteins of *Chlamydia trachomatis. Infect. Immun. 38*:1181-1189.

Newhall, W. J. and Jones, R. B. (1983). Disulfide-linked oligomers of the major outer membrane proteins of chlamydiae. *J. Bacteriol. 154*:998-1001.

Nurminen, M., Leinonen, M., Saikku, P., and Makela, P. H. (1983). The genus-specific antigen of *Chlamydia*: Resemblance to the lipopolysaccharide of enteric bacteria. *Science 220*:1279-1281.

Nurminen, M., Rietschel, E. T., and Brade, H. (1984). Notes: Chemical characterization of *Chlamydia trachomatis* lipopolysaccharide. *Infect. Immun. 48*:573-575.

Peeling, R., Maclean, I. W., and Brunham, R. C. (1984). In vitro neutralization of *Chlamydia trachomatis* with monoclonal antibody to an epitope on the major outer membrane protein. *Infect. Immun. 46*:484-488.

Sacks, D. L. and MacDonald, A. B. (1979). Isolation of a type-specific antigen from *Chlamydia trachomatis* by sodium dodecyl sulfate-polyacrylamide gel electrophoresis. *J. Immunol. 122*:136-139.

Schachter, J. (1984). Biology of *Chlamydia trachomatis*. In *Sexually Transmitted Diseases* (K. K. Holmes, P. A. Mardh, P. F. Sparling, and P. J. Wiesner, eds.). McGraw-Hill, New York, pp. 243-257.

Schachter, J. and Caldwell, H. D. (1980). Chlamydiae. *Ann. Rev. Microbiol. 34*: 285-309.

Schacther, J. and Dawson, C. R. (1978). *Human Chlamydial Infections*. PSG Publishing, Massachusetts.

Schachter, J., Hill, E. C., King, E. B., Coleman, U. R., Jones, P., and Meyer, K. F. (1975). *Chlamydial* infection in women with cervical dysplasia. *Am. J. Obstet. Gynecol. 123*:753-755.

Stamm, W. E. and Holmes, K. K. (1984). *Chlamydia trachomatis* infection of the adult. In *Sexually Transmitted Diseases* (K. K. Holmes, P. A. Mardh, P. F. Sparling, and P. J. Wiesner, eds.). McGraw-Hill, New York, pp. 258-270.

Stamm, W. E., Tam, M., Koester, M., and Cles, L. (1983). Detection of *Chlamydia trachomatis* inclusions in McCoy cell cultures with fluorescein-conjugated monoclonal antibodies. *J. Clin. Microbiol. 17*:666-668.

Stephens, R. S. (1983). Immunoclassification of *Chlamydia trachomatis* isolates. Doctoral Dissertation, University of Washington, pp. 57-60.

Stephens, R. S. and Kuo, C.-C. (1984). *Chlamydia trachomatis* species-specific epitope detected on mouse biovar outer membrane protein. *Infect. Immun. 45*:790-791.

Stephens, R. S., Kuo, C.-C., Newport, G., and Agabian, N. (1985). Molecular cloning and expression of *Chlamydia trachomatis* major outer membrane protein antigens in *Escherichia coli. Infect. Immun. 47*:713-718.

Stephens, R. S., Kuo, C.-C., and Tam, M. R. (1982a). Sensitivity of immunofluorescence with monoclonal antibodies for detection of *Chlamydia trachomatis* inclusions in cell culture. *J. Clin. Microbiol. 16*:4-7.

Stephens, R. S., Kuo, C.-C., Tam, M. R., and Nowinski, R. C. (1982b). Monoclonal antibodies to *Chlamydia trachomatis*. In *Chlamydial Infections* (P.-A. Mardh, K. K. Holmes, J. D. Oriel, P. Piot, and J. Schachter, eds.). Elsevier Biomedical Press, New York, pp. 329-332.

Stephens, R. S., Tam, M. R., Kuo, C.-C., and Nowinski, R. C. (1982c). Monoclonal antibodies to *Chlamydia trachomatis*: Antibody specificities and antigen characterization. *J. Immunol. 128*:1083-1089.

Sweet, R. L., Schachter, J., and Robbie, M. O. (1983). Failure of β-lactam antibiotics to eradicate *Chlamydia trachomatis* in the endometrium despite apparent clinical cure of acute salpingitis. *J. Am. Med. Assoc. 250*:2641-2645.

Tam, M. R., Stamm, W. E., Hansfield, H. H., Stephens, R. S., Kuo, C.-C., Holmes, K. K., Ditsenberger, K., Krieger, M., and Nowinski, R. C. (1984). Culture-independent diagnosis of *Chlamydia trachomatis* using monoclonal antibodies. *N. Engl. J. Med. 310*:1146-1150.

Tam, M. R., Stephens, R. S., Kuo, C.-C., Holmes, K. K., Stamm, W. E., and Nowinski, R. C. (1982). Use of monoclonal antibodies to *Chlamydia trachomatis* as immunodiagnostic reagents. In *Chlamydial Infections* (P.-A. Mardh, K. K. Holmes, J. D. Oriel, P. Piot, and J. Schachter, eds.). Elsevier Biomedical Press, New York, pp. 317-320.

Terho, P., Matikainen, M. T., Arstila, P., and Treharne, J. (1982). In *Chlamydial Infections* (P.-A. Mardh, K. K. Holmes, J. D. Oriel, P. Piot, and J. Schachter, eds.). Elsevier Biomedical Press, New York, pp. 321-324.

Thomas, B. J., Evans, R. J., Hutchinson, G. R., and Taylor-Robinson, D. (1977). Early detection of chlamydial inclusions combining the use of cycloheximide-treated McCoy cells and immunofluorescence staining. *J. Clin. Microbiol. 6*: 285-292.

Thompson, E. E. and Washington, A. E. (1983). Epidemiology of sexually transmitted *Chlamydia trachomatis* infections. *Epidemiol. Rev. 5*:96-123.

Todd, W. J. and Storz, J. (1975). Ultrastructural cytochemical evidence for the activation of lysosomes in the cytocidal effect of *Chlamydia psittaci*. *Infect. Immun. 12*:638-646.

Wang, S.-P. and Grayston, J. T. (1970). Immunologic relationship between genital TRIC, lymphogranuloma venereum, and related organisms in a new microtiter indirect immunofluorescence test. *Am. J. Ophthalmol. 70*:367-370.

Wang, S.-P. and Grayston, J. T. (1982). Micro-immunofluorescence antibody responses in *Chlamydia trachomatis* infection. A review. In *Chlamydial Infections* (P.-A. Mardh, K. K. Holmes, J. D. Oriel, P. Piot, and J. Schachter, eds.). Elsevier Biomedical Press, New York, pp. 301-316.

Wang, S.-P., Kuo, C.-C., Barnes, R. C., Stephens, R. S., and Grayston, J. T. (1985). Immunotyping of *Chlamydia trachomatis* with monoclonal antibodies. *J. Infect. Dis. 152*:791-800.

Wang, S.-P., Kuo, C.-C., and Grayston, J. T. (1973). A simplified method for immunological typing of trachoma-inclusion conjunctivitis-lymphogranuloma venereum organisms. *Infect. Immun. 7*:356-360.

Wolner-Hansen, P., Westrom, L., and Mardh, P. A. (1980). Perihepatitis in chlamydial salpingitis. *Lancet 1*:901-902.

SIX

Immunological Diagnosis of
Chlamydia trachomatis Infection

Cho-chou Kuo
University of Washington
Seattle, Washington

Milton R. Tam
Genetic Systems Corporation
Seattle, Washington

I. DISEASES AND EPIDEMIOLOGY

The diseases caused by *Chlamydia trachomatis* fall into three main categories:
ocular, respiratory, and urogenital infections. *Chlamydia trachomatis* can initially
colonize the mucous membranes including the conjunctiva, nasopharynx, rectum,
urethra, and cervix (Moulder et al., 1984), after which the infection can then
spread to affect the deeper organ systems. There are 15 antigenically distinctive
serovars of *C. trachomatis*. The major disease syndromes produced by the 12
trachoma serovars of *C. trachomatis* (serovars A-K and Ba) are trachoma, conjunctivitis, pneumonia in infants under 6 months of age (Beem and Saxon, 1977),
urethritis (Holmes et al., 1975), epididymitis (Berger et al., 1978), mucopurulent
cervicitis (Brunham et al., 1984), pelvic inflammatory disease (PID) (Mardh et al.,
1977), perihepatitis (Muller-Schoop et al., 1978), and proctitis (Quinn et al.,
1981). Tubal infertility (Moore et al., 1982) and ectopic pregnancy (Svensson
et al., 1985) as secondary effects of PID have been implicated as complications
that can arise from *C. trachomatis* infection. Although endemic trachoma is mostly caused by serovars A, B, Ba, and C and genital infections by serovars D through
K, definite microbiological and virulence markers for differentiating ocular and
genital strains do not exist (Grayston and Wang, 1975; Kuo et al., 1983; Wang et
al., 1977). All trachoma serovars have the potential of inducing any of the mentioned diseases or syndromes. The geographical distribution of serovars seen today is probably the result of thousands of years of selective pressures by socioeconomic and environmental factors, rather than by differences in the inherent
pathogenesis of the organisms. The other three serovars of *C. trachomatis* (L1,
L2, and L3) can produce lymphogranuloma venereum (LGV), a distinct sexually
transmitted disease (STD) syndrome involving the inguinal lymph nodes and the
efferent lymphatics. Lymphogranuloma venereum is still endemic in certain parts
of Africa such as Ethiopia (Perine et al., 1980) and Nigeria (Osoba, personal communication). The prevalence of infection produced by LGV is far less than that
of the trachoma strains. A spectrum of diseases that can be caused by *C. trachomatis* is presented in Table 1.

Trachoma is a potentially blinding, chronic follicular conjunctivitis that has
been prevalent in Africa, the Middle East, and Asia, especially in areas with a hot,
arid climate where sanitation is minimal. The incidence and severity of trachoma
has decreased greatly throughout the world during the past 30 years as a result
of improvement in hygienic conditions and living standards. Trachoma is now
the major cause of preventable blindness in northern and sub-Sahara Africa and
in the Middle East. Pockets of blinding trachoma still exist in parts of Africa,
North India, Southeast Asia, Australia, the Pacific Islands, and Latin America.
The World Health Organization has estimated that trachoma affects 400 million
people worldwide (World Health Organization Statistics Report, 1971).

Table 1 Clinical Spectrum of *C. trachomatis* Infection

Biovar	Organ system	Disease or syndrome
Trachoma	Ocular	Trachoma
		Conjunctivitis in newborns, children, and adults
	Respiratory	Pneumonia in infants and in normal (?) or immunosuppressed adults
		Nasopharyngitis in infants
		Otitis media in infants (?)
	Genital: male	Urethritis
		Epididymitis
		Prostatitis (?)
	female	Mucopurulent cervicitis
		Urethral syndrome
		Endometritis
		Salpingitis (PID)
		Ectopic pregnancy
		Tubal infertility
		Peritonitis and perihepatitis (Fitz-Hugh-Curtis syndrome)
		Vaginal asymptomatic carriage in infants
	Others	Proctitis
		Reiter's syndrome (?)
		Childhood myocarditis (?)
		Endocarditis (?)
		Cervical dysplasia (?)
LGV	Lymphatic	Lymphogranuloma venereum

In the developed countries of Europe and North America, chlamydial infection has surpassed gonorrhea as the most common STD (Holmes, 1984; *Morbidity and Mortality Weekly Report*, 1985; Thompson and Washington, 1983). For example, an estimated 3 million new cases occur each year in the United States alone (Thompson and Washington, 1983). This may be an underestimate by as much as threefold because chlamydial infection is not reportable in the United States. In England and Wales, where most cases of nongonococcal urethritis (NGU) are reportable, the incidence has nearly doubled from 1970 to 1980; about half of the cases of NGU reported have been caused by *C. trachomatis* (Thompson and Washington, 1983). A similar increase in the incidence of NGU has been documented in the United States in the period between 1975 and 1983, based on the data obtained from several metropolitan STD clinics (Thompson and Washington, 1983). Recent studies in developing and underdeveloped countries have also revealed that *C. trachomatis* infections are common among the prevalent STDs (Forsey et al., 1982; Osoba, 1981). The risk of genital *C. trachomatis* infection is inversely related to age and socioeconomic factors but is positively correlated with the number of sex partners (*Morbidity and Mortality Weekly Report*, 1985).

Studies in the United States have reported the prevalence of cervical *C. trachomatis* infection among pregnant women to vary from 2 to 37%, with most studies reporting infection rates of 8-12% (*Morbidity and Mortality Weekly Report*, 1985). The risk of infants acquiring chlamydial infection, by passing through the infected cervical canal of the mother at birth, has been estimated to be 60-70% (Schachter and Dawson, 1981). For these infants, the sites of colonization are the conjunctiva, nasopharynx, oropharynx, rectum, and vagina. Approximately 25-50% of these exposed infants will develop conjunctivitis and 10-20% will develop pneumonia.

II. CONVENTIONAL DIAGNOSTIC METHODS

Laboratory diagnosis of *C. trachomatis* infection has been based on (1) isolation of the organism in egg or tissue culture from clinical specimens, (2) cytological methods in which intracellular inclusion bodies are demonstrated by microscopy in scrapings, and (3) serological methods that detect antibodies to chlamydial organisms.

A. Isolation

Isolation of organisms is the definitive method for diagnosis of chlamydial infection. However, isolation has relied on culturing the organisms in eggs or mammalian cells because chlamydiae are obligate intracellular bacteria. Such culture methods are technically difficult, labor-intensive, cumbersome, and expensive, and therefore, have not been widely adopted as routine tests performed in general clinical laboratories.

1. Egg Culture

Trachoma agents were first isolated in the yolk sacs of embryonated chicken eggs by T'ang et al. (1957). The standard method uses 7-day old embryonated eggs into which specimens are inoculated. Yolk sac membranes are harvested when the eggs are killed by the growth of chlamydiae, or if the eggs survive, on day 12 or day 13, before hatching (Wang and Grayston, 1964). Smears are then made from the yolk sac membranes onto microscope slides and the chlaymdial organisms identified by Macchiavello stain. Non-LGV "genital" *C. trachomatis* strains have been reported as generally more difficult to grow and therefore harder to isolate in egg culture (Kuo et al., 1975) than are ocular "trachoma" strains. Egg culture is not recommended for routine isolation of *C. trachomatis*, because cell culture is more sensitive and dependable (Gordon et al., 1969).

2. Cell Culture

The introduction of the cell culture method by Gordon and Quan (1965) has replaced the more cumbersome egg culture technique for the routine isolation of chlamydiae. Cell lines commonly used for the isolation of *C. trachomatis* include McCoy (Gordon and Quan, 1965), HeLa 229 (Kuo et al., 1972), and BHK-21 (Blyth and Taverne, 1974). The sensitivity of cell culture for the isolation of chlamydiae is enhanced by pretreatment of cells with polycations (DEAE-dextran) (Kuo et al., 1972), centrifugation of the inoculum onto the cell monlayer (Gordon and Quan, 1965), and incorporation of antimetabolites such as cycloheximide (Ripa and Mardh, 1977) or cytochalasin B (Sompolinsky and Richmond, 1974) into the culture medium. Cultures can be performed in small vials (Gordon and Quan, 1965; Kuo et al., 1972) or in microtiter plates (Yoder et al., 1981) if larger numbers of specimens are handled. For the detection and identification of chlamydial inclusions, vial coverslips or the microtiter wells containing cell monolayers are fixed and stained with iodine, Giemsa, or fluorescein-isothiocyanate (FITC)-labeled antibody 48-72 hr after inoculation, depending upon the staining method. Some factors affecting the sensitivity of isolation include specimen collection, transportation and storage, whether vial or microtiter plate culture systems are used, and the cell line used. Ideally, the specimens should be kept at 4°C if cultures can be inoculated within 24 hr; otherwise they should be placed at −65°C or below as soon as possible. The sensitivity of isolation has been shown to range from 60 to 80% depending upon the laboratory and the culture system used (*Morbidity and Mortality Weekly Report*, 1985). The isolation rate also depends upon the stage of the disease; in trachoma it ranges from 86% in the acute form to 33% in the chronic stage (Kuo et al., 1977). When conventional methods are used, two-thirds of the positive samples are usually obtained in the initial inoculation and the remaining one-third in a subsequent cell culture passage (Stamm et al., 1983; Stephens et al., 1982a). Because a second passage is often performed, the cell culture diagnosis may take from 2 to 7 days.

B. Cytology and Detection of Inclusions

Trachoma agents were first discovered by Halberstaedter and von Prowazek (1907). They succeeded in transmitting trachoma from infected patients to experimental primates, finding cytoplasmic inclusions in the conjunctival epithelial cells of both the patients and infected animals (Halberstaedter and von Prowazek, 1907). In 1909 and 1910, similar inclusions were discovered in the conjunctiva of newborn infants, in female genital epithelium of the mother of a baby with conjunctivitis, and also in male nongonococcal urethritis, suggesting a causal relationship between trachoma, inclusion conjunctivitis, and genital infection (Lindner, 1910).

The inclusions, termed Halberstaedter and von Prowazek bodies after their discoverers, have become the principal microscopic diagnostic features of chlamydial infections. Demonstration of inclusions was the only diagnostic method for *C. trachomatis* infection until the availability of egg culture methods in 1957. Conjunctival, urethral, and cervical scrapings are obtained with metal or wooden spatulas and fixed with absolute methanol. For detection of chlamydial inclusions the specimens have, in the past, been stained with Giemsa, with iodine, or by immunofluorescence (IF) using conventional antiserum in one- or two-step methods. The advantages to these methods are the simplicity of their procedures, particularly if light microscopy is used. If iodine or Giemsa stain is used, disadvantages include poor sensitivity and difficulty of interpretation owing to artifacts, such as glycogen inclusions in cervical epithelial cells, or pigment granules (melanin granules) and nuclear extrusions in conjunctival cells (Yoneda et al., 1975). Inclusion detection in smears by these methods is relatively insensitive. When staining methods were compared with cell culture, the rate was found to be from only 20-60% as sensitive using specimens from patients with trachoma and neonatal conjunctivitis (Darougar et al., 1980; Rowe et al., 1979; Sandstrom et al., 1984). Recent studies with Papanicolaou-stained cervical smears suggest that the inflammatory pattern may be useful as a screening test to select patients for confirmation of infection (Kiviat et al., 1985a; Kiviat et al., 1985b). The Papanicolaou method used alone, however, is not satisfactory for diagnosis because the inherent specificity of the method is low. If this screening method to define patients at high risk is followed up by cell culture isolation or by a direct method, this two-step approach may then have considerable value for diagnosis of *C. trachomatis* infection (Kiviat et al., 1985b).

C. Serology

Several serological tests have been developed for the diagnosis of chlamydial infection. These tests involve complement-fixation (CF), indirect fluorescent antibody (FA), and enzyme-linked immunosorbent assays (ELISA). Although serological tests have been shown to be useful to establish chlamydial infection, diagnosis by serology is generally not definitive without culture confirmation. In some cases, however, serology is often of diagnostic value, such as in the demonstration of specific IgM antibody in infant pneumonia (Schachter et al., 1982; Wang and Grayston, 1984) or of high-titered IgG antibody in PID (Wang and Grayston, 1984), and in the Fitz-Hugh-Curtis syndrome (perihepatitis) (Muller-Schoop et al., 1978). Serology is of less diagnostic value for STD clinic patients because chlamydial antibody is common in such populations (Wang et al., 1977).

1. Complement-Fixation Test

The CF test detects genus-specific antibodies against both *C. psittaci* and *C. trachomatis*. The CF test is less sensitive than FA tests and is generally useful only for detection of psittacosis and LGV infection (Meyer et al., 1965). A CF titer of 10 or higher is considered positive, a titer present in more than 80% of LGV cases (Schachter et al., 1969).

2. Immunofluorescence Test

The specificity of the indirect immunofluorescence (IF) test depends upon the antigen used. Because the genus-specific antigens are more accessible to antibodies in inclusions and reticulate bodies, the test is genus-specific (detects antibodies to both *C. trachomatis* and *C. psittaci*) when infected cells are used (Richmond and Caul, 1975) or reticulate bodies (Yong et al., 1979) are used, but type-specific when elementary bodies of several *C. trachomatis* immunotypes are used, as in the microimmunofluorescence (micro-IF) test of Wang and Grayston (1970).

Immunoglobulin M, IgG, and local secretory antibody can be detected by using immunoglobulin class-specific fluorescein conjugates in the IF test (Wang et al., 1977). The micro-IF test of Wang and Grayston (1970) is a useful, sensitive assay that has been used to detect antichlamydial antibody in serum as well as in tears. For example, tear antibody is a good indicator of disease activity in trachoma (Grayston et al., 1977; Wang et al., 1977). In addition, tear antibody is usually detected in infants with *C. trachomatis* infection after 3-5 weeks of age, regardless of the site of infection, in 75% of asymptomatic infections and 100% of pneumonia cases (Wang and Grayston, 1984). About 60% of the patients attending STD clinics have demonstrable micro-IF serum antibody titers (Wang et al., 1977). In one study with genital chlamydial infection, the micro-IF antibody titers were, on an average, fivefold higher in females than in males, with geometric mean titers (GMTs) of 101 versus 21, respectively (Wang et al., 1977). In another study with laboratory-confirmed cases of STD, antibodies to *C. trachomatis* were demonstrated in 100% of females but in only 81% of males (Wang and Grayston, 1984). Transplacental maternal antibody can produce measurable serum antibody in neonates and young infants. The GMT of the micro-IF antibody in cord blood of babies whose mothers were cervical culture-positive averaged 22 with an upper limit (2 SD) of 512 (S.P. Wang and T.A. Bell, unpublished data). Demonstration of IgM antibody has been suggested as diagnostic of infantile *C. trachomatis* pneumonia (Schachter et al., 1982). Studies by Wang however, showed that IgM antibody could be demonstrated in only 70% of culture-proven cases of chlamydial pneumonia (Wang and Grayston, 1984). The micro-IF test is also useful in the investigation of diseases in which a chlamydial cause has not been proved (Grayston et al., 1981; Muller-Schoop et al., 1978). Unfortunately, micro-IF, a sensitive and specific serological test of real diagnostic value in seroepidemiological studies, is labor-intensive, complicated, and requires the preparation and use of elementary bodies representing multiple serovars. Its use has been limited to a few research laboratories in the world.

3. Enzyme-Linked Immunosorbent Assay

Enzyme-linked immunosorbent assay (ELISA) serology was first applied to chlamydiae by Lewis et al. (1977), but it was not until 1982 that interest in it was renewed, which results in a number of studies on ELISA serology for *C. trachomatis*. These studies used either intact chlamydial organisms (Jones et al., 1983; Lewis et al., 1977; Mahony et al., 1983; Saikku et al., 1983), or solubilized antigens (Duc-Goiran et al., 1983; Mahoney et al., 1983) of serovar L2. These studies showed a comparable sensitivity between ELISA and IF serology, in which increases or decreases in antibody titers could be demonstrated. However, there continues to be a lack of standardization, which is essential for consistent interpretation, in the test procedures. Factors that need to be standardized among laboratories performing ELISA serology include use of standardized serotypes of elementary body or reticulate body antigens, concentration of antigens used, endpoints of positive versus negative samples, definition of other criteria for determining whether a test is positive or negative, and the determination of background values or natural antibody titers in normal persons. Therefore, unless a defined *C. trachomatis* antigen can be mass-produced, such as by recombinant DNA technology, and then standardized and made widely available for use, ELISA serology for diagnosis of *C. trachomatis* will remain of little value.

III. NEW DIAGNOSTIC METHODS

Methods of rapid diagnosis by direct detection of microbial antigens or nucleic acids in clinical specimens or tissue samples have evolved rapidly in recent years. This has been due to the advances in both bioengineering and genetic engineering in combination with application of newer immunochemical and genetic techniques.

A. Antigen Detection with Monoclonal Antibodies

In 1982 we reported the development of monoclonal antibodies (MAbs) against *C. trachomatis* and characterized the antibody specificities and the recognized antigens (Stephens et al., 1982a,b,c). Subsequently, several reports describing other *C. trachomatis* MAbs and their specificities have appeared (Caldwell and Hitchcock, 1984; Clark et al., 1982; Matikainen and Terho, 1983; Rosen et al., 1983). The detailed description of the production and characterization of *C. trachomatis*-specific MAbs can be found in Chap. 5. Antibody specificities of MAbs to *C. trachomatis* demonstrate serovar, subspecies, species, and genus reactions. We have developed serotyping methods for *C. trachomatis* isolates using serovar- and subspecies-specific MAbs in indirect FA (Wang et al., 1985) and dot ELISA tests (Barnes et al., 1985). We have applied *C. trachomatis*-specific MAbs for the immunohistological identification of *C. trachomatis* organisms in tissue sections from humans (Klotz et al., 1983) and experimental animals (Patton et al., 1983).

A genus-specific MAb specific for LPS is useful for the identification of both *C. trachomatis* and *C. psittaci* inclusions during cell culture isolation. Although we have used IF staining, others (Thornley et al., 1985) have used a reverse passive hemagglutination assay. The use of a genus-specific MAb has potential value in the direct detection of *C. psittaci* antigen in clinical material from humans and animals.

An exciting development in the immunodiagnosis of *C. trachomatis* infection has been the rapid identification of extracellular organisms in smears with FITC-conjugated species-specific MAbs (Bell et al., 1984; Nowinski et al., 1983; Tam et al., 1984). The test can be performed when a culture facility is not available. When compared with culture isolation, the sensitivity and specificity of the culture-independent test is over 90%. Because the test can be performed within 30 min, it could be used as an office test while patients are waiting. Limitations of the test include the requirement for a high-quality fluorescence microscope, trained personnel, and possible fatigue if large numbers of samples are read at one time. The use of *C. trachomatis* MAbs in the immunodiagnosis of *C. trachomatis* will be described in more detail in Sect. IV.

B. Antigen Detection by Enzyme-Linked Immunosorbent Assay

The antigen capture assays using ELISA has been shown to have considerable sensitivity for the direct detection of *C. trachomatis* in clinical specimens. We have assessed the use of a species-specific MAb for the direct detection of chlamydial antigens utilizing a two-site immunoenzymometric assay (Stephens et al., 1982b). Chlamydial antigen was captured on microtiter wells precoated with rabbit hyperimmune antichlamydial serum and the absorbed antigens were detected by ELISA using a species-specific MAb (Fig. 1). The maximum sensitivity was 3 ng of protein antigen which, as determined by particle counts in electron microscopy, represented approximately $2\text{-}4 \times 10^4$ chlamydial particles per well. This represented a value of 2.5 times the average of background values. Clinical samples that contained more than 1×10^2 inclusion-forming units per well, as determined by cell culture, were readily detected by ELISA. The apparent discrepancy between the number of chlamydial particles and inclusion-forming units detected was probably due to the substantial proportion of nonviable chlamydial particles present in some clinical samples. Improvements in sensitivity may be obtained by experimenting with different methods of solublization of chlamydial antigens from chlamydial elementary bodies and with use of different antibody systems to capture antigens.

A similar test using polystyrene beads to capture nonspecifically sodium deoxycholate-solubilized chlamydial antigens has been introduced for direct diagnosis

ELISA Antigen Capture Assay

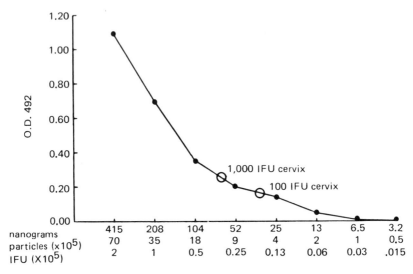

2.1 X conjugate control = 0.032

Fig. 1 Two-site immunoenzymometric assay. Anti-L2 rabbit immunoglobulin (4 mg/ml) was adsorbed to wells of microtiter plates. Dilutions of purified chlamydial EBs, which had been characterized for protein content, number of particles, and inclusion-forming units (IFU), were added to the wells and incubated. Wells were washed and 40 μg/ml of MAb 1H8 (species-specific) was added. Immune reactions were detected with peroxidase-conjugated antiserum. The endpoint was calculated as 2.5 times the background values of negative controls. Clinical samples of cervical origin with known IFU were also assayed (*Source*: courtesy of R. S. Stephens, Monoclonal antibodies to *Chlamydia trachomatis*, Ph.D. Thesis, University of Washington, Seattle, Washington, 1983).

of *C. trachomatis* infection (Amortegui and Meyer, 1985; Jones et al., 1984). The captured antigens are detected by an ELISA method using rabbit anti-*C. trachomatis* serum, which probably detects multiple antigens, including genus-specific antigens. Studies with patients attending STD and family-planning clinics showed sensitivities of 80-82% and specificities of 98% when compared with cell culture isolation. The isolation rates for *C. trachomatis* in these clinics were 9-20%. The advantages to this test are that the reading is objective and a relatively large number of specimens can be screened at one time. However, this test takes 5-6 hr to perform and is not optimal for testing individual or even small numbers of specimens that arrive at the laboratory sporadically and that require immediate test results. Also, ELISA tests provide no information about specimen adequacy, such as can be obtained with smears. Whether or not this test will be sufficiently sensitive and specific for the screening of low-prevalence populations has yet to be shown.

C. Diagnosis with DNA Probes

Diagnosis of C. trachomatis by DNA hybridization is still experimental. Preliminary reports describing the use of cloned C. trachomatis genomic or plasmid DNA as a DNA probe have appeared recently and have demonstrated some promising results for the detection of chlamydial DNA in cultured and swab specimens (Hyypia et al., 1984; Palva et al., 1984). The advantages of the DNA hybridization method are that a cloned DNA probe can be made absolutely specific to C. trachomatis, clinical specimens can be shipped to central laboratories at ambient temperatures, and the test is independent of culture and should be applicable for all types of clinical specimens. The disadvantages are that, at present, radioisotopes must be used for the detection of chlamydial DNA and the test is not rapid; the autoradiographic technique now used usually requires an overnight exposure or more. Also, a high degree of sensitivity and specificity of the DNA hybridization technique for diagnosis of C. trachomatis in routine clinical specimens has yet to be proved. The application of the DNA probe method as a routine test will be limited unless radioisotopes can be replaced with other detection systems such as an ELISA test. This would simplify and shorten the test procedure and would allow a much wider acceptance than one that is based on the use of radioisotopes.

IV. IMMUNODIAGNOSIS WITH MONOCLONAL ANTIBODIES

Monoclonal antibody (MAb) techniques are now widely practiced and the diagnostic potential of MAbs for the immunological identification of viruses, bacteria, fungi, and parasites in tissues, exudates, or body fluids has become apparent. Monoclonal antibodies specific to C. trachomatis have become available (Stephens et al., 1982c). We have introduced an MAb-based immunological diagnostic method, using IF as the assay system, for C. trachomatis that is rapid, sensitive, and specific (Bell et al., 1984; Nowinski et al., 1983; Tam et al., 1984). These tests will be described in this section. We anticipate that other assay systems utilizing MAbs, such as the preliminary report using an ELISA-based assay (Caul and Paul, 1985), will be developed enabling the rapid, precise, and semiautomated diagnosis of C. trachomatis.

A. Detection of Inclusions in Cell Culture

For the cell culture isolation of C. trachomatis, the general practice is to stain coverslips containing cell monolayers with Giemsa or iodine at 72 hr after inoculation and to scan the coverslips for inclusions under light microscopy (Gordon

Table 2 Number of Chlamydia-Positive Specimens Detected by Giemsa or Iodine Staining in Comparison with IF Staining Using MAbs for Cell Culture Isolation of *C. trachomatis*

		No. of positive specimens[a]			
	Culture system:	Vial[b] ($n = 115$)		Microtiter plate[c] ($n = 878$)	
Cell culture passages	Staining:	IF	Giemsa[d]	IF	Iodine
1		38	23	129	70
2		1[e]	13	2[f]	42

[a]Urethral and cervical specimens.
[b]HeLa 229 cell culture.
[c]McCoy cell culture.
[d]Three additional positives by either rescanning or a third passage.
[e]<10 inclusions per coverslip.
[f]<20 inclusions per well.
Source: [c]Stamm et al., 1983; [b]Stephens et al., 1982a.

and Quan, 1965; Kuo et al., 1972; Ripa and Mardh, 1977). If no inclusions are found, the cells are harvested at 72 hr, passaged for a second time onto new cell monolayers, and after an additional 72 hr stained with the same methods for detection of inclusions. The isolation attempt is regarded as negative if no inclusions are detected on the second passage. In all, the culture diagnosis may take from 3 to 7 days.

We have compared the sensitivity of inclusion detection by staining with FITC-conjugated MAbs that recognize *C. trachomatis* species-specific antigens, with that of Giemsa (Stephens et al., 1982a) and iodine staining methods (Stamm et al., 1983). We have used either the vial or microtiter plate culture system for the diagnosis of genital infection in patients attending STD clinics (Table 2). Staining was done on day 2 postinoculation for IF and on day 3 postinoculation for Giemsa and iodine, because the results of staining with IF on day 2 was found to be comparable with day 3. With the method of vial culture using HeLa 229 cells, the comparison of 115 genital specimens showed that the Giemsa method detected 23 positive samples (64% of the positives) in the first passage compared with 38 positive specimens (97%) by the IF method in the first passage ($p <$ .0005). The Giemsa method produced 13 additional positive results in the second passage (36%), while IF produced only one additional positive result (3%) (Stephens et al., 1982a). The single specimen missed by the IF method on first passage contained less than 10 inclusions on the coverslip. Three additional positive results were obtained with the Giemsa method, either by rescanning the coverslips or by a third cell passage. The number of inclusions counted by IF averaged twice as many as with the Giemsa method and averaged threefold higher in coverslips containing fewer than 200 inclusions. In addition, the time required to scan coverslips stained with FITC-labeled MAb averaged 5 min as compared with average of 12 min for Giemsa-stained coverslips.

Similar results were seen when IF staining was compared with iodine staining using microtiter plates (Stamm et al., 1983). Among 878 urethral and cervical specimens tested in parallel, the IF method detected eight times as many inclusions per monolayer, identified a higher proportion of positive specimens in the first passage (98 versus 62%; $p < .01$), and improved the overall sensitivity (98% of total positive specimens detected versus 84%; $p < .01$). Improved sensitivity was most evident in specimens with a low number of inclusions. Furthermore, 30% less time was required for scanning IF-stained coverslips than required for iodine-stained coverslips.

These two studies showed that the IF method could be used routinely as a single-passage detection technique for chlaymdial isolation with a loss of only 2-3% of the positives. Elimination of the second passage would halve the number of cultures, reduce reporting time, and save a considerable amount of technician time as well.

B. Direct Antigen Detection in Clinical Samples

Direct detection of chlamydial genital infection by iodine, Giemsa, or IF staining of chlamydial inclusions in patient specimens has been shown to be insensitive. Hence, cell culture isolation has been the method of choice for the confirmation of chlamydial infection. However, such methods are expensive and technically difficult to perform and are thus practiced in far too few diagnostic laboratories to meet the clinical needs for most communities. To develop a more rapid test, we have used the same FITC-labeled MAb to detect extracellular chlamydial organisms in patients' specimens (Tam et al., 1984) [Fig. 2 (see Plate I, facing p. 204)]. Examination of urethral or cervical smears (Fig. 2D) by fluorescence microscopy demonstrated a characteristic pattern of staining in chlamydia-infected patients. Extracellular elementary bodies were observed as discrete, evenly fluorescent, smooth-edged disks approximately 300 nm in diameter. They were stained apple-green against a background of counterstained epithelial and inflammatory cells and cellular debris. We also observed slightly larger particles that appeared evenly stained, like the elementary bodies, or with a peripheral "halo" stain. These we interpreted as immature forms and replicative forms (reticulate bodies) derived from ruptured chlamydial inclusions. Only a few specimens contained patient cells with intact intracytoplasmic chlamydial inclusions.

The direct IF test was compared with cultures from specimens obtained from men and women attending an STD clinic (Table 3). The cultured specimens, stained with either FITC-labeled MAb or iodine, revealed a prevalence of infection of 23%

Table 3 Comparison of Culture Results and the Direct Slide Test for Diagnosis of Chlamydial Infection

	Pattern of reaction							
---	A	B	C	D	E	F	G	H
Direct slide test	+	–	+	+	–	–	–	+
Culture-antibody stain	+	–	–	+	+	–	+	–
Culture-iodine stain	+	–	–	–	+	+	–	+

	No. of patients with reaction pattern							
---	A	B	C	D	E	F	G	H
Men	117	468	13	5	5	5	8	2
Women	65	225	6	2	3	1	0	1
Total	182	693	19	7	8	6	8	3

Source: from Tam et al., 1984. *N. Engl. J. Med., 310*:1146-1150; reproduced with permission.

in the men and 22% in the women. For 926 patients, agreement among the three diagnostic tests was observed in 94% of the specimens tested. If MAb-stained cultures were considered to be the reference method (100% "correct" diagnosis), the sensitivity of the direct IF test was 92% and the specificity was 97%. If iodine-stained cultures were considered to be the reference method, then the sensitivity of the direct IF test was 93% and specificity 96%. The direct IF test is a rapid, sensitive method in which results can be obtained in 30-45 min.

In a subsequent multicenter trial (Stamm et al., 1984), a close correlation between the direct IF method and culture was also found. The direct smear had a sensitivity of 89% and specificity of 99% for 595 women with cervicitis, and a sensitivity of 86% and specificity of 99% for 225 asymptomatic, pregnant women screened while attending prenatal or abortion clinics.

In studying a population of lower prevalence, 27 positive specimens were identified among 401 asymptomatic women (6.7%) attending a family-planning clinic (Uyeda et al., 1984). Direct IF tests performed in parallel with cultures stained with FITC-labeled MAb resulted in a sensitivity of 96% and a specificity of more than 99%.

The direct IF method can also be applied to extragenital sites [Fig. 2A,B,C (see Plate I, facing p. 204)]. In a study of infants with purulent conjunctivitis, we found a 100% correlation of the direct test when compared with MAb-stained cultures for diagnosis of chlamydial conjunctivitis in 16 of 39 infants. Positive smears were also obtained from 12 of 14 culture-positive, and four of 16 culture-negative nasopharyngeal samples from the same infants with chlamydial conjunc-

PLATE I
(*Chapter 6*)

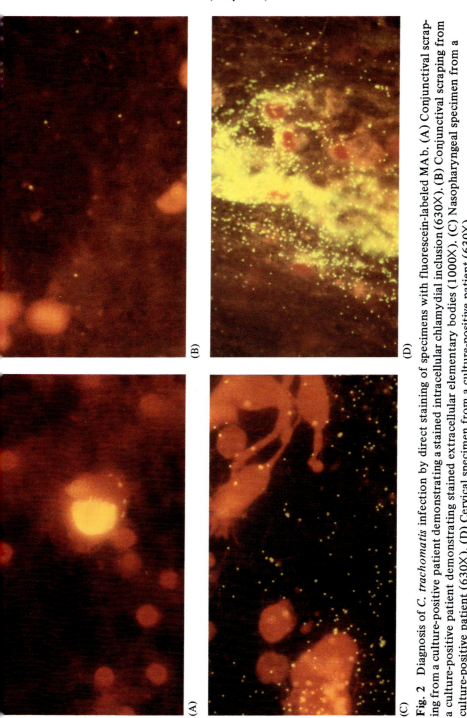

(B)

(D)

(A)

(C)

Fig. 2 Diagnosis of *C. trachomatis* infection by direct staining of specimens with fluorescein-labeled MAb. (A) Conjunctival scraping from a culture-positive patient demonstrating a stained intracellular chlamydial inclusion (630X). (B) Conjunctival scraping from a culture-positive patient demonstrating stained extracellular elementary bodies (1000X). (C) Nasopharyngeal specimen from a culture-positive patient (630X). (D) Cervical specimen from a culture-positive patient (630X).

PLATE II
(*Chapter 7*)

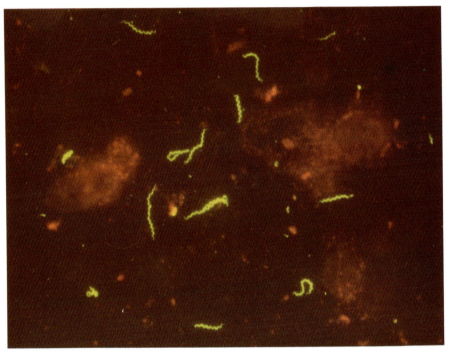

Fig. 3 Direct MAb identification of *T. pallidum* in exudate from a primary chancre (*Source*: Reprinted with permission from Lukehart et al., 1985).

tivitis. For this application, the direct IF method affords excellent sensitivity and specificity with regard to culture and is a convenient, rapid method that can supplant traditional Giemsa stain, a popular cytologic method in the past. The disadvantages of the Giemsa method, which identifies intracytoplasmic inclusions, have been a lack of sensitivity—only 20-60% as sensitive as culture (Darougar et al., 1980; Sandström et al., 1984; Yoneda et al., 1975), the delicate task of scraping the infant's conjunctival surface with a sharp spatula, and the several hours required for cytological staining and reading the smear.

Chlamydial organisms were also detected in secretions of the respiratory tract of infants with pneumonia (Friis et al., 1984). In this study two of 41 nasopharyngeal and laryngeal aspirates from infants and children were positive for *C. trachomatis* by both direct IF stain and culture. The two infants also had high titers of IgM antibodies to *C. trachomatis*. None of these three diagnostic methods were positive in the other 39 infants or the young children with symptoms of pneumonia who were tested.

In summary, the findings suggest that the direct IF test can be used for detection of chlamydiae for genital or extragenital infection in high-prevalence or symptomatic and low-prevalence or asymptomatic patient populations. Discrepancies between the direct IF test and culture results may appear in samples characterized by low numbers of chlamydial particles on slides or few inclusion-forming units in culture and are thus probably due to sampling error. Chlamydial particles with typically stained morphology are sometimes observed as false-positives in culture-negative specimens. These may represent specimens from patients who are truly infected with *C. trachomatis*, but from whom viable organisms were not recovered because the sample contained substances inhibitory to the growth of chlamydiae in cell culture or because the chlamydiae have failed to survive transport conditions to the laboratory.

V. CONCLUSIONS

Culture-independent tests utilizing both monoclonal and polyclonal antibody reagents are already accepted and are being used for the diagnosis of chlamydial infections. The FA and ELISA methods demonstrated a favorable degree of sensitivity and specificity when compared with reference culture methods. The direct tests required from less than an hour to perform for FA, to 5-6 hr for ELISA. These tests represent major advancements in diagnoses that previously required from 2 to 7 days to perform. Moreover, the use of these tests will permit laboratories not versed in mammalian cell culture to perform rapid diagnostic testing. This increased availability should facilitate case detection and contact tracing, which would have a positive impact on disease control. In addition, rapid differential diagnosis of infection will now be possible. Because chlamydial infection

and other diseases such as gonorrhea may be transmitted simultaneously and share
similar clinical manifestations, it will be possible to differentiate a single from a
multiple infection by parallel testing of direct specimens with the appropriate
reagents.

REFERENCES

Amortegui, A. J. and Meyer, M. P. (1985). Enzyme immunoassay for detection
   of *Chlamydia trachomatis* from the cervix. *Obstet. Gynecol. 65*:523-526.
Barnes, R. C., Wang, S. P., Kuo, C. C., and Stamm, W. E. (1985). Rapid immunotyping of *Chlamydia trachomatis* with monoclonal antibodies in a solid-phase
   enzyme immunoassay. *J. Clin. Microbiol. 22*:609-613.
Beem, M. O. and Saxon, E. M. (1977). Respiratory-tract colonization and a distinctive pneumonia syndrome in infants infected with *Chlamydia trachomatis. N. Engl. J. Med. 296*:306-310.
Bell, T. A., Kuo, C. C., Stamm, W. E., Tam, M. R., Stephens, R. S., Holmes, K.
   K., and Grayston, J. T. (1984). Direct fluorescent monoclonal antibody
   stain for rapid detection of infant *Chlamydia trachomatis* infections. *Pedi-
   atrics 74*:224-228.
Berger, R. E., Alexander, E. R., Monda, G. D., Ansell, J., McCormick, G., and
   Holmes, K. K. (1978). *Chlamydia trachomatis* as a cause of acute "idio-
   pathic" epididymitis. *N. Engl. J. Med. 298*:301-304.
Blyth, W. A. and Taverne, J. (1974). Cultivation of TRIC agents: A comparison
   between the use of BHK-21 and irradiated McCoy cells. *J. Hyg. 72*:121-128.
Brunham, R. C., Paavonen, J., Stevens, C. E., Kiviat, N., Kuo, C. C., Critchlow,
   C. W., and Holmes, K. K. (1984). Mucopurulent cervicitis—the ignored counterpart in women of urethritis in men. *N. Engl. J. Med. 311*:1-6.
Caldwell, H. D. and Hitchcock, P. J. (1984). Monoclonal antibody against a genus-
   specific antigen of *Chlamydia* species: Location of the epitope on chlamydial lipopolysaccharide. *Infect. Immun. 44*:306-314.
Caul, E. O. and Paul, I. D. (1985). Monoclonal antibody based ELISA for detecting *Chlamydia trachomatis. Lancet 1*:279.
Clark, R. B., Nachamkin, I., Schatzki, P. F., and Dalton, H. P. (1982). Localization of distinct surface antigens on *Chlamydia trachomatis* HAR-13 by immune electron microscopy with monoclonal antibodies. *Infect. Immun. 38*:
   1273-1278.
Darougar, S., Woodland, R. M., Jones, B. R., Houshmand, A., and Farahmandian,
   H. A. (1980). Comparative sensitivity of fluorescent antibody staining of
   conjunctival scrapings and irradiated McCoy cell culture for the diagnosis of
   hyperendemic trachoma. *Br. J. Ophthalmol. 64*:276-278.
Duc-Goiran, P., Raymond, J., Leaute, J. B., and Orfila, J. (1983). Use of the enzyme-linked immunosorbent assay for detection of antibodies to *Chlamydia
   trachomatis. Eur. J. Clin. Microbiol. 2*:32-38.

Forsey, T., Darougar, S., Dines, R. J., Wright, D. J. M., and Friedman, P. S. (1982). Chlamydia genital infection in Addis Ababa, Ethiopia. *Br. J. Vener. Dis. 58*: 370-373.

Friis, B., Kuo, C. C., Wang, S. P., Mordhorst, C. H., and Grayston, J. T. (1984). Rapid diagnosis of *Chlamydia trachomatis* pneumonia in infants. *Acta Pathol. Microbiol. Immunol. Scand. Sect. B. 92*:139-143.

Gordon, F. B., Harper, I. A., Quan, A. L., Treharne, J. D., Dwyer, R. St. C., and Garland, J. A. (1969). Detection of chlamydia (Bedsonia) in certain infections of man. I. Laboratory procedures: Comparison of yolk sac and cell culture for detection and isolation. *J. Infect. Dis. 120*:451-462.

Gordon, F. B. and Quan, A. L. (1965). Isolation of the trachoma agent in cell culture. *Proc. Soc. Exp. Biol. Med. 118*:354-359.

Grayston, J. T., Mordhorst, C. H., and Wang, S. P. (1981). Childhood myocarditis associated with *Chlamydia trachomatis* infection. *J. Am. Med. Assoc. 246*: 2823-2827.

Grayston, J. T. and Wang, S. P. (1975). New knowledge of chlamydiae and the diseases they cause. *J. Infect. Dis. 132*:87-105.

Grayston, J. T., Yeh, L. J., Wang, S. P., Kuo, C. C., Beasley, R. P., and Gale, J. L. (1977). Pathogenesis of ocular *Chlamydia trachomatis* infections in humans. In *Nongonococcal Urethritis and Related Infections* (H. Hobson and K. K. Holmes, eds.). American Society for Microbiology, Washington, DC, pp. 113-125.

Halberstaedter, L. and von Prowazek, S. (1907). Uber Zelleinschlusse parasitarer Natur beim Trachom. *Arb. Kaiserlichen Gesundheitsamte 26*:44-47.

Holmes, K. K. (1984). Sexually transmitted diseases: Past, present, and future. 1983 ADL lecture, Center for Disease Control, U.S. Department of Health and Human Services, Epidemiology Program Office, Atlanta, Ga.

Holmes, K. K., Handsfield, H. H., Wang, S. P., Wentworth, B. B., Turck, M., Anderson, J. B., and Alexander, E. R. (1975). Etiology of nongonococcal urethritis. *N. Engl. J. Med. 292*:1199-1205.

Hyypia, T., Larsen, S. H., Stahlberg, T., and Terho, P. (1984). Analysis and detection of chlamydial DNA. *J. Gen. Microbiol. 130*:3159-3164.

Jones, M. F., Smith, T. F., Houglum, A. J., and Herrman, J. E. (1984). Detection of *Chlamydia trachomatis* in genital specimens by the Chlamydiazyme test. *J. Clin. Microbiol. 20*:465-467.

Jones, R. B., Bruins, S. C., and Newhall, W. J. (1983). Comparison of reticulate and elementary body antigens in detection of antibodies against *Chlamydia trachomatis* by an enzyme-linked immunosorbent assay. *J. Clin. Microbiol. 17*:466-471.

Kiviat, N. B., Paavonen, J. A., Brockway, J., Critchlow, C. W., Brunham, R. C., Stevens, C. E., Stamm, W. E., Kuo, C. C., DeRouen, T., and Holmes, K. K. (1985a). Cytologic manifestations of cervical and vaginal infections, I. Epithelial and inflammatory cellular changes. *J. Am. Med. Assoc. 253*:989-996.

Kiviat, N. B., Peterson, M., Kinney-Thomas, E., Tam, M., Stamm, W. E., and Holmes, K. K. (1985b). Cytologic manifestations of cervical and vaginal infections, II. Confirmation of *Chlamydia trachomatis* infection by direct immunofluorescence using monoclonal antibodies. *J. Am. Med. Assoc. 253*: 997-1000.

Klotz, S. A., Drutz, D. J., Tam, M. R., and Reed, K. H. (1983). Hemorrhagic proctitis due to lymphogranuloma venereum serogroup L2. Diagnosis by fluorescent monoclonal antibody. *N. Engl. J. Med. 308*:1563-1565.

Kuo, C. C., Wang, S. P., and Grayston, J. T. (1975). Comparative infectivity of trachoma organisms in HeLa 229 cells and egg cultures. *Infect. Immun. 12*: 1078-1082.

Kuo, C. C., Wang, S. P., and Grayston, J. T. (1977). Growth of trachoma organisms in HeLa 229 Cell Culture. In *Nongonococcal Urethritis and Related Infections* (D. Hobson and K. K. Holmes, eds.). American Society for Microbiology, Washington, DC, pp. 328-336.

Kuo, C. C., Wang, S. P., Holmes, K. K., and Grayston, J. T. (1983). Immunotypes of *Chlamydia trachomatis* isolates in Seattle, Washington. *Infect. Immun. 41*:865-868.

Kuo, C. C., Wang, S. P., Wentworth, B. B., and Grayston, J. T. (1972). Primary isolation of TRIC organisms in HeLa 229 cells treated with DEAE-dextran. *J. Infect. Dis. 125*:665-668.

Lewis, V. J., Thacker, W. L., and Mitchell, S. H. (1977). Enzyme-linked immunosorbent assay for chlamydial antibodies. *J. Clin. Microbiol. 6*:507-510.

Lindner, K. (1910). Zur Aetiologie der gonokokkenfreien Urethritis. *Wien. Klin. Wochenschr. 23*:283-284.

Mahony, J. B., Schachter, J., and Chernesky, M. A. (1983). Detection of antichlamydial immunoglobulin G and M antibodies by enzyme-linked immunosorbent assay. *J. Clin. Microbiol. 18*:270-275.

Mardh, P.-A., Ripa, T., Svensson, L., and Westrom, L. (1977). *Chlamydia trachomatis* infection in patients with acute salpingitis. *N. Engl. J. Med. 296*:1377-1379.

Matikainen, M.-T. and Terho, P. (1983). Immunochemical analysis of antigenic determinants of *Chlamydia trachomatis* by monoclonal antibodies. *J. Gen. Microbiol. 129*:2343-2350.

Meyer, K. F., Eddie, B., and Schachter, J. (1965). Psittacosis-lymphogranuloma venereum agents. In *Diagnostic Procedures for Viral and Rickettsial Infections* (E. H. Lennette and N. J. Schmidt, eds.). American Public Health Association, New York, pp. 869-903.

Moore, D. E., Spadoni, L. R., Foy, H. M., Wang, S. P., Daling, J. R., Kuo, C. C., Grayston, J. T., and Eschenbach, D. A. (1982). Increased frequency of serum antibodies to *Chlamydia trachomatis* in infertility due to distal tubal disease. *Lancet 2*:574-577.

Morbidity and Mortality Weekly Report (1985). *Chlamydia trachomatis* infections, policy guidelines for prevention and control. Suppl. *34*(35), The Massachusetts Medical Society, Boston.

Moulder, J. W., Hatch, T. P., Kuo, C. C., Schachter, J., and Storz, J. (1984). Genus I. *Chlamydia* Jones, Rake and Stearns 1945,55. In *Bergey's Manual of Systematic Bacteriology* (N. R. Krieg, ed.). Vol. 1, Williams & Wilkins, Baltimore, pp. 729-739.

Muller-Schoop, J. W., Wang, S. P., Munzinger, J., Schlapfer, H. U., Knoblauch, M., and Ammann, R. W. (1978). *Chlamydia trachomatis* as possible cause of peritonitis and perihepatitis in young women. *Br. Med. J. 1*:1022-1024.

Nowinski, R. C., Tam, M. R., Goldstein, L. G., Stong, L., Kuo, C. C., Corey, L., Stamm, W. E., Handsfield, H. H., Knapp, J. S., and Holmes, K. K. (1983). Monoclonal antibodies for diagnosis of infectious diseases in humans. *Science 219*:637-644.

Osoba, A. O. (1981). Sexually transmitted diseases in tropical Africa: A review of the present situation. *Br. J. Vener. Dis. 57*:89-94.

Palva, A., Jousimies-Somer, H., Saikku, P., Vaananen, P., Soderlund, H., and Ranki, M. (1984). Detection of *Chlamydia trachomatis* by nucleic acid sandwich hybridization. *FEMS Microbiol. Lett. 23*:83-89.

Patton, D. L., Halbert, S. A., Kuo, C. C., Wang, S. P., and Holmes, K. K. (1983). Host response to primary *Chlamydia trachomatis* infection of the fallopian tube in pig-tailed monkeys. *Fert. Steril. 40*:829-840.

Perine, P. L., Andersen, A. J., Krause, D. W., Awoke, S., Wang, S. P., Kuo, C. C., and Holmes, K. K. (1980). Diagnosis and treatment of lymphogranuloma venereum in Ethiopia. In *Current Chemotherapy and Infectious Disease* (J. D. Nelson and C. Grassi, eds.). American Society for Microbiology, Washington, DC, pp. 1280-1282.

Quinn, T. C., Goodell, S. E., Mkrtichian, E., Schuffler, M. D., Wang, S. P., Stamm, W. E., and Holmes, K. K. (1981). *Chlamydia trachomatis* proctitis. *N. Engl. J. Med. 305*:195-200.

Richmond, S. J. and Caul, E. O. (1975). Fluorescent antibody studies in chlamydial infections. *J. Clin. Microbiol. 1*:345-352.

Ripa, K. T. and Mardh, P.-A. (1977). Cultivation of *Chlamydia trachomatis* in cycloheximide-treated McCoy cells. *J. Clin. Microbiol. 6*:328-331.

Rosen, A., Persson, K., and Klein, G. (1983). Human monoclonal antibodies to a genus-specific chlaymdial antigen, produced by EBV-transformed B Cells. *J. Immunol. 130*:2899-2902.

Rowe, D. S., Aicardi, E. Z., Dawson, C. R., and Schachter, J. (1979). Purulent ocular discharge in neonates: Significance of *Chlamydia trachomatis*. *Pediatrics 63*:628-632.

Saikku, P., Paavonen, J., Vaananen, P., and Vaheri, A. (1983). Solid-phase enzyme immunoassay for chlamydial antibodies. *J. Clin. Microbiol. 17*:22-27.

Sandström, K. I., Bell, T. A., Chandler, J. W., Kuo, C. C., Wang, S. P., Grayston, J. T., Foy, H. M., Stamm, W. E., Cooney, M. K., Smith, A. L., and Holmes, K. K. (1984). Microbial causes of neonatal conjunctivitis. *J. Pediatr. 105*: 706-711.

Schachter, J. and Dawson, C. R. (1981). Chlamydial infections, a worldwide problem: Epidemiology and implications for trachoma therapy. *Sex. Transm. Dis. 8*:167-174.

Schachter, J., Grossman, M., and Azimi, P. H. (1982). Serology of *Chlamydia trachomatis* in infants. *J. Infect. Dis. 146*:530-535.

Schachter, J., Smith, D. E., Dawson, C. R., Anderson, W. R., Deller, J. J., Jr., Hoke, A. W., Smartt, W. H., and Meyer, K. F. (1969). Lymphogranuloma venereum. I. Comparison of the Frei test, complement fixation test, and isolation of the agent. *J. Infect. Dis. 120*:372-375.

Sompolinsky, D. and Richmond, S. J. (1974). The growth of *Chlamydia trachomatis* in McCoy cells treated with cytochalasin B. *Appl. Microbiol. 28*:912-914.

Stamm, W. E., Harrison, H. R., Alexander, E. R., Cles, L. D., Spence, M. R., and Quinn, T. C. (1984). Diagnosis of *Chlamydia trachomatis* infections by direct immunofluorescence staining of genital secretions. A multicenter trial. *Ann. Intern. Med. 101*:638-641.

Stamm, W. E., Tam, M., Koester, M., and Cles, L. (1983). Detection of *Chlamydia trachomatis* inclusions in McCoy cell cultures with fluorescein-conjugated monoclonal antibodies. *J. Clin. Microbiol. 17*:666-668.

Stephens, R. S., Kuo, C. C., and Tam, M. R. (1982a). Sensitivity of immunofluorescence with monoclonal antibodies for detection of *Chlamydia trachomatis* inclusions in cell culture. *J. Clin. Microbiol. 16*:4-7.

Stephens, R. S., Kuo, C. C., Tam, M. R., and Nowinski, R. C. (1982b). Monoclonal antibodies to *Chlamydia trachomatis*. In *Chlamydial Infections* (P.-A. Mardh, K. K. Holmes, J. D. Oriel, P. Piot, and J. Schachter, eds.). Elsevier Biomedical, Amsterdam, pp. 329-332.

Stephens, R. S., Tam, M. R., Kuo, C. C., and Nowinski, R. C. (1982c). Monoclonal antibodies to *Chlamydia trachomatis*: Antibody specificities and antigen characterization. *J. Immunol. 128*:1083-1089.

Svensson, L., Mardh, P.-A., Ahlgren, M., Nordenskjold, F. (1985). Ectopic pregnancy and antibodies to *Chlamydia trachomatis*. *Fert. Steril. 44*:313-317.

Tam, M. R., Stamm, W. E., Handsfield, H. H., Stephens, R. S., Kuo, C. C., Holmes, K. K., Ditzenberger, K., Krieger, M., and Nowinski, R. C. (1984). Culture-independent diagnosis of *Chlamydia trachomatis* using monoclonal antibodies. *N. Engl. J. Med. 310*:1146-1150.

T'ang, F., Chang, H., Huang, Y., and Wang, K. (1957). Studies on the etiology of trachoma with special reference to isolation of the virus in chick embryo. *Chin. Med. J. 75*:429-447.

Thompson, S. E. and Washington, A. E. (1983). Epidemiology of sexually transmitted *Chlamydia trachomatis* infections. *Epidemiol. Rev. 5*:96-123.

Thornley, M. J., Zamze, S. E., Byrne, M. D., Lusher, M., and Evans, R. T. (1985). Properties of monoclonal antibodies to the genus-specific antigen of *Chlamydia* and their use for antigen detection by reverse passive haemagglutination. *J. Gen. Microbiol. 131*:7-15.

Uyeda, C. T., Welborn, P., Ellison-Birang, N., Shunk, K., and Tsaouse, B. (1984). Rapid diagnosis of chlamydial infections with the MicroTrak direct test. *J. Clin. Microbiol. 20*:948-950.

Wang, S. P. and Grayston, J. T. (1964). Egg infectivity assay of trachoma virus. *Proc. Soc. Exp. Biol. Med. 115*:587-591.

Wang, S. P. and Grayston, J. T. (1970). Immunologic relationship between genital TRIC, lymphogranuloma venereum, and related organisms in a new microtiter indirect immunofluorescence test. *Am. J. Ophthalmol. 70*:367-374.

Wang, S. P. and Grayston, J. T. (1984). Micro-immunofluorescence serology of *Chlamydia trachomatis*. In *Medical Virology III* (L. M. de la Mazas and E. M. Peterson, eds.). Elsevier, New York, pp. 87-118.

Wang, S. P., Grayston, J. T., Kuo, C. C., Alexander, E. R., and Holmes, K. K. (1977). Serodiagnosis of *Chlamydia trachomatis* infection with the micro-immunofluorescence test. In *Nongonococcal Urethritis and Related Infections* (D. Hobson and K. K. Holmes, eds.). American Society for Microbiology, Washington, DC, pp. 237-248.

Wang, S. P., Kuo, C. C., Barnes, R. C., Stephens, R. S., and Grayston, J. T. (1985). Immunotyping of *Chlamydia trachomatis* with monoclonal antibodies. *J. Infect. Dis. 152*:791-800.

World Health Organization Statistics Report. (1971). Geneva: World Health Organization, *24*:248-329.

Yoder, B. L., Stamm, W. E., Koester, C. M., and Alexander, E. R. (1981). Microtest procedure for isolation of *Chlamydia trachomatis*. *J. Clin. Microbiol. 13*:1036-1039.

Yoneda, C., Dawson, C. R., Daghfous, T., Hoshiwara, I., Jones, P., Messadi, M., and Schachter, J. (1975). Cytology as a guide to the presence of chlamydia inclusions in Giemsa-stained conjunctival smears in severe endemic trachoma. *Br. J. Ophthalmol. 59*:116-124.

Yong, E. C., Chinn, J. S., Caldwell, H. D., and Kuo, C. C. (1979). Reticulate bodies as single antigen in *Chlamydia trachomatis* serology with microimmunofluorescence. *J. Clin. Microbiol. 10*:351-356.

SEVEN

Diagnostic Potential of Monoclonal Antibodies Against *Treponema pallidum*

Sheila A. Lukehart
Sharon A. Baker-Zander
University of Washington
School of Medicine
Seattle, Washington

I. BIOLOGY OF *TREPONEMA PALLIDUM*

A. Classification

Treponemes are helically shaped, tightly coiled bacteria, 0.10-0.18 μm in diameter and 6-20 μm in length. The *Treponema* are members of the order, Spirochaetales, which also include the *Leptospira* and *Borrelia*.

Four species are pathogenic for humans: *T. pallidum* ssp. *pallidum* (syphilis), *T. pallidum* ssp. *pertenue* (yaws), *T. pallidum* ssp. *endemicum* (endemic syphilis or bejel), and *T. carateum* (pinta). *Treponema paraluiscuniculi*, which is not pathogenic for humans, causes venereal spirochetosis in rabbits. These species are morphologically indistinguishable, microaerophilic (Fieldsteel et al., 1981; Smibert, 1984) and noncultivable. Studies of DNA homology show virtual genetic identity between *T. pallidum* ssp. *pallidum* and *T. pallidum* ssp. *pertenue* (Table 1) (Miao and Fieldsteel, 1980); there has been a single report of plasmid DNA in the Nichols strain of *T. pallidum* ssp. *pallidum* (Norgard and Miller, 1981).

Table 1 Genetic Relationships Between *T. pallidum* ssp. *pallidum* and Other Species of Treponemes

	Mol % G+C content	% DNA homology with *T. pallidum* subsp. *pallidum*
T. pallidum subsp. *pallidum*	52.4-53.7	100
T. pallidum subsp. *pertenue*	ND[a]	100
T. phagedenis	38-39	<5
T. refringens	41.5	<5

[a]Not done.

Source: Miao and Fieldsteel, 1978 and 1980.

The numerous nonpathogenic treponemes, which are cultivable anaerobes found in the flora of humans and animals, include *T. phagedenis, T. refringens, T. denticola,* and *T. vincentii.* The nonpathogens tested show essentially no DNA homology with pathogenic treponemes (Miao and Fieldsteel, 1978; Nath, 1983).

B. Morphology and Physiology

Morphologically, these organisms consist of an outer membrane containing protein, carbohydrate, and lipid (mainly phospholipid and glycolipid) surrounding periplasmic flagella or axial filaments. These organelles are believed to be responsible for the bacteria's characteristic corkscrew motility and lie between the outer membrane and the peptidoglycan layer (Hovind-Hougen, 1983; Smibert, 1984).

The pathogenic treponemes are microaerophilic. Oxygen utilization by *T. pallidum* has been reported (Barbieri and Cox, 1981; Cox and Barber, 1974) and is glucose-dependent. Oxidative phosphorylation occurs (Lysko and Cox, 1978); glucose is metabolized via both the Embden-Meyerhof-Parnas and the hexose monophosphate pathways (Schiller and Cox, 1977). Oxidation of pyruvate occurs in the presence of oxygen (Barbieri and Cox, 1979).

Although replication of *T. pallidum* ssp. *pallidum,* Nichols strain, has been achieved in growth media containing mammalian tissue culture cells (Fieldsteel et al., 1981; Norris, 1982), in vitro maintenance of *T. pallidum* has not been successful. Growth of these organisms in rabbit testes is still requisite; the estimated generation time is approximately 33 hr (Cumberland and Turner, 1949). The outer envelope of pathogenic treponemes is coated by a loosely associated layer of glycosaminoglycans (mucopolysaccharide); its origin, whether treponemal or host derived, remains unclear (Christiansen, 1963; Fitzgerald and Johnson, 1979; Fitzgerald et al., 1985; van der Sluis et al., 1985; Strugnell et al., 1984a; Strugnell et al., 1984b; Turner and Hollander, 1957; Wos and Wicher, 1985; Zeigler et al., 1976). Host-derived serum proteins, including albumin and immunoglobulin, are also present on its surface (Alderete and Baseman, 1979; Logan, 1974).

II. EPIDEMIOLOGY OF SYPHILIS

Syphilis is a sexually transmitted infection with worldwide distribution. Because the accuracy of prevalence data from individual countries is dependent upon the sophistication of the health care infrastructure, case-finding efforts, reporting practices, and other less-defined social factors, reliable estimates of the worldwide burden of syphilis are lacking. Until recent decades, syphilis was an extremely common disease even in developed nations. Various autopsy studies conducted in the United States in the first half of the twentieth century revealed a prevalence of 5-10% (Rosahn, 1947; Symmers, 1916) with 25% of the population affected in certain low socioeconomic groups (Olanksky et al., 1954). The initiation of widespread education and control efforts, in conjunction with the introduction of highly efficacious penicillin therapy, resulted in a dramatic decrease in the incidence of syphilis in the mid-1950s. In the past two decades, the incidence of early syphilis has increased slightly or remained steady in most countries (World Health Organization, 1982). The reported prevalence of primary and secondary syphilis in developed countries is two to 12 cases per 100,000 population (World Health Organization, 1982); in the United States, 30-35 cases of syphilis of all stages are reported annually per 100,000 population (U. S. Department of Health and Human Services, 1986).

In developing nations, syphilis is a major public health problem, with seropositivity rates in pregnant women in parts of Africa ranging from 10-30%. Congenital syphilis is a major cause of prematurity, stillbirth, infant morbidity, and neonatal death in these nations (Ratnam et al., 1982).

As with most sexually transmitted diseases, the peak prevalence of infection is in young adults, ages 15-34 years. The populations most affected by syphilis have changed dramatically in developed countries in the past 20 years. In the United States, the percentage of early syphilitic male patients who named a male sexual contact rose from 38% in 1969 to 70% in 1979, with a resulting change in the male/female ratio for early syphilis from 1.5:1 to 3.4:1. In the United Kingdom, the proportion of early syphilis cases acquired by homosexual contact rose from 42.4% in 1971 to 54% in 1977 (British Cooperative Clinical Group. 1980). Early epidemiological studies of patients with acquired immunodeficiency syndrome (AIDS) reflected this trend: 68% of homosexual AIDS patients had serological evidence of past syphilis, compared with 6% of heterosexual patients with AIDS (Guinan et al., 1984; Jaffe et al., 1983). In developed countries, then, syphilis has become a disease that disproportionately affects the homosexual and bisexual male population. The activities of bisexual individuals result in the involvement of females in community outbreaks as well.

The prevalence of symptomatic tertiary syphilis has decreased markedly in the antibiotic era, and the classic late manifestations of syphilis (gummas, aneurysms, tabes dorsalis, paresis) are rarely seen in developed nations. There have been reports, however, that central nervous system involvement may be increasing in prevalence (Chap. 8) but that the manifestations may be changing to more subtle, ill-defined syndromes than seen before the advent of antibiotics (Hotson, 1981).

III. PATHOGENESIS OF SYPHILIS

Syphilis is transmitted by direct, usually sexual, contact; the organisms rapidly penetrate mucous membranes or abraded skin where they multiply locally as well as disseminate throughout the body via the lymphatic and circulatory systems. *Treponema pallidum* attaches to the surface of mammalian cells in vitro, and this attachment is believed to play an important role in pathogenesis (Fitzgerald et al., 1975; Fitzgerald et al., 1977; Fitzgerald, 1983; Hayes et al., 1977). After a period of 10-90 days (average 3-6 weeks), the infectious primary lesion (chancre) appears at the site of inoculation. The chancre first appears as a small painless papule which quickly ulcerates producing an ulcer with an indurated, well-circumscribed border. Atypical lesions may resemble other ulcerative conditions of the genitalia, for example herpes or chancroid. The lesion heals spontaneously in 2-8 weeks. Within 1-3 months, the maculopapular rash of secondary syphilis appears on the trunk, extremities, and, uniquely, on the palms and soles. Papules around the vulva and perianal region become hypertrophic (condylomata lata) and, as they ulcerate, are often infectious; motile treponemes are frequently isolated from them. Primary and secondary syphilis are commonly accompanied by regional or generalized lymphadenopathy; secondary syphilis may also present with fever, malaise, and headache. Symptoms spontaneously resolve after 2-10 weeks, but may recur in 25% of patients during the first year. The patient is potentially infectious throughout the primary and secondary stages.

Untreated patients then enter a period of latency in which they are not infectious or symptomatic but continue to exhibit seropositivity in treponemal serological tests. Latency may persist for the lifetime of the patient or, in approximately 30% of untreated persons, progress to the late manifestations, including neurological (asymptomatic or symptomatic), cardiovascular, or gummatous syphilis.

The organism can cross the placenta, and fetal infection with *T. pallidum* ssp. *pallidum* can occur during any stage of infection in the mother, resulting in spontaneous abortion, stillbirth, prematurity, or congenital syphilis.

IV. EXPERIMENTAL MODELS OF SYPHILIS

Experimental infection of the rabbit with *T. pallidum* ssp. *pallidum* mimics some aspects of human syphilis (Collart et al., 1971; Turner and Hollander, 1957). Intradermal inoculation results in the appearance of a papular lesion that ulcerates and then heals spontaneously. The incubation period is inversely related to the number of organisms introduced. Intratesticular inoculation produces a nonulcerative orchitis that also resolves spontaneously. Latent infection persists for the life of the animal, and virulent organisms can be recovered from lymph nodes years after initial infection. True secondary or late manifestations are rarely, if ever, seen in the rabbit model. Multiple primary chancres, considered by some investigators to be the experimental equivalent of secondary syphilis, can be produced on the cooler parts of the rabbit's body by intravenous inoculation of *T. pallidum*. In fact, this infection is probably more analogous to congenital syphilis, which is a severe disseminated primary infection, rather than acquired secondary syphilis in which the host's immune system has already been sensitized. The intradermal inoculation of other animals, including chimpanzees (Brown et al., 1970), inbred hamsters (Schell et al., 1980) and guinea pigs (Pavia and Niederbuhl, 1985; Pierce et al., 1983) with *T. pallidum* has also proved useful in the study of the host response to infection.

V. HOST RESPONSE TO SYPHILIS INFECTION

A. Humoral Immune Response

Traditionally, the humoral immune response to treponemal infection has been measured by serological tests, including flocculation methods using nontreponemal cardiolipin-lecithin antigens [rapid plasma reagin (RPR), venereal disease research laboratory (VDRL) tests] and by immunofluorescence (fluorescent treponemal antibody absorption; FTA-ABS) or hemagglutination methods directed against antigens of *T. pallidum* ssp. *pallidum*, Nichols strain (Chap. 8). Both IgM and IgG antitreponemal antibodies are detectable in primary syphilis, and both continue to be produced throughout the course of the disease. Except in early primary syphilis, IgG reaches far higher titers than IgM.

Serum from humans and infected rabbits can immobilize and neutralize *T. pallidum* in the presence of complement (Bishop and Miller, 1976b; Nelson and Mayer, 1949); IgG has been shown to be the treponemicidal factor (Blanco et al., 1984). Passive administration of immune rabbit serum to uninfected recipients delays and alters the development of lesions following challenge, but protection is not complete (Bishop and Miller, 1976a; Graves and Alden, 1979; Perine et al., 1973; Sepetjian et al., 1973; Titus and Weiser, 1979; Turner et al., 1973; Weiser et al., 1976). In hamsters, immune serum confers complete protection against infection with *T. pallidum* ssp. *endemicum* (Azadegan et al., 1983) but only partial protection against infection with *T. pallidum* ssp. *pertenue* (Schell et al., 1978). Immune serum provides only incomplete protection against *T. pallidum* ssp. *pallidum* infection in guinea pigs (Pavia et al., 1985).

B. Cellular Immune Response

Examination of hematoxylin and eosin-stained sections of human syphilitic lesions reveals extensive infiltration by mononuclear cells, including lymphocytes, histiocytes, and large numbers of plasma cells (Johnson, 1972). In the experimental model, infection with *T. pallidum* ssp. *pallidum* results in a vigorous immune response with lymphoid hyperplasia and local infiltration by sensitized T cells (Lukehart et al., 1980a; Lukehart et al., 1981; Sell et al., 1980a; Sell et al., 1980b).

Numerous investigators have examined the cellular arm of the immune response using lymphocyte blast transformation, lymphokine release assays, and adoptive transfer. These studies have shown that T lymphocytes are sensitized to treponemal antigens early in infection (Lukehart et al., 1980b) and release soluble macrophage-activating factors (Lukehart, 1982). The phagocytosis of *T. pallidum* has been demonstrated in vitro (Lukehart and Miller, 1978) and in vivo (Lukehart et al., 1981; Sell et al., 1982). Despite the fact that humoral and cellular immunity are long-lived (Baker-Zander and Sell, 1980), some treponemes evade the immune response, resulting in persistent latent infection. The mechanism of *T. pallidum*'s ability to escape this early and vigorous immune response is unclear, but it may involve sequestration in immunologically privileged sites or the masking of antigens by bacterial or host-derived substances. A complete review of the host response to *T. pallidum* infection is available for the interested reader (Schell and Musher, 1983).

VI. ANTIGENIC ANALYSIS

A. Immunological Cross-Reactivity

Despite a lack of DNA homology between pathogenic and nonpathogenic treponemes, substantial immunological cross-reactivity exists between these organisms (Cannefax and Garson, 1959; Deacon and Hunter, 1962), and a protein component of *T. phagedenis* has been used for serodiagnosis of syphilis (Cannefax and Garson, 1959; D'Allessandro and Dardanoni, 1953). Immunization of experimental animals with nonpathogenic treponemes or their extracts, however, fails to confer any degree of protection against challenge with *T. pallidum* (Al-Samarrai and Henderson, 1976; Gelperin, 1951; Hindersson et al., 1985; Miller et al., 1963; Izzat et al., 1970).

Immunological cross-reactivity between *T. pallidum* ssp. *pallidum* and *T. pallidum* ssp. *pertenue* has been shown by the presence of similar serological cross-agglutination and immobilization titers in rabbits infected with these subspecies (Khan et al., 1951; Turner and Hollander, 1957) and by immunofluorescence reactivity (Al-Samarrai and Henderson, 1977). These similarities prevent the differentiation of syphilis, yaws, bejel, and pinta on the basis of serological testing alone.

Challenge experiments have shown varying degrees of cross-immunity between the pathogenic treponemes. Rabbits infected with *T. pallidum* ssp. *pallidum* or immunized with gamma-irradiated *T. pallidum* ssp. *pallidum* vaccine (Miller, 1973; Turner and Hollander, 1957) are only partially resistant to challenge with *T. pallidum* ssp. *pertenue*; infection with *T. pallidum* ssp. *pertenue* provides even less protection against challenge with *T. pallidum* ssp. *pallidum* (Turner and Hollander, 1957). In contrast, hamsters infected with either subspecies exhibit complete protection against symptomatic infection with heterologous organisms (Schell et al., 1982). In humans there are several early observations of concurrent syphilis and yaws infection, suggesting that little or no protection is afforded by one for the other. Yet, it is commonly accepted that syphilis is seldom seen in areas in which yaws is prevalent (Chesney, 1926).

Cross-immunity between different strains of *T. pallidum* ssp. *pallidum* is even less clearly defined. In rabbits differing degrees of cross-protection between the Nichols strain and two other patient-derived strains have been observed (Magnuson et al., 1951).

B. Early Antigenic Studies

Historically, studies of the antigenic nature of *T. pallidum* have focused on efforts to identify antigens of *T. pallidum* or *T. phagedenis* biotype Reiter which could be used for improved diagnostic methods or vaccine preparations. Proteins extracted from the Reiter treponeme were shown to react with sera from syphilis and yaws patients (D'Alessandro and Dardanoni, 1953; DeBruijn, 1959; Cannefax and Garson, 1959; Hardy et al., 1975) but, when injected into rabbits, failed to elicit antibodies capable of immobilizing *T. pallidum*. Both heat-stable and heat-labile antigens of *T. pallidum* have been described (Metzger and Podwinska, 1968; Miller et al., 1966). Attempts to extract polysaccharide antigens have met with limited success (Christiansen, 1964; Nell and Hardy, 1966), but Miller et al. (1969), extracted a heat-stable polysaccharide from the Nichols strain that reacted with sera from homologously infected rabbits. It did not, however, react with sera from patients with syphilis, suggesting its strain-specificity.

C. Molecular Characterization of Antigens

1.   Identification of Antigenic Molecules Using Polyvalent Antisera

Despite these early efforts, very little information about the molecular nature of treponemal antigens was forthcoming until the advent of newer technologies including sodium dodecyl sulfate-polyacrylamide gel electrophoresis (SDS-PAGE), two-dimensional gel electrophoresis, immunoblotting, radioimmunoprecipitation (RIP), and gene cloning.

The SDS-PAGE and immunoblotting methods have been employed by several investigators to examine the SDS-denatured polypeptide antigens of *T. pallidum*. Pooled immune rabbit sera (Baker-Zander and Lukehart, 1983; Hanff et al., 1983a; Lukehart et al., 1982; Penn et al., 1985) or sera from patients with secondary or early latent syphilis (Baker Zander et al., 1985; Hanff et al., 1982; Hensel et al., 1985) have initially been used to establish the antigenic profile of the organism (Fig. 1). As many as 22 treponemal molecules with molecular weights between 115,000 and 12,000 have been identified; eight polypeptides display strong reactivity with antibody, suggesting they may be major antigens, including a molecule with an approximate molecular weight 47,000. On the basis of RIP,

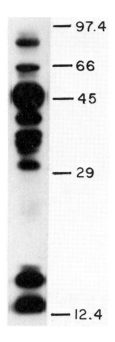

— 97.4

— 66

— 45

— 29

— l2.4

Fig. 1 Antigenic profile of *T. pallidum*, Nichols strain, as revealed by autoradiography with pooled syphilitic rabbit sera and ^{125}I-labeled protein A. Treponemes were disrupted by sonication, solubilized in 1% SDS, and electrophoresed on 12.5% polyacrylamide gels before electrophoretic transfer onto nitrocellulose paper for reaction with antibody and ^{125}I-labeled protein A. Twenty-two antigenic molecules were identified; positions of molecular weight standards are shown.

this molecule has been shown to have a surface location (Stamm and Bassford, 1985). Two-dimensional electrophoresis, consisting of isoelectric focusing followed by SDS-PAGE, has revealed approximately 60-70 antigenic treponemal molecules (Norris and Sell, 1984; Thornburg and Baseman, 1983).

2. Common Versus Pathogen-Specific Antigens

On the basis of the reactivities of normal (nonsyphilitic) human sera, four to 12 *T. pallidum* antigens are believed to share antigenic determinants with the Reiter treponeme (Baker-Zander et al., 1985; Baughn et al., 1983; Hanff et al., 1983b; Hensel et al., 1985; Limberger and Charon, 1985). Cross-absorption studies (Lukehart et al., 1982), using antisera raised against both *T. pallidum* and the Reiter treponeme, show five proteins with common antigenic determinants. Five of 40 Reiter treponemal proteins cross-react with human syphilitic sera by crossed-immunoelectrophoresis (Strandberg-Pedersen et al., 1980) indicating the presence of common determinants.

Treponema pallidum has also been shown to contain antigens in common with both pathogenic and nonpathogenic strains of *T. hyodysenteriae* and with pathogenic species of *Leptospira* and *Borrelia* (Baker-Zander and Lukehart, 1984). Some of these antigens also cross-react with the Reiter treponeme, suggesting the presence of group-specific antigens common to the order Spirochaetales.

Studies using polyclonal antibodies against *T. pallidum* have detected at least three molecules with pathogen-specific determinants (Jones et al., 1984; Lukehart et al., 1982). One is the 47,000- to 48,000-mol. wt. molecule that appears to contain both common and specific determinants, and two pathogen-specific molecules of 14,000 and 12,000 mol. wt. A 37,000-mol. wt. molecule may also contain both common and pathogen-specific determinants (Lukehart et al., 1982). Other molecules with common and/or pathogen-specific determinants have also been reported (Baughn et al., 1983; Hanff et al., 1983b; Moskophidis and Muller, 1984a,b; Penn et al., 1985).

3. Species and Strain Comparisons

The antigenic profiles of *T. pallidum* ssp. *pallidum* and *T. pallidum* ssp. *pertenue* have been compared using sera from rabbits with experimental syphilis or yaws (Baker-Zander and Lukehart, 1983; Stamm and Bassford, 1985; Thornburg and Baseman, 1983) or sera from patients with yaws (Baseman and Hayes, 1980) and the profiles of both organisms are virtually identical; minor differences in molecular weights were detected, but no unique polypeptides were identified.

Virtual molecular identity has also been seen with *T. carateum* by reacting sera from patients with pinta against *T. pallidum* antigens in the immunoblotting method (Fohn, Wignall, Baker-Zander, and Lukehart, unpublished observations). *Treponema pallidum* ssp. *pallidum* has also been shown to possess nearly complete antigenic identity with molecules of *T. paraluiscuniculi* (Baker-Zander and Lukehart, 1984).

Only minor differences between the Nichols strain of *T. pallidum* ssp. *pallidum* and other recently isolated strains have been detected using RIP (Stamm and Bassford, 1985) or immunoblotting (Lukehart and Baker-Zander, unpublished observations).

4. Location and Function of Antigenic Molecules

Immunoprecipitation of surface ^{125}I-labeled *T. pallidum* using immune rabbit sera or human syphilitic sera has detected outer membrane polypeptides with reported molecular weights of 89,500, 59,000, 42,500, 29,500, and 25,500 (Alderete and Baseman, 1980; Alderete and Baseman, 1981; Baseman and Hayes, 1980); some were avidly associated with host serum proteins (Alderete and Baseman, 1979). Other cell surface proteins and four extracellular protein antigens also have been described (Moskophidis and Muller, 1984b; Stamm and Baseford, 1985).

Mammalian cell-binding capabilities have been attributed to three of the outer membrane molecules (89,500, 37,000, and 32,000 mol. wt.) (Baseman and Hayes,

1980). These molecules also bind fibronectin (Peterson et al., 1983), and anti-
fibronectin antisera or purified fibronectin binding-domain can block the binding of [^{35}S] methionine-labeled treponemal molecules to cell monolayers (Peterson et al., 1983; Thomas et al., 1985a,b). The nature of fibronectin binding to
whole organisms has also been examined (Fitzgerald et al., 1984; Steiner and
Sell, 1985).

5. Humoral Response During Infection

Antibody responses of humans with syphilis to individual treponemal antigens
have been characterized (Baker-Zander et al., 1985; Baker-Zander et al., 1986;
van Eijk and van Embden, 1982; Hanff et al., 1982; Hensel et al., 1985; Moskophidis and Muller, 1984a). The IgG and IgM reactivity in patients with primary
syphilis is variable, but generally the number of molecules recognized by antibodies and the intensity of reactivity directly reflect the duration of clinical
symptoms (Baker-Zander et al., 1985). In secondary and early latent syphilis,
more uniform and intense staining of the full profile of treponemal antigens is
apparent. Therapeutic intervention at any stage of the disease causes a generalized
loss of antibody against individual antigens; the rate and degree of this loss is in-
verse proportional to the duration of symptoms and the stage of the disease before therapy (Baker-Zander et al., 1986).

Sera from individuals with biological false-positive tests for syphilis contain
antibodies that bind weakly to several common treponemal antigens (Baker-
Zander et al., 1985; Hanff et al., 1982; Hensel et al., 1985). Sera from persons
who have had sexual contact with individuals with infectious syphilis also display IgG reactivity to treponemal antigens; it is more intense than that seen in
normal sera and displays a broad range of reactivities, similar to those seen in
primary syphilis (Baker-Zander et al., 1985).

The ontogeny of the immune response to treponemal antigens in experimental syphilis has also been examined (Baughn et al., 1983; Hanff et al., 1983a;
Lukehart et al., 1986). Reactivity against the 37,000- and 47,000-mol. wt. molecules develops soon after inoculation, and antibodies against the full complement
of treponemal antigens are rapidly generated thereafter. Curative therapy early
in infection results in lower antibody titers, but does not interfere with the development of IgG antibody directed against the major treponemal antigens (Lukehart et al., 1986). Some of these antigens can also be detected as components
of the circulating immune complexes in sera obtained from rabbits with disseminated syphilis following intravenous inoculation of *T. pallidum* (Baughn et al.,
1983).

D. Gene Cloning

Several laboratories have successfully cloned genes for *T. pallidum* that encode
immunogenic proteins and these genes have been expressed in *Escherichia coli*

(van Embden et al., 1983; Fehniger et al., 1984; Hansen et al., 1985; Norgard and Miller, 1983; Stamm et al., 1982; Stamm et al., 1983; Walfield et al., 1982). Major protein antigens with molecular weights of 39,000, 35,000, 25,000 (Stamm et al., 1983), 44,000 (Norgard and Miller, 1983), 46,000 and 44,000 (van Embden et al., 1983), and 90,000 (Fehniger et al., 1984) have been reported. Partial DNA sequences of genes encoding two immunologically unrelated protein antigens with molecular weights of 44,000 and 35,000 have been determined (Hansen et al., 1985).

VII. PRODUCTION AND CHARACTERIZATION OF MONOCLONAL ANTIBODIES TO *TREPONEMA PALLIDUM*

Antigenic analysis of noncultivable organisms, such as *T. pallidum*, is technically difficult for several reasons. Because *T. pallidum* must be extracted from infected rabbit tissue, the acquisition of a sufficient quantity of bacteria is very costly and labor-intensive. In addition to treponemes, these extracts contain various amounts of host tissue, including erythrocytes, lymphocytes, spermatozoa, loosely and avidly associated serum proteins, and other noncellular material. Although gross cellular debris can be removed by differential centrifugation, the removal of bacteria-associated rabbit serum proteins has proved difficult. Vigorous washing and treatment with detergents has been avoided because of the risk of inadvertently removing the outer envelope or other antigenic material. Purification by Percoll density-gradient centrifugation (Hanff et al., 1984) is effective for removing loosely associated material but is probably not effective in removing all rabbit material.

Despite these technical difficulties, an impressive amount of information concerning the antigenic structure of *T. pallidum* has been amassed in the past 5 years. The recent development of hybridoma technology has provided useful tools for the identification and characterization of the nature, location, and functional properties of *T. pallidum* antigens. The following discussion will include strategies in the production and selection of *T. pallidum* monoclonal antibodies (MAbs), and their respective current and future contributions to the examination of treponemal antigens and to improved methods for the diagnosis of syphilis.

A. Production of Monoclonal Antibodies

A number of laboratories have produced MAbs with specificity for *T. pallidum*; only six, however, have published their results. This discussion will be limited to these published reports.

1. Immunization

The intended use of MAbs can, in some circumstances, suggest the optimal method for immunization of the mice whose lymphocytes will be used for hybridoma production. If the antibodies will be used to define antigens expressed during natural infection, the best method for producing such antibodies would, theoretically, be active infection of the mice. Unfortunately, that method is not optimal for syphilis. Infection of mice with *T. pallidum* results in self-limited asymptomatic disease accompanied by a poor humoral immune response (Saunders and Folds, 1985). Therefore, effective antibody production is accomplished by administering the bacteria using a standard immunization and boosting protocol, as for an inert antigen.

This immunizing preparation will also contain some contaminating rabbit testis material, and the immunized mouse will produce rabbit-reactive clones that may subsequently be confused with antitreponemal antibodies. Because the treponemal preparations used for screening also contain contaminating rabbit tissue, careful interpretation of these results is essential. Various methods for minimizing rabbit contamination of treponemal suspensions have been employed: differential centrifugation, density-gradient centrifugation, and continuous particle electrophoresis. The degree of purity obtained by these methods is variable and the benefits of increased purity must be weighed against the resultant reduced yield and potential damage to, or loss of, labile treponemal surface antigens. The use of intact, freshly isolated virulent *T. pallidum* by two laboratories was an attempt to preserve, at the cost of purity, loosely associated outer envelope antigens (Robertson et al., 1982; Saunders and Folds, 1983). In contrast, continuous particle electrophoresis-purified *T. pallidum* was used as the immunizing suspension by Lukehart et al. (1985) in an attempt to eliminate contaminating rabbit tissue. The laboratories that employed density-gradient centrifugation techniques for purification chose a moderate course (van Embden et al., 1983; Moskophidis and Muller, 1985; Thornburg and Baseman, 1983; Thornburg et al., 1985). Given the published data concerning the range of antigenic specificities of the MAbs produced with these various preparations, there is little, if any, apparent advantage in one purification method over another. Although the laboratories using less-purified treponemal suspensions reported a slightly higher rate of rabbit-reactive clones, this did not appear to affect the production of antitreponemal antibodies. All clones must ultimately be tested for reactivity against rabbit tissue, and rabbit-reactive clones can then be eliminated. This point will be discussed in screening strategies (Sect. VII.A.2).

The route of immunization, duration of immunization, and total dose of *T. pallidum* varied among the six laboratories. Although each laboratory included at least one intraperitoneal injection, there was no obvious advantage to other combinations of immunization routes. The duration of immunization varied from

24 days to 5 months, with a median of 6-8 weeks; no advantage in terms of numbers of clones or subclasses of immunoglobulins produced was apparent with
longer immunization schedules. The total number of *T. pallidum* used for immunization ranged from 7×10^7 to 1.2×10^9, with no clear benefit obtained
with larger inocula. All laboratories reported the production of numerous antibody-producing clones, except van Embden et al. (1983), who reported a total of
three clones from three separate fusions. This laboratory immunized with the lowest
number of organisms and was the only one that did not employ complete Freund's
adjuvant (CFA). In contrast, Lukehart et al. (1985) used a similar number of immunizing organisms, with CFA, and reported a high yield of *T. pallidum* clones.

All six laboratories employed standard fusion methodologies. Spleen cells
from the immunized mice were mixed with myeloma cells at ratios ranging from
4:1 to 10:1. In all studies, fusion was facilitated using polyethylene glycol (PEG),
and fusion products were selected in hypoxanthine, aminopterin, thymidine (HAT)
medium.

2. Screening Methods and Strategies

Enzyme-linked immunosorbent assay (ELISA) and solid phase radioimmunoassay,
which both use a 96-well configuration, have been used extensively for screening
the large numbers of wells required for MAb production. Most laboratories used
sonicated *T. pallidum* preparations in a single method for all screening assays. The
exception was Lukehart et al. (1985) who used a double-screening method at
each step, with initial identification of positive wells by ELISA and confirmation
by indirect immunofluorescence (IF) of whole organisms. Clearly, the screening
method should reflect the intended use of the antibodies: if immunofluorescence
is a desired application, IF screening should be performed early; a similar ration-
ale is appropriate if reactivity in immunoblotting is desired.

All putative antitreponemal antibodies must be tested for reactivity to normal rabbit testicular tissue (NRT). The stage at which this screening occurs, however, may affect the yield of the fusion. Primary fusion wells frequently contain
many hybridoma clones, and the use of a negative selection method (such as
screening against NRT) at this stage may result in the inadvertent loss of valuable
anti-*T. pallidum* clones. Hence, a positive-selection method (such as IF screening
with purified *T. pallidum*) in which reactivity is also based upon morphological
criteria, is useful. This confirms the presence of a desired clone in a primary well
and defers the elimination of rabbit-reactive clones to a later stage in which fewer
clones are represented in a single well.

B. Characterization of Monoclonal Antibody Reactivity to *Treponema pallidum* and Related Organisms

1. Reactivity with Nonpathogenic Treponemes

The antigenic cross-reactivity of the pathogenic and nonpathogenic treponemes
is well established and the preliminary identification of molecules containing

common and/or pathogen-specific determinants has been accomplished using polyvalent antisera (Section VI.C.). Monoclonal antibodies also provide useful tools for these analyses because they are inherently monospecific and circumvent the potential shortcomings of the absorption steps required with polyvalent antisera.

Four laboratories have reported the production of antitreponemal MAbs that recognize a determinant common to pathogenic and nonpathogenic treponemes as determined by ELISA, IF, or RIA (Lukehart et al., 1985; Moskophidis and Muller, 1985; Robertson et al., 1982; Saunders and Folds, 1983). The molecular specificities of such antibodies were examined by Lukehart et al. (1985) who showed, by immunoblotting, that antibody C2-1, that reacted with *T. pallidum*, four nonpathogenic treponemes, and two related spirochetes, identifies a 47,000- to 48,000-mol. wt. molecule of *T. pallidum*. A molecule with an identical apparent molecular weight was also shown to have pathogen-specific antigenic determinants (Sect. VI.C.2 and VII.B.2) (Table 2). This finding supports the hypothesis, based on results of studies with extensively absorbed polyvalent antisera, that both common and specific determinants reside on the 47,000- to 48,000-mol. wt. molecule (Lukehart et al., 1982). Preliminary two-dimensional electrophoresis studies indicate that both determinants are indeed found on a single molecule, rather than two comigrating molecules (Fohn, Baker-Zander, and Lukehart, unpublished results).

Table 2 Characterization of *T. pallidum* Antigens by MAb

Mol. wt.	Common determinant	Pathogen-specific determinant	Surface location	Immobilization
102,000	?[g]	+[g]	+[g]	+[g]
84,000		?[g]	+[g]	
45-48,000	+[a]	+[a-f]	+[c-f]	+[c,f]
44,000		+[b,f]	+[f]	+[f]
37,000		+[a]		
33,000		+[f]		+[f]
24,000		+[g]	+[g]	+[g]
15,500		+[f]		+[f]
12,000		+[a]		

Sources:
[a]Lukehart et al., 1985.
[b]van Embden et al., 1982.
[c]Jones et al., 1984.
[d]Marchitto et al., 1984.
[e]Thornburg et al., 1985.
[f]Moskophidis and Muller, 1985.
[g]Marchitto et al., 1986.

Antibody G2-1 (Lukehart et al., 1985) also reacts, as shown by ELISA and IF, with *T. pallidum*, four nonpathogenic treponemes, and two related spirochetes. Because it does not react in immunoblotting assays, the molecular specificity of this antibody is not yet known. These two antibodies, both IgM, fail to react against *Chlamydia trachomatis*-infected HeLa cells (Stephens et al., 1982); therefore, they appear to recognize a spirochete group determinant and not common bacterial or mammalian cell antigens.

2. Pathogen-Specific Monoclonal Antibodies

Most investigators have concentrated their efforts on those antibodies that react with only the pathogenic treponemes.

a. Range of Reactivity

Subspecies Differentiation: Many of these pathogen-specific antibodies have been examined for reactivity against *T. pallidum* ssp. *pertenue* and *T. pallidum* spp. *endemicum*. As described in Sect. I.A., the subspecies of *T. pallidum* have virtually total DNA homology but have shown little antigenic heterogeneity by immunological methods that use polyvalent antisera. Cross-protection studies, however, have suggested antigenic differences. Because of their exquisite sensitivity, the greatest promise for the serotyping of the subspecies lies with MAbs. Three laboratories have examined their antibodies for reactivity with other *T. pallidum* subspecies. Thornburg and Baseman (1983) reported identical binding, as shown by immunoblotting, of a MAb directed at a 45,000-mol. wt. molecule (probably the 47,000-48,000 molecule referred to earlier in this chapter) with both *T. pallidum* ssp. *pallidum* and *T. pallidum* ssp. *pertenue*. They also demonstrated by lactoperoxidase-catalyzed iodination that this molecule was less exposed on the surface of intact *T. pallidum* ssp. *pertenue* compared with *T. pallidum* ssp. *pallidum*. Marchitto and coworkers (1984) examined two MAbs directed against the 47,000-mol. wt. molecule for reactivity with *T. pallidum* ssp. *pertenue* and *T. pallidum* ssp. *endemicum* by RIA, immunoblotting, and surface-binding assays. Although both antibodies reacted equally well with all three organisms in RIA and immunoblotting assays, the surface-binding assays revealed significantly lower binding of these antibodies to *T. pallidum* ssp. *pertenue* than to *T. pallidum* ssp. *pallidum*. The authors hypothesized that, although the determinant was found in all subspecies, its orientation on the surface differed between organisms, altering its availability for antibody binding, consistent with the findings of Thornburg and Baseman (1983).

Preliminary studies in our laboratory (unpublished results) support this hypothesis. Differential IF reactivity of five MAbs has been shown with *T. pallidum* ssp. *pallidum* and *T. pallidum* ssp. *pertenue*. Although fluorescence was apparent at high antibody concentrations with both organisms, the intensity of the fluorescence differed. Upon titration of the antibodies, strong reactivity persisted against *T. pallidum* ssp. *pallidum*, whereas reactivity to *T. pallidum* ssp. *pertenue* disappeared. When these same antibodies were tested by ELISA and RIA using sonicated organisms, equivalent reactivity was found, supporting the hypothesis that determinants may be present in both organisms but are altered in the degree of surface exposure in intact *T. pallidum* ssp. *pertenue*.

Recognition of Different Strains of *T. pallidum* ssp. *pallidum*: All anti-*T. pallidum* MAbs that have been reported were produced against the Nichols strain of *T. pallidum* ssp. *pallidum*. This strain, which has been passaged in rabbits since its isolation in 1915, remains the antigen source for current serological tests for syphilis. Cross-protection studies, however, have shown minor antigenic differences between different strains of *T. pallidum* ssp. *pallidum*. The value of MAbs produced against one strain for diagnostic purposes or for the identification of relevant antigens is dependent upon the reactivity of those antibodies with modern "street strains." Two laboratories have reported the reactivities of their MAbs with strains other than the immunizing strain. Lukehart et al. (1985) demonstrated that the IF reactivity of 13 antibodies against four recently isolated (fewer than five passages in rabbits) strains of *T. pallidum* was comparable with that observed with the Nichols strain. Eight antibodies described by Saunders and Folds (1983) reacted equally well with the Street 14 and Nichols strains of *T. pallidum*.

The H9-1 antibody produced by Lukehart et al. (1985) has also been used for the identification of *T. pallidum* organisms that have never been passaged in rabbits. Treponemes have been identified by IF with this antibody in lesion exudates from patients in the United States, Canada (Sect. IX.A.), Zambia, and Kenya (unpublished results), indicating that the determinant defined by H9-1 on the 47,000- to 48,000-mol. wt. molecule has been highly conserved from 1915 to the present. Marchitto et al. (1986) have also recently reported the IF reactivity of several of their antibodies with treponemes in impression smears of human genital ulcers.

b. Identification and Characterization of Pathogen-Specific Antigens. As described in Sect. VI.C., 22 antigenic molecules of *T. pallidum* have been defined by various authors using SDS-PAGE and immunoblotting; even more antigens may be visible by two-dimensional gel electrophoresis. Monoclonal antibodies with specificities for many of these major antigens have been reported (see Table 2).

The 47,000- to 48,000-Molecular Weight Antigen: All laboratories who examined the molecular specificities of their MAbs reported production of antibodies with reactivity against the immunodominant 47,000- to 48,000-mol. wt. molecule. Although the published molecular weights for this molecule range from 45,000 to 48,000, most investigators agree that this molecule contains one or more pathogen-specific determinants, based on studies with MAbs and absorbed polyclonal antisera. By use of MAbs, this molecule has been demonstrated on the surface of *T. pallidum* by immunoelectron microscopy (Marchitto et al., 1984; Walker, Bishop, and Lukehart, unpublished results), surface-binding assays (Marchitto et al., 1984), and RIP of lactoperoxidase-catalyzed surface iodinated treponemal antigens (Jones et al., 1984; Moskophidis and Muller, 1985). Monoclonal antibodies to pathogen-specific determinants on the 47,000- to 48,000-mol. wt. molecule can immobilize or neutralize *T. pallidum* in the presence of complement (Jones et al., 1984; Moskophidis and Muller, 1985). Additionally, there is preliminary evidence that a MAb directed against this molecule can block the attachment of viable *T. pallidum* to eukaryotic cells in tissue culture (reported in Jones et al., 1984).

Other Pathogen-Specific Antigens Defined by Monoclonal Antibodies: Lukehart and coworkers (1985) also described MAbs with specificity for molecules with relative molecular weights of 37,000 and 12,000. Moskophidis and Muller (1985) produced MAbs with reactivity for the 15,500-, 33,000-, and 44,000-mol. wt. molecules; antibodies against each of these molecules were reactive in the *T. pallidum* immobilization test (TPI). Marchitto et al. (1986) recently reported antibodies against 102,000-, 84,000-, and 24,000-mol. wt. molecules; MAbs directed against the 102,000- and 24,000-mol. wt. molecules were reactive in the TPI test. Although they also reported antibodies with specificities for the 29,000-, 32,000-, and 52,000- to 54,000-mol. wt. molecules, these data were unconvincing because of the poor quality of the negative controls.

VIII. LIMITATIONS IN EXISTING METHODS FOR DIAGNOSIS OF SYPHILIS

Syphilis diagnosis is currently based upon several criteria: history, clinical presentation, serological testing, and identification of *T. pallidum* in lesions or tissues. None of these methods alone is sensitive and specific in all stages of disease, and frequently the findings for each criterion must be synthesized by the clinician into a "best-guess" diagnosis. Culture diagnosis can be used for herpes simplex virus and *Haemophilus ducreyi*, two other common causes of genital ulceration, but it is not available for *T. pallidum*. Although syphilis is responsible for 20% of genital ulcer disease in the United States and Europe, it must be considered in the differential diagnosis of all genital ulcerations. Syphilis also must be considered in the evaluation of many other seemingly disparate clinical presentations including skin rashes, persistent headaches, visual or hearing abnormalities, dementia, and other neurological abnormalities, aortitis, and liver or kidney dysfunction.

A. History

Although a history of exposure to syphilis, or a history of unexplained ulceration or rash, is often helpful in directing diagnostic efforts, historical information is often unreliable; lack of corroborating historical evidence should never eliminate the consideration of syphilis in any patient.

B. Clinical Presentation

Syphilis has been called "the great imitator" because of the myriad clinical manifestations attributed to *T. pallidum* infection. The most common manifestation of primary syphilis is a painless ulcerative lesion, or chancre. While these lesions are characteristically single, well-circumscribed, and indurated, atypical presentations are common, and clinical impression may be misleading. In an evaluation of the specificity of the diagnosis of penile ulceration that is based on clinical presentation alone, the accuracy for diagnosis of syphilis was 78% among well-trained clinicians in a sexually transmitted disease clinic (Chapel et al., 1977). In other settings where syphilis is less frequently observed, this value would undoubtedly be lower. Rectal chancres may be painful and superinfected and may cause symptoms of proctitis. Vaginal or cervical chancres are usually asymptomatic and are not recognized. The rash of secondary syphilis may be confused with other dermatological conditions including eczema, pityriasis rosea, tinea versicolor, and psoriasis. It may also be so subtle as to be unrecognized by the patient or clinician. Condylomata lata may be easily confused with genital warts (condylomata acuminata). Latent syphilis may persist for decades and lack any clinical manifestation, whereas tertiary syphilis may involve virtually any organ of the body, including the central nervous system. There are few, if any, clinical manifestations that are specific for tertiary syphilis.

C. Serological Testing

The currently available methods for serological diagnosis of syphilis are discussed in detail in Chap. 8. There are several points concerning the sensitivity and specificity of these tests that warrant consideration here as well. As shown in Table 3,

Table 3   Reactivity of Serological Tests in Untreated Syphilis

	Stage of disease, % positive			
	Primary	Secondary	Latent	Late
VDRL, RPR	59-87	100	73-91	37-94
FTA-ABS	86-100	99-100	96-99	96-100
MHA-TP	64-87	96-100	96-100	94-100

Source: Modified (with permission) from Jaffe, H. (1984). Management of the reactive serology. In *Sexually Transmitted Diseases* (Holmes, K. K., Mardh, P. A., Sparling, P. F., and Weisner, P. J., eds.). McGraw-Hill, New York.

the nontreponemal screening tests (RPR, VDRL) may be insensitive in stages of syphilis other than secondary. This is a particular diagnostic problem in early primary syphilis when cardiolipin antibodies may not yet have been produced. The standard practice of repeating a nonreactive serological test after 1-3 weeks in patients with suspect lesions is not ideal because of the risk of transmission to others during that interval. Empirical therapy for such patients is also undesirable.

The treponemal tests (FTA-ABS, MHA-TP) are more sensitive than the nontreponemal tests in latent and tertiary disease but have variable sensitivities in primary syphilis. While the FTA-ABS is more sensitive than the VDRL and RPR in the primary stage, the specificity of this test decreases when it is used for routine screening, and its use for this purpose is not recommended. The hemagglutination tests are less sensitive than the VDRL and RPR in primary syphilis. Another confounding factor in the interpretation of the treponemal serological tests is that they frequently remain reactive after adequate therapy, making it extremely difficult to assess possible reinfection (Chap. 8 Sect. III).

D. Microscopic Identification of *Treponema pallidum* in Lesions

Even when serological testing can be used for the diagnosis of syphilis, the delay in obtaining the result from the laboratory may range from days to a week or more; such a delay is particularly unfortunate in patients with potentially infectious (primary and secondary) lesions. Hence, the rapid identification of *T. pallidum* in the clinic or physician's office can help establish an early diagnosis so that therapy can be initiated. The standard method for the identification of *T. pallidum* in primary or secondary lesions is darkfield microscopic examination of exudate obtained from the lesion. This method involves the identification of a motile, spiral-shaped organism with morphology and motility characteristic of *T. pallidum* (Fig. 2). The specificity of darkfield microscopy is solely dependent upon the skill of the microscopist in distinguishing *T. pallidum* from the numerous commensal spirochetes that are found in the normal flora of the genital and rectal mucosal surfaces. Even a skilled microscopist should not attempt to perform a darkfield examination of oral lesions because of the similar-appearing nonpathogenic treponemes found there.

Although a positive test is useful in establishing a diagnosis of syphilis, darkfield-negative lesions may still be treponemal. The sensitivity of the darkfield examination, which has been shown to be 74% in primary syphilis (Daniels and Ferneyhough, 1977), can be affected by the common practice among patients of self-treatment with antibiotics or antibacterial ointments, by the natural resolution of the lesion, or by interference with microscopic identification by refractile tissue debris and erythrocytes. There are relatively few well-trained darkfield microscopists or darkfield microscopes except in STD clinics; therefore, the practical application of this test for most syphilis patients is limited.

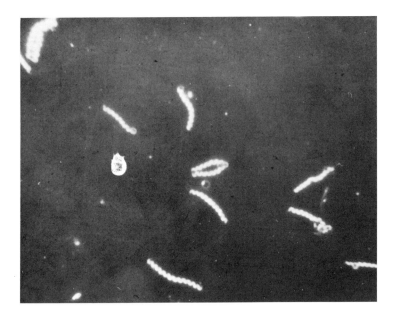

Fig. 2   Darkfield microscopic appearance of *T. pallidum* ssp. *pallidum* (*Source*: courtesy of Dr. James N. Miller).

A laboratory-based alternative to darkfield microscopy uses polyvalent rabbit anti-*T. pallidum* antiserum to detect treponemes in lesion exudate by direct fluorescent antibody staining (DFA-TP test) (Edwards, 1962). Because polyvalent antisera raised against *T. pallidum* contain antibodies that react with antigens common to the pathogenic as well as nonpathogenic treponemes, the antiserum used for the DFA-TP test is extensively absorbed with nonpathogenic treponemes in an effort to obtain a specific reagent (Jue et al., 1967; Kellogg and Mothershed, 1969; Wilkinson and Cowell, 1971).

Both darkfield microscopy and the DFA-TP test can be used for the evaluation of lesions in primary or secondary syphilis or those of the nasal mucosa (syphilitic rhinitis) or skin in early congenital syphilis. Cerebrospinal fluid and other body fluids (aqueous humor, endolymph) have also been examined for *T. pallidum* using darkfield and immunofluorescence microscopy (Davis and Sperry, 1978; Smith and Israel, 1967). The sensitivity and specificity of these tests in body fluids have been questioned (Brown, 1969; Montenegro et al., 1969) but have not been evaluated in a controlled study.

E. Identification of *Treponema pallidum* in Tissues

Diagnosis of syphilis is occasionally made or confirmed by identification of *T. pallidum* in tissue specimens. Silver staining, the standard method for identification of spirochetes in tissue, has been used to identify treponemes in placental tissue, lesion biopsy material, aorta, heart, liver, and brain. When the possibility of syphilis is highly suspected, silver staining can be useful, but caution must be exercised when only a few organisms are seen or when stained forms are not classic spirochetes. Many normal tissue components, such as collagen, are also stained and may be easily confused for spiral organisms.

Immunohistochemical methods, such as immunofluorescence (Al-Samarrai and Henderson, 1977; Yobs et al., 1964) or immunoperoxidase (Beckett and Bigbee, 1979) staining using polyvalent rabbit anti-*T. pallidum* antiserum, have been described for the identification of *T. pallidum* in tissue specimens; these methods, however, have been primarily confined to research laboratories, but they have the advantage over silver staining of immunological specificity. Immunofluorescence staining has been used for the identification of *T. pallidum* in lymph nodes of patients before and after therapy (Yobs et al., 1965) and for examination of the progression and resolution of primary infection in the rabbit model (Baker-Zander and Sell, 1980; Lukehart et al., 1980a; Sell et al., 1980b; Sell et al., 1982).

IX. USE OF MONOCLONAL ANTIBODIES FOR THE DETECTION OF *TREPONEMA PALLIDUM*

Detection of *T. pallidum* is used primarily in the evaluation of suspicious genital ulceration or skin rashes. If organisms can be identified, a definitive diagnosis can be made, even in the absence of reactive serology. Because of the limitations of existing methods and the difficulties encountered in distinguishing pathogenic from nonpathogenic treponemes, MAbs, with their inherent specificity, promise to be extremely useful tools in this aspect of syphilis diagnosis.

They have several potential advantages over standard darkfield microscopy: (1) Motile treponemes are not required for identification. Accurate differentiation of *T. pallidum* from commensal spirochetes by darkfield microscopy is dependent upon the examination of actively motile organisms, thus specimens must be examined within 10-30 min. Furthermore, treponemes that are readily accessible on the surface of the lesion are usually nonmotile and cannot be evaluated accurately by darkfield microscopy; they are still evaluable by immunological methods. (2) The specificity of the test is inherent. Accurate interpretation of darkfield microscopic findings is dependent upon the very specialized expertise of the microscopist. Detection methods based upon MAb reactions are inherently as specific as the antibody reagent, and accurate interpretation of results can be accomplished by laboratory personnel with minimal training. Oral lesions, which cannot be evaluated by darkfield microscopy, can be accurately examined using pathogen-specific MAbs. (3) The test could be widely available. Because darkfield microscopes are rarely available except in specialty clinics, many physicians must choose either to make a diagnosis based on only clinical presentation and serological testing or to refer their patient to a STD clinic for evaluation. The availability of a sensitive and specific laboratory-based treponemal detection method would provide the clinician with a valuable diagnostic tool. Although MAb-based detection methods are unlikely to replace the rapid, inexpensive darkfield microscope in STD clinics, they have an important potential role for private physicians.

A. Direct Immunofluorescence

Lukehart et al. (1985) first described the identification of *T. pallidum* in lesion exudate using a fluorescein-labeled pathogen-specific MAb [Fig. 3 (see Plate II, facing p. 205)] and this method has been evaluated for the detection of *T. pallidum* in two reported clinical trials. Monoclonal antibody H9-1, which is specific for the 47,000- to 48,000-mol. wt. antigen of *T. pallidum*, has been shown by ELISA and immunofluorescence to react with *T. pallidum* subspecies but not with the nonpathogenic *T. phagedenis* biotype Reiter, *T. denticola, T. refringens,* or *T. vincentii,* nor with the related spirochetes *Leptospira interrogans* and *Borrelia recurrentis.* For this test, the antibody is partially purified from mouse ascites fluid by ammonium sulfate precipitation and conjugated with fluorescein isothiocyanate. The reagent is stable in the refrigerator or freezer for many months. Lesion exudate collected on a microscope slide, as for darkfield microscopy, is air-dried and fixed in acetone for 2-10 min, then transported to a laboratory where immunofluorescent staining and microscopic examination can be performed easily within 30 min. The addition of Evans blue counterstain to the antibody allows a greater contrast between the stained cellular debris (red) and the brightly fluorescent treponemes (green).

At the Seattle-King County STD clinic, 61 patients with genital ulcerations or skin rashes were evaluated for syphilis using the direct MAb test (Hook et al., 1985). Treponemes were identified by MAb staining in all 30 (100%) patients with syphilis, whereas darkfield microscopy was positive in 29 of 30 (97%). Of the 31 patients who did not have syphilis, spirochetes were identified by darkfield microscopy in seven (23%); specimens from these patients were negative for *T. pallidum* using the MAb test. In five of these seven patients, commensal spirochetes were identified by staining with another MAb, C2-1, which recognizes an antigenic determinant common to all spirochetes tested to date (Lukehart et al., 1985). In this study, the MAb test was 100% sensitive and specific for *T. pallidum* compared with the final diagnosis that was based on standard methods. In a similar evaluation of 128 patients at the Alberta STD clinic (Romanowski et al., 1984), the MAb test was positive in 73% of syphilis patients,

compared with 79% for darkfield microscopy; the Mab test and darkfield microscopy were 100% specific in this study.

As with any antigen detection method, the sensitivity of the test depends
upon the quality of the specimen collected. In syphilitic lesions, where the number of organisms is variable depending upon the stage of evolution of the lesion
and the use of antibacterial substances by the patient, single specimens may not
be adequate. Darkfield microscopic examination is not considered to be negative
until multiple slides have been examined on several separate occasions (U.S. Department of Health, Education, and Welfare, 1969). Similarly, multiple specimens
should be collected for Mab staining to ensure maximum sensitivity. All slides
need not be examined, however; the identification of a single organism on any
slide is sufficient for diagnosis.

B. Solid Phase Immunoblot Assay

Norgard et al. (1984) described a solid phase immunoblot assay for the detection
of *T. pallidum* using MAbs. Specimens were air-dried onto nitrocellulose filter
paper and *T. pallidum* was detected using MAb, ^{125}I-labeled rabbit antimouse
IgG, and autoradiography. Three MAbs were able to detect 10^3 treponemes, and
one antibody could detect as few as 500 organisms with a 2- to 4-day autoradiography period. The antibodies with the highest sensitivity were specific for the
47,000-mol. wt. antigen. The specificity of this method was examined using *T.
phagedenis* biotype Reiter, *Haemophilus ducreyi, Neisseria gonorrhoeae,* herpes
simplex virus type 2, and normal rabbit tissue. This test was developed using *T.
pallidum* extracted from infected rabbit tissue, but the sensitivity and specificity
of the method in clinical specimens has not been examined. Because 500 organisms appear to be the lower level of detectability in this assay, even after prolonged
autoradiographic exposure, its applicability in a clinical setting is questionable.

X. POTENTIAL VALUE OF MONOCLONAL ANTIBODIES IN DIAGNOSIS OF SYPHILIS

The most obvious direct application of Mab in the diagnosis of syphilis is the
identification of *T. pallidum* in material from lesions or tissues. To date, *T. pallidum* in clinical specimens has been examined using only direct or indirect immunofluorescence. This methodology is fast, sensitive, and specific and is applicable to early infectious and congenital syphilis, as well as to any biopsy or autopsy tissue. At present, such reagents are only available in research laboratories.
If they should become commercially available, perhaps in combination with MAbs
for the detection of other genital ulcer pathogens, the applicability would be wide.
The ability of a physician to collect material from an ulcer on two or three wells
of a slide and to learn, within a day, whether the patient had syphilis or herpes

or both, would be an important practical advance in the diagnosis of genital ulcer disease.

A major diagnostic problem in syphilis is the identification of sensitive and specific criteria for confirming central nervous system involvement (Chap. 8, Sect. IV.C). A sensitive method for the detection of treponemal antigens in body fluids, particularly CSF is needed. The solid phase immunoblot assay described by Norgard et al. (1984) might be applicable to body fluids if the sensitivity could be increased 10- to 100-fold. The development of an assay for capturing and detecting *T. pallidum* organisms as well as particulate or soluble treponemal antigens should be pursued using a combination of polyvalent antisera (capture) and MAbs (specific detection).

XI. OTHER POTENTIAL USES OF MONOCLONAL ANTIBODIES TO *TREPONEMA PALLIDUM*

Monoclonal antibodies with specificities for antigens of *T. pallidum* can provide excellent tools for elucidating and characterizing the location and relationships of these antigens. As described earlier, information has already been accumulated regarding the degree of surface exposure of shared antigens of *T. pallidum* ssp. *pallidum* and *T. pallidum* ssp. *pertenue*. This type of information may provide insight into the differences in pathogenic mechanisms of the subspecies.

More importantly, MAbs can be used in affinity chromatography techniques to purify pathogen-specific antigens in quantities sufficient to provide reagents for diagnostic use, with resulting improved sensitivity and specificity. These purified antigens can also be used for characterization of the host humoral and cellular immune response, and ultimately, for vaccine development.

ACKNOWLEDGMENTS

The authors thank Sally Post for excellent manuscript preparation. This work was supported by Public Health Grants AI 18988 and NS 23677 from the National Institutes of Health.

REFERENCES

Alderete, J. F. and Baseman, J. B. (1979). Surface-associated host proteins on virulent *Treponema pallidum*. *Infect. Immun. 26*:1048-1056.
Alderete, J. F. and Baseman, J. B. (1980). Surface characterization of virulent *Treponema pallidum*. *Infect. Immun. 30*:814-823.
Alderete, J. F. and Baseman, J. B. (1981). Analysis of serum IgG against *Treponema pallidum* protein antigens in experimentally infected rabbits. *Br. J. Vener. Dis. 57*:302-308.

Al-Samarrai, H. T. and Henderson, W. G. (1976). Immunity in syphilis: Studies in active immunity. *Br. J. Vener. Dis.* *52*:300-308.

Al-Samarrai, H. T. and Henderson, W. G. (1977). Immunofluorescent staining of *Treponema pallidum* and *Treponema pertenue* in tissue fixed by formalin and embedded in paraffin wax. *Br. J. Vener. Dis.* *53*:1-11.

Azadegan, A. A., Schell, R. F., and LeFrock, J. L. (1983). Immune serum confers protection against syphilitic infection on hamsters. *Infect. Immun.* *42*: 42-47.

Baker-Zander, S. A., Hook, III, E. W., Bonin, P., Handsfield, H. H., and Lukehart, S. A. (1985). Antigens of *Treponema pallidum* recognized by IgG and IgM antibodies during syphilis in humans. *J. Infect. Dis.* *151*:264-272.

Baker-Zander, S. A. and Lukehart, S. A. (1983). Molecular basis of immunological cross-reactivity between *Treponema pallidum* and *Treponema pertenue*. *Infect. Immun.* *42*:634-638.

Baker-Zander, S. A. and Lukehart, S. A. (1984). Antigenic cross-reactivity between *Treponema pallidum* and other pathogenic members of the family Spirochaetaceae. *Infect. Immun.* *46*:116-121.

Baker-Zander, S. A., Roddy, R. E., Handsfield, H. H., and Lukehart, S. A. (1986). IgG and IgM antibody reactivity to antigens of *Treponema pallidum* following treatment of syphilis. *Sex. Transm. Dis.* *13*:214-220.

Baker-Zander, S. A. and Sell, S. (1980). A histopathologic and immunologic study of the course of syphilis in the experimentally infected rabbit. Demonstration of long-lasting cellular immunity. *Am. J. Pathol.* *101*:387-414.

Barbieri, J. T. and Cox, C. D. (1979). Pyruvate oxidation by *Treponema pallidum*. *Infect. Immun.* *25*:157-163.

Barbieri, J. T. and Cox, C. D. (1981). Influence of oxygen on respiration and glucose catabolism by *Treponema pallidum*. *Infect. Immun.* *31*:992-997.

Baseman, J. B. and Hayes, E. C. (1980). Molecular characterization of receptor binding proteins and immunogens of virulent *Treponema pallidum*. *J. Exp. Med.* *151*:573-586.

Baughn, R. E., Adams, C. B., and Musher, D. M. (1983). Circulating immune complexes in experimental syphilis: Identification of treponemal antigens in isolated complexes. *Infect. Immun.* *42*:585-593.

Beckett, J. H. and Bigbee, J. W. (1979). Immunoperoxidase localization of *Treponema pallidum*. *Arch. Pathol. Lab. Med.* *103*:135-138.

Bishop, N. H. and Miller, J. N. (1976a). Humoral immunity in experimental syphilis. I. The demonstration of resistance conferred by passive immunization. *J. Immunol.* *117*:191-196.

Bishop, N. H. and Miller, J. N. (1976b). Humoral immunity in experimental syphilis. II. The relationship of neutralizing factors in immune serum to acquired resistance. *J. Immunol.* *117*:197-207.

Blanco, D. R., Miller, J. N., and Hanff, P. A. (1984). Humoral immunity in experimental syphilis: The demonstration of IgG as a treponemicidal factor in immune rabbit serum. *J. Immunol.* *133*:2693-2697.

British Cooperative Clinical Group (1980). Homosexuality and venereal disease in the United Kingdom. *Br. J. Vener. Dis.* *56*:6-11.

Brown, B. C. (1969). Spiral organisms in body fluids. *Am. J. Ophthalmol. 68*: 945-949.

Brown, W. J., Kuhn, U. S. G., Tolliver, E. A., and Norins, L. C. (1970). Experimental syphilis in the chimpanzee. Immunoglobulin class of early antibodies reactive with *Treponema pallidum. Br. J. Vener. Dis. 46*:198-200.

Cannefax, G. R. and Garson, W. (1959). The demonstration of a common antigen in Reiter's treponeme and virulent *Treponema pallidum. J. Immunol. 82*:198-200.

Chapel, T. A., Brown, W. J., Jeffries, C., and Stewart, J. A. (1977). How reliable is the morphological diagnosis of penile ulcerations? *Sex. Transm. Dis. 4*: 150-152.

Chesney, A. M. (1926). Immunity in syphilis. *Medicine 5*:463-547.

Christiansen, A. H. (1964). Studies on the antigenic structure of *T. pallidum*. 5. Attempts to isolate polysaccharide antigen from Nichols' pathogenic strain. *Acta Pathol. Microbiol. Scand. 61*:141-149.

Christiansen, S. (1963). Protective layer covering pathogenic treponemata. *Lancet 1*:423-425.

Collart, P., Franceschini, P., and Durel, P. (1971). Experimental rabbit syphilis. *Br. J. Vener. Dis. 47*:389-400.

Cox, C. D. and Barber, M. K. (1974). Oxygen uptake by *Treponema pallidum. Infect. Immun. 10*:123-127.

Cumberland, M. C. and Turner, T. B. (1949). The rate of multiplication of *Treponema pallidum* in normal and immune rabbits. *Am. J. Syph. Gon. Vener. Dis. 33*:201-212.

D'Allesandro, G. and Dardanoni, L. (1953). Isolation and purification of the protein antigen of the Reiter treponeme. A study of its serologic reactions. *Am. J. Syphilol. 37*:137-150.

Daniels, K. C. and Ferneyhough, H. S. (1977). Specific direct fluorescent antibody detection of *Treponema pallidum. Health Lab. Sci. 14*:164-171.

Davis, L. E. and Sperry, S. (1978). Bell's palsy and secondary syphilis: CSF spirochetes detected by immunofluorescence. *Ann. Neurol. 4*:378-380.

Deacon, W. E. and Hunter, E. F. (1962). Treponemal antigens as related to identification and syphilis serology. *Proc. Soc. Exp. Biol. 110*:352-356.

DeBruijn, J. H. (1959). Investigations into the antigenic structure of the Reiter strain of *Treponema pallidum*. II. The complex nature of the protein fraction. *Antonie Leeuwenhoek J. Microbiol. 25*:41-45.

Edwards, E. A. (1962). Detecting *Treponema pallidum* in primary lesions by the fluorescent antibody technique. *Public Health Rep. 77*:427-430.

Eijk, R. V. W. van and Embden, J. D. A. van (1982). Molecular characterization of *Treponema pallidum* proteins responsible for the human immune response to syphilis. *Antonie Leeuwenhoek J. Microbiol. 48*:486-487.

Embden, J. D. van, Donk, H. J. van der, Eijk, R. V. van, Heide, H. G. van der, De Jong, J. A., Olderen, M. F. van, Osterhaus, A. D., and Schouls, L. M. (1983). Molecular cloning and expression of *Treponema pallidum* DNA in *Escherichia coli* K-12. *Infect. Immun. 42*:187-196.

Fehniger, T. E., Walfield, A. M., Cunningham, T. M., Radolf, J. D., Miller, J. N., and Lovett, M. A. (1984). Purification and characterization of a cloned protease-resistant *Treponema pallidum*-specific antigen. *Infect. Immun. 46*: 598-607.

Fieldsteel, A. H., Cox, D. L., and Moeckli, R. A. (1981). Cultivation of virulent *Treponema pallidum* in tissue culture. *Infect. Immun. 32*:908-915.

Fitzgerald, T. J. (1983). Attachment of treponemes to cell surfaces. In *Pathogenesis and Immunology of Treponemal Infection* (R. F. Schell and D. M. Musher, eds.). Marcel Dekker, New York, pp. 195-228.

Fitzgerald, T. J. and Johnson, R. C. (1979). Surface mucopolysaccharides of *Treponema pallidum*. *Infect. Immun. 24*:244-251.

Fitzgerald, T. J., Johnson, R. C., Miller, J. N., and Sykes, J. A. (1977). Characterization of the attachment of *Treponema pallidum* (Nichols strain) to cultured mammalian cells and the potential relationship of attachment to pathogenicity. *Infect. Immun. 18*:467-478.

Fitzgerald, T. J., Miller, J. N., Repesh, L. A., Rice, M., and Urquhart, A. (1985). Binding of glycosaminoglycans to the surface of *Treponema pallidum* and subsequent effects on complement interactions between antigen and antibody. *Genitourin. Med. 61*:13-20.

Fitzgerald, T. J., Miller, J. N., and Sykes, J. A. (1975). *Treponema pallidum* (Nichols strain) in tissue cultures: Cellular attachment, entry, and survival. *Infect. Immun. 11*:1133-1140.

Fitzgerald, T. J. and Repesh, L. A. (1985). Interactions of fibronectin with *Treponema pallidum*. *Genitourin. Med. 61*:147-155.

Fitzgerald, T. J., Repesh, L. A., Blanco, D. R., and Miller, J. N. (1984). Attachment of *Treponema pallidum* to fibronectin, laminin, collagen IV, and collagen I, and blockage of attachment by immune rabbit IgG. *Br. J. Vener. Dis. 60*:357-363.

Gelperin, A. (1951). Immunochemical studies of the Reiter spirochete. *Am. J. Syphilol. 35*:1-13.

Graves, S. and Alden, J. (1979). Limited protection of rabbits against infection with *Treponema pallidum* by immune rabbit sera. *Br. J. Vener. Dis. 55*:399-403.

Guinan, M. E., Thomas, P. A., Pinsky, P. F., Goodrich, J. T., Selik, R. M., Jaffe, H. W., Haverkos, H. W., Noble, G., and Curran, J. W. (1984). Heterosexual and homosexual patients with the acquired immunodeficiency syndrome. A comparison of surveillance, interview, and laboratory data. *Ann. Intern. Med. 100*:213-218.

Hanff, P. A., Bishop, N. H., Miller, J. N., and Lovett, M. A. (1983a). Humoral immune response in experimental syphilis to polypeptides of *Treponema pallidum*. *J. Immunol. 131*:1973-1977.

Hanff, P. A., Fehniger, T. E., Miller, J. N., Lovett, M. A. (1982). Humoral immune response in human syphilis to polypeptides of *Treponema pallidum*. *J. Immunol. 129*:1287-1291.

Hanff, P. A., Miller, J. N., and Lovett, M. A. (1983b). Molecular characterization of common treponemal antigens. *Infect. Immun. 40*:825-828.

Hanff, P. A., Norris, S. J., Lovett, M. A., and Miller, J. N. (1984). Purification of *Treponema pallidum*, Nichols strain, by Percoll density gradient centrifugation. *Sex. Transm. Dis. 11*:275-286.

Hansen, E. B., Pederson, P. E., Schouls, L. M., Severin, E., and Embden, J. D. A. van (1985). Genetic characterization and partial sequence determination of a *Treponema pallidum* operon expressing two immunogenic membrane proteins in *Escherichia coli. J. Bacteriol. 162*:1227-1237.

Hardy, Jr., P. H., Fredericks, W. R., and Nell, E. E. (1975). Isolation and antigenic characteristics of axial filaments from the Reiter treponeme. *Infect. Immun. 11*:380-386.

Hayes, N. S., Muse, K. E., Collier, A. M., and Baseman, J. B. (1977). Parasitism by virulent *Treponema pallidum* of host cell surfaces. *Infect. Immun. 17*: 174-186.

Hensel, U., Wellensiek, H. J., and Bhakdi, S. (1985). Sodium dodecyl sulfate-polyacrylamide gel electrophoresis immunoblotting as a serological tool in the diagnosis of syphilitic infections. *J. Clin. Microbiol. 21*:82-87.

Hindersson, P., Peterson, C. S., and Axelson, N. H. (1985). Purified flagella from *Treponema phagedenis* biotype Reiter does not induce protective immunity against experimental syphilis in rabbits. *Sex. Transm. Dis. 12*:124-127.

Hook, III, E. W., Roddy, R. E., Lukehart, S. A., Hom, J., Holmes, K. K., and Tam, M. R. (1985). Detection of *Treponema pallidum* in lesion exudate with a pathogen-specific monoclonal antibody. *J. Clin. Microbiol. 22*:241-244.

Hotson, J. R. (1981). Modern neurosyphilis: A partially treated chronic meningitis. *West. J. Med. 135*:191-200.

Hovind-Hougen, K. (1983). Morphology. In *Pathogenesis and Immunology of Treponemal Infection* (R. F. Schell and D. M. Musher, eds.). Marcel Dekker, New York, pp. 3-28.

Izzat, N. N., Dacres, W. G., Knox, J. M., and Wende, R. (1970). Attempts at immunization against syphilis with avirulent *Treponema pallidum. Br. J. Vener. Dis. 46*:451-453.

Jaffe, H. W., Choi, K., Thomas, P. A., Haverkos, H. W., Auerbach, D. M., Guinan, M. E., Rogers, M. F., Spira, T. J., Darrow, W. W., Kramer, M. A., Friedman, S. M., Monroe, J. M., Friedman-Kien, A. E., Laubenstein, L. J., Marmor, M., Safai, B., Dritz, S. K., Crispi, S. J., Fannin, S. L., Orkwis, J. P., Kelter, A., Rushing, W. R., Thacker, S. B., and Curran, J. W. (1983). National case-control study of Kaposi's sarcoma and *Pneumocystis carinii* pneumonia in homosexual men: Part 1, Epidemiologic results. *Ann. Intern. Med. 99*:145-151.

Johnson, W. C. (1972). Venereal diseases and treponemal infections. In *Dermal Pathology* (J. H. Graham, W. C. Johnson, and E. B. Helwig, eds.). Harper and Row, Hagerstown, pp. 371-385.

Jones, S. A., Marchitto, K. S., Miller, J. N., and Norgard, M. V. (1984). Monoclonal antibody with hemagglutination, immobilization, and neutralization activities defines an immunodominant, 47,000 mol wt, surface-exposed immunogen of *Treponema pallidum* (Nichols). *J. Exp. Med. 160*:1404-1420.

Jue, R., Puffer, J., Wood, R. M., Schochet, G., Smartt, W. H., and Keterer, W. A. (1967). Comparison of fluorescent and conventional darkfield methods for the detection of *Treponema pallidum* in syphilitic lesions. *Am. J. Clin. Pathol.* *47*:809-811.

Kellogg, D. S. and Mothershed, S. M. (1969). Immunofluorescent detection of *Treponema pallidum*. *J. Am. Med. Assoc.* *207*:938-941.

Khan, A. S., Nelson, Jr., R. A., and Turner, T. B. (1951). Immunological relationship among species and strains of virulent treponemes as determined with the treponemal immobilization test. *Am. J. Hyg.* *53*:296-316.

Limberger, R. J. and Charon, N. W. (1985). Periplasmic flagellar proteins of *Treponema phagedenis*. Abstract D99, *Abstr. Ann. Meet. Am. Soc. Microbiol.*

Logan, L. C. (1974). Rabbit globulin and antiglobulin factors associated with *Treponema pallidum* grown in rabbits. *Br. J. Vener. Dis.* *50*:421-427.

Lukehart, S. A. (1982). Activation of macrophages by products of lymphocytes from normal and syphilitic rabbits. *Infect. Immun.* *37*:64-69.

Lukehart, S. A., Baker-Zander, S. A., and Gubish, Jr., E. R. (1982). Identification of *Treponema pallidum* antigens: Comparison with a nonpathogenic treponeme. *J. Immunol.* *129*:833-838.

Lukehart, S. A., Baker-Zander, S. A., Lloyd, R. M. C., and Sell, S. (1980a). Characterization of lymphocyte responsiveness in early experimental syphilis. II. Nature of cellular infiltration and *Treponema pallidum* distribution in testicular lesions. *J. Immunol.* *124*:461-467.

Lukehart, S. A., Baker-Zander, S. A., Lloyd, R. M. C., and Sell, S. (1981). Effect of cortisone administration on host-parasite relationships in early experimental syphilis. *J. Immunol.* *127*:1361-1368.

Lukehart, S. A., Baker-Zander, S. A., and Sell, S. (1980b). Characterization of lymphocyte responsiveness in early experimental syphilis. I. In vitro response to mitogens and *Treponema pallidum* antigens. *J. Immunol.* *124*:454-460.

Lukehart, S. A., Baker-Zander, S. A., and Sell, S. (1986). Characterization of the humoral immune response to antigens of *Treponema pallidum* following experimental infection and therapy in rabbits. *Sex. Transm. Dis.* *13*:9-15.

Lukehart, S. A. and Miller, J. N. (1978). Demonstration of the in vitro phagocytosis of *Treponema pallidum* by rabbit peritoneal macrophages. *J. Immunol.* *121*:2014-2024.

Lukehart, S. A., Tam, M. R., Hom, J., Baker-Zander, S. A., Holmes, K. K., and Nowinski, R. C. (1985). Characterization of monoclonal antibodies to *Treponema pallidum*. *J. Immunol.* *134*:585-592.

Lysko, P. G. and Cox, C. D. (1978). Respiration and oxidative phosphorylation in *Treponema pallidum*. *Infect. Immun.* *21*:462-473.

Magnuson, H. J., Thompson, F. A., and McLeod, C. P. (1951). Relationship between treponemal immobilizing antibodies and acquired immunity in experimental syphilis. *J. Immunol.* *67*:41-48.

Marchitto, K. S., Jones, S. A., Schell, R. F., Holmans, P. L., and Norgard, M. V. (1984). Monoclonal antibody analysis of specific antigenic similarities among pathogenic *Treponema pallidum* subspecies. *Infect. Immun.* *45*:660-666.

Marchitto, K. S., Selland-Grossling, C. K., and Norgard, M. V. (1986). Molecular specificities of monoclonal antibodies directed against virulent *Treponema pallidum*. *Infect. Immun. 51*:168-176.

Metzger, M. and Podwinska, J. (1968). A study of the heat-labile antigen of *Treponema pallidum*. *Arch. Immunol. Ther. Exp. 16*:888-894.

Miao, R. and Fieldsteel, A. H. (1978). Genetics of *Treponema*: Relationship between *Treponema pallidum* and five cultivable treponemes. *J. Bacteriol. 133*:101-107.

Miao, R. M. and Fieldsteel, A. H. (1980). Genetic relationship between *Treponema pallidum* and *Treponema pertenue*, two noncultivable human pathogens. *J. Bacteriol. 141*:427-429.

Miller, J. N. (1973). Immunity in experimental syphilis. VI. Successful vaccination of rabbits with *Treponema pallidum*, Nichols strain, attenuated by gamma-irradiation. *J. Immunol. 110*:1206-1215.

Miller, J. N., DeBruijn, J. H., Bekker, J. H., and Onvlee, P. C. (1966). The antigenic structure of *Treponema pallidum*, Nichols strain: I. The demonstration, nature and location of specific and shared antigens. *J. Immunol. 96*: 450-456.

Miller, J. N., DeBruijn, J. H., Bekker, J. H., and Onvlee, P. C. (1969). The antigenic structure of *Treponema pallidum*, Nichols strain: II. Extraction of a polysaccharide antigen with "strain-specific" serologic activity. *J. Bacteriol. 99*:132-135.

Miller, J. N., Whang, S. I., and Fazzan, F. P. (1963). Studies on immunity in experimental syphilis. I. Immunologic response of rabbits immunized with Reiter protein antigen and challenged with virulent *Treponema pallidum*. *Br. J. Vener. Dis. 39*:195-198.

Montenegro, E. N. R., Nicol, W. G., and Smith, J. L. (1969). Treponemalike forms and artifacts. *Am. J. Ophthalmol. 68*:197-205.

Moskophidis, M. and Muller, F. (1984a). Molecular analysis of immunoglobulins M and G immune response to protein antigens of *Treponema pallidum* in human syphilis. *Infect. Immun. 43*:127-132.

Moskophidis, M. and Muller, F. (1984b). Molecular characterization of glycoprotein antigens on surface of *Treponema pallidum*: Comparison with nonpathogenic *Treponema phagedenis* biotype Reiter. *Infect. Immun. 46*:867-869.

Moskophidis, M. and Muller, F. (1985). Monoclonal antibodies to *Treponema pallidum*: Monoclonal antibodies directed against immunodominant surface-exposed protein antigens of *Treponema pallidum*. *Eur. J. Clin. Microbiol. 4*: 473-477.

Nath, K. (1983). Restriction analysis of DNA from *Treponema pallidum*, the causative agent of syphilis. *Mol. Gen. Genet. 191*:126-131.

Nell, E. E. and Hardy, P. H. (1966). Studies on the chemical composition and immunologic properties of a polysaccharide from the Reiter treponeme. *Immunochemistry 3*:233-245.

Nelson, Jr., R. A. and Mayer, M. M. (1949). Immobilization of *Treponema pallidum* in vitro by antibody produced in syphilitic infection. *J. Exp. Med. 89*:369-393.

Norgard, M. V. and Miller, J. N. (1981). Plasmid DNA in *Treponema pallidum* (Nichols): Potential for antibiotic resistance by syphilis bacteria. *Science 213*:553-555.

Norgard, M. V. and Miller, J. N. (1983). Cloning and expression of *Treponema pallidum* (Nichols) antigen genes in *Escherichia coli. Infect. Immun. 42*: 435-445.

Norgard, M. V., Selland, C. K., Kettman, J. R., and Miller, J. N. (1984). Sensitivity and specificity of monoclonal antibodies directed against antigenic determinants of *Treponema pallidum* Nichols in the diagnosis of syphilis. *J. Clin. Microbiol. 20*:711-717.

Norris, S. J. (1982). In vitro cultivation of *Treponema pallidum*: Independent confirmation. *Infect. Immun. 36*:437-439.

Norris, S. J. and Sell, S. (1984). Antigenic complexity of *Treponema pallidum*: Antigenicity and surface localization of major peptides. *J. Immunol. 133*: 2686-2692.

Olansky, S., Simpson, L., and Schuman, S. H. (1954). Untreated syphilis in the male Negro: Environmental factors in the Tuskegee Study. *Public Health Rep. 69*:691-698.

Pavia, C. S. and Niederbuhl, C. J. (1985). Experimental *Treponema pallidum* infection in inbred guinea pigs: Development of lesions and formation of antibodies. *Genitourin. Med. 61*:75-81.

Pavia, C. S., Niederbuhl, C. J., and Saunders, J. (1985). Antibody-mediated protection of guinea-pigs against infection with *Treponema pallidum*. *Immunology 56*:195-202.

Penn, C. W., Bailey, M. J., and Cockayne, A. (1985). The axial filament antigen of *Treponema pallidum. Immunology 54*:635-641.

Perine, P. L., Weiser, R. S., and Klebanoff, S. J. (1973). Immunity to syphilis. I. Passive transfer in rabbits with hyperimmune serum. *Infect. Immun. 8*:787-790.

Peterson, K. M., Baseman, J. B., and Alderete, J. F. (1983). *Treponema pallidum* receptor binding proteins interact with fibronectin. *J. Exp. Med. 157*:1958-1970.

Pierce, C. S., Wicher, K., and Nakeeb, S. (1983). Experimental syphilis: Guinea pig model. *Br. J. Vener. Dis. 59*:157-168.

Ratnam, A. V., Din, S. N., Hira, S. K., Bhat, G. J., Wacha, D. S. A., Rukmini, A., and Mulenga, R. C. (1982). Syphilis in pregnant women in Zambia. *Br. J. Vener. Dis. 58*:355-358.

Robertson, S. M., Kettman, J. R., Miller, J. N., and Norgard, M. V. (1982). Murine monoclonal antibodies specific for virulent *Treponema pallidum* (Nichols). *Infect. Immun. 36*:1076-1085.

Romanowski, B., Forsey, E., Prasad, E., Lukehart, S. A., Tam, M. R., and Hook, III, E. W. (1987). Fluorescent monoclonal antibody detection for *Treponema pallidum. Sex. Transm. Dis.* (in press).
       search, Brighton, England.

Rosahn, P. D. (1947). Autopsy studies in syphilis. *J. Vener. Dis. Inform. Suppl. 21*:1-67.

Saunders, J. M. and Folds, J. D. (1983). Development of monoclonal antibodies that recognize *Treponema pallidum*. *Infect. Immun. 41*:844-847.

Saunders, J. M. and Folds, J. D. (1985). Humoral response of the mouse to *Treponema pallidum*. *Genitourin. Med. 61*:221-229.

Schell, R. F., Azadegan, A. A., Nitskansky, S. G., and LeFrock, J. L. (1982). Acquired resistance of hamsters to challenge with homologous and heterologous virulent treponemes. *Infect. Immun. 37*:617-621.

Schell, R. F., LeFrock, J. L., and Babu, J. P. (1978). Passive transfer of resistance to frambesial infection in hamsters. *Infect. Immun. 21*:430-435.

Schell, R. F., LeFrock, J. L., Chan, J. K., and Bagasra, O. (1980). LSH hamster model of syphilitic infection. *Infect. Immun. 28*:909-913.

Schell, R. F. and Musher, D. M. (eds.) (1983). *Pathogenesis and Immunology of Treponemal Infection*. Marcel Dekker, New York, pp. 1-392.

Schiller, N. L. and Cox, C. D. (1977). Catabolism of glucose and fatty acids by virulent *Treponema pallidum*. *Infect. Immun. 16*:60-68.

Sell, S., Baker-Zander, S. A., and Lloyd, R. M. C. (1980a). T-cell hyperplasia of lymphoid tissues of rabbits infected with *Treponema pallidum*: Evidence for a vigorous immune response. *Sex. Transm. Dis. 7*:74-84.

Sell, S., Baker-Zander, S. A., and Powell, H. C. (1982). Experimental syphilitic orchitis in rabbits. Ultrastructural appearance of *Treponema pallidum* during phagocytosis and dissolution by macrophages in vivo. *Lab. Invest. 46*:355-364.

Sell, S., Gamboa, D., Baker-Zander, S. A., Lukehart, S. A., and Miller, J. N. (1980b). Host response to *Treponema pallidum* in intradermally-infected rabbits: Evidence for persistence of infection at local and distant sites. *J. Invest. Dermatol. 75*:470-475.

Sepetjian, M., Salussola, D., and Thivolet, J. (1973). Attempt to protect rabbits against experimental syphilis by passive immunization. *Br. J. Vener. Dis. 49*: 335-337.

Sluis, J. J., van der, Dijk, G., van, Boer, M., Stolz, E., and Joost, T., van (1985). Mucopolysaccharides in suspensions of *Treponema pallidum* extracted from infected rabbit testes. *Genitourin. Med. 61*:7-12.

Smibert, R. M. (1984). Genus III. *Treponema*. In Bergey's Manual of Systematic Bacteriology (N. R. Krieg, ed.), Vol. 1. Williams & Wilkins, Baltimore, pp. 49-57.

Smith, J. L. and Israel, C. W. (1967). Spirochetes in the aqueous humor in seronegative ocular syphilis. *Arch. Ophthalmol. 77*:474-477.

Stamm, L. V. and Bassford, Jr., P. J. (1985). Cellular and extracellular protein antigens of *Treponema pallidum* synthesized during in vitro incubation of freshly extracted organisms. *Infect. Immun. 47*:799-807.

Stamm, L. V., Folds, J. D., and Bassford, Jr., P. J. (1982). Expression of *Treponema pallidum* antigens in *Escherichia coli* K-12. *Infect. Immun. 36*:1238-1241.

Stamm, L. V., Kerner, Jr., T. C., Bankaitis, V. A., and Bassford, Jr., P. L. (1983). Identification and preliminary characterization of *Treponema pallidum* protein antigens expressed in *Escherichia coli*. *Infect. Immun. 41*:709-721.

Steiner, B. M. and Sell, S. (1985). Characterization of the interaction between fibronectin and *Treponema pallidum. Curr. Microbiol. 12*:157-162.

Stephens, R. S., Tam, M. R., Kuo, C., and Nowinski, R. C. (1982). Monoclonal antibodies to *Chlamydia trachomatis*: Antibody specificities and antigen characterization. *J. Immunol. 128*:1083-1089.

Strandberg-Pedersen, N., Axelsen, N. H., Jorgensen, B. B., and Sand-Petersen, C. (1980). Antibodies in secondary syphilis against five of forty Reiter treponeme antigens. *Scand. J. Immunol. 11*:629-633.

Strugnell, R. A., Handley, C. J., Drummond, L., Faine, S., Lowther, D. A., and Graves, S. R. (1984a). Polyanions in syphilis: Evidence that glycoproteins and macromolecules resembling glycosaminoglycans are synthesized by host tissues in response to infection with *Treponema pallidum. Br. J. Vener. Dis. 60*:75-82.

Strugnell, R. A., Handley, C. J., Lowther, D. A., Faine, S., and Graves, S. R. (1984b). *Treponema pallidum* does not synthesize in vitro a capsule containing glycosaminoglycans or proteoglycans. *Br. J. Vener. Dis. 60*:8-13.

Symmers, D. (1916). Anatomic lesions in late acquired syphilis: A study of 314 cases based on the analysis of 4,880 necroposies at Bellevue Hospital. *J. Am. Med. Assoc. 66*:1457-1462.

Thomas, D. D., Baseman, J. B., and Alderete, J. F. (1985a). Fibronectin mediates *Treponema pallidum* cytadherence through recognition of fibronectin cell-binding domain. *J. Exp. Med. 161*:514-525.

Thomas, D. D., Baseman, J. B., and Alderete, J. F. (1985b). Putative *Treponema pallidum* cytadhesins share a common functional domain. *Infect. Immun. 49*:833-835.

Thornburg, R. W. and Baseman, J. B. (1983). Comparison of major protein antigens and protein profiles of *Treponema pallidum* and *Treponema pertenue. Infect. Immun. 42*:623-627.

Thornburg, R. W., Morrison-Plummer, J., and Baseman, J. B. (1985). Monoclonal antibodies to *Treponema pallidum*: Recognition of a major polypeptide antigen. *Genitourin. Med. 61*:1-6.

Titus, R. G. and Weiser, R. S. (1979). Experimental syphilis in the rabbit: Passive transfer of immunity with immunoglobulin G from immune serum. *J. Infect. Dis. 140*:904-913.

Turner, T. B., Hardy, Jr., P. H., Newman, B., and Nell, E. E. (1973). Effects of passive immunization on experimental syphilis in the rabbit. *Johns Hopkins Med. J. 133*:241-251.

Turner, T. B. and Hollander, D. H. (1957). *Biology of the Treponematoses.* World Health Organization, Geneva, pp. 1-278.

U.S. Department of Health, Education, and Welfare. (1969). *Manual of Tests for Syphilis.* U.S. Government Printing Office, Washington, pp. 1-81.

U.S. Department of Health and Human Services. (1986). *Annual Summary 1984: Reported Morbidity and Mortality in the United States.* HHS Pub No. (CDC) 86-8241, pp. 124-129.

Walfield, A. M., Hanff, P. A., and Lovett, M. A. (1982). Expression of *Treponema pallidum* antigens in *Escherichia coli. Science 216*:522-523.

Weiser, R. S., Erickson, D., Perine, P. L., and Pearsall, N. N. (1976). Immunity to syphilis: Passive transfer in rabbits using serial doses of immune serum. *Infect. Immun. 131*:1402-1407.

Wilkinson, A. E. and Cowell, L. P. (1971). Immunofluorescent staining for the detection of *Treponema pallidum* in early syphilitic lesions. *Br. J. Vener. Dis. 47*:252-254.

World Health Organization (1982). Treponemal infections. Technical report series 674, World Health organization, Geneva.

Wos, S. M. and Wicher, K. (1985). Antigenic evidence for host origin of exudative fluids in lesions of *Treponema pallidum*-infected rabbits. *Infect. Immun. 47*:228-233.

Yobs, A. R., Brown, L., and Hunter, E. F. (1964). Fluorescent antibody technique in early syphilis. *Arch. Pathol. 77*:220-225.

Yobs, A. R., Olansky, S., Rockwell, D. H., and Clarke, Jr., J. W. (1965). Do treponemes survive adequate treatment of late syphilis? *Arch. Dermatol. 91*:379-389.

Zeigler, J. A., Jones, A. M., Jones, R. H., and Kubica, K. M. (1976). Demonstration of extracellular material at the surface of pathogenic *T. pallidum* cells. *Br. J. Vener. Dis. 52*:1-8.

EIGHT

Serological Diagnosis of Syphilis: Current Methods

Anton F. H. Luger
Ludwig Boltzmann Institut
für Dermato-Venerologische Serodiagnostik
University of Vienna
Vienna, Austria

Serological methods remain the mainstay for the diagnosis of syphilis at all stages, other than, perhaps, the very early stages of the disease and provide the sole means to detect asymptomatic (latent) infections.

I. TESTS USING LIPOIDAL ANTIGENS

The "antigen" used in 1906 by Wassermann et al. in their first test for the detection of circulating antibodies in patients with syphilis, was an extract from the livers of cadavers of neonates with congenital syphilis which contained numerous *Treponema pallidum*. Later it became evident that it was not the *T. pallidum* antigen that reacted in the complement fixation test with the serum antibodies of patients with syphilis but rather lipoidal substances that can be extracted from mammalian tissues.

In 1941 Mary Pangborn isolated and purified a diphospholipid called cardiolipin from ox hearts. This substance is originally inert but becomes a serologically active antigen after the addition of lecithin and cholesterol and reacts with "reagins" or "Wassermann antibodies" in the sera of patients with syphilis. These reagins are autoantibodies directed against substances in the mitochondrial membranes (Doniach, 1976; Luger and Caterall, 1981). The identification of mitochondrial cardiolipin in patients with syphilis suggests that *T. pallidum* interacts not only with mammalian cell membranes but also with intracellular organelles (Wicher and Wicher, 1983). On the other hand, the mitochondrial cardiolipin antibodies are not identical with the Wassermann antibodies (Wicher and Wicher, 1983).

Although many assays utilizing lipoidal antigens have been used, the most generally accepted method now recommended by the World Health Organization (1982), was developed in 1946 by Harris and coworkers in the Venereal Disease Research Laboratories, Centers for Disease Control (CDC), Atlanta, Georgia. All other tests including complement fixation, Kline, Kolmer, Mazzini, Meinicke, give less reliable results and have been discontinued in most laboratories.

A. Venereal Disease Research Laboratory Test

The antigen consists of 0.03% cardiolipin with 0.9% cholesterol and 0.21% lecithin. The mixture in saline solution decomposes after some hours and, therefore, must be freshly prepared daily.

Lipoidal antibodies in the serum cause a macroscopically visible flocculation on mixing with the antigen. Microscopic examination at low magnification may be helpful in doubtful cases. A quantitative evaluation of the circulating antibodies can be obtained by serially doubling the serum dilutions. The highest dilution that can be classified as reactive is reported as the titer.

The specificity and sensitivity differ during the various stages of the disease but the Venereal Disease Research Laboratory (VDRL) test results are better than those given by other assays using lipoidal antigens. The concordance rate with tests applying *T. pallidum* antigens (e.g., *T. pallidum* hemagglutination assay, TPHA; and fluorescent treponemal antibody absorption, FTA-ABS), however, is about 90% in the early disease stages but as low as 29-43% during late latency (Larsen et al., 1984; Luger, 1987).

1. Reactivity During Treated and Untreated Infection

The VDRL test usually becomes reactive between 4 and 5 weeks after infection. Spontaneous reversal from reactivity to nonreactivity may occur in about 25-40% of untreated syphilitics during late latency (Hart, 1986). Sera from about 30% of patients with cardiovascular syphilis or with neurosyphilis are nonreactive in the VDRL test. An estimated 1% of patients with secondary syphilis will have a negative result if undiluted serum is used in the test procedure, which on further dilutions of the serum will become positive (the prozone phenomenon) (Rhodes and Luger, 1986).

Following adequate treatment, the VDRL test becomes nonreactive after an interval that is related to the time span between infection and therapy. Sera from patients who received therapy within 3 months of infection become nonreactive within the following 6-12 months. Reactivity may persist up to 60 months if treatment is given later in the early stage. Sera from 18% of patients who are treated for secondary syphilis are still reactive after 30-35 years. Sera from 56% of patients who are treated during the late phase became nonreactive within 5 years. The mean period of reactivity after treatment is 4 months for primary syphilis, 13 months for early latent disease, 17 months for the secondary stage, and 60 months for latent infections of indeterminate duration (Luger et al., 1983). Generally, after treatment of early syphilis the titer declines approximately four-fold at 3 months and eightfold at 6 months (Braun et al., 1985). A sustained four-fold or more increase in titer indicates reinfection or treatment failure.

2. Nonspecific Reactivity (Biological False-Positive Results)

Biological false-positive (BFP) results may occur in 0.25-0.86% of all sera examined (Larsen et al., 1984; Luger et al., 1983) and in 4.8-8.1% of all reactive samples (Luger et al., 1983) and are mainly caused by autoantibodies of the IgM class (rheumatoid factors). The total IgM concentration in the sera of patients with BFP reactions are usually twice as high as in nonreactive controls.

Biological false-positive VDRL results occur mostly in patients with autoimmune disorders (14% of all BFP reactions) and in diseases with an increased turnover of nucleic acid, as in infectious mononucleosis, malaria, psittacosis, and other bacterial infections, e.g., in viral pneumonia, malignant tumors, and in leprosy. The BFP results found during pregnancy apparently do not exceed the prevalence in nonpregnant females, but women at gestation are regularly tested with the VDRL test, and consequently more (transient) BFP reactions are discovered.

Later investigations revealed that the anticardiolipin antibody might be part of the anti-DNA antibodies in systemic lupus erythematosus (SLE) (Koike et al., 1984a,b). Sera from 41.7% of patients with SLE had the anticardiolipin antibody, and a separate antibody against VDRL antigen was also detected. The anti-DNA antibody, which reacted with the common antigenic determinants of nucleic acids, could bind to cardiolipin but failed to bind to other phospholipids including VDRL antigen. Among SLE patients, the prevalence of antibody against VDRL antigens was 29.2% IgG and 25% IgM. The occurrence of these antibodies correlated with BFP reactions in the VDRL test (Koike et al., 1984b).

3. Advantages and Disadvantages of the Venereal Disease Research Laboratory Test

The VDRL test can be accomplished in any laboratory with basic equipment, the method is easy to perform, and does not require specially skilled or qualified personnel. The results are reliable and can be obtained within 40 min. The reagents and the method are standardized, and results from different laboratories should be comparable. The VDRL test performance can be readily monitored by internal quality control (Wasley, 1985) and by participation in external quality control schemes. Finally, the VDRL test is the least expensive of all nontreponemal antigen tests (Larsen et al., 1984).

The disadvantages compared with results of the tests using *T. pallidum* antigen are the low sensitivity and specificity, the BFP reactions, and the prozone phenomenon. A further disadvantage is that the antigen must be prepared fresh daily and the sera must be heat-inactivated before testing. Heat inactivation, however, is now favored by many laboratories as it inactivates the viruses associated with AIDS.

B. Variations of the Venereal Disease Research Laboratory Test

1. Minor Variations in Performance

The test can be carried out in tubes, although this is seldom done. Inactivation can be omitted in the standard VDRL test; this simplifies the method, but the agreement rate with the original method is only 84%.

2. Unheated Serum Reagin Test

The unheated serum reagin (USR) assay uses a stabilized antigen that differs slightly from the VDRL reagent; it need not be prepared daily and is only a little more expensive. The test is carried out with unheated serum, all other steps are the same as in the standard VDRL test. Although the results agree well with the VDRL test, the sensitivity and the specificity are a little lower.

3. Rapid Plasma Reagin Test

The rapid plasma reagin (RPR) assay, which is another variant of the VDRL test, is performed with unheated serum on a small plastic card and is therefore sometimes called the rapid plasma reagin card (RPRC) test.

The antigen is cardiolipin, and the method is the same as that of the VDRL. Charcoal particles are added to the antigen resulting in a dark-colored flocculation with reactive sera that can be recognized easily without a microscope.

Specificity, sensitivity, onset, and decline of reactivity are almost identical with the VDRL slide test. The advantage over the VDRL test is simplicity. The test can be performed without laboratory equipment (Watson, 1985), and the results are available within 5 min. Reactive findings should be checked by tests using *T. pallidum* antigen. Its disadvantages are a lower sensitivity (the agreement rate with reactive VDRL results is 98%) (Fischer et al., 1984) and somewhat higher costs.

4. Automated Reagin Test

The automated reagin (ART) test, an automated version of the RPR card test, requires the use of an autoanalyzer that samples a measured portion of each test serum, mixes it with RPR antigen and deposits it on a strip of filter paper. The results of photometric reading are printed on a record form.

This procedure is the most expensive of all VDRL variants but its use is advantageous when large numbers of samples with a low rate of reactivity must be screened, e.g., in blood banks (Larsen et al., 1984).

5. Reagin Screen Test

The reagin screen test (RST) is a variant using a stabilized RPR antigen with the lipid-soluble diazo dye Sudan Black B instead of charcoal. The method is the same as that of the RPR, and the results are identical.

6. Toluidine Red Unheated Serum Test

The toluidine red unheated serum test (TRUST) has been developed by Pettit et al. (1983) in the Centers for Disease Control, Atlanta, Georgia, to replace or to supplement the RPR test whose reagents soon decompose during storage in hot climates, may not be easily obtainable, or may be too costly to be used in developing countries (Larsen and D'Costa, 1986). The method is identical with the RPR, but the antigen remains stable over a period of approximately 6 months at room temperature (26-31°C) and toluidine red paint pigment is used instead of charcoal to aid in the visualization of the test (Larsen et al., 1984; Larsen and D'Costa, 1986; Pettit et al., 1983).

A comparative evaluation of VDRL, RPR, TRUST, and FTA-ABS test results revealed no differences between VDRL, RPR, and TRUST findings insofar as the sensitivity (98.4%), the specificity (98.6%), and the reproducibility (98.2%) are concerned (Parham et al., 1984). Quantitative agreement within a dilution between TRUST and RPR was 92.3% but averaged at only 50% between TRUST and RPR versus VDRL (Parham et al., 1984). In a comparison of the TRUST using finger-prick blood and manual rotation, 96% agreement with the VDRL slide test was found (Larsen and D'Costa, 1986).

Further advantages or disadvantages may be reported after more experience is available.

II. TESTS USING *TREPONEMA PALLIDUM* ANTIGEN

Well-defined or selected antigenic components of *T. pallidum* are not yet generally available, therefore, the entire organism or fragments of it are used as antigens. Nevertheless, the specificity and sensitivity of these tests are close to optimal, the respective values vary between 95 and 99.9%, and allow a precise diagnosis of syphilis. On the other hand, the reactivity persists for years or decades after adequate therapy because these highly sensitive methods detect specific IgG antibodies even at unusually low levels.

A. *Treponema pallidum* Immobilization Test

As developed in 1949 by Nelson and Mayer, the *T. pallidum* immobilization (TPI) test was the yardstick of syphilis serology for almost a quarter of a century, but it was gradually replaced in the early 1970s by the hemagglutination assay which offered greater sensitivity and specificity and was much cheaper and easier to perform. Because of its shortcomings the TPI test is no longer used in routine serology or as a confirmatory test (World Health Organization, 1982).

B. Fluorescent Treponemal Antibody Absorption Test

The fluorescent treponemal antibody absorption test, an indirect immunofluor-escence method, was introduced into syphilis serology by Deacon et al. (1957) and subsequently improved by the introduction of an absorption stage (Hunter et al., 1964). *Treponema pallidum*, harvested from rabbit orchitis and acetone-fixed on slides, is used as antigen; careful purification from host testicular and serum components ensures better results (Hanff et al., 1984). As the sera of most normal individuals contain antibodies against nonpathogenic treponemes (Larsen et al., 1984), it is necessary to absorb these before testing by diluting the test serum 1:5 in sorbent (an extract of Reiter treponemes). The slide–fixed *T. pallidum* –is then incubated with the serum. Antibodies to *T. pallidum* bind to the surface of the treponemes. After rinsing, a fluorescein isothiocyanate-labeled antihuman globulin from rabbits is added, it binds to the human immunoglobulin, and after rinsing can be visualized using a fluoroscence microscope.

The intensity of fluorescence is classified by the symbols: – (nonreactive), ± (borderline), +, ++, +++, and ++++ (reactive at different degrees). A quantitative evaluation of antibody activity can be undertaken using serial trebling dilutions of sera starting at 1:5. As high titers persist for years after treatment, quantitation is generally not helpful, and for practical purposes scoring a 1:5 dilution as reactive or nonreactive is adequate.

All reagents, the antigen, the sorbent, and the conjugate are commercially available. Lyophilized treponemes can be stored for a long period without loss of antigenic quality.

1. Sensitivity and Specificity

When reagents are of good quality and the test is properly controlled, the sensitivity and specificity are high. An evaluation of four different kits revealed considerable differences among them. The ability to detect reactive serum samples varied from 82.5 to 95% and nonreactive samples from 80.9 to 96.4%. The reproducibility averaged 42%. These results show that a standard for use in the manufacture of FTA-ABS reagents is essential (Beebe and Nouri, 1984).

False reactivity may result from inefficient binding of nonspecific group antibodies in the absorption step or by "rheumafactors" in autoimmune disorders, hepatic cirrhosis, balanitis, herpes genitalis, and others. The reports on the occurrence of false-reactive findings during pregnancy and in diabetic patients are controversial.

The overall prevalence of false reactivity is low; it was found in 3.2% of 500 patients with collagen diseases and rheumatoid arthritis, in 0.7% of patients with various skin diseases, and in 6-10% of all FTA-ABS reactive samples. False-nonreactive results may occur in about 0.03% of samples from hospitalized patients (Luger et al., 1983).

The use of a biotin-avidin system in the FTA method increased the sensitivity for the detection of IgG antibodies by 15,000 times and for IgM antibodies by 3000 times compared with the conventional method (Berntsson, 1985). The effect of the increased sensitivity on the specificity of the test remains to be evaluated.

2. Reactivity During Treated and Untreated Infection

The onset of reactivity can be expected during the third week of infection. The test never becomes negative in untreated patients, and reactivity may still be observed years after successful therapy of early infections. In one study 20 of 23 patients (87%) with primary syphilis and all 53 patients with secondary syphilis were reactive in the FTA-ABS test 30-35 years after adequate treatment.

3. Advantages and Disadvantages of the Fluorescent Treponemal Antibody Absorption Test

The FTA-ABS test becomes reactive 1-2 weeks before all other assays, and its high specificity and sensitivity make it the most reliable test available for use in sera from doubtful cases.

The performance of the FTA-ABS test, however, requires highly trained personnel; it is time-consuming, the reading of results is tiresome, the whole procedure is expensive, and preferably it should, therefore, be used as a confirmatory test in samples showing reactivity in other assays.

C. *Treponema pallidum* Hemagglutination Assay

The first practicable hemagglutination assays for the diagnosis of syphilis were developed by Rathlev (1965) and by Tomizawa and Kasmatsu (1966). Generally, the TPHA and its variants, the microhemagglutination test with *T. pallidum* antigen (MHA-TP) and the automated version (AMHA-TP) use reagents produced by Fujirebio, Japan, whereas the hemagglutination treponemal test for syphilis (HTTS) is performed with products from Difco in the United States (Larsen et al., 1984).

Formalized sheep erythrocytes are coated with an ultrasonicate of *T. pallidum*, which has been harvested from rabbit orchitis, and purified. Absorbing diluent, containing extracts of sheep and beef erythrocyte membranes, Reiter treponemes, rabbit testicular tissue, and serum is added. After 30-min incubation, antigen-coated red cells are added. The absorbing diluent binds nonspecific group antibodies and agglutinins leaving only specific antibodies against *T. pallidum* to agglutinate the sensitized erythrocytes during a second incubation. Sera are usually screened at a 1:80 dilution. Quantitative tests can be performed with serial doubling dilutions from 1:80 to greater than 1:5120.

Heat inactivation is unnecessary. Comparative evaluation of test results after use of heated versus unheated sera showed a 99.2% agreement.

Reading of results is simple. A preliminary classification is possible after an incubation of 3-4 hr at room temperature, but the final reading should be made after 18 hr.

A result is classified as reactive if agglutination occurs at a dilution of > 1:80 but agglutination at a dilution of 1:40 is considered negative.

1. Specificity and Sensitivity

The TPHA test is, at present, the most sensitive and the most specific method for the detection of antibodies to *T. pallidum*. In both aspects the hemagglutination test is superior to the FTA-ABS (except during the third to fourth week of infection) and to the VDRL. In relation to all samples examined the margin of error is between 0.008% false-nonreactive and 0.07% false-reactive findings (Luger, 1981).

False-nonreactive results may occur in very early infection. False-reactive results may be caused by heteroagglutination (0.02% of all sera examined) or to genus-specific (group) antibodies (0.04% of all sera).

2. Reactivity During Untreated and Treated Infection

The onset of reactivity depends upon the IgM-binding capacity of the reagents. The sooner after infection of the rabbit the treponemes are harvested for antigen production the less IgG coating occurs and the better is the IgM sensitivity. Generally, reactivity is detectable during the fourth week of infection. Low titers (up to 320 or 640) can be found in very early or very late syphilis or many years after effective treatment. Persistently high titers, however, do not always reflect activity of the disease. Rarely, a decline in reactivity can be observed after effective treatment at the beginning of primary syphilis. If therapy is started at a later stage, the TPHA will invariably remain positive for life, although a rapid fall in titer may occur rarely after treatment for secondary infection.

3. Advantages and Disadvantages of the Test

The test can be easily carried out by personnel who have received minimal training in laboratories with basic equipment. The TPHA test now gives the most reliable results in syphilis serology.

The reagents, however, are rather expensive and the quality may vary even in batches from the same manufacturer. As standardization is far from ideal, internal quality control and proficiency testing is very important.

D. Variants of the *Treponema pallidum* Hemagglutination Test

1. Microhemagglutination Test with Treponema pallidum Antigen

The microhemagglutination test with *T. pallidum* antigen (MHA-TP) is performed on 96-well polystyrene microtiter plates with the TPHA reagents, but it requires less serum, one-sixteenth of the absorbing diluent, and less than one-sixth of the antigen. Using serial doubling dilutions of sera, quantitative evaluation is possible. Final results can be read after an incubation of only 4 hr. The MHA-TP is much less expensive and gives results that are equivalent to the TPHA.

2. Automated Microhemagglutination Assay with Treponema pallidum Antigen

A partial automation of the MHA-TP test by filling all 96 wells at once and by performing the dilutions in a processor saves personnel time and secures precision. The machines are, however, expensive, but their use is cost-effective in laboratories processing more than 200 samples daily. The results do not differ from those of the THPA or the MHA-TP.

3. Hemagglutination Treponemal Test for Syphilis

In the hemagglutination treponemal test for syphilis (HTTS), glutaraldehyde-stabilized turkey erythrocytes are used as carriers for *T. pallidum* antigen. The procedure is the same as that for the MHA-TP. The results are similar, agreement with the FTA-ABS being 93.9-96.6% (Friedly et al., 1983; Moyer et al., 1984). False nonreactivity occurs mainly during the primary and late latent disease stages (Larsen et al., 1984; Moyer et al., 1984).

4. *Microcapsule Agglutination Test for* Treponema pallidum *Antibodies*

The microcapsule agglutination test for *T. pallidum* antibodies (MCA-TP) uses chemically stable plastic microcapsules coated with *T. pallidum* antigen instead of the erythrocytes used in the MHA-TP test. The IgM reactivity and the sensitivity in detecting cases of primary syphilis is reportedly superior to the MHA-TP test (Kobayashi et al., 1983).

5. *Microhemagglutination Test with* Treponema pallidum *Antigen with Fingerprick Blood*

One of the major difficulties of blood collection in remote areas is the storage of samples and transport to the laboratory. A new method has been described by Larsen and D'Costa (1986). Fingerprick blood is spotted onto Ropaco No 1023 = 038 filter paper, air-dried, and then transported in a slide box. In the laboratory, a disk 5 mm in diameter is punched out and placed in a well of a microtiter plate containing 0.1 ml of absorbing diluent. The disk is soaked for at least 1 hr or preferably overnight; serial dilutions of the eluate are prepared, the second dilution being equivalent to a final dilution of 1:160 in the MHA-TP. The agreement with the MHA-TP is 99.5% (Larsen et al., 1984).

A similar assay has been reported by Müller and Keil (1984) and can be used for the examination of blood stains (Keil et al., 1984).

E. Enzyme-Linked Immunosorbent Assay with *Treponema pallidum* Antigen

The enzyme-linked immunosorbent assay (ELISA) was first described by Veldkamp and Visser in 1975. It is performed in polystyrene microtiter plates. Although several variants have been developed by the use of different antigens and conjugates, in principle the method is the same in all versions.

Originally an ultrasonicate of *T. pallidum* was used as antigen, but this was replaced by preparations from flagella or from the axial filament of Reiter treponemes (Schmidt and Schonwald, 1984). At present, extracts of protein fractions of *T. pallidum* are used most widely (Borobio et al., 1985; Farshy et al., 1984; Farshy et al., 1985; Morrison-Plummer et al., 1983; Pospisil, 1983; Stevens and Schmitt, 1985). The ELISA method is highly sensitive and specific, depending upon the type of reagents used. The agreement with the MHA-TP is between 93.1 and 98.5% (Farshy et al., 1984; Schmidt and Schonwald, 1984). The future looks promising for its use in the diagnosis of syphilis (Larsen et al., 1984).

Antigen fixed to the wells of microtiter plates is incubated with serum for 30-60 min. Antibodies bind to the antigen. After rinsing, a conjugate consisting of an antihuman IgG, from goats or from pigs, labeled with an enzyme, usually horseradish peroxidase (HRP) or alkaline phosphatase, is added. After a further incubation and rinsing of the respective substrate, o-phenylenediamine (for peroxidase) or p-nitrophenylphosphate (for alkaline phosphatase) is added and the color reaction measured.

The reading is facilitated by simultaneous measuring at 492 nm (measure beam) and at 600 nm (reference beam). Finally, the degree of turbidity can be registered (measure beam), and eventual sources of error (e.g., resulting from dimness of the test plate) can be eliminated through an electronic evaluation system comparing the results of the measure beam with those of the reference beam. The result is automatically printed on the record slip, and by measuring the absorbance, a quantitative evaluation is possible.

A measurement of antitreponemal IgG and IgM is possible in one assay by adding two different conjugates: alkaline phosphatase-labeled antihuman IgG and peroxidase-labeled antihuman IgM followed by the sequential application of two distinct substrates (Farshy et al., 1984).

1. Syphilis BioEnza Bead Test

The BioEnza Bead test uses *T. pallidum* antigen bound to the surface of ferrous metal beads that can be transported for washing and for transfer to other wells of microtiter plates containing serum (first step), conjugate (second step), and substrate (third step), by a magnetic device. The agreement rate with the VDRL, the ART, and FTA-ABS ranged from 93 to 99.5% (Stevens and Schmitt, 1985). In another study, using the same reference test, the sensitivity was 75% and the specificity 98.1% (Borobio et al., 1985).

III. ASSESSMENT OF TREATMENT STATUS

A common and difficult clinical problem is the significance of positive serological tests for syphilis in a patient who does not give a clear history of adequate treatment. The serological methods described previously are adequate as screening tests, but the results do not permit differentiation of treated and untreated disease. For this purpose, tests based on the detection of specific IgM have been developed.

A. Humoral Immune Response to Infections with
Treponema pallidum

Within a short time after treponemes have established themselves in the host, local multiplication and dissemination occur. The inflammatory response essentially consists of swelling and proliferation of endothelial cells and a perivascular infiltrate composed of lymphoid cells and many plasma cells, probably indicating local antibody production (Rice and Fitzgerald, 1985). There is also an influx of plasma components including complement and IgG.

1. Immunoglobulin M Antibodies

The first demonstrable sign of a humoral immune response of the human host to infection with *T. pallidum* is the production of antibodies of the IgM class that can be detected in the serum toward the end of the second week of infection. Immunoglobulin M synthesis through memory cells does not occur, and therefore, the production of these particular immunoglobulins is terminated soon after the elimination of the antigen.

A reactive IgM test in untreated patients is proof of active disease and indicates the need for treatment. The titers of specific IgM decline rapidly after adequate therapy of early syphilis and reactivity ceases within 3-9 months; reactivity may be found from 1 to 1.5 years after treatment of late disease (Eichmann et al., 1986; Luger, 1983a; Müller and Wollemann, 1985). The mean period of IgM reactivity after effective therapy of primary and early-latent syphilis is 2-4 months. The respective values are 3-4 months for the secondary stage and for latent infections of indeterminant duration (Luger, 1987). Comparable findings were reported for yaws (Schmidt et al., 1985). The results in late disease, particularly in neurosyphilis, may be impaired by the rather frequent occurrence of autoantibodies (Luger, 1983a, 1987) which may produce false reactivity. On the other hand, competitive inhibition of IgM production by high tiers of IgG may cause false-nonreactive results (Müller and Wollemann, 1985).

The reappearance of IgM reactivity after repeated nonreactivity strongly suggests reinfection. Persistence of reactivity after therapy indicates treatment failure, provided reactivity caused by autoantibodies of the IgM class (Luger, 1983a) can be excluded.

The large IgM molecules (molecular weight around 900,000) migrate in the ultracentrifuge at 19S units. Because of their size, they cannot pass the intact placenta and cannot cross the undisturbed blood/cerebrospinal fluid (CSF) barrier.

Immunoglobulin M reactivity of the serum of the newborn is proof of prenatal infection (i.e., congenital syphilis), and the detection of antitreponemal IgM in the CSF indicates neurosyphilis, provided the blood/CSF function is within normal limits (Luger, 1983b).

Immunoglobulin M antibodies with a molecular weight of about 150,000 that migrate as 7S units in the ultracentrifuge have been found rather frequently (82-92%) at high titers in the sera of patients with early syphilis. The titers decrease later, but the antibodies persist at low titers over a long period (Tanaka et al., 1984). Patients with late disease did not show any appreciable change in the 7S IgM titer even after adequate treatment. The implication of these findings is not yet clear.

2. Immunoglobulin G Antibodies

The molecular weight of IgG antibodies is between 145,000 and 160,000 and they migrate as 7S units in the ultracentrifuge. Immunoglobulin G production begins soon after that of IgM synthesis and becomes detectable in the serum around the fourth to fifth week after infection. The titers peak within the first year of the disease (Hart, 1986), usually during the secondary stage, and titers decrease as the disease becomes latent.

Low-level IgG synthesis is continued by memory cells for years or for life after elimination of the antigen. The detection of antitreponemal IgG, therefore, does not permit any conclusions concerning the activity of the disease or on the efficacy of treatment.

The comparatively small IgG molecules can easily pass the placenta and the blood/CSF barrier, and their appearance in the serum of newborns or in the CSF is not proof of congenital syphilis or of involvement of the CNS.

3. Immunoglobulin A Antibodies

Immunoglobulin A antibodies of molecular weight 160,000-390,000 migrate in the ultracentrifuge as 7S to 11S units. The significance of these immunoglobulins has not yet been sufficiently investigated. Antitreponemal IgA in the CSF may favor the development of neurosyphilis as it may competitively inhibit IgG and consequently block the complement cascade, thereby interfering with essential mechanisms of protective immunity (Gschnait et al., 1981).

B. Methods for the Selective Detection of Immunoglobulin M Antibodies to *Treponema pallidum*

The detection of IgM antibodies to *T. pallidum* is essential for the diagnosis of congenital syphilis or of reinfection and indicates the need for treatment. A reduction in IgM reactivity can be considered proof of successful therapy. There is now some 8 years experience with two tests for specific IgM, the 19S-IgM-FTA-ABS and the IgM solid phase hemadsorption (SPHA) tests, the results of which complement each other. The fluorescence method indicates reactivity earlier in the primary stage, whereas the solid phase method may yield more specific results later in the course of the disease. The agreement rate between the two assays is around 84.2% (Gschnait, 1983). The specificity is about 70-97% in the 19S-IgM-FTA-ABS (Luger, 1983a; Merlin et al., 1985; Müller and Wollemann, 1985) and between 97.4 and 99% in the IgM-SPHA test (Gschnait, 1983; Merlin et al., 1985; Sato et al., 1984). The sensitivity is 92% in the 19S-IgM-FTA-ABS (Merlin et al., 1985) and 92-97.6% (Merlin et al., 1985; Sato et al., 1984) in the IgM-SPHA. A persistence of reactivity after adequate treatment may occur in both tests (Baker-Zander et al., 1986; Larsen et al., 1984; Luger, 1983a) and may be caused by autoantibodies of the IgM class.

The 19S IgM molecules are rather labile and may be broken by the influence of enzymes or by increased temperature, e.g., 56°C for 30 min. (Müller, 1982). Titers in the specific antitreponemal IgM test decrease with the duration of storage. The IgM content of deeply frozen samples (in liquid nitrogen containers) remains stable, but a decrease of one to two dilutions can be expected at each thawing. Transport of samples for IgM testing preferably should be performed in a frozen condition, but the decrease of IgM reactivity remains within reasonable limits if serum samples are carried in plastic tubes within Styropore boxes and are stored in a refrigerator at 6-8°C at intervals between periods of shipping.

1. Immunoglobulin M Fluorescent Treponemal Antibody Absorption Test

The first attempt to identify IgM antibodies against *T. pallidum* was with a fluorescein isothiocyanate-labeled antihuman IgM instead of the antihuman globulin conjugate in the FTA-ABS test. Approximately 15-35% of results were falsely positive because of several sources of error (Luger, 1983a).

False nonreactivity occurred through competitive inhibition of IgM by IgG when IgG was at high titer. The receptors on the surface of *T. pallidum* are occuppied or overlaid by IgG before the larger IgM molecules can react. Also, a surplus of IgG can inhibit IgM production (Moskophidis and Müller, 1984).

False reactivity may be caused by IgM antibodies to immunoglobulins of the IgG class (rheumafactors). The prevalence of such factors in syphilitic patients increases with the duration of infection: they were found in 1 of 13 sera from patients with primary syphilis, in 3 of 13 samples from patients with secondary stage syphilis, and in 10 of 27 specimens from patients with latent disease (Cerny et al., 1985a).

2. 19S Immunoglobulin M Fluorescent Treponemal Antibody Absorption Test

An attempt to eliminate the sources of error in the IgM-FTA-ABS test was made by the separation of the IgM from the IgG class of immunoglobulins. The IgM fraction can be isolated from the serum by gel filtration, by electrophoresis, or by ultracentrifugation. The introduction of a fully automated method using high-performance liquid chromatography (HPLC) with electronic surveillance, yields an optimal 19S IgM fraction without contamination by low-molecular-weight 7S IgM or by 7S IgG (Luger, 1983a).

The sensitivity and specificity is high. Reactivity begins toward the end of the second week of infection and disappears soon after effective treatment (Borobio et al., 1985).

False reactivity may be found in up to 3.4% of all reactive samples and false nonreactivity occurs in 3.6% of all specimens that are reactive in other assays. The latter is observed mostly during the secondary stage of the disease and in about 3% of patients with late syphilis (Müller and Wollemann, 1985; Schroter et al., 1983).

As the performance of the 19S-IgM-FTA-ABS test is expensive and requires specially equipped laboratories and highly qualified personnel, its use should be limited to selected cases of problem sera. With the introduction of HPLC, however, laboratories handling large numbers of reactive sera may be able to use this method routinely for evaluating specimens with positive results in screening tests.

3. Immunoglobulin M Solid Phase Hemadsorption Test

The IgM solid phase hemadsorption test (IgM-SPHA) was developed by Schmidt in 1980 in the course of studies to find a simple and inexpensive method for the detection of antitreponemal IgM.

The wells of polystyrene microtiter plates are coated with a μ chain-specific serum (anti-IgM). The patients serum is then added and incubated for 30 min. After rinsing, the MHA-TP test is performed as indicated in Sect. II.D.1. Serum IgM binds to the walls of the wells and antitreponemal IgM reacts with the TPHA antigen.

The reagents used are the same as those of the MHA-TP test. A result is classified as reactive if agglutination occurs at a dilution $\geq 1:8$; $1:4$ is a borderline finding, and the result is negative if agglutination is observed at a dilution $1:2$ or below. The sensitivity of the SPHA is around 96% and the specificity is 97.4% when compared with other IgM assays (Merlin et al., 1985).

False nonreactivity is observed in about 8% of all reactive sera and occurs at low IgM titers, particularly in the early primary stage. This is in accordance with the somewhat delayed onset of reactivity in the TPHA test during the first weeks of infection and is probably due to a low IgM binding capacity of the TPHA antigen or later to competitive inhibition of IgM at increasingly high titers of IgG.

False reactivity may occur in about 1% of all reactive samples and can be caused by rheumafactors or circulating immune complexes. This occurs mainly in patients with late neurosyphilis (Luger, 1983a, 1987), probably for reasons similar to those causing false reactivity in the 19S-IgM-FTA-ABS test.

The advantages of the SPHA over the 19S-IgM-FTA-ABS test are its simplicity and low cost. Also, the IgM-SPHA is superior to the VDRL in the assessment of treatment and in the diagnosis of reinfections (Eichmann et al., 1983; Meyer and Futh, 1984).

In untreated patients, a reactive result indicates the need for therapy, but a nonreactive result does not exclude such a need with the same high degree of probability. When there is doubt, nonreactive SPHA results should be checked by the 19S-IgM-FTA-ABS test, particularly if other evidence (e.g., high VDRL titers) suggest active disease.

4. Treponema pallidum-Specific Immunoglobulin M Hemagglutination Test

Erythrocytes coated with an antihuman IgM bind IgM antibodies from the serum of the patient. Antitreponemal IgM reacts in a second step with erythrocytes coated with *T. pallidum* antigen. When compared with the 19S-IgM-FTA-ABS test, the sensitivity of the test was found to be 99.7% and the specificity 97.6% (Sato et al., 1984).

5. Immunoglobulin M Enzyme-Linked Immunosorbent Assay

The IgM ELISA is similar to the ELISA method for the detection of IgG antibodies (Lee et al., 1986; Muller, 1983). The antigen is adsorbed to the walls of the wells of polystyrene microtiter plates and serial dilutions of the serum are added. After incubation and rinsing, the conjugate, HRP-labeled antihuman IgM is added, and after further incubation and rinsing the wells are filled with the substrate *o*-phenylenediamine. The reaction is stopped by addition of oxalic acid and the plates are read spectrophotometrically at 490 nm.

A modification of the test uses polystyrene beads as carriers for the antigen (Müller, 1983). Before testing, absorption of the sera with aggregated IgG is recommended to eliminate false results through rheumafactors. The specificity is about 98% (Lee et al., 1986; Muller and Moskophidis, 1984), the sensitivity varies between 93 and 98% depending upon the stage of the disease (Müller and Moskophidis, 1984), the 19S-IgM-FTA-ABS serving as standard in the evaluations of Müller and Moskophidis (1984).

The advantage of the ELISA method over the 19S-IgM-FTA-ABS test is that the method is simple and can be partly or fully automated. Furthermore, the use of whole serum instead of the isolated IgM faction leads to substantial savings in time and money. The IgM-SPHA test is still much less expensive and much simpler to perform, but the IgM ELISA technique apparently offers higher sensitivity.

6. CAPTIA Syphilis-M Monoclonal Antibody
Enzyme-Linked Immunosorbent Assay

The CAPTIA Syphilis-M test (Mercia Diagnostics) depends upon IgM capture: rabbit antibodies against human IgM (μ chain-specific) are coated on the inner surfaces of microtiter wells. When test sera, diluted 1:50, are incubated in the wells a portion of the total IgM is captured. Unbound antibodies and other serum proteins are removed by washing. Specific antitreponemal IgM within the total bound IgM is then detected by adding a freshly prepared tracer system. The tracer is prepared by mixing highly purified *T. pallidum* antigen, biotinylated MAb reactive with an epitope on the 37,000-mol. wt. axial filament, and streptavidin-HRP conjugate. After incubation and washing to remove excess, tracer-bound HRP is detected by adding tetramethylbenzidine substrate. Because the HRP is indirectly bound to the specific antitreponemal IgM through the streptavidin-biotinylated MAb-*T. pallidum* antigen, the intensity of the blue reaction product is directly proportional to the amount of anti-*T. pallidum* IgM in the original serum.

The test is not subject to interference by rheumafactors or by competition from antitreponemal IgG. Although a comprehensive evaluation is required the

Table 1 Indications for Different Types of Serological Tests

	Tests using	
Indication	Lipoidal antigens	*T. pallidum* antigen
Screening diagnosis	VDRL or RPR	TPHA (MHA-TP, AMHA-TP)
Confirmation of diagnosis (in case of discrepant results)		FTA-ABS
Activity of infection	Quantitative	IgM-SPHA
Response to treatment	VDRL or RPR	19S-IgM-FTA-ABS
		IgM ELISA

Source: World Health Organization (1982).

test is potentially a highly sensitive and specific method for detecting antitreponemal IgM, particularly during the first weeks of infection (Luger et al., 1987, Figs. 3 and 4, and Table 3).

IV. APPLICATION OF TESTS IN ROUTINE SYPHILIS SEROLOGY

The indications for the use of the various serological tests are summarized in Table 1.

A. Screening

The considerable increase of latent, or atypical infections requires the application of serological screening for syphilis at every possible opportunity. It should always be undertaken in hospitalized patients, in pregnant women, and in persons at risk of venereal infections (Aho, 1984; Coester et al., 1984; World Health Organization, 1982). Screening during pregnancy has proved to be of economic advantage in a cost-benefit evaluation (Stray-Pedersen, 1983).

Generally, the VDRL test is used for screening. This assay, however, failed to identify 64% of reactive samples, mainly those from individuals in the stage of late latency (Luger et al., 1987). A careful examination of 53 persons with nonreactive VDRL, but with reactive AMHA-TP results at routine screening, revealed mesaortitis in four and neurosyphilis in two patients (Luger et al., 1987). In another study, only half of the 97 patients with syphilitic aortitis (diagnoses confirmed at autopsy) were reactive in the VDRL test (Gormsen, 1984). These observations concern highly selected groups and are not representative, but they emphasize the importance of using the MHA-TP or the AMHA-TP for routine testing (Luger et al., 1987). The use of the MHA-TP or AMHA-TP eventually combined with the VDRL, is therefore suggested for syphilis screening in industrialized countries (Luger, 1987; World Health Organization, 1982).

Cardiovascular syphilis and mesaortitis do not occur in areas where yaws occurs and are very rarely observed in endemic areas of nonvenereal "endemic" syphilis. therefore, screening by only the VDRL is sufficient in such regions.

The MHA-TP or the VDRL with fingerprick blood may be applied in areas where the storage and transportation of blood specimens are difficult.

B. Confirmation

All reactive results in the MHA-TP and/or VDRL tests should be checked by the FTA-ABS test (World Health Organization, 1982) to exclude false-positive findings resulting from rheumafactors or other autoantibodies.

Reactivity in the MHA-TP and in the FTA-ABS tests is proof of syphilis, provided the same result is obtained from two samples taken on two different occasions. The second examination is recommended to avoid technical errors, although such mistakes only rarely occur in well-organized laboratories.

1. Activity of Syphilitic Infection

Active disease and the need for treatment is indicated by VDRL titers greater than 16, which may increase on repeated examinations, and by reactivity in the specific IgM tests (19S-IgM-FTA-ABS, IgM-SPHA, IgM-ELISA).

2. Success of Treatment

The success of treatment is indicated by the rapid decline in titers in the IgM tests, the VDRL titers show slower regression. A reversal to nonreactivity in the IgM tests can be considered as a sign of cure.

3. Reinfection

Reinfection has to be assumed when the IgM tests become reactive again after they have reverted to nonreactivity following treatment.

C. Diagnosis of Neurosyphilis

The incidence of neurosyphilis has increased during the past decade in most industrialized countries (Gomez and Aviles, 1984; Moskophidis and Müller, 1985). The diagnosis has become increasingly difficult because atypical forms apparently prevail (Dose et al., 1984; Harper, 1985; Moskophidis and Müller, 1985; Risse et al., 1985; Sachs, 1985; Schmidt et al., 1985; Simon, 1985) although other investigators did not observe essential deviations from the classic symptoms (Talbot and Morton, 1985). The performance of lumbar puncture or of cisternal puncture is essential in all patients with reactive serum tests but no history of infection with

T. pallidum (Bruke and Schaberg, 1985), particularly if these findings persist un-changed after treatment (Harper, 1985).

The serological diagnosis of neurosyphilis by examination of the CSF has changed fundamentally during the past years by the introduction of new mea-surements that enable a precise evaluation of involvement of the CNS.

The traditional diagnostic criteria of neurosyphilis have proved inadequate. The result of the colloidal reactions, the gold sol and mastic graphs are not suf-ficiently precise and reproducibility is poor.

Abnormal findings in the Dattner-Thomas formula (cell count $> 5 \times 10^6$/L and total protein above 0.45 g/L) indicate inflammation without indicating its causation.

The CSF VDRL test is nonreactive in 30-47% (Hammerstrom and Zimmer, 1985; Muller and Wollemann, 1985; Sequeira, 1983) of patients with active neuro-syphilis, and therefore, this test cannot be used as an indicator of CNS involve-ment.

Undiluted (unabsorbed) fluid is used in the first step of the IgM-SPHA test and may also be employed in the FTA test to increase its sensitivity (Jaffe, 1984; Rhodes and Luger, 1986). Separation of the immunoglobulin classes from CSF is impracticable because quantities are too small. The 19S-IgM-FTA-ABS, there-fore, cannot be performed on the CSF. The IgM-SPHA is classified as reactive if agglutination occurs with undiluted fluid. Quantitative evaluations are based on serial doubling of dilutions: the TPHA and the MHA-TP tests are considered posi-tive at a titer of $\geqslant 10$ dilutions.

A reactive finding in the CSF-MHA-TP or in the CSF-FTA-ABS is irrelevant for the diagnosis of neurosyphilis because IgG antibodies can pass the intact blood/ CSF barrier and may therefore have been transferred passively from the serum.

On the other hand a nonreactive CSF-TPHA or MHA-TP and/or FTA-ABS test result excludes neurosyphilis almost with certainty.

An important factor for the evaluation of all CSF findings is the blood/CSF barrier function which is indicated by the formula:

$$\text{Albumin quotient} = \frac{\text{CSF albumin (mg/dl)} \times 10^3}{\text{serum albumin (mg/dl)}}$$

Normal values vary between 3 and 8 (Luger et al., 1981). Another method for the evaluation of the blood/CSF barrier function is the determination of adenovirus antibodies in the CSF by an ELISA assay (Cerny et al., 1985b). About 89% of normal individuals examined in Atlanta, Georgia, have such antibodies in the serum but not in the CSF in detectable amounts. The identification of adeno-virus antibodies in the CSF, therefore, indicates either contamination with periph-eral blood or damaged blood/brain barrier function. The detection of antitrepon-emal IgM in the CSF and a nonreactive CSF adenovirus antibody test is, therefore, indicative of active neurosyphilis. Antibody production within the CSF is derived from the IgG quotient:

$$\text{The IgG quotient} = \frac{\text{CSF IgG (mg/dl)} \times 10^3}{\text{serum IgG (mg/dl)}}$$

Values > 1.5 indicate local antibody production within the CSF but do not permit conclusions to be drawn about the antigen that stimulated the synthesis.

The search for a specific factor for the identification of neurosyphilis led to the introduction of the TPHA index which is calculated by the formula: CSF TPHA-titer/albumin quotient.

Values above 100 are strongly suggestive and above 500 are proof of neurosyphilis, provided the albumin quotient does not exceed a limit of 20 (Dose et al., 1984; Luger et al., 1981). Extreme disorders of the blood/CSF barrier at albumin quotient values above 20 may cause false-nonreactive results in the TPHA index. A modification of the TPHA index has been suggested by Stockli (1982) who proposed the formula:

$$\frac{\text{CSF TPHA-titer/serum TPHA-titer}}{\text{albumin quotient}}$$

Normal values are below 2. Elevated or high serum TPHA titers, which occur almost regularly in neurosyphilis cannot be reproduced exactly and the difference between 5120 and 10,240, for example, can seriously interefere with the results of the modified TPHA-index.

A further factor, the TPA-index, has been introduced by Moskophidis and Müller (1985) and Müller and Moskophidis (1983) and compares the anti-*T. pallidum* IgG titers in the CSF with findings in the serum:

$$\frac{\text{TPHA-IgG titer per mg total IgG CSF}}{\text{TPHA-IgG titer per mg total IgG serum}}$$

normal values are between 0.5 and 2.

The detection of IgM antibodies to *T. pallidum* in the CSF by the IgM-SPHA (Luger et al., 1981; Luger, 1983b) or by the different ELISA assays (Luger, 1983b; Moskophidis and Müller, 1985) in patients with normal blood/CSF barrier function is indicative of neurosyphilis.

Immunoglobulin A antibodies to *T. pallidum* were found in some CSF samples and might play a role in the pathogenesis of neurosyphilis because it seems to compete with IgG at the receptor sites of the target organism (Gschnait et al., 1981). Immunoglobulin A does not cause cytotoxicity by activating the classic complement pathway; therefore, the simultaneous presence of IgA and IgG can, in fact, decrease the antibacterial effect of IgG. The importance of the occurrence of IgA antibodies in the CSF remains to be established (Gschnait et al., 1981).

In summary, the diagnosis of neurosyphilis can be established by a TPHA index above 100, by a TPA index above 2, and by reactivity in the CSF-IgM-SPHA or in the CSF-IgM-ELISA tests. The results in the IgM assays are relevant even at a disturbed blood/brain barrier because antitreponemal IgM derived from peripheral blood would still indicate active disease and the need for treatment regardless of CNS involvement. The effectiveness of treatment is first indicated by a restoration of the normal CSF cytology and chemistry (Michel et al., 1983) and by a decrease of the CSF-IgM-titers with reversal to nonreactivity.

The further development of tests using MAbs should simplify the performance and improve the reliability of tests to detect specific anti-*T. pallidum* IgM. Such tests could become routine for assessing treatment status and monitoring the efficacy of treatment. The diagnosis of neurosyphilis may also be improved by developing tests for treponemal antigen in CSF that combine polyclonal antibodies for antigen capture with MAbs for specific detection.

REFERENCES

Aho, K. (1984). Screening for syphilis. *Eur. J. Sex. Transm. Dis.* 2:25-26.

Baker-Zander, S. A., Roddy, R. E., Handsfield, H. H., and Lukehart, S. A. (1986). IgG and IgM antibody reactivity to antigens of *Treponema pallidum* after treatment of syphilis. *Sex. Transm. Dis.* 13:214-220.

Beebe, J. L. and Nouri, N. J. (1984). Comparative evaluation of commercial fluorescent treponemal antibody absorbed test kits. *J. Clin. Microbiol.* 19: 789-793.

Berntsson, E. (1985). Increased sensitivity of the fluorescent treponemal antibody absorption test with biotin/avidin: A comparison with conventional FTA-ABS. *Acta Dermato-Venereol.* 65:89-91.

Borobio, M. V., Alvarez-Dardet, C., and Gallardo, R. M. (1985). Evaluation of a solid-phase enzyme immunoassay in the diagnosis of syphilis. *Eur. J. Sex. Transm. Dis.* 2:231-233.

Braun, S. T., Zaidi, A., Larsen, S. A., and Reynolds, G. H. (1985). Serological response to syphilis treatment. A new analysis of old data. *J. Am. Med. Assoc.* 253:1296-1299.

Bruke, J. M. and Schaberg, D. R. (1985). Neurosyphilis in the antibiotic area. *Neurology 35*:1368-1371.

Cerny, E. H., Farshy, C. E., Hunter, E. F., and Larsen, S. A. (1985a). Rheumatoid factor in syphilis. *J. Clin. Microbiol.* 22:89-94.

Cerny, E. H., Hambie, E. A., Lee, F., Farshy, C., and Larsen, S. A. (1985b). Adenovirus ELISA for the evaluation of Cerebrospinal fluid in patients with suspected neurosyphilis. *Am. J. Clin. Pathol.* 84:505-508.

Coester, C. H., Bienzle, U., Hoffmann, H. G., Koehn, E., and Guggenmoos-Holzmann, I. (1984). Syphilis, hepatitis A and hepatitis B seromarkers in homosexual men. *Klin. Wochenschr.* 62:810-813.

Deacon, W. E., F·lcone, V. H., and Harris, A. (1957). A fluorescent test for treponemal antibodies. *Proc. Soc. Exp. Biol. Med. 96*:477-480.

Doniach, D. (1976). Autoantibodies in syphilis and chronic biologic false positive reactions. In *Sexually Transmitted Diseases* (R. D. Catterall and C. S. Nicol, eds.). Academic Press, New York, pp. 210-214.

Dose, D., Heise, H., Ratz, K. H., Blatz, R., and Thielebeule, U. (1984). Liquordiagnostik bei Syphilis. *Z. Hautkr. 59*:101-106.

Eichmann, A., Butling, M., and Meyer, J. C. H. (1986). The SPHA Test in the diagnosis of syphilis. Results in various stages of untreated syphilis. *Eur. J. Sex. Transm. Dis. 3*:95-98.

Eichmann, A., Meyer, J. C., Schmid, E., Luger, A., and Schmidt, B. L. (1983). Zur Spezifitat und Sensitivitat des Solid-Phase-Haemadsorptions (SPHA)-Testes: Eine Untersuchung bei behandelten und unbehandelten Syphilitikern. *Z. Hautkr. 58*:1369-1388.

Farshy, C. E., Hunter, E. F., Helsel, L. O., and Larsen, S. A. (1985). Four step enzyme-linked immunosorbent assay for detection of *Treponema pallidum* antibody. *J. Clin. Microbiol. 21*:387-389.

Farshy, C. E., Junter, E. F., Larsen, S. A., and Cerny, E. H. (1984). Double conjugate enzyme linked immunosorbent assay for immunoglobulins G and M against *T. pallidum*. *J. Clin. Microbiol. 20*:1109-1113.

Fischer, G. S., Kleger, B., and Colavita, M. T. (1984). Reactivity of Dade rapid plasma reagin card test with low-titer sera. *J. Clin. Microbiol. 19*:435.

Friedly, G., Zartarian, M. V., Wood, J. C., Floyd, C. M., Peterson, E. M., and de la Maza, L. M. (1983). Hemagglutination treponemal test for syphilis. *J. Clin. Microbiol. 18*:775-778.

Gomez, E. A. and Aviles, M. (1984). Neurosyphilis in community mental health clinics: A case series. *J. Clin. Psychiatry 45*:127-129.

Gormsen, H. (1984). Postmortem diagnosis of syphilitic aortitis, including serological verification on postmortem blood. *Forensic Sci. Int. 24*:51-56.

Gschnait, F. (1983). Erfahrungen mit dem SPHA-test. *Hautarzt 34*:(Suppl. 6): 154.

Gschnait, F., Schmidt, B. L., and Luger, A. (1981). Cerebrospinal fluid immunoglobulins in neurosyphilis. *Br. J. Vener. Dis. 57*:238-240.

Hammerstrom, D. C. and Zimmer, B. (1985). The role of lumbar puncture in the evaluation of dementia: The University of Pittsburgh Study. *J. Am. Geriatr. Soc. 33*:397-400.

Hanff, P. A., Norris, S. J., Lovett, M. A., and Miller, J. N. (1984). Purification of *Treponema pallidum*, Nichols strain, by Percoll density gradient centrifugation. *Sex. Transm. Dis. 11*:275-286.

Harper, P. (1985). Criteria for undertaking lumbar puncture in the assessment of syphilis. *Genitourin. Med. 61*:66-67.

Harris, A., Rosenberg, A. A., and Riedel, L. M. (1946). A microflocculation test for syphilis using cardiolipin antigen. *J. Vener. Dis. Inform. 27*:169-175.

Hart, G. (1986). Syphilis tests in diagnostic and therapeutic decision making. *Ann. Intern. Med. 104*:368-376.

Hunter, E. F., Deacon, W. E., and Meyer, P. E. (1964). An improved FTA test for syphilis, the absorption procedure (FTA-ABS). *Public Health Rep. 79*: 410-412.

Jaffe, H. W. (1984). Management of the reactive serology. In *Sexually Transmitted Diseases* (K. K. Holmes, P. A. Mardh, P. F. Sparling, and P. J. Wiesner, eds.). McGraw-Hill, New York, pp. 313-318.

Kobayashi, S., Yamaya, S. I., Sugahara, T., and Matuhasi, T. (1983). Microcapsule agglutination test for *T. pallidum* antibodies. A new serodiagnostic test for syphilis. *Br. J. Vener. Dis. 59*:1-7.

Keil, W., Muller, G., and Nitschke, H. (1984). Erste Erfahrungen mit dem *Treponema-pallidum*-Haemagglutinations-(TPHA)-test an Blutspuren. *Z. Rechtsmed. 91*:247-253.

Koike, T., Maruyama, H., Funaki, H., Tomioka, H., and Hoshida, S. (1984a). Specificity of mouse hybridoma antibodies to DNA. II. Phospholipid reactivity and biological false positive serological test for syphilis. *Clin. Exp. Immunol. 57*:345-350.

Koike, T., Sueishi, M., Funaki, H., Tomioka, H., and Yoshida, S. (1984b). Antiphospholipid antibodies and biological false positive serological test for syphilis in patients with systemic lupus erythematosus. *Clin. Exp. Immunol. 56*: 193-199.

Larsen, S. A. and D'Costa, J. F. (1986). Laboratory tests and serologic surveillance for yaws and other diseases and conditions. *Southeast Asian J. Trop. Med. Public Health 17 (Suppl. No. 4)*:70-77.

Larsen, S. A., McGrew, B. E., Hunter, E. F., and Creighton, E. T. (1984). Syphilis serology and darkfield microscopy. In *Sexually Transmitted Diseases* (K. K. Holmes, P. A. Mardh, P. F. Sparling, and P. J. Wiesner, eds.). McGraw-Hill, New York, pp. 875-888.

Lee, J. B., Farshy, C. E., Hunter, E. F., Hambie, E. A., Wobig, G. H., and Larsen, S. A. (1986). Detection of IgM in Cerebrospinal fluid from syphilis patients by an enzyme-linked immunosorbent assay. *J. Clin. Microbiol. 24*:736-740.

Luger, A. (1981). Diagnosis of syphilis. *Bull. WHO. 59*:647-654.

Luger, A. (1983a). Die IgM Diagnostik in der Syphilisserologie. *Wien. Klin. Wochenschr. 95*:843-847.

Luger, A. (1983b). Neurosyphilis. *Internist 24*:576-581.

Luger, A. (1987). Syphilisserologie heute. In *Fortschritte der Dermatologie und Venerologie*. Springer, Berlin, (in press).

Luger, A. and Catterall, R. D. (1981). Immunologie der Syphilis. In *Dermatologie in Klinik und Praxis* (G. W. Korting, eds.), Vol. 4. G. Thieme, Stuttgart, New York, pp. 44-79.

Luger, A., Marhold, I., and Schmidt, B. L. (1987). Diagnostische Neuheiten— Syphilisserologie. *Schrifttum und Praxis* (in press).

Luger, A., Schmidt, B. L., Steyrer, K., and Schonwald, E. (1981). Diagnosis of neurosyphilis by examination of the cerebrospinal fluid. *Br. J. Vener. Dis. 57*:232-237.

Luger, A., Schmidt, B. L., Steyrer, K., and Wider, G. (1983). Screening for syphilis with the AMHA TP test. *Eur. J. Sex. Transm. Dis. 1*:25-27.

Merlin, S., Andre, J., Alacque, B., and Paris-Hamelin, A. (1985). Importance of specific IgM antibodies in 116 patients with various stages of syphilis. *Genitourin. Med. 61*:82-87.

Meyer, K. G. and Futh, U. (1984). Der solid phase haemadsorptions (SPHA)-test bei Syphilis Reinfektionen. *Z. Hautkr. 59*:739-748.

Michel, D., Blanc, A., Laurent, B., Foyatier, N., and Portafaix, M. (1983). Etude biologique, psychometrique et tomodensitometrique de la neurosyphilis traitee. *Rev. Neurol. (Paris) 139*:737-743.

Morrison-Plummer, J., Alderete, J. F., and Baseman, J. B. (1983). Enzyme-linked immunosorbent assay for the detection of serum antibody to outer membrane proteins of *Treponema pallidum. Br. J. Vener. Dis. 59*:75-79.

Moyer, N. P., Hudson, H. D., and Hausler, W. J. (1984). Evaluation of the haemagglutination treponemal test for syphilis. *J. Clin. Microbiol. 19*:849-852.

Moskophidis, M. and Müller, F. (1984). Molecular analysis of immunoglobulins M and G immune response to protein antigens of *Treponema pallidum* in human syphilis. *Infect. Immun. 43*:127-132.

Moskophidis, M. and Müller, F. (1985). Immunologie der Neurosyphilis: Intrathekale Synthese *T. pallidum* spezifischer IgG and IgM Antikorper. *Immun. Infekt. 13*:91-98.

Müller, F. (1982). Der 19S (IgM)-FTA-ABS Test in der Serodiagnostik der Syphilis. *Immun. Infekt. 10*:23-34.

Müller, F. (1983). Der *Treponema pallidum*-IgM-enzyme-linked immunosorbent-Assay (TP-IgM-ELISA). Nachweis erregerspezifischer IgM Antikorper im Serum und Liquor cerebrospinalis bei Syphilis Patienten mit und ohne Beteiligung des Zentralnervensystems an der Infektion. *Z. Hautkr. 58*:1689-1708.

Müller, G. and Keil, W. (1984). Durchführung des TPHA-Tests mit Trockenblutproben. *Dermatol. Monatsschr. 170*:332-335.

Müller, G. and Moskophidis, M. (1983). Estimation of the local production of antibodies to *T. pallidum* in the central nervous system of patients with neurosyphilis. *Br. J. Vener. Dis. 59*:80-84.

Müller, F. and Moskophidis, M. (1984). Evaluation of an enzyme immunoassay for IgM antibodies to *T. pallidum* in men. *Br. J. Vener. Dis. 60*:288-292.

Müller, F. and Wollemann, G. (1985). Analysis of specific immunoglobulin M immune response to *Treponema pallidum* before and after penicillin treatment of human syphilis. *Eur. J. Sex. Transm. Dis. 2*:67-72.

Nelson, R. A. and Mayer, M. M. (1949). Immobilization of *Treponema pallidum* in vitro by antibody produced by syphilitic infection. *J. Exp. Med. 89*:369-393.

Pangborn, M. C. (1941). A new serologically active phospholipid from beef heart. *Proc. Soc. Exp. Biol. Med. 48*:484-486.

Parham, C. E., Pettit, D. E., Larsen, S. A., Hambie, E. A., Perryman, M. W., and McGrew, B. E. (1984). Interlaboratory comparison of the toluidine red unheated serum test antigen preparation. *J. Clin. Microbiol. 20*:434-437.

Pettit, D. E., Larsen, S. A., Harbec, P. S., Feeley, J. C., Parham, C. E., Cruce, D. D., Hambie, E. A., and Perryman, M. W. (1983). Toluidine red unheated serum test, a nontreponemal test for syphilis. *J. Clin. Microbiol. 18*:1141-1145.

Pospisil, L. (1983). A simplified ELISA method for syphilis. *Dermatologica 167*: 105-108.

Rathlev, T. (1965). Hemagglutination tests utilizing antigens from pathogenic and apathogenic *Treponema pallidum. WHO/VDT/RES 77.65*. WHO, Geneva.

Rhodes, A. R. and Luger, A. (1986). Syphilis and other treponematoses. In *Dermatology in General Medicine* (T. B. Fitzpatrick, A. Z. Eisen, K. Wolff, I. M. Freedberg, and K. F. Austen, eds.), Vol. 2, 3rd Ed. McGraw-Hill, pp. 2395-2452.

Rice, M. and Fitzgerald, T. J. (1985). Detection of functional characterization of early appearing antibodies in rabbits with experimental syphilis. *Can. J. Microbiol. 31*:62-67.

Risse, A., Rhode, A., and Marneros, A. (1985). Erscheingungsformen der progressiven Paralyse. *Dtsch. Wochenschr. 110*:202-205.

Sachs, B. (1985). Zur gegenwaritigen Rolle der Neuroles in der Differential diagnose neuropsychiatrischer Krankheitsbilder. *Psychiatr. Neurol. Med. Psychol. 37*:416-420.

Sato, T., Kubo, E., Yokota, M., Kayashima, T., and Tomizawa, T. (1984). *T. pallidum* specific IgM haemagglutination test for serodiagnosis of syphilis. *Br. J. Vener. Dis. 60*:364-370.

Schmidt, B. L. (1980). Solid phase hemadsorption: A method for rapid detection of *Treponema pallidum*-specific IgM. *Sex. Transm. Dis. 7*:53-58.

Schmidt, B. L., Hutapea, N. O., Gschnait, F., Steinmetz, G., and Luger, A. (1985). The value of *Treponema pallidum* specific IgM tests for the diagnosis of latent yaws. *Eur. J. Sex. Transm. Dis. 2*:171-173.

Schmidt, B. L. and Schonwald, E. (1984). Die Elisa-Technik in der Syphilis-serologie (Erfahungsbericht). *Wien. Klin. Wochenschr. 96*:178-182.

Schröter, R., Wirth, H., and Petzoldt, D. (1983). Tertiaersyphilis der Haut mit biologisch falsch negativem 19S-(IgM)FTA-ABS Test. *Hautarzt 34*:332-334.

Sequeira, P. J. L. (1983). Serological diagnosis of untreated early syphilis. Importance of the differences in THA, TPHA and VDRL test titers. *Br. J. Vener. Dis. 59*:145-150.

Simon, R. P. (1985). Neurosyphilis. *Arch. Neurol. 42*:606-613.

Stevens, R. W. and Schmitt, M. E. (1985). Evaluation of an enzyme-linked immunosorbent assay for treponemal antibody. *J. Clin. Microbiol. 21*:399-402.

Stöckli, H. R. (1982). Diagnostik und Therapie der Neuroles heute. *Schweiz. Rundschau Med. (Praxis) 71*:1853-1859.

Stray-Pedersen, B. (1983). Economic evaluation of maternal screening to prevent congenital syphilis. *Sex. Transm. Dis. 10*:167-172.

Talbot, M. D. and Morton, R. (1985). Neurosyphilis: The most common things are most common. *Genitourin. Med. 61*:95-98.

Tanaka, S., Suzuki, T., Shimada, K., and Nishioka, K. (1984). Low molecular weight-IgM antibody in syphilis detected by *Treponema pallidum* immune adherence (TPIA) test. *Med. Microbiol. Immunol. 173*:155-165.

Tomizawa, T. and Kasamatsu, S. (1966). Haemagglutination tests for diagnosis of syphilis. A preliminary report. *Jpn. J. Med. Sci. Biol. 19*:305-338.

Veldkamp, J. and Visser, A. M. (1975). Application of the enzyme-linked immunosorbent assay (ELISA) in the serodiagnosis of syphilis. *Br. J. Vener. Dis. 51*:227-231.

Wasley, G. D. (1985). Internal quality control in serological test for syphilis. *Genitourin. Med. 61*:88-94.

Wassermann, A., Neisser, A., and Bruck, C. (1906). Eine serodiagnostische Reaktion bei Syphilis. *Dtsch. Med. Wochenschr. 32*:745-746.

Watson, P. A. (1985). The use of screening tests for sexually transmitted diseases in a Third World community a feasibility study in Malawi. *Eur. J. Sex. Transm. Dis. 2*:63-65.

Wicher, K. and Wicher, V. (1983). Immunopathology of syphilis. In *Pathogenesis and Immunology of Treponemal Infection* (R. F. Schell and D. M. Musher, eds.). Marcel Dekker, New York, pp. 139-159.

World Health Organization (1982). Treponemal infections, Report of a WHO Scientific Group. Technical Report Series No. 674, WHO, Geneva.

NINE

Immunological Diagnosis
of Trichomoniasis

John P. Ackers and Alexander Yule
London School of Hygiene
and Tropical Medicine
London, England

I. INTRODUCTION

Trichomoniasis is by far the most common protozoan infection in Europe and North America, and although in the Third World its importance is overshadowed by more lethal parasitic diseases, the actual prevalence there is even higher. It has also been claimed to be the world's most common sexually transmitted disease (Sun, 1982). Because it is never fatal, there is a common tendency to underrate the importance of this disease, but wherever it occurs trichomoniasis causes pain and deep distress, particularly to women. It is also suspiciously (but probably not causally) linked to carcinoma of the cervix and has been suggested as a cause of a low birth-weight in babies (Hardy et al., 1984). Because once diagnosed almost all cases of the infection can be treated successfully, there is a considerable need for inexpensive, rapid diagnostic tests that do not rely on a high level of expertise in the operator. After many false starts it now seems that immunological methods may be about to provide just this.

Trichomoniasis is caused by infection with the flagellate protozoon *Trichomonas vaginalis*. In women the infection is most commonly found in the vagina, the urethra, and the paraurethral glands; the organism does not, as a rule, ascend into the uterine cavity or the fallopian tubes (Catterall, 1972). Parasitemia does not occur, and dissemination beyond the lower urogenital tract is extremely rare. In males the most common site of infection is the urethra, although evidence (Gardener and Culberson, 1985) suggests that penetration of the stroma of the prostate may occur.

Some 25% of infected women are completely asymptomatic. Most of those with symptoms complain of vaginal discharge, and up to a half notice vulvovaginal soreness or irritation. Dysuria or urinary frequency is reported by about 25% of infected women and dyspareunia is common (Rein, 1985). The majority of infected men are completely asymptomatic; the remainder usually have urethral discharge (normally slight) and dysuria.

One of the most common methods of making a presumptive diagnosis of trichomoniasis is simply based on the presence of a purulent frothy vaginal discharge—essentially as described by Donne in 1836. Although certainly common in infected women, this clinical finding is far from adequate for making a correct diagnosis. In an important report Fouts and Kraus (1980) showed that 88% of 131 infected women would not have been identified; conversely 29% of women with frothy leukorrhea were not infected with *T. vaginalis*. The existence of asymptomatic trichomoniasis in a substantial proportion of infected women was again confirmed, and it seems unlikely that any combination of clinical symptoms will ever be an adequate substitute for laboratory investigations.

II. EPIDEMIOLOGY OF TRICHOMONIASIS

The sexual transmissibility of *T. vaginalis* is now universally accepted, and for at least 40 years it has been widely believed that most infections are so acquired (Catterall and Nicol, 1960; Trussell, 1974; Whittington, 1957; Willcox, 1960). Cases of neonatal trichomoniasis, however, have been reported. Al Salihi and colleagues (1974) found three cases among 984 newborn babies in New Jersey. Transmission to the baby, however, does not necessarily occur even from mothers infected at the time of delivery. In another study none of 14 female babies delivered to infected mothers harbored the parasite (Bramley, 1976). The organism is believed to be able to establish itself because the baby's vaginal epithelium is under the influence of maternal estrogen; as the hormone levels decline the infection usually resolves spontaneously. Because, however, infections are known in both prepubertal girls and postmenopausal women, it cannot be true that *T. vaginalis* can only persist in the vagina when the latter is under the influence of adult levels of estrogen.

Komorowska and Kurnatowska (1983) reported that the prevalence of trichomoniasis in a group (size not specified) of Polish girls was similar (about 0.8%) in newborns and in those aged 3 weeks to 10 years old, rising to about 4% in those aged 10-16 years. There was a strong correlation between infection in the girls and in one or the other of their parents. The authors regard this as evidence for transmission by the shared use of sanitary fittings. There is at least the possibility, however, that sexual abuse was responsible. Jones et al. (1985) reported trichomoniasis in four sexually abused girls, two of whom were premenarchal. Infections in postmenopausal women are also well documented; in fact the age distribution of the infection is unusual and very different from that of gonorrhea. The latter infection has a pronounced peak in the late teens and twenties (*Genitourin. Med.*, 1985; Nielsen, 1973) declining rapidly thereafter. Cases of trichomoniasis, on the other hand, while showing a peak in the years of greatest sexual activity, subsequently remain at a lower but more or less constant level until declining in women over 50. In at least two surveys a smaller secondary peak was found in women aged around 45 years old (Lipinski, 1983; Nielsen, 1973). The explanation for this bimodal distribution is not known, but it is possible that the second peak represents the recrudescence of long-standing asymptomatic infections. Some evidence that untreated infections with this parasite are not particularly short-lived comes from the work of Bogus-Rozkowska and Zablotniak (1966) who reported that the incidence of infection in male and female prisoners did not decline with an increase in time spent in custody—at least up to 2 years. Taken at face value this evidence would also seem to cast doubt on the suggestion, frequently invoked to explain the relative rarity of positive findings in men, that in males the infection is very transitory.

The possibility that some infections may be acquired without sexual contact has been repeatedly raised since Whittington (1957) showed that four of 30 female patients left infective material on toilet seats after using them and that organisms in vaginal material artificially applied to such seats remained viable for 30-45 min. The actual importance of this or other routes of nonsexual transmission (such as shared towels or clothing) is almost impossible to assess, but it is generally regarded as very slight (Honigberg, 1978).

III. CURRENT DIAGNOSTIC METHODS AND THEIR LIMITATIONS

In this section we describe methods based upon direct detection of the organism—either microscopically or by culture—together with a few miscellaneous techniques. Detailed instructions for taking suitable specimens are included in standard textbooks or in reviews such as those by Brown (1972) or Catterall (1972).

A. Microscopic Methods

1. Wet Films

The traditional wet-film examination still has a great deal to recommend it. A good microscope is far from inexpensive, but that apart, the equipment required is not expensive and is widely available. The sample needs to be examined fairly soon after being taken from the patient, which is a disadvantage, but the corollary is that a result can be obtained within a few minutes, and it is not necessary for the patient to be present on a second occasion. Finally, a living, motile trichomonad is quite unmistakable, and a positive diagnosis can be made with absolute confidence. Both phase-contrast and normal illumination have been used, but the former does not seem to have any overwhelming advantages. The chief disadvantage of the method is its limited sensitivity; studies comparing wet-film examination with culture methods have repeatedly found 20-30% more infections with the latter technique.

Most workers who have employed wet film examination have relied on the distinctive motility of trichomonads to pick them out among the cellular debris, but occasionally vital staining has been tried to enhance the sensitivity of the method. The various dyes that have been used are described by Honigberg (1978), who also mentions those that have been employed to distinguish living from dead organisms; however, neither method is used much today.

2. Fixed and Stained Preparations

In our experience *T. vaginalis* becomes much more difficult to identify when it is dead because the characteristic flagella and undulating membrane are far less visible. However, the use of fixed and stained films for diagnosis is a technique employed by many workers with great success. Of the dyes employed, the various Romanowsky stains are probably the most popular, having been employed by many of the authors listed by Honigberg (1978) and Kariks (1983). In general, those who employed it were very satisfied with the method, but we found that it was easy to overstain the organisms, producing nothing but a dark, featureless blob. We were, however, able to produce satisfactory slides for demonstration purposes by fixing the undried organisms with osmium tetroxide vapor and staining them for 20-40 min with dilute Giemsa (Neva et al., 1961), but this method is far too cumbersome for routine use. Other stains that have been recommended include periodic acid-Schiff (Rodriguez-Martinez, 1973), gentian violet (Teras and Kaarma, 1969), and the Gram stain which is not, however, generally useful (Jirovec and Petru, 1968). The stains most studied have been the fluorescent dye acridine orange and the Papanicolaou stain.

Acridine orange staining has been claimed to be even more sensitive than culture by some workers (Fripp et al., 1975; Juranyi and Kleeberg, 1973; Mason et al., 1976) but not by others (Ghosh and Douglass, 1983; Martin et al., 1963); the method suffers from the disadvantage that an expensive fluorescence microscope is needed. Papanicolaou staining was an obvious method to try: not only is it widely available but as smears taken from infected women are prone to show apparently suspicious atypical cellular hyperplasia (Frost, 1967; Honigberg, 1978) the ability to diagnose infection with *T. vaginalis* in routine cervical smears would be clearly valuable. Results, however, have been mixed. Some investigators have found the method useful: Summers and Ford (1972) found trichomonads in an extremely high proportion (72%) of male contacts when using the stain on prostatic fluid samples, but other investigators have found it very difficult to make a positive identification using this technique and suspect that it yields many false-positive results (Perl, 1972).

3. Fluorescent Antibody Staining

Fluorescent antibody staining is considered in Sect. VII.

B. Culture

Although a few investigators have found examination of fresh or stained films to be as good as (or even better than) culture as a diagnostic tool, there is almost complete agreement that culturing of specimens will yield more positive results than any other method. Because the final diagnosis is made by visual examination of a copious number of living organisms, the accuracy of the method may be regarded as perfect; if necessary, carefully stained films may be examined to differentiate between the three human trichomonads. The only serious disadvantages of using culture for routine diagnosis are the time taken to obtain a positive result and the not inconsiderable expense involved in preparing and handling large quantities of serum-rich media. In our experience most cultures become positive within 2 days, but as a few specimens (often taken from male patients) do not show visible growth for 10-12 days (Wilson and Ackers, 1980) it is unwise to discard them after less than 7 days incubation. For our most critical work, therefore, we keep cultures for 2 weeks before discarding them.

Numerous culture media have been devised for the axenic growth of *T. vaginalis* and there is no doubt that many of them are perfectly satisfactory. In our own work we have used either modified Lumsden's medium (Ackers et al., 1975), Hollander's medium (1976) (both fluid and solid), and more recently, modified Diamond's medium (Diamond, 1957). The last has become probably the most widely used medium worldwide and is obviously highly satisfactory. Hollander's solid medium appears to be capable of growing discrete colonies from single organisms with high efficiency, and the Lumsden medium has the advantage that it contains an indicator. The color change from purple to yellow caused by the production of lactic and other organic acids by the growing trichomonads makes the rapid checking of large numbers of samples easy. Many other media are used by different clinics and research groups with complete success. Details of some but by no means all can be found in reviews by Taylor and Baker (1968), Honigberg (1978) and Diamond (1983). Antibacterial and sometimes antifungal agents are included in all media currently used for clinical diagnosis to prevent overgrowth of the parasites; it seems generally agreed that penicillins are not inhibitory and may be used in any desired amount, but it is probably wise to keep the concentration of other antibiotics down to the minimum effective level. A discussion of the possible undesirable effects of antibiotics on the phenotype of *T. vaginalis* in culture is given by Honigberg (1970).

C. Miscellaneous Met:10ds

Trichomonas vaginalis is known to contain high levels of putrescine (White et al., 1983), and Chen et al. (1982) showed that diamines could be detected in a high percentage of women with trichomonal vaginitis and in those with nonspecific vaginitis. In an earlier study (Nunn et al., 1974) it was shown that four *N*-nitrosamines were present in pooled vaginal discharge from black women infected with *T. vaginalis* but not in uninfected women. Although these results are interesting and could be important in view of the frequently reported correlation between infection with *T. vaginalis* and cervical carcinoma, neither has yet been developed as a routine diagnostic tool.

D. Conclusions

For the present, a combination of wet-film examination, for speed and accuracy, and culture (which will detect 20-30% more cases) seem to be the optimum diagnostic protocol. In the experience of most workers, fixed and stained films lose the immediacy of the wet-film examination without attaining the sensitivity of culture techniques.

IV. ANTIGENIC STRUCTURE

This section deals with the grosser serological differences that have been known for some time, whereas the more detailed knowledge of specific parasite components derived from studies using monoclonal antibodies (MAb) are considered in Sects. VII and VIII.

The first attempts at antigenic analysis of *T. vaginalis* were concerned with establishing the organism as a valid species, distinct from other human trichomonads. In early work, Tokura (1935) showed that trichomonads were antigenic in experimental animals and that agglutination tests with the resulting sera could distinguish between *T. vaginalis* and *Pentatrichomonas hominis*. After bacteria-free cultivation had been achieved, unambiguous antigenic differences between *T. vaginalis* and *Tritrichomonas foetus* were shown by a number of workers, whose results are summarized by Honigberg (1970, 1978). Another important early report was that of Kott and Adler (1961) who showed the existence of both unique and common antigens in the three human species of trichomonad: *T. vaginalis, T. tenax,* and *P. hominis.*

Later work was more concerned with the demonstration of antigenic differences between different isolates of the same species—in almost all cases *T. vaginalis*. These antigenically defined populations were referred to as serotypes. The existence of serotypes among isolates of *T. vaginalis* was first reported by Schoenherr in 1956, but the most extensive investigations have been by the Estonian group of Teras and his collaborators (Teras, 1965, 1966). These authors reported the presence of four serotypes among several hundred clinical isolates and demonstrated that the results were consistent whether they were determined by agglutination, indirect hemagglutination, or complement fixation (Teras et al., 1966). Kott and Adler (1961) had already found even more heterogeneity, detecting no fewer than eight different serotypes among only 23 isolates. The Estonian group subsequently claimed that the existence of serotypes was also shown by the results of attempts to develop serodiagnostic tests, and that these tests were satisfactory only if the full range of locally occurring serotypes were included in the test antigen. It is interesting, therefore, that this serotype specificity has not been apparent in some more recently described diagnostic tests. Studies employing indirect fluorescence (Mason, 1979), an enzyme-linked immunosorbent assay (ELISA) (Street et al., 1982), and direct agglutination (Ackers, 1987) have failed to show higher titers or more positive results when sera from infected women were tested with homologous rather than heterologous antigen. It may well be, however, that the total polyclonal response, which is what these tests measure, is dominated by antibodies directed against common determinants.

In recent years, several groups have again returned to the question of the antigenic diversity of *T. vaginalis.* By use of quantitative fluorescent antibody methods Su-Lin and Honigberg (1983) examined five cloned strains and determined the relative amounts of common antigen present in each by measuring the reduction in fluorescence (compared with unabsorbed homologous rabbit antiserum) when the staining serum was absorbed with homologous and heterologous antigen. The results showed that each strain possessed unique antigens as well as antigens shared with the other strains examined.

Subsequently, Alderete (1983) examined the total trichloracetic acid precipitable proteins of five strains of the parasite by electrophoresis in sodium dodecyl sulfate polyacrylamide gels (SDS-PAGE). A complex pattern of protein bands was seen, covering a range of molecular weights from 20,000 to 200,000 but, apart from small variations in intensity, there were no significant differences among the five strains; the pattern of bands from *Tritrichomonas foetus* was, however, considerably different. Radioimmunoprecipitation was then used to discover which bands were recognized as immunogens by rabbits. It was shown that almost the same patterns were obtained with both heterologous and homologous sera; a change in pattern was not seen when organisms were reexamined after 1 year in laboratory culture. A similar result was reported by Delachambre (1980) using the relatively insensitive technique of precipitation in gel. Both of these findings were in contrast with the results reported for *T. gallinae* and *Histomonas meleagridis* (Dwyer, 1974). Further details of specific parasite antigens recognized by monoclonal antibodies (MAbs) will be given in Sect. VIII, but in an important report Krieger and coworkers (1985) described the geographical variation among isolates of *T. vaginalis* from various areas of the United States.

The whole field is once again the subject of intensive research, but two conclusions now appear to be reasonably firmly established: (1) *T. vaginalis* isolates possess a large number of common antigens and a much smaller number that are shared with other Trichomonadidae; and (2) antibodies raised against *T. vaginalis* recognize not only common but also strain-specific antigens. Whether this represents genuine antigenic diversity or merely variability in the immune response of the host is not yet clear.

Not all antigens present on the surface of *T. vaginalis* are necessarily of parasite origin. It has long been suspected that trichomonads obtained by in vitro culture will possess medium components bound to their surface; absorption of many different components has now been demonstrated directly (Peterson and

Alderete, 1982). Interestingly, although most molecules can be removed by simple washing, others including a_1-antitrypsin, a_2-macroglobulin, lactoferrin, and lipoproteins appear to be firmly bound (Peterson and Alderete, 1983, 1984a,b). Although these bound molecules may have nutritional or protective, rather than immunological functions, there is no doubt, as they have elicited MAbs, that absorbed medium components are antigenic (Torian et al., 1984). The extent to which *T. vaginalis* grown in vivo in its normal host possess bound human proteins has not yet been discovered, but it seems likely that they are present. To what extent, if any, such proteins assist the parasite's survival by conferring upon it a degree of "immunological invisibility" is unknown.

V. SEROLOGICAL AND LOCAL ANTIBODY RESPONSES TO INFECTION

The profusion of antibody-based diagnostic tests that follow is proof that infected women and men do produce antibodies against *T. vaginalis*; that none of these tests are in widespread clinical use shows equally clearly that this response, if present, may not be particularly powerful. In addition, any study of induced antiparasitic antibodies is further complicated by the preexistence of natural serum antibodies.

A. Natural Antibodies

The occurrence of agglutinating and (complement-mediated) lytic factors in the sera of humans who have not been exposed to *T. vaginalis* has been recognized for many years—ever since it became necessary to define the lower limit of positivity of diagnostic tests based on serum antibody detection. In general, and depending upon the technique used, titers from 20 to 160 were regarded as nonspecific (Honigberg, 1970). Although the activity was and is generally assumed to be due to antibody and was normally regarded as a nuisance, an attempt to study the phenomenon in its own right was made by Reisenhoffer (1963). She studied the lytic and agglutinating activities of a wide variety of sera against *T. vaginalis*. Her conclusions for human sera were, first, that unheated serum had a powerful lytic activity that did not depend upon age, sex, or previous or current infection with the parasite, and second, that heating the sera for 30 min at 56°C reduced but did not abolish the activity. The agglutinating activity of human serum was modest, but that of bovine serum much greater. Low agglutinin titers (not exceeding 4) were also reported by Tatsuki (1957) and were found in our own (unpublished) work. Nigesen, however, when developing an agglutination test, regarded all titers up to 160 as resulting from natural antibody (Honigberg, 1970). A major study by Samuels and Chun-Hoon (1964) of agglutinins in heat-inactivated sera was chiefly concerned with *T. augusta*. They noted, however,

that when sera were active against a number of trichomonad species, including
T. vaginalis, activity against one species could be absorbed out with organisms
of that species without affecting the titers against the others. This specificity
convinced the authors that the agglutination observed was due to antibodies, and
this opinion has not been challenged since. Most, if not all, of the previously reported lytic activity in unheated serum would now, however, probably be attributed to the alternative pathway activation of complement (Gillin and Sher, 1981;
Holbrook et al., 1982).

The origin of these natural antibodies in human and other sera is not known,
but it has been attributed to cross-reaction with components of the normal flora,
infection with commensal trichomonads, or genetic predisposition (Samuels and
Chun-Hoon, 1964). In humans, in whom infections with *T. tenax* and *P. hominis*
are relatively rare, particularly in youth, the first explanation is perhaps the most
probable (Ackers and Lumsden, 1978). The antibody's role, if any, in host defense mechanisms is not known, but specific natural antibody is known to be able
to play a stimulatory role in the activation of complement by the alternative
pathway and may thus contribute to the effectiveness of that potent antitrichomonal system (Gillin and Sher, 1981).

B. Induced Antibody Formation

Although the existence of specific serum antibody in at least some cases of human
trichomoniasis is undoubted, there is very little evidence that it has any affect on
the parasite in vivo. In fact, examination of an exhaustive survey (Honigberg,
1970) of the older results of attempts to develop serodiagnostic tests reveals that
two of the three most-used techniques (complement fixation and indirect hemagglutination) give a higher percentage of positive results in patients with chronic
long-lasting infections; only agglutination tests gave similar results with acute and
chronic cases. The interpretation of all such results is complicated by the need to
allow for preexisting natural antibody, but to the extent that new, specific antibody is formed, it is clearly ineffective in eliminating the infection. More recent
serological tests confirm the existence of serum antibody of the IgM, IgG, and
IgA classes, but not of the IgE class; however, their function in protective immunity is unknown. Chipperfield and Evans (1972) showed that an increase in
the number of IgM-, IgG-, and IgA-secreting plasma cells occurred in the endocervix following infection with *T. vaginalis, Neisseria gonorrhoeae,* and *Candida
albicans*; the greatest increase in IgM-bearing cells was found in patients with
trichomoniasis.

It has been long appreciated that if antibody produced in response to infection with a noninvasive organism, such as *T. vaginalis*, is to have any effect on
the parasite, then it must do so within the lumen of the genitourinary tract. Such
antibody may be either synthesized locally or derived from the serum. In the last

10 years, the presence of antitrichomonal antibody in the cervicovaginal secretions has been demonstrated by radioimmunoassay (Ackers et al., 1975), ELISA (Alderete, 1984; Street et al., 1982) and immunofluorescence (Su, 1982) methods. In general, IgG and IgA antibodies were detected in most, but by no means in all, infected women; specific IgM, or IgE, or both, was found either in only a small percentage or not at all. The last result is rather surprising considering the findings of Chipperfield and Evans (1972) and suggests that a large part of the detected antibody could have been derived from the serum. Although in our original work we suggested the existence of a possible correlation between the presence of local antibody and low numbers of parasites (Ackers et al., 1975), the effect was far from definite. Samples containing some of the highest detected levels of antibody had no apparent harmful effects on cultured organisms in vitro (Ackers, unpublished). Again, if local antibody is an effective defense mechanism, its presence could explain the rarity of symptomatic trichomoniasis in men. We were, however, unable to find significant amounts of specific antibody in either infected men or male contacts of infected women (Ackers et al., 1978). If, in fact, locally synthesized IgA antibody is important in host defense, it may possibly be by a recently described mechanism whereby specific IgA potentiates the effect of opsonization by IgG on the phagocytosis of target cells by human peripheral blood polymorphonuclear leukocytes (Goldstine et al., 1983).

Although outside the scope of this review, it is clear that even though there undoubtedly is an immune response to *T. vaginalis* in infected men and women, there is little or no evidence for any effect on the parasite in vivo; clinical experience leaves no doubt that repeated infections in the same patient are common. The usefulness, or otherwise, of these responses as the basis of diagnostic methods is considered in the following section.

VI. ANTIBODY-BASED DIAGNOSTIC METHODS

It would be extremely useful, particularly for population surveys, to have a means of diagnosing trichominiasis (and other sexually transmitted diseases) from a blood sample, thus avoiding the intimate examinations necessary to obtain specimens for culture of direct microscopy. The lack of such a test is the fundamental reason we do not have accurate figures for the prevalence of trichomoniasis in unselected populations. It is, therefore, not surprising that, over the years, much effort has been devoted to developing a serodiagnostic test; so far with disappointing results.

The problem does not lie in the detection of the antibody but, rather, in the failure of some infected patients to make a sufficiently virogous antibody response. Consequently, low limits have to be set for negative results, and these then tend to overlap with the levels of natural antibody found in some uninfected individuals.

In 1970, Honigberg published a comprehensive review of the immunological aspects of trichomonads in general, which included summaries of virtually all of the work carried out up to that point on the serodiagnosis of *T. vaginalis* infections. Reasonably promising results with a complement fixation test were obtained by Hoffman and coworkers (1963). Even better results were reported by Jaakmees et al. (1966) who found that sera from all infected patients, both men and women, were positive, as were 28 of 40 female contacts and four of five male contacts. All control sera were negative. Results from direct agglutination tests were also impressive. Teras and his colleagues (1966) reported that sera from 96% of infected women and 84% of infected men were positive. The minimum titer considered significant was high (320) but values of up to half this were found in uninfected controls. These high titers of presumably natural agglutinins are in contrast with the low values found by Tatsuki (1957) and Reisenhoffer (1963). Indirect hemagglutination tests were first applied to trichomoniasis patients by McEntegart (1952) who found that sera from 84% of infected women were reactive. Subsequently Hoffman (1966) reported positive results from 90% of infected women but from only 55% of infected men. Disappointingly, however, Lanceley and McEntegart (1953) had already studied five male volunteers experimentally inoculated intraurethrally with cultured *T. vaginalis*; three definitely became infected but none developed detectable levels of antibody.

Although little new work was published in the following decade, more recently interest has reappeared, mostly in applying newer or more convenient methods of detecting antitrichomonal antibody. Thus, the ELISA technique has been used widely (Ackers et al., 1983; Alderete, 1984; Cogne et al., 1985; Garber et al., 1986; Street et al., 1982), immunofluorescence (IFAT) was employed by Mason (1979), and indirect hemagglutination (IHA) by Mathews and Healy (1983) and Yano and coworkers (1983). Mathews and Healy also evaluated precipitation in gel and Cogne et al. (1985) directly compared ELISA, IFAT, and IHA, finding that ELISA correlated best with past or present infection. Lukasic et al. (1977) also described a coated particle (carbon) agglutination test. Some of these authors were more interested in the fundamentals of the host immune response rather than in possible diagnostic tests, but the results of the others are summarized in Table 1. It is extremely difficult to compare tests carried out by different investigators on diverse groups of patients, but the following conclusions might be warranted: First, if the results from the control groups can be taken at face value (most consist of children) many uninfected women possess significant levels of antibody, which suggests that the tests are not particularly specific, or that past infections produce long-lasting seroconversion, or that the diagnostic methods used are missing a considerable number of low-level infections. The results of Cogne and coworkers (1985) lend some support to the second suggestion because nine of 14 women infected at an unstated time in the past gave a positive result. Second, it still seems clear that none of the tests described have

Table 1 Results of Some Recent Attempts to Develop a Serodiagnostic Test for Human Trichomoniasis

Assay method[a]	Ref.[d]	Positive results reported with (%)				
		Infected women	Uninfected women	Infected men	Uninfected men	Controls[b]
ELISA	1	33/41 (81)	23/168 (14)	ND	ND	3/99 (3)
ELISA	2	ND	ND	0/3	1/96 (1)	ND
ELISA	3	22/22 (100)	29/59[c] (49)	2/3	ND	0/50 (0)
IHA	4	138/178 (78)	35/72 (49)	ND	ND	ND
IHA	3	15/22 (68)	8/59[c] (13)	1/3	ND	0/30 (0)
PG	4	76/178 (43)	45/181 (25)	ND	ND	ND
IFA	5	48/52 (92)	25/148 (17)	ND	ND	1/30 (3)
IFA	3	19/22 (86)	22/59[c] (37)	1/3	ND	0/30 (0)
IFA	6	4/10 (40)	0/6	ND	ND	ND

[a]ELISA, enzyme-linked immunosorbent assay; IHA, indirect hemagglutination; PG, precipitation in gel; IFA, immunofluorescence assay; ND, not done.
[b]An arbitrary distinction is drawn between "uninfected" persons, defined as those who are at risk but uninfected at the time of the study, and "controls" who are persons most unlikely ever to have been infected.
[c]Sex not defined, but the majority female.
[d]References: 1, Street et al. (1982); 2, Ackers et al. (1983); 3, Cogne et al. (1985); 4, Mathews and Healey (1983); 5, Mason (1979); 6, Yano et al. (1983).

Table 2 Results of Four Recent Studies of Local Antitrichomonal Antibody in Women

| Assay method[a] | Ref.[b] | Positive results reported with (%) | | Antibody class |
		Infected women	Apparently uninfected women	
RIA	1	22/29 (76)	8/19 (42)	IgA
ELISA	2	30/40 (73)	41/100 (41)	IgA or IgG or both
IFA	3	17/24 (71)	7/30 (22)	IgG
IFA	4	9/30 (30)	ND[a]	IgA

[a]RIA, radioimmunoassay; ELISA, enzyme-linked immunosorbent assay; IFA, immunofluorescence assay; ND, not done.
[b]References: 1, Ackers et al. (1975); 2, Street et al. (1982); 3, Su (1982); 4, Martinotti et al. (1982).

yet achieved the combination of specificity and sensitivity that would make sero-diagnosis a reliable and routine procedure. Third, with the possible exception of the ELISA test of Cogne and coworkers, the particularly disappointing results previously found with samples from men are seen again in the few samples in-cluded in the results in Table 1. Finally, and in contrast with the earlier reports (particularly from the Estonian group of Teras and his coworkers) that empha-sized the serotype-specific nature of human serum antibody responses to *T. vag-inalis*, there is no evidence in the more recent reports for a higher frequency of positive results when sera are tested against homologous rather than heterologous antigen.

As a powerful serum antibody response to a luminal parasite, such as *T. vaginalis*, is unlikely to occur in all patients, it seemed useful to look for local antibody in servicovaginal secretions. The techniques used and the samples taken are too diverse to summarize easily but, in general, where the class of antibody present has been determined, specific IgG has been found more often than IgA (Street et al., 1982; Su, 1982). The results of four recent studies of infected women are shown in Table 2; results from a group of women unlikely ever to have been at risk are not available. As with the serum antibody tests, it is clear that more infected than uninfected women give positive results but also that the test is, if anything, less sensitive and specific than one based on serum antibody. As before, there was no improvement in sensitivity when homologous rather than heterologous antigen was used (Ackers et al., 1975; Street et al., 1982; Su, 1982).

VII. PRODUCTION AND CHARACTERIZATION OF POLYCLONAL ANTISERA AND MONOCLONAL ANTIBODIES

Clearly, serodiagnostic tests for *T. vaginalis* have not attained the specificity and sensitivity required for clinical use and, given the limited host immune response to the parasite, it is unlikely that this situation will alter. The immunological de-tection of *T. vaginalis* antigen (or whole organisms) appears more promising, and much current research is directed toward the identification of key parasite anti-gens and to the production of suitable monoclonal and polyclonal reagents.

A. Polyclonal Antisera

1. Immunization Schedules

Whereas *T. vaginalis* elicits only a limited serum antibody response in its human host, immunization of experimental animals has produced antisera of sufficiently high titer to allow antigen analysis by radioimmunoprecipitation and immuno-blotting techniques and for diagnostic use. Rabbits have been widely employed and published immunization regimens have used both intramuscular and subcutaneous routes, or a combination of these. We (Yule et al., 1987) have found that intramuscular immunization with 2×10^6 organisms (derived from axenic culture) in Freund's complete adjuvant followed by two boosts of the same dose in incomplete adjuvant, at intervals of 14 days, with bleeding 7 days after the last boost, produces antisera of sufficient quality for antigen detection by enzyme immunoassay. Maintenance of this regimen results in further increases in antibody concentration and affinity (Yule and Carney, unpublished observation).

Torian et al. (1984) used the regimen of Cooney and Kenny (1970) in which rabbits were primed intramuscularly with previously frozen *T. vaginalis* (initial dose of 1.65 mg protein in 1 ml incomplete adjuvant) and boosted intravenously after 21 days with increasing doses (0.1, 0.2, 0.3, and 0.4 ml) at intervals of 3-4 days. Alderete (1983) found no amplification of the antibody response in rabbits by boosting intravenously with formalin-fixed organisms after primary immunization by the intramuscular route. Bennet et al. (1980) used sustained subcutaneous immunization of approximately 3×10^7 organisms twice weekly for a period of 12 weeks to produce antisera for use in an indirect immunoperoxidase technique.

Because *T. vaginalis* has the ability to bind medium-derived serum components to its surface (Peterson and Alderete, 1982), organisms require repeated washing with phosphate-buffered saline (PBS) or Tris-buffered saline (TBS) before use in immunization. As a further precaution, Torian et al. (1984) cultured organisms in a medium dialysate supplemented with an "agamma" rabbit serum fraction. When producing rabbit antisera for use in immunodiagnosis, we (Yule et al., 1987) routinely immunize with PBS-washed organisms cultured in a yeast extract-free medium (Meyer's HSP-1 medium; Meyer, 1976) supplemented with homologous serum to minimize the risk of provoking a medium component-directed antibody response that could potentially cross-react with other antigens present in the urogenital tract.

2. Detection and Characterization

Serological methods used to detect the human immune response against *T. vaginalis* have also been applied to the assessment of serum antibody responses in challenged animals. The earlier methods of direct agglutination and passive hemagglutination (Kott and Adler, 1961) have been largely superseded by ELISA and immunofluorescence assay (IFA) methods. Microtiter plate-based ELISAs using both ethanol-fixed trichomonads and aqueous trichomonal protein extracts as antigens have been described by Alderete (1984) for the detection of immunized rabbit (and infected mouse and human) serum responses. We (Yule and Ackers, unpublished observations) found a twofold increase in the ELISA optical density values obtained with immune rabbit sera when whole cells were replaced with a soluble antigen fraction prepared by repeated slow freezing and thawing of pelleted *T. vaginalis*. Nonionic detergent (Nonidet P40- NP40) lysates of whole cells have also proved suitable as antigen in ELISA (Yule and Ackers, unpublished observations) and can be coated directly onto polystyrene microtiter plates without removing the detergent from the preparation.

Characterization of the antigenic specificity of polyclonal antisera has been performed using radioimmunoprecipitation of detergent (Zwittergent 3-12)-extracted antigens, direct parasite agglutination, and IFA of motile parasites (Alderete, 1983). In evaluating antisera for diagnostic use an indirect inhibition enzyme immunoassay, in which known numbers of trichomonads or other test material are preincubated with a selected concentration of rabbit anti-*T. vaginalis* antiserum, is convenient for determining the degree of cross-reactivity with a number of *T. vaginalis* isolates and for confirming the absence of reactivity with medium-derived components (Yule and Ackers, 1985).

B. Monoclonal Antibodies

1. Immunization Schedules

Trichomonas vaginalis readily elicits an antibody response in mice, and standard fusion protocols using hypoxanthine, aminopterin, thymidine (HAT) selection and the murine myeloma cell lines NS/1 (Krieger et al., 1985; Torian et al., 1984), P3-X63-Ag8-653 (Chang et al., 1986; Yule and Ackers, unpublished data), and SP2/0-Ag14 (Alderete et al., 1986) have been successful in producing monoclonal antibodies (MAbs). We (Yule and Ackers, unpublished data) and others (Chang et al., 1986; Torian et al., 1984) have used combined intraperitoneal and intravenous immunization with between 8×10^5 and 1×10^7 live organisms per injection, whereas Krieger et al. (1985) used only the intraperitoneal route. Intraperitoneal immunization with a nonionic detergent (NP40) lysate of whole trichomonads (0.2 mg protein per immunization) has also been used (Yule and Ackers, unpublished data). Alderete et al. (1986) have used subcutaneous infection of mice to generate a MAb against a selected surface glycoprotein antigen associated with antigenic heterogeneity.

2. Detection and Characterization

As in the polyclonal antibody responses, ELISA and IFA have been widely applied to the detection of anti-*T. vaginalis* MAbs. The ELISA is particularly suited to the large number of screening tests involved in MAb production, and microtiter plate assays using either live, formalin-fixed (Torian et al., 1984), ethanol-fixed (Alderete et al., 1986), or sonicated organisms (Krieger et al., 1985) have been described. Chang et al. (1986) applied an indirect-binding radioimmunoassay utilizing live parasites in free suspension. To safeguard against the inadvertent selection of hybridomas secreting antibodies directed against medium-derived components, we (Yule and Ackers, unpublished work) and Torian et al. (1984) cultured organisms intended for use in screening in a medium (HSP-1) (Meyer, 1976) that did not share components with the medium in which the immunizing isolates were grown (TYM or TYI-S-33) (Diamond, 1957, 1978).

As they allow some discrimination between intracellular and extracellular antibody binding, indirect IFA methods have proved particularly useful in the characterization of antitrichomonal Mabs. Both formalin-fixed (Connelly et al., 1985; Krieger et al., 1985; Torian et al., 1984) and acetone-fixed organisms (Chang et al., 1986; Yule and Ackers, unpublished work) have been employed. Motile parasites have also been used in IFA (Alderete et al., 1986; Torian et al., 1984) to demonstrate parasite surface antigen-directed antibodies. Connelly et al. (1985) used direct parasite agglutination for the same purpose. Further characterization of the antigens defined by monoclonal antibodies has been performed by immunoblotting (Connelly et al., 1985; Torian et al., 1984), periodate or protease treatment of whole cells bound to microtiter plates followed by ELISA (Alderete et al., 1986; Connelly et al., 1985; Torian et al., 1984), and radioimmunoprecipitation (Alderete et al., 1986). Torian and his colleagues found that three antibodies were unreactive in immunoblotting; however, the corresponding antigens could be affinity-isolated from detergent (Triton X-100) extracts of *T. vaginalis* eluted through MAb-bearing Sepharose immunoabsorbent columns (Connelly et al., 1985).

VIII. DETECTION OF *TRICHOMONAS VAGINALIS* ANTIGEN WITH POLYCLONAL ANTISERA AND MONOCLONAL ANTIBODIES

A. Current Status of *Trichomonas vaginalis* Immunodiagnosis

At the time of writing, the application of *T. vaginalis* antigen detection to clinical diagnosis is still very much in its infancy. Past attempts have concentrated on the immunocytochemical localization of trichomonads with peroxidase or fluorescein-labeled antibody, and the recent availability of Mabs to *T. vaginalis* has lead to renewed interest in IFA as a diagnostic method. However, IFA and immunoperoxidase methods require subjective evaluation of a specimen by microscopic examination. Accurate diagnosis, therefore, depends upon not only the selection of suitable reagents but also upon the skill and experience of the operator and the quality of sample preparation. We have concentrated our efforts on the detection of trichomonal antigen by more objective means and have developed an enzyme immunoassay (EIA) for this purpose.

In addition to the question of what constitutes the most appropriate immunodiagnostic technique for urogenital trichomoniasis, the more basic question of *T. vaginalis* antigenic heterogeneity and its relevance to the production and selection of suitable diagnostic reagents requires consideration. Available evidence suggests that heterogeneity should not present a problem in polyclonal-based assay systems because, given the number of highly immunogenic *T. vaginalis* proteins recognized by polyclonal antisera (Alderete, 1983), it is probable that a rabbit antiserum raised against one isolate will also react with all others. By using rabbit antisera raised against a single isolate, O'Hara et al. (1980) successfully detected organisms by an immunoperoxidase method in each of 22 urine cytological preparations obtained from 22 *T. vaginalis*-infected patients. We (Yule and Ackers, 1985) raised rabbit antisera against a combination of two isolates and found comparable levels of inhibition between the immunizing isolates and eight other isolates in an indirect inhibition EIA.

Published reports indicate that antigenic heterogeneity requires more careful consideration in the selection of MAbs for diagnostic use. Torian et al. (1984) found different patterns of reactivity in IFA and ELISA with MAbs prepared in mice immunized with either one or two isolates; eight antibodies showed identical patterns with four isolates but were unreactive with a further five isolates, whereas one antibody reacted with all *T. vaginalis* isolates tested, as well as with isolates of *T. gallinae, Tritrichomonas foetus,* and *Giardia lamblia.* In a larger study (Krieger et al., 1985), mice were immunized with a combination of four isolates obtained from the same geographical area. Nine of the resulting MAbs were examined by IFA for reactivity with 88 isolates obtained from five geographical areas of the United States. Each isolate reacted with at least one antibody, with the individual reactivities of antibodies ranging between 22 and 76% of isolates; five antibodies detected more than 60% of isolates, whereas four "narrowly reactive" antibodies demonstrated differences in the antigenic composition of isolates obtained from different geographical areas.

Little is now known of the specific components that mediate antigenic heterogeneity in *T. vaginalis.* The reactivity of eight isolate-specific MAbs was abolished by periodate treatment, suggesting that their corresponding antigens were carbohydrate (Torian et al., 1984). In a further study, each of three of these antibodies (Connelly et al., 1985) was found to recognize a 115 kd component, and one or more components of 59-64 kd. These antigens were expressed on the surface of three of four isolates that were tested by direct agglutination and could not be isolated on an immunoabsorbent column from an extract of the nonreactive isolate. It has been proposed (Alderete et al., 1985) that heterogeneity is dependent upon the surface disposition of high-molecular-weight proteinaceous antigens that are synthesized, but not externalized, by all *T. vaginalis* isolates. Studies with a MAb (Alderete et al., 1986) suggest that a major surface glycoprotein of 267 kd may be implicated in antigenic heterogeneity, although of seven isolates examined, one possessed a cross-reactive 170-kd antigen, rather than a 267-kd antigen.

B. Polyclonal Antisera

1. Immunoperoxidase Staining

O'Hara et al. (1980) evaluated an earlier indirect immunoperoxidase (IP) technique (Bennet et al., 1980) for the detection of *T. vaginalis* in cytological preparations. Trichomonads were easily identified on low-power microscopic examination by their dark-brown, granular, appearance. In a direct comparison using duplicate cervical smears obtained from 100 patients, *T. vaginalis* was detected by both Papanicolaou staining and IP staining in four smears, and in a further 16 smears by IP only. Additionally, organisms were successfully identified in urine cytological preparations and in previously Papanicolaou-stained cervical smears. The authors demonstrated the value of immunoperoxidase staining as a means of unequivocally identifying trichomonads in unusual sites by confirming their presence in fluid from a renal cyst. More recently, Gardner and Culberson (1985) applied the technique to the identification of otherwise unrecognizable *T. vaginalis* organisms in histological sections of human prostate.

2. Immunofluorescence Assay

Surprisingly, few attempts using polyclonal antisera have been made to apply the immunofluorescence assay (IFA) to the diagnosis of *T. vaginalis* infection. McEntegart et al. (1958) were unsuccessful in applying a globulin fraction of immune rabbit serum directly conjugated to fluorescein isothiocyanate to the detection of *T. vaginalis* in vaginal smears because of high levels of nonspecific staining. In a short abstract, Hayes and Kotcher (1960) reported the comparison of a direct IFA procedure that used rabbit antiserum with established techniques for detecting *T. vaginalis* in vaginal secretions. Of 225 specimens examined, 33.3% were positive for *T. vaginalis* by wet-mount examination, 13% by Papanicolaou staining, 40% by culture, and 39.6% by direct IFA. By use of immune rabbit serum absorbed with rat liver powder Karbowski (1966) demonstrated the use of direct IFA to detect *T. vaginalis* antigens in histological sections of experimentally infected mice.

3. Antigen-Detecting Enzyme Immunoassay

The enzyme immunoassay (EIA) currently used in our laboratory is the "tandem" type, and uses the same rabbit antibody fraction, affinity-purified on a Sepharose-*T. vaginalis* NP40 detergent lysate column, for both antigen capture and antigen detection. The clinical applicability of the assay was evaluated using duplicate vaginal swabs obtained from women attending a local STD clinic (Yule et al., 1987). Of 482 women tested, 44 (9.13%) were culture-positive for *T. vaginalis* infection; antigen was detected in 41 of these women by EIA (8.51% of those tested). In an additional nine culture-negative women, antigen was also detected at concentrations comparable with those found in the culture-positive women. Examination of their clinical histories indicated that five of these women had vaginal symptoms suggestive of *T. vaginalis* infection at the time of sampling, whereas four women were completely asymptomatic. This suggests the possibility of culture failure in at least some of these cases and illustrates the difficulty of selecting a suitable reference method when assessing diagnostic tests for infectious agents.

The three culture-positive samples in which antigen was not detected by EIA required a full 6 days incubations before organisms were observed, which would suggest that only small quantities of trichomonal antigen were originally present. As separate swabs were taken for culture and antigen collection, differences in the quantity of vaginal material collected may have contributed to the failure of EIA to detect antigen in these three samples. No significant differences were found between one of these isolates and several isolates from samples positive by EIA on testing by inhibition assay and immunoblotting, indicating that EIA failure was not due to antigenic variation between isolates.

The overall results of our study indicate that EIA is an appropriate diagnostic test for *T. vaginalis* infection. With culture as the reference method, the sensitivity of EIA was 93.2% with a specificity of 97.5%. The predictive value of a positive test was 82%, and the predictive value of a negative test was 99.3%.

C. Monoclonal Antibodies

1. Immunofluorescence Assay

To date, the few published accounts concerning the use of MAbs for the detection of *T. vaginalis* in clinical specimens have all applied IFA techniques. Torian et al. (1985) found a nucleus-specific antibody to be useful in diagnosis. Krieger et al. (1985) combined two MAbs that were broadly reactive against isolates from different geographical areas and successfully detected trichomonads in vaginal smears from each of 10 culture-positive patients. By using a mixture of three MAbs we (Yule and Ackers, unpublished data) detected organisms in a urethral swab from the culture-negative male contact of an infected woman.

Chang et al. (1986), using a combination of three antibodies specific for cytoplasm, nuclei, and flagella, directly compared an IFA with wet-mount examination and found a correlation of 96.1% between the methods. Of 231 clinical specimens examined, 34 were found positive by both methods and 188 negative by both methods; one specimen was positive by wet-mount examination but negative by IFA, which was attributed to possible poor sample preparation. An additional eight specimens were positive by IFA but negative by wet-mount examination, although these were not confirmed by culture.

D. Future Prospects

Further analysis of the antigenic structure of *T. vaginalis* through its dissection by polyclonal antibodies and MAbs will contribute enormously to improved diagnostic tests for this common parasitic infection. A logical approach is the identification and characterization of the trichomonal antigens present in all cases of urogenital trichomoniasis and the generation of MAbs to these disease markers. Preliminary studies indicate that a limited number of major antigens of between 80 and 45 kd appear to be common in infected women (Yule and Ackers, unpublished data). The development of an effective means of diagnosing *T. vaginalis* infection in men has long been neglected, and highly sensitive immunodiagnostic tests could aid greatly in this task, as well as furthering our understanding of the epidemiology of trichomoniasis.

Ideally, a diagnostic test for *T. vaginalis* should combine the sensitivity of culture with the speed and simplicity of wet-film examination, allowing treatment to be initiated at the patient's first attendance. Antigen-detecting immunoassays with short time-courses suitable for "sideroom" use are currently under evaluation.

REFERENCES

Ackers, J. P. (1987). Immunologic aspects of human trichomoniasis. In *Trichomonads Parasitic in Humans* (B. M. Honigberg, ed.). Springer-Verlag, New York, (in press).

Ackers, J. P., Catterall, R. D., Lumsden, W. H. R., and McMillan, A. (1978). Absence of detectable local antibody in genito-urinary tract secretions of male contacts of women infected with *Trichomonas vaginalis. Br. J. Vener. Dis. 54*:168-171.

Ackers, J. P. and Lumsden, W. H. R. (1978). Immunology of genito-urinary trichomoniasis. *Bull. Mem. Soc. Med. Paris* September 1978, 109-113.

Ackers, J. P., Lumsden, W. H. R., Catterall, R. D., and Coyle, R. (1975). Antitrichomonal antibody in the vaginal secretions of women infected with *Trichomonas vaginalis. Br. J. Vener. Dis. 51*:319-323.

Ackers, J. P., McMillan, A., Street, D. A., and Taylor-Robinson, D. (1983). Trichomonal antibody in male homosexuals. *Lancet 1*:880.

Alderete, J. F. (1983). Antigenic analysis of several pathogenic strains of *Trichomonas vaginalis. Infect. Immun. 39*:1041-1047.

Alderete, J. F. (1984). Enzyme linked immunosorbent assay for detecting antibody to *Trichomonas vaginalis*: Use of whole cells and aqueous extract as antigen. *Br. J. Vener. Dis. 60*:164-170.

Alderete, J. F., Suprun-Brown, L., and Kasmala, L. (1986). Monoclonal antibody to a major surface glycoprotein immunogen differentiates isolates and subpopulations of *Trichomonas vaginalis. Infect. Immun. 52*:70-75.

Alderete, J. F., Suprun-Brown, L., Kasmala, L., Smith, J., and Spence, M. (1985). Heterogeneity of *Trichomonas vaginalis* and discrimination among isolates and subpopulations with sera of patients and experimentally infected mice. *Infect. Immun. 49*:463-468.

Al-Salihi, F. L., Curran, J. P., and Wang, J.-S. (1974). Neonatal *Trichomonas vaginalis*. Report of three cases and review of the literature. *Pediatrics 53*: 196-200.

Bennett, B. D., Bailey, J., and Gardner, W. A. (1980). Immunocytochemical identification of trichomonads. *Arch. Pathol. Lab. Med. 104*:247-249.

Bogusz-Rozkowska, D. and Zablotniak, R. (1966). Trichomonadosis in inmates of penal institutions. *Wiad. Parazytol. 12*:342-345. (In Polish, English summary).

Bramley, M. (1976). Study of female babies of women entering confinement with vaginal trichomoniasis. *Br. J. Vener. Dis. 52*:58-62.

Brown, M. T. (1972). Trichomoniasis. *Practitioner 209*:639-644.

Catterall, R. D. (1972). Trichomonal infection of the genital tract. *Med. Clin. N. Am. 56*:193-213.

Catterall, R. D. (1983). Epidemiology of human trichomoniasis. *Wiad. Parazytol. 29*:87-92.

Catterall, R. D. and Nicol, C. S. (1960). Is trichomonal infection a venereal disease? *Br. Med. J. 1*:1177-1179.

Chang, T. H., Tsing, S. Y., and Tzeng, S. (1986). Monoclonal antibodies against *Trichomonas vaginalis*. *Hybridoma 5*:43-51.

Chen, K. C. S., Amsel, R., Eschenbach, D. A., and Holmes, K. K. (1982). Biochemical diagnosis of vaginitis: Determination of diamines in vaginal fluid. *J. Infect. Dis. 145*:337-345.

Chipperfield, E. J. and Evans, B. A. (1972). The influence of local infection on immunoglobulin formation in the human endocervix. *Clin. Exp. Immunol. 11*:219-213.

Cogne, M., Brasseur, P., and Ballet, J. J. (1985). Detection and characterization of serum antitrichomonal antibodies in urogenital trichomoniasis. *J. Clin. Microbiol. 21*:588-592.

Connelly, R. J., Torian, B. E., and Stibbs, H. H. (1985). Identification of a surface antigen of *Trichomonas vaginalis*. *Infect. Immun. 49*:270-274.

Cooney, M. K. and Kenny, G. E. (1970). Immunogenicity of rhinoviruses. *Proc. Soc. Exp. Biol. Med. 133*:645-650.

Delachambre, D. (1980). Etude critique comparee des antigenes de deux clones d'une meme souche d'un Flagelle parasite (*Trichomonas vaginalis*). *Ann. Parasitol. (Paris) 55*:1-11.

Diamond, L. S. (1957). The establishment of various trichomonads of animals and man in axenic cultures. *J. Parasitol. 43*:488-490.

Diamond, L. S. (1983). Lumen dwelling protozoa: *Entamoeba*, trichomonads and *Giardia*. In *In Vitro Cultivation of Protozoan Parasites* (J. B. Jansen, ed.). CRC Press, Boca Raton, pp. 65-109.

Diamond, L. S., Harlow, D. R., and Cunick, C. C. (1978). A new medium for the axenic cultivation of *Entamoeba histolytica* and other *Entamoeba*. *Trans. R. Soc. Trop. Med. Hyg.* 72:431-432.

Donne, A. (1836). Animalcules observe dans les matieres purulentes et le produit de secretions des organes genitaux de l'homme et de la femme. *C. R. Hebd. Seances Acad. Sci.* 3:385-386.

Dwyer, D. M. (1974). Analysis of the antigenc relationships among *Trichomonas, Histomonas, Dientamoeba,* and *Entamoeba* III. Immunoelectrophoresis technics. *J. Protozool.* 21:139-145.

Fouts, A. C. and Kraus, S. J. (1980). *Trichomonas vaginalis*: Reevaluation of its clinical presentation and laboratory diagnosis. *J. Infect. Dis.* 141:137-143.

Fripp, P. J., Mason, P. R., and Super, H. (1975). A method for the diagnosis of *Trichomonas vaginalis* using acridine orange. *J. Parasitol.* 61:966-967.

Frost, J. K. (1967). Gynecologic and obstetric exfoliative cytopathology. In *Novak's Gynecologic and Obstetric Pathology* (E. R. Novak and J. D. Woodruff, eds.). W. B. Saunders, Philadelphia, pp. 595-628.

Garber, G. E., Procter, E. M., and Bowie, W. R. (1986). Immunogenic proteins of *Trichomonas vaginalis* as demonstrated by the immunoblot technique. *Infect. Immun.* 51:250-253.

Gardner, W. A. and Culberson, D. E. (1985). Histopathological correlates of male trichomoniasis. *Abstr. Int. Symp. Trichomonads and the Trichomoniases, Prague.* p. 79.

Genitourin. Med. (1985). Sexually transmitted diseases: Extract from the report of the Chief Medical Officer of the Department of Health and Social Security for the year 1985. 61:204-207.

Ghosh, H. K. and Douglass, G. R. (1983). Comparison of wet mounts, stained smears and culture for detecting *Trichomonas* in vaginitis. *Med. J. Aust. 1*: 404.

Gillin, F. D. and Sher, A. (1981). Activation of the alternative complement pathway by *Trichomonas vaginalis. Infect. Immun.* 34:268-273.

Goldstine, S. N., Tsai, A., Kemp, C. J., and Fanger, M. W. (1983). Role of IgA antibody in phagocytosis by human polymorphonuclear leucocytes. In *The Secretory Immune System* (J. R. McGhee and J. Mestecky, eds.). New York Academy of Sciences, New York, p. 824.

Hardy, P. H., Hardy, J. B., Nell, E. E., Graham, D. A., Spence, M. R., and Rosenbaum, R. C. (1984). Prevalence of six sexually transmitted disease agents among pregnant inner-city adolescents and pregnancy outcome. *Lancet 2*: 333-337.

Hayes, B. S. and Kotcher, E. (1960). Evaluation of techniques for the demonstration of *Trichomonas vaginalis. J. Parasitol. 46(suppl.)*:45.

Hoffman, B. (1966). An evaluation of the use of the indirect hemagglutination method in the serodiagnosis of trichomonas. *Wiad. Parazytol. 12*:392-397.

Hoffman, B., Kazanowska, W., Kilczewski, W., and Krach, J. (1963). Serologic diagnosis of trichomonas infection. *Med. Dosw. Mikrobiol. 15*:91-99. (In Polish, English summary).

Holbrook, T. W., Boackle, R. J., Vessley, J., and Parker, B. W. (1982). *Tricho-monas vaginalis*: Alternative pathway activation of complement. *Trans. R. Soc. Trop. Med. Hyg. 76*:473-475.

Hollander, D. H. (1976). Colonial morphology of *Trichomonas vaginalis* in agar. *J. Parasitol. 62*:826-828.

Honigberg, B. M. (1970). Trichomonads. In *Immunity to Parasitic Animals* (G. J. Jackson, R. Herman, and L. Singer, eds.), Vol. 3. Appleton-Century-Crofts, New York, pp. 469-550.

Honigberg, B. M. (1978). Trichomonads of importance in human medicine. In *Parasitic Protozoa* (J. P. Krier, eds.), Vol. 2. Academic Press, New York, pp. 276-454.

Jaakmees, H. P., Teras, J. K., Roigas, E. M., Nigesen, U. K., and Tompel, H. J. (1966). Complement-fixing antibodies in the blood serum of men infested with *Trichomonas vaginalis*. *Wiad. Parazytol. 12·*378-384.

Jirovec, O. and Petru, M. (1968). *Trichomonas vaginalis* and trichomoniasis. *Adv. Parasitol. 6*:117-188.

Jones, J. G., Yamauchi, T., and Lambert, B. (1985). *Trichomonas vaginalis* in-festation in sexually abused girls. *Am. J. Dis. Child. 139*:846-847.

Juranyi, R., Vag, J., and Kleeberg, V. S. (1973). Fluorescence method in the diagnosis of trichomonadosis in young girls. *Wiad. Parazytol. 19*:433-435.

Kariks, J. (1983). A convenient method for detecting trichomonas vaginitis. *Med. J. Aust. 2*:540.

Karbowski, J. (1966). The value of the direct immunofluorescence method in the investigation of experimental trichomonadosis in mice. *Wiad. Parazytol. 12*:304-311.

Komorowska, A. and Kurnatowska, A. (1983). Epidemiological aspects of trich-omonadosis in girls. *Wiad. Parazytol. 29*:107-110.

Kott, H. and Adler, S. (1961). A serological study of *Trichomonas* species para-sitic in man. *Trans. R. Soc. Trop. Med. Hyg. 55*:333-344.

Krieger, J. N., Holmes, K. K., Spence, M. R., Rein, M. F., McCormack, W. M., and Tam, M. R. (1985). Geographic variation among isolates of *Tricho-monas vaginalis*: Demonstration of antigenic heterogeneity by using mono-clonal antibodies and the indirect immunofluorescence technique. *J. Infect. Dis. 152*:979-984.

Lanceley, F. and McEntegart, M. G. (1953). *Trichomonas vaginalis* in the male; the experimental infection of a few volunteers. *Lancet* 668-671.

Lipinski, A. (1983). Age of the women with vaginal trichomonadosis. *Wiad. Par-azytol. 29*:77-78.

Lukasic, M., Dynia, J., and Kosmiderski, S. (1977). An attempt to diagnose tricho-monadosis by means of carbonate [*sic*] agglutination reaction. *Wiad. Para-zytol. 23*:590-592. (In Polish, English summary).

Martin, R. D., Kaufman, R. H., and Burns, M. (1963). *Trichomonas vaginalis* vaginitis. *Am. J. Obstet. Gynecol. 87*:1024-1027.

Martinotti, M. G., Pugliese, A., Savoia, D., Perego, R., and Martinetto, P. (1982). Ricerca di IgA specifiche anti-*Trichomonas vaginalis* nel secreto vaginale mediante immunofluorescencza indiretta. *G. Batteriol. Virol. Immunol. 75*: 189-195.

Mason, P. R. (1979). The diagnosis of *Trichomonas vaginalis* infection by the indirect fluorescence antibody test. *J. Clin. Pathol. 32*:1211-1215.

Mason, P. R., Super, H., and Fripp, P. J. (1976). Comparison of four techniques for the routine diagnosis of *Trichomonas vaginalis* infection. *J. Clin. Pathol. 29*:154-157.

Mathews, H. M. and Healy, G. R. (1983). Evaluation of two serological tests for *Trichomonas vaginalis* infection. *J. Clin. Microbiol. 17*:840-843.

McEntegart, M. G. (1952). The application of haemagglutination technique to the study of *Trichomonas vaginalis* infections. *J. Clin. Pathol. 5*:275-280.

McEntegart, M. G., Chadwick, C. S., and Nairn, R. C. (1958). Fluorescent antisera in the detection of serological varieties of *Trichomonas vaginalis*. *Br. J. Vener. Dis. 34*:1-3.

Meyer, E. A. (1976). *Giardia lamblia*: Isolation and axenic cultivation. *Exp. Parasitol. 39*:101-105.

Neva, F. A., Malone, M. F., and Myers, B. R. (1961). Factors influencing the intracellular growth of *Trypanosoma cruzi* in vitro. *Am. J. Trop. Med. Hyg. 10*:141-149.

Nielsen, R. (1973). *Trichomonas vaginalis* II. Laboratory investigations in trichomoniasis. *Br. J. Vener. Dis. 49*:531-535.

Nunn, J. R., Harington, J. S., Allsobrook, A. J. R., Du Plessis, L. S., and Nunn, A. J. (1974). *N*-nitrosamines in the human vaginal vault. *S. Afr. J. Med. Sci. 39*:179-182.

O'Hara, C. M., Gardner, W. A., and Bennett, B. D. (1980). Immunoperoxidase staining of *Trichomonas vaginalis* in cytologic material. *Acta Cytol. 24*: 448-451.

Perl, G. (1972). Errors in the diagnosis of *Trichomonas vaginalis* infection as observed among 1199 patients. *Obstet. Gynecol. 39*:7-9.

Peterson, K. M. and Alderete, J. F. (1982). Host plasma proteins on the surface of pathogenic *Trichomonas vaginalis*. *Infect. Immun. 37*:755-762.

Peterson, K. M. and Alderete, J. F. (1983). Acquisition of a_1-antitrypsin by a pathogenic strain of *Trichomonas vaginalis*. *Infect. Immun. 40*:640-646.

Peterson, K. M. and Alderete, J. F. (1984a). Selective acquisition of plasma proteins by *Trichomonas vaginalis* and human lipoproteins as a growth requirement for this species. *Mol. Biochem. Parasitol. 12*:37-48.

Peterson, K. M. and Alderete, J. F. (1984b). Iron uptake and increased intracellular enzyme activity follow host lactoferrin binding by *Trichomonas vaginalis* receptors. *J. Exp. Med. 160*:398-410.

Rein, M. F. (1985). *Trichomonas vaginalis*. In *Principles and Practice of Infectious Diseases*, 2nd ed. (G. L. Mandel, R. G. Douglas, and J. E. Bennett, eds.). John Wiley & Sons, New York, pp. 1556-1558.

Reisenhoffer, V. (1963). Uber die Beeinflussung von *Trichomonas vaginalis* durch verschiedene Sera. *Arch. Hyg. Bakteriol. 146*:628-635.

Rodriguez-Martinez, H. A., Rosales, M. de la L., Galloso de Bello, L., and Ruiz-Moreno, J. A. (1973). Adequate staining of *Trichomonas vaginalis* by McManus periodic acid-Schiff stain. *Am. J. Clin. Pathol. 59*:741-746.

Samuels, R. and Chun-Hoon, H. (1964). Serological investigations of trichomonads. I. Comparisons of "natural" and immune antibodies. *J. Protozool. 11*: 36-46.

Schoenherr, K. E. (1956). Serological investigations of trichomonads. *Z. Immunitaetsforsch. Allerg. Klin. Immunol. 113*:83-94.

Street, D. A., Taylor-Robinson, D., Ackers, J. P., Hanna, N. F., and McMillan, A. (1982). Evaluation of enzyme-linked immunosorbent assay for the detection of antibody to *Trichomonas vaginalis*. *Br. J. Vener. Dis. 58*:330-333.

Su, K. E. (1982). Antibody to *Trichomonas vaginalis* in human cervicovaginal secretions. *Infect. Immun. 37*:852-857.

Su-Lin, K.-Y. and Honigberg, B. M. (1983). Antigenic analysis of *Trichomonas vaginalis* strains by quantitative fluorescent antibody methods. *Z. Parasitenkd. 69*:161-181.

Summers, J. L. and Ford, M. L. (1972). The Papnicolaou smear as a diagnostic tool in male trichomoniasis. *J. Urol. 107*:840-842.

Sun, T. (1982). Trichomoniasis, In *Pathology and Clinical Features of Parasitic Diseases*. Masson Publishing, New York, pp. 87-94.

Tatsuki, T. (1957). Studies on *Trichomonas vaginalis*. II. Immunoserological reactions of *Trichomonas vaginalis* by sera and colostra from women infected therewith. *Nagasaki Igakkai Zasshi 32*:983-993. (In Japanese, English summary).

Taylor, A. E. R. and Baker, J. R. (1968). *The Cultivation of Parasites In Vitro*. Blackwell Scientific, Oxford, pp. 77-119.

Teras, J. K. (1965). On the varieties of *Trichomonas vaginalis*. *Proc. 2nd Int. Congr. Protozool.* pp. 197-198.

Teras, J. K. (1966). Differences in the antigenic properties within strains of *Trichomonas vaginalis*. *Wiad. Parazytol. 12*:357-363.

Teras, J. K. and Kaarma, H. (1969). The efficiency of microscopic, culture and serological diagnostic methods in the different clinical forms of genitourinary trichomonadosis. *Wiad. Parazytol. 15*:359-361.

Teras, J. K., Jaakmees, H., Nigesen, U., Roigas, E., and Tompel, H. (1966). On the agglutinogenic properties of *Trichomonas vaginalis*. *Wiad. Parazytol. 12*: 370-377.

Tokura, N. (1935). Biologische und immunologische Untersuchungen uber die menschenparasitaren Trichomonaden. *Igaku Kenkyu 9*:1-13.

Torian, B. E., Connelly, R. J., Stephens, R. S., and Stibbs, H. H. (1984). Specific and common antigens of *Trichomonas vaginalis* detected by monoclonal antibodies. *Infect. Immun. 43*:270-275.

Torian, B. E., Connelly, R. J., Barnes, R. C., and Kenny, G. E. (1985). Antigens of *Trichomonas vaginalis* and *Tritrichomonas foetus* characterized by monoclonal antibodies. *Abstr. Int. Symp. Trichomonads and Trichomoniasis, Prague*, p. 23.

Trussell, R. E. (1947). *Trichomonas vaginalis and Trichomoniasis.* Charles C. Thomas, Springfield Ill.

White, E., Hart, D., and Sanderson, B. E. (1983). Polyamines in *Trichomonas vaginalis. Mol. Biochem. Parasitol. 9*:309-318.

Whittington, M. J. (1957). Epidemiology of infections with *Trichomonas vaginalis* in the light of improved diagnostic methods. *Br. J. Vener. Dis. 33*:80-91.

Willcox, R. R. (1960). Epidemiological aspects of human trichomoniasis. *Br. J. Vener. Dis. 36*:167-174.

Wilson, A. and Ackers, J. P. (1980). Urine culture for the detection of *Trichomonas vaginalis* in men. *Br. J. Vener. Dis. 56*:46-48.

Yano, A., Yui, K., Aosai, F., Kojima, S., Kawana, T., and Ovary, Z. (1983). Immune response to *Trichomonas vaginalis* IV. Immunochemical and immunobiological analyses of *T. vaginalis* antigen. *Int. Arch. Allergy Appl. Immunol. 72*:150-157.

Yule, A. and Ackers, J. P. (1985). Development of enzyme immunoassays for the detection of *Trichomonas vaginalis* antigen. *Abstr. Int. Symp. Trichomonads and Trichomoniasis, Prague,* p. 32.

Yule, A., Gellan, M. C. A., Oriel, J. D., and Ackers, J. P. (1987). Detection of *Trichomonas vaginalis* antigen in women by enzyme immunoassay. *J. Clin. Pathol. 40*:566-568.

TEN

Intestinal Protozoal Infection

Alexander McMillan
The Royal Infirmary
Edinburgh, Scotland

I. INTRODUCTION

Although the sexual transmission of enteric pathogens probably plays a small part in their global epidemiology, it is of some importance in temperate climates. As oral-anal intercourse with multiple partners is practiced widely by sexually active homosexual men, they are at particular risk for the acquisition of these organisms including the protozoa *Entamoeba histolytica* and *Giardia intestinalis*. Indeed many studies, the results from some of which are presented in Table 1, indicate the increased prevalence of these parasites in this population group.

As infected individuals may suffer prolonged periods of ill-health and be sources of infection to others, the detection and treatment of these men are important. The standard methods of stool examination are difficult and considerable technical expertise is needed for the accurate identification of the intestinal protozoa. With the aim of improving diagnostic methods for these organisms, other tests based on the detection of protozoal antibodies, or antigens, or both, have been developed. These are considered in the following sections.

II. *ENTAMOEBA HISTOLYTICA*

A. Life Cycle

There are three stages in the life cycle of *E. histolytica*: the trophozoite, precyst, and cyst. The latter is the infective form of *E. histolytica*. After ingestion, excystation occurs in the ileum resulting in four-nucleated amebae that divide further yielding up to eight small amebae, each containing a single nucleus. These grow and the trophozoites colonize the large intestine. Before the formation of the cyst, the trophozoite become sluggish, extrudes ingested food, rounds up and secretes a cell wall (Alback and Booden, 1978).

B. Pathology

Amebiasis, the condition of harboring *E. histolytica* with or without clinical manifestations, has been classified (World Health Organization Expert Committee, 1969) into asymptomatic and symptomatic. The latter category is subdivided into intestinal amebiasis, which presents as dysentery, nondysenteric colitis, ameboma, and amebic appendicitis, and extraintestinal amebiasis, including hepatic abscess formation and cutaneous disease.

The most common histological finding in patients with symptomatic amebiasis is nonspecific proctitis (Pittman and Hennigar, 1974; Prathap and Gilman, 1970). Although trophozoites may be seen in the surface exudate, amebae are not found in the crypts or tissues. Early invasive lesions are associated with small interglandular foci of epithelial cell destruction, but later there is ulceration extending through the muscularis mucosae into the submucosa ("flask ulcers"). Amebae are found in and around the necrotic tissue of these lesions. An uncommon complication of intestinal amebiasis is ameboma, a single lesion that results

Table 1 Prevalence of Intestinal Protozoa in Homosexual Men

City (country) studied	Number of men tested	Number (%) of stools containing:							Ref.
		Entamoeba histolytica	Entamoeba hartmanni	Entamoeba coli	Endolimax nana	Iodamoeba butschlii	Giardia intestinalis	Dientamoeba fragilis	
New York (USA)	89	18 (20)	NS	12 (13)	10 (11)	4 (5)	11 (12)	1 (1)	William et al. (1978)
Glasgow (UK)	118	4 (4)	NS	NS	NS	1 (1)	2 (2)	0 (0)	McMillan (1980)
Toronto (Canada)	200	54 (27)	NS	NS	NS	NS	26 (13)	NS	Keystone et al. (1980)
New York (USA)	51	10 (20)	NS	NS	NS	NS	2 (4)	NS	Phillips et al. (1981)
San Francisco (USA)	150	54 (36)	53 (35)	57 (38)	58 (39)	63 (42)	7 (5)	2 (1)	Ortega et al. (1984)
London (UK)	83	10 (12)	4 (5)	21 (25)	18 (22)	3 (4)	7 (8)	0 (0)	Chin and Gerken (1984)
Edinburgh (UK)	310	30 (10)	3 (1)	30 (10)	16 (5)	5 (2)	19 (6)	0 (0)	McMillan (1984) (unpublished)
San Francisco (USA)	508	145 (29)	127 (25)	108 (21)	192 (38)	68 (13)	29 (6)	7 (1)	Markell et al. (1984)

NS, not stated.

from the destructive changes produced by the ameba and the host's response, with the production of inflammation and granulation tissue without fibrosis (Brandt and Tamayo, 1970). Hematogenous dissemination of amebae from the intestine may result in abscess formation in the liver and, rarely, in other organs. At the time of presentation, few individuals with amebic hepatic abscess have colitic symptoms and amebae are seldom found in the feces. Although the latent period between the time of infection and the development of the abscess generally ranges between 8 and 20 weeks (Knobluck and Mannweiler, 1983), it can be much longer.

C. Pathogenicity

As most individuals infected with *E. histolytica* are asymptomatic, the existence of virulent and avirulent strains of the ameba has been postulated. Indeed, based on the ability of axenically grown amebae to produce hepatic abscesses in hamsters, virulent and avirulent strains are known to exist (Mattern and Keister, 1977). McGowan et al. (1982) isolated a head-labile cytotoxin from highly virulent strains of *E. histolytica* and showed that avirulent strains produced little, if any, of this cytotoxin. In 1978, Sargeaunt and colleagues reported an electrophoretic isoenzyme analysis of *E. histolytica*, and since then have recognized some 22 isoenzyme patterns (zymodemes) (Editorial, *Lancet*, 1985): he considers that nine of these 22 zymodemes are associated with tissue invasiveness.

In a study of 52 isolates of *E. histolytica* from homosexual men who attended three STD clinics in the United Kingdom, Sargeaunt et al. (1983) did not identify amebae with zymodemes associated with pathogenicity. Conflicting data on the significance of *E. histolytica* in homosexual men have been reported by McMillan et al. (1984) and Goldmeier et al. (1986). Although the former group of workers showed a significant association between the presence of *E. histolytica* and proctitis, the latter authors found no difference in the prevalence of inflammatory changes in the rectum and of amebic infection. Neither group found either histological or serological evidence of tissue invasion.

As invasive amebiasis has been reported, however, in homosexual men (Burnham et al., 1980; Meyers et al., 1977; Thompson et al., 1983; Ylvisaker and McDonald, 1980), the conclusion reached by Golmeier et al. (1986) that *E. histolytica* is not a pathogen in homosexual men must be treated with caution. In this population, the host response may be more important than infection with a particular strain of the organism.

D. Detection of *Entamoeba histolytica* in Feces by Microscopy and Culture

The most definitive test for amebiasis is the identification of the organism in feces or tissues. In warm saline-mount preparations of fresh diarrheal stool, or rectal exudate, trophozoites are 15-30 μm in size and exhibit unidirectional movement with the sudden extrusion of finger-shaped pseudopodia (lobopodia). Unless erythrocytes are seen within the cytoplasm of the trophozoite, it is difficult to differentiate with certainty *E. histolytica* from the nonpathogenic amebae that are found in the intestine. Stool samples are best examined within 15 min of passage, but if this is not possible, a specimen may be collected into polyvinyl alcohol (PVA) fixative (Brooke and Goldman, 1949) in which cysts and trophozoites are well preserved. Microscopy of Schaudinn-fixed smears of feces that have been stained with a modification of Gomori's trichrome stain or iron-hematoxylin (Lumsden and McMillan, 1987) is essential for the characterization of amebic trophozoites. Even then, differentiation can be difficult.

Trophozoites are seldom found in formed stool samples, but cysts may be seen in iodine-stained wet preparations. As few cysts per unit weight of feces may be excreted, a method for the concentration of cysts is usually routinely employed. A modification of the Ridley and Hagwood (1956) formol-ether method has proved useful in our laboratory. Up to 80% of infections will not be identified unless this procedure is undertaken (McMillan and McNeillage, 1984). It should be emphasized that the differentiation of cysts of *E. histolytica* from those of nonpathogenic amebae is often difficult, if not impossible, for the inexperienced observer. Furthermore, the passage of cysts is often intermittent and the ingestion of antimicrobial agents, kaolin, barium sulfate, bismuth salts, and antimalarial drugs may interfere with cyst excretion.

By relying on the results of examination by direct microscopy and after cyst concentration of a single stool sample, more than 50% of infections with *E. histolytica* will not be identified. At least six examinations on different occasions are necessary to recognize 90% of infections (Sawitz and Faust, 1942).

Although cultivation of *E. histolytica* is not undertaken in many routine microbiology laboratories, there is little doubt that the diagnostic yield is higher than if only microscopical methods are used (McMillan and McNeillage, 1984; Robinson, 1968). Various media have been tried but Robinson's has proved most useful (Robinson, 1968). For best results, the media should be inoculated within a few hours of passage of the stool sample. Cultivation, however, is time-consuming and as nonpathogenic amebae also grow, differentiation of *E. histolytica* trophozoites from these by stained smear microscopy is essential.

As trophozoites within the surface exudate and in the tissues of a routinely processed colonic biopsy specimen are found in only about 50% of cases of amebic colitis, this procedure lacks sensitivity as a diagnostic method.

As the detection of *E. histolytica* in fecal material or in histological sections of rectal mucosa from patients with intestinal amebiasis can be difficult, and as amebae are not commonly found in cases of hepatic amebic abscesses, immunological methods for the identification of infected individuals have been developed. Before detailing these tests, it is useful to consider what is known of the antigenic composition of *E. histolytica*.

E. Antigenic Analysis of *Entamoeba histolytica*

The characterization of the antigenic composition of *E. histolytica* is important for the development and improvement of diagnostic tests. For this purpose, the protozoa must be cultivated. As it is difficult, if not impossible, to separate the relevant antigens, polyxenic cultures that are useful in the laboratory diagnosis of amebiasis are of limited value. Cocultivation of *E. histolytica* with another known organism (monoxenic cultivation), such as *Trypanosoma cruzi* or *Crithidia* sp., was developed so that more precise biochemical and immunological investigation could be undertaken. A major advance, however, in the search for a source of better defined material was the successful axenic cultivation of several strains of *E. histolytica* by Diamond (1968).

Several strains of *E. histolytica*, e.g., HK-9 and NIH 200, that were isolated from individuals who had been infected in Korea, have been used extensively in immunological investigation. It should be remembered, however, that antigenic changes in those organisms may have occurred during repeated subculture (Bos, 1978). Also, the proteins of the animal serum used in the culture medium adhere to the plasma membrane of the trophozoites even after thorough washing.

Detailed analysis of the antigens against which serum antibodies are produced in experimental animals and man have been reported. In an immunoelectrophoretic (IEP) analysis of sera obtained from Canadian-American Indians and South Africans living in endemic areas, Krupp (1977) used as antigens sonicates of *E. histolytica* strains NH 200 and K9 that had been grown axenically. Very simple patterns with on average four or five antigen/antibody arcs, a few of which were common to all positive sera, were obtained. She identified 14 antigens that reacted with sera from patients from different localities. The presence of common antigens was confirmed by Ishaq and Pudma (1980) who studied by IEP the reactions of antigens obtained from these strains against homologous and heterologous rabbit antisera. However, as some arcs developed with only one or two strains, they deduced that 70% of the antigens extracted were strain-specific.

A careful study of the reactivity of rabbit and human sera with a sonicate of two axenized strains (HK9 and HT31) of *E. histolytica* was reported by Chang et al. (1979). By two-dimensional IEP (2D-IEP) up to 32 precipitin peaks were noted with each strain tested against the homologous rabbit antiserum. When heterologous antisera were used, there were fewer peaks with HT-31 and more peaks with HK9 sonicates than seen when these were reacted with homologous antisera. By gel filtration on Sephadex G-200, three and four major protein fractions were separated from the sonicates of HT-31 and HK9 strains, respectively.

Sawhney and colleagues (1980) fractionated a sonicate of *E. histolytica* (strain NIH:200) on Sephadex G-200 and obtained three major fractions. From a consideration of the gel filtration results, they calculated that the molecular weight of the protein in the supernate varied between 1450 and 65,000. Although sera raised in rabbits against each fraction agglutinated erythrocytes that had been coated with the respective fraction, the main activity was found among the higher-molecular-weight proteins. They calculated that this fraction, which contained glycoprotein, had potential for use in serodiagnosis.

An elegant study by Kettis et al. (1983) showed that in the whole extracts of *E. histolytica* strains HK-9 and NIH-200, more than 60 polypeptide bands, ranging in molecular weight from 9000 to 200,000 could be distinguished by sodium dodecyl sulfate polyacrylamide gel electrophoresis (SDS-PAGE).

When whole amebae extract, from eight sera from patients with amebiasis, was absorbed on the IgG fractions bonded to CNBr-activated Sepharose 4-B, seven polypeptide bands, all staining with periodic acid-Schiff (PAS) were shown by SDS-PAGE.

Because absorption of rabbit hyperimmune or human amebic sera with whole amebae extinguished the precipitin lines as shown by gel immunodiffusion or counterimmunoelectrophoresis, it was likely that the relevant antigenic determinants were accessible on the cell surface.

After labeling intact trophozoites with ^{125}I these were solubilized and run on SDS-PAGE. Autoradiography showed 12 iodinated bands, ranging in molecular weight from 9000 to more than 150,000, but the most prominent was the 88,000-mol. wt. band. All corresponding bands stained with PAS, thus indicating the presence of carbohydrate.

Similar findings on the major surface-labeled polypeptides were reported by Aley et al. (1980) who found that preincubation of amebae with concanavalin A stabilized the plasma membrane and maintained it in large sheets during homogenization. These workers also noted that the plasma membrane was enriched with cholesterol to a molar ratio of 0.87 with phospholipid. They also found a high proportion of the phosphonolipid, ceramide aminoethyl phosphonate, in the plasma membrane. Another piece of evidence indicating that surface antigens are important in the induction of amebic antibodies is that IgG purified from the sera of patients with amebiasis binds to the surface of cultivated *E. histolytica* as shown by immunofluorescence and immune electron microscopy (O'Shea and Feria Velasco, 1974). Incubation of trophozoites with specific antiserum induces a polar redistribution of surface components with accumulation at the uroid region—"capping" (Calderon et al., 1980). During the capping process, newly exposed antigens appear on the surface of the trophozoite.

Amebic antigens may also be located in the cytoplasm of the organism and antigens have been obtained from lysosomal and ribosomal fractions (Arroyo-Begovich, 1978).

F. Immunological Tests

1. Serological Tests

a. Complement Fixation Test. The complement fixation (CF) test was the first serological test to be described for the diagnosis of amebiasis (Izar, 1914; Scalas,

Table 2 Serologic Tests in Amebiasis

| Test | Percentage of patients whose sera gave positive results in that test (number of patients tested) | | | | Ref. |
	Amebic dysentery	Extraintestinal amebiasis	Symptomless cyst passage	No evidence of current amebic infection	
Complement fixation	90 (92)	100 (20)	28 (101)	0 (0)	Kessel et al. (1965)
	63 (30)	84 (37)	11 (19)	0 (19)	Thompson et al. (1968)
	65 (188)	83 (272)	7 (14)	0 (21)	Krupp and Powell (1971)
	85 (61)	83 (12)	58 (33)	NS	Juniper et al. (1972)
Gel diffusion	88 (231)	97 (151)	40 (51)	0 (248)	Maddison et al. (1965)
	54 (41)	80 (49)	0 (19)	0 (12)	Thompson et al. (1968)
	95 (206)	99 (288)	39 (18)	8 (92)	Krupp and Powell (1971)
	86 (63)	88 (16)	52 (27)	NS	Juniper et al. (1972)
Indirect hemagglutination	84 (133)	100 (35)	65 (140)	1 (101)	Kessel et al. (1965)
	82 (83)	97 (110)	9 (70)	0.2 (807)	Milgram et al. (1966)

Method					Reference
Indirect immunofluorescence	90 (41)	100 (48)	58 (19)	17 (12)	Thompson et al. (1968)
	81 (206)	98 (288)	28 (18)	11 (103)	Krupp and Powell (1971)
	NS	100 (12)	NS	0 (20)	Garcia et al. (1982)
	89 (26)	80 (5)	55 (20)	35 (17)	Goldman (1966)
	72 (32)	88 (33)	NS	0 (94)	Boonpucknavig and Nairn (1967)
Latex agglutination	27 (40)	98 (6)	14 (37)	1 (270)	Jeanes (1969)
	54 (142)	100 (412)	25 (94)	1 (227)	Ambroise-Thomas (1976)
	96 (100)	98 (100)	NS	5 (100)	Morris and Powell (1970)
	59 (41)	88 (74)	NS	4 (227)	Ambroise-Thomas (1974)
Enzyme-linked immunosorbent assay (ELISA)	63 (8)	100 (18)	50 (26)	0 (15)	Bos and Van der Eijk (1976)
	57 (7)	100 (5)	NS	NS	Ambroise-Thomas et al. (1978)
	NS	100 (53)	NS	4 (693)	Yang and Kennedy (1979)
	NS	92 (12)	0 (14)	0 (340)	Speiser (1980)

NS, not stated.

1921). Although the specificity of the test seems to be high, when the amebae used for antigen preparation have been grown in axenic or monoxenic media, the sensitivity of the CF test in the diagnosis of invasive amebiasis is significantly lower than that of other tests (Table 2).

As more recently developed tests have improved sensitivity and specificity, the CF test is now rarely used.

b. Indirect Immunofluorescent Antibody Test. The detection by immunofluorescence of serum antibodies against *E. histolytica* was first described by Goldman (1966). Table 2 indicates the results obtained in the indirect immunofluorescent antibody (IFA) test on the sera of patients with different clinical forms of amebaisis, and as may be seen, the specificity of the test is high with the exception of one study by Goldman (1966). The majority of patients with extraintestinal disease have serum antibody detectable at high titer. Unfortunately, the sensitivity of the test is much lower in patients with disease confined to the intestine; when present, antibodies are detectable at significantly lower titers than those found in patients with hepatic abscesses (Ambroise-Thomas, 1974). Low-titered antibody is generally found in only about 15% of asymptomatic cyst excreters. Interestingly, in a recent study (Jackson et al., 1985) each of 17 asymptomatic carriers of strains of *E. histolytica* that were believed to be pathogenic were seropositive in the IFA and the gel diffusion tests; only seven of 33 asymptomatic individuals who carried (presumed) nonpathogenic strains were seropositive.

The preponderant class of antibody detected in the IFA test is IgG, but specific IgM together with IgG may be found in a small proportion of patients (Boonpucknavig and Nairn, 1967).

After successful treatment the antibody titer declines rapidly but generally does not become negative until about 12 months later (Ambroise-Thomas, 1976). The use of a solid phase indirect immunofluorescent assay was described by Walls and Wilson (1983). Preliminary data suggested that there was good correlation between the results of the test and the indirect hemagglutination (IHA) test in the diagnosis of invasive amebiasis.

The principal use of the IFA is in the diagnosis of hepatic amebic abscess and in assessing efficacy of treatment.

c. Enzyme-Linked Immunosorbent Assay. A lyophilized complete antigen prepared from axenically cultivated *E. histolytica* strain HK-9 was first used in an enzyme-linked immunosorbent assay (ELISA) test for amebiasis by Bos and colleagues (1976). Excellent correlation with the results of the IFA test were reported (Ambroise-Thomas et al., 1978; Speiser, 1980; Yang and Kennedy, 1979) but the ELISA titers were higher. After successful treatment, there is a gradual decrease in the ELISA titers, paralleling those in the IFA test. With its ease of application to the analysis of many serum samples, the ELISA test has been used in seroepidemiological studies of invasive amebiasis (Bos et al., 1980). Although the sensitivity of the test in the diagnosis of hepatic disease is high (see Table 2), antibodies are not detected regularly in the sera of patients with intestinal infection.

d. Indirect Hemagglutination Assay. An indirect hemagglutination assay (IHA) for serum antibodies was described by Kessel and colleagues (1961) using tanned red cells treated with an extract of monoxenically cultivated (with *Trypanosoma cruzi*) *E. histolytica*. The results of several studies (see Table 2) have clearly shown the value of the IHA test in the diagnosis of hepatic abscess and, to a lesser degree, that of amebic dysentery.

The titer of the IHA test usually peaks 4 weeks after the onset of the clinical features of hepatic amebic abscess (Knoblock and Mannweiler, 1983) but, although the titer generally decreases after 6 months of successful treatment, the test may remain positive in up to 90% of patients for 2 or more years (Krupp and Powell, 1971; Stamm et al., 1976). Hence, the test may be of limited value in the diagnosis of infection in endemic areas but has been used widely in seroepidemiological studies.

Antibodies are not detectable in the sera of at least half of the individuals with nondysenteric amebic colitis or in asymptomatic cyst passers.

e. Gel Diffusion Precipitin Test. One of the most simple tests to be used in the serodiagnosis of amebiasis is double diffusion in agar gel (GDP). The antigen is the supernatant from axenically cultivated amebae that have been disrupted by ultrasound and repeatedly frozen and thawed. In positive tests, at least two precipitin lines develop between the antigen and serum-containing wells. Although the sensitivity of the test is high in the diagnosis of extraintestinal amebiasis, a much lower proportion of sera from patients with infection confined to the intestinal lumen contain antibody detectable by this test (see Table 2).

Two years after successful treatment of amebic abscess or dysentery, 60 and 80%, respectively, of individuals are still seropositive in the test (Krupp and Powell, (1971).

A disadvantage of the test for field studies is that the results are not available for about 48 hr. However, the use of cellulose acetate membrane instead of agar allows reading within 4 hr, and the results show excellent correlation with these of agar gel diffusion (Stamm and Phillips, 1977).

f. Latex Agglutination Test. Application of the latex agglutination (LA) test to the serodiagnosis of amebiasis was described by Morris and Powell (1970). Latex particles were sensitized with antigen prepared from axenically cultivated *E. histolytica*. The results obtained on testing sera from patients with hepatic amebic abscesses and dysentery were excellent (see Table 2). Ambroise-Thomas (1974) reported the use of a commercial LA test (Seramoeba Kit, Miles Laboratories) and found that the sensitivity of the test was a little lower than that of the

IFA test with which it was compared. The LA test, however, detected antibodies in the sera of patients with dysenteric colitis more frequently than the IFA test. Cross-reactions were noted with the sera from patients with syphilis and hepatic cirrhosis.

When sera that were positive by IHA, GDP, LA, and IFA were absorbed with sensitized red cells, the IHA and LA tests became negative, but the GDP test and IFA tests were unaffected (Stamm et al., 1973). This indicated that the antibodies concerned in the latter two tests were similar but differed from those detected by the IFA and GDP tests.

As with the IFA test, the LA assay often remains positive years after successful treatment (Stamm et al., 1976).

g.   Immunoelectrophoresis.   The application of immunoelectrophoresis to the serology of amebiasis was first described by Maddison et al. (1965). Although Savanat and Chaicumpa (1969) found that this method was more sensitive than gel diffusion, antibodies were detected in only four of six patients with amebic colitis. With immunoelectrophoresis of fractions of amebic sera separated by gel filtration they noted that most of the antibody activity was associated with the IgG class. Although the method has proved useful in the analysis of the antigenic composition of *E. histolytica*, it is time-consuming and has been largely replaced as a diagnostic test by counterimmunoelectrophoresis (CIEP).

h.   Counter Immunoelectrophoresis Precipitin (One-Dimensional Double Electroimmunodiffusion).   In the CIEP test, antigen and the serum under test are placed in wells cut in agar gel or applied directly to a cellulose acetate membrane and separated by a suitable distance. When a current is passed through the gel, a precipitin line(s) develops (usually within 30 min) at a point intermediate between their origins if the serum contains antibody.

Krupp (1974) found that CIEP was 10 times more sensitive than agar gel diffusion in the detection of serum antibodies against *E. histolytica*. The number of arcs seen corresponded to the complexity of the pattern on immunoelectrophoresis with which the test was compared.

By CIEP, antibodies are found in the sera of almost all patients with hepatic abscess (Garcia et al., 1982; Sheehan et al., 1979). Within 3 months of successful treatment, the titer in the CIEP test decreased. Few patients with intestinal infection have a detectable antibody response.

From this brief review it is clear that serological tests have a major role in the diagnosis of extraintestinal amebiasis, particularly hepatic abscesses. The sensitivity of the various tests in the detection of disease confined to the intestinal tract, however, is low. As the majority of homosexual men with amebiasis do not have invasive disease (Goldmeier et al., 1986; McMillan et al., 1984), the use of these tests in the identification of infected individuals is limited. Hence, the application of immunological tests for the detection of amebic antigen in serum or in fecal samples is of particular interest.

2. Detection of Amebic Trophozoites by Immunofluorescence and Immunoperoxidase Methods

Because the differentiation of trophozoites of *E. histolytica* from other amebae that have been cultured in Robinson's and other media is often difficult, immunofluorescent antibody methods for the correct identification of these organisms have been described. Goldman (1953) showed that *E. histolytica* could be demonstrated in fixed preparations of cultured amebae by immunofluorescence using rabbit antiserum. Trophozoites in smears of feces preserved in polyvinyl alcohol or fixed in Schaudinn's fluid are easily identified by direct immunofluorescence (Parelkar and Stamm, 1973). Similarly, trophozoites can be detected in tissue biopsies (Parelkar et al., 1971). Although these initial results were encouraging, fluorescent antibody methods require the use of expensive microscopes, and there are problems in the specificity. As a result, few laboratories use direct immunofluorescence as a diagnostic procedure.

Immunoperoxidase methods, however, offer certain advantages over immunofluorescence. They are applicable to fixed tissue, allow accurate localization of antigen, and the preparations are permanent.

Using an indirect immunoperoxidase method with rat antiserum, trophozoites have been shown in routine histological sections and cytological preparations of colonic mucosa (Kobayashi et al., 1985).

3. Detection of Circulating Antigens in Amebiasis

As serological tests for *E. histolytica* may be of limited value in areas of the world with a high prevalence of amebiasis, the detection of amebic antigens in the serum reflecting current infection would offer advantages. Two solid phase sandwich radioimmunoassays, one using rabbit and the other human antiamebic affinity purified antibody, have been described (Pillai and Mohimen, 1982). Although antigens were not detected in whole serum, by use of the latter method, they were found in polyethylene glycol (PEG) precipitates of the sera of each of 21 patients with untreated amebiasis (11 had untreated colonic disease and 10 had hepatic abscesses), but they were found in only one of 22 control subjects. Preliminary experiments had shown that this system could detect as little as 40 ng of a soluble amebic protein mixture. A "sandwich" between rabbit antibodies, however, failed to detect amebic antigen in the precipitated immune complexes. This suggested that the circulating antigens were of restricted heterogeneity and that the antigenic determinant on the protein was antigenic in humans but not in rabbits.

A simple radioimmunoprecipitation assay for the detection of circulating amebic antigens was also reported (Pillai and Mohimen, 1982). Diluted serum was incubated with ^{125}I-labeled affinity-purified rabbit antiserum against *E. histolytica*. After 18 hr, PEG was added and the radioactivity measured in the precipitate.

As wide experience has not yet been gained on the application of these methods to the diagnosis of amebiasis, their use now remains experimental.

4. Detection of Amebic Antigens in Feces

Root et al. (1978) described an ELISA method for the detection of amebic antigens in feces. The IgG fraction of serum (whose antibody source was not stated) containing antibodies reactive with *E. histolytica* was absorbed onto 13 mm diameter disks mounted on polystyrene slides. A suspension of feces in buffer solution was prepared and the slide agitated in the slurry for 12-16 hr. After thorough washing, peroxidase-labeled antiamebic IgG was added to each disk and the slide incubated for 2 hr at 20°C. After this procedure the disk was washed in buffer and the substrate (3-amino-5-ethylcarbazole) added. The inclusion of disks that had not been treated with IgG enabled the detection of any nonspecific reaction caused by the presence of endogenous peroxidase. These workers showed that the method had a sensitivity of 0.23 μg/ml of strain HK9 antigen. Cross-reactivity with other amebic antigens was not found. This method formed the basis of a commercial kit (Immunozyme *E. histolytica* Reagent Kit, Millipore Corporation, Bedford, Massachusetts).

Doubts about the specificity of the system, however, were raised by Palacios et al. (1978) who noted that although 155 of 159 fecal specimens, containing trophozoites and cysts of *E. histolytica*, were ELISA-positive, only 307 of 562 microscopy-negative samples were ELISA-negative.

The Immunozyme *E. histolytica* kit (Millipore Corporation) was used for the detection of amebic antigen in the feces of 113 homosexual men in San Francisco, and the results were compared with those of microscopy (Randall et al., 1984). They found that only seven of the 12 samples that contained *E. histolytica* trophozoites gave positive results in the test.

Another ELISA method that utilized plastic microtiter plates that had been coated with specific rabbit anti-*E. histolytica* immunoglobulin was described by Grundy (1982). In a model system this method was more sensitive than that of Root and colleagues; as little as 0.15 μg/ml of *E. histolytica* (strain HK9) protein was detected. There was, however, little reactivity with stool samples that contained only cystic forms of the ameba. To explain this finding, it was suggested that the antigenic composition of the cyst surface may differ from the trophozoite material used in the immunization of the rabbits for the preparation of the immunosorbent.

To circumvent the problems of sensitivity and specificity inherent in the previous test system, a double-antibody indirect ELISA test using a combination of monoclonal and polyclonal antibodies was described by Ungar et al. (1985). However, details of the development of the MAb have not been published. Polystyrene microtiter plates were coated with an MAb produced to the HK9 strain (Synbiotex Corporation, San Marcos, California). After incubation with a suitably diluted feces sample, rabbit antiserum against strain HK9 was added followed, after appropriate washes, by an alkaline phosphatase-labeled goat antirabbit serum. Eighteen of 22 specimens containing *E. histolytica* trophozoites or cysts and only three of 186 microscopy-negative samples gave positive results. The ELISA test results were negative on specimens containing other species of amebae. Microscopy-positive specimens that had been preserved in formalin or polyvinyl alcohol gave negative results, and it was shown that the antigenicity of the specimen varied with storage at 4°C beyond 48 hr or by repeated freezing and thawing.

Although the authors conclude that this is a rapid and cost-effective diagnostic test, further experience with its use is necessary before firm conclusions can be drawn.

III. GIARDIA INTESTINALIS

Giardia intestinalis (*G. lamblia*) is a common cause of diarrhea in the tropics and, less frequently, in temperate areas. In addition many infected individuals, if not most, are asymptomatic. Malabsorption is common in symptomatic patients (Wright et al., 1977) and resolves after antigiardia treatment. Variable degrees of mucosal damage induced by giardia are found in patients with malabsorption but although the organism may be detected within the jejunal lumen or within the crypts (Ridley and Ridley, 1976), invasion of the epithelium is rare (Saha and Ghosh, 1977). Although usually self-limiting (Rendtorff, 1954), the infection can become protracted with chronic ill-health. However, the immunological mechanisms involved in resolution of the infection are not clear (Editorial, *Lancet*, 1982).

As there may be differences in virulence among strains of *G. intestinalis* (Owen, 1980), parasitic factors may also be important in the pathogenesis of the infection.

A. Life Cycle

The various aspects of the life cycle are well reviewed by Kulda and Nohynkova (1978). There are two stages in the life cycle of *G. intestinalis*: the trophozoite and the cyst. The trophozoites are pear shaped, measuring 12-15 μm in length, 6-8 μm wide, and 2-4 μm thick, and are rounded anteriorly, pointed posteriorly, and concave ventrally. On the ventral aspect is a circular adhesion disk about 6 μm in diameter which forms a dome-shaped concave chamber. This is the organelle of attachment to host cells. From a kinetosomal complex situated in the midline between the two oval nuclei arise eight flagella, two of which emerge anterolaterally, two posterolaterally, two ventrally, and two caudally.

The striated disk that supports the domed chamber of the adhesive disk arises from the fusion of two rows of supranuclear microtubules which undergo helicoidal spiraling. Extensive cross-linking with neighboring microtubules results in a robust cytoskeleton.

The oval cysts, which measure 8-12 by 7-10 μm, have a homogeneous wall up to 0.5 μm thick that is closely apposed to the cell membrane. Chitin is an important structural component of the cell wall (Ward et al., 1985). There are two to four nuclei, kinetosomes, the axonemes of the flagella, microtubules, and ribosomes.

Trophozoites of *G. intestinalis* inhabit the duodenum and jejunum where they divide by binary fission. They attach by their adhesive disk to the columnar epithelial cells of the lumen and crypts. The cysts are the infective stage of the giardia; trophozoites do not survive outside the body and are passed only in diarrheal stools. Shortly after the cyst wall is formed during transit through the distal jejunum and colon nuclear division occurs, and two to four nucleated cysts are passed in the feces. After reaching the duodenum and jejunum of the new host, excystation occurs with the release of two trophozoites.

B.   Detection of *Giardia intestinalis* Trophozoites or Cysts

1.   In Feces

In freshly passed or PVA-preserved fluid stools, the trophozoites of *G. intestinalis* may be found by microscopy of a saline mount or trichrome-stained preparation. Cysts are not always detectable in trophozoite-containing diarrheal stools; however, in the formed feces from patients with giardiasis cysts but not trophozoites are found. Methods for the concentration of cysts from feces (e.g., that of Ridley and Hagwood, 1956) should be employed routinely in the diagnostic laboratory (McMillan and McNeillage, 1984) because these often double the detection rate. The rate of excretion of cysts varies from patient to patient and is often intermittent (Danciger and Lopez, 1975). The value of examination of multiple fecal samples was shown in a study of 670 confirmed cases of giardiasis (Wolfe, 1978). Seventy-six percent, 90%, and 97% of infections were identified by examination of first, second, and third specimens; a further 1.7% were found in the fourth or subsequent specimens. As in amebiasis, ingestion of several substances can interfere with cyst excretion, and this should be considered when interpreting the results of parasitological examination (Sect. II.D.).

Although excystation and subsequent cultivation of cysts of *G. intestinalis* has been described (Bhatia and Warhurst, 1981), the method is difficult to reproduce and does not lend itself to routine use in the diagnosis of giardiasis.

2.   In Duodenojejunal Aspirates or Biopsy Specimens

As cyst excretion in the feces is often intermittent but trophozoites are always present in the upper small intestine, it is not surprising that examination of duodenal and jejunal aspirates is a more sensitive diagnostic test than microscopy of feces (Kamath and Murugasu, 1974). Occasionally, however, organisms are found in the feces but not in jejunal aspirate. The use of Enterotest (Health Development

Corporation, Palo Alto, California) for sampling duodenojejunal contents mini-mizes discomfort to the patient.

Occasionally trophozoites are not detected in the duodenojejunal aspirates but are found in jejunal biopsies (Kamath and Murugasu, 1974). Because many serial sections may have to be examined before trophozoites are seen, micro-scopy of Giemsa-stained impression smears is preferred.

A preliminary report on the culture of trophozoites from duodenal aspirates gave encouraging results and suggested that this method, using a modification of Diamond's medium, might be useful in diagnosis (Gordts et al., 1984).

C. Isoenzyme and Restriction Endonuclease Analysis of *Giardia intestinalis*

Because many individuals infected with *G. intestinalis* are asymptomatic but oth-ers have transient or persistent gastrointestinal symptoms, the existence of viru-lent and avirulent strains has been postulated. Unlike *E. histolytica*, animal models for the study of virulence are not helpful. Isoenzyme analysis of amebic isolates shows a limited number of patterns and certain zymodemes have been related to pathogenicity (Sect. II.C.). Similar studies on five isolates of giardia were reported by Bertram et al. (1983), and three patterns were distinguished.

A comprehensive study by restriction endonuclease analysis of DNA from giardia isolates from human and animals was undertaken by Nash and colleagues (1985). By agarose electrophoresis of Hind III-restricted DNA fragments, two major groups of 15 isolates could be distinguished. On Southern blot analysis nine different banding patterns among these isolates were visualized. Although one common pattern was found in six isolates, the others were unique, some of the patterns differing markedly from the others. The authors concluded that this method of analysis might be useful in epidemiological investigations. The question of the existence of virulent strains, however, remains unanswered.

D. Antigenic Composition of *Giardia intestinalis*

The first major study of the antigenic composition of *G. intestinalis* was reported by Smith et al. (1982). An SDS-PAGE analysis of solubilized trophozoites of four giardia strains (designated WB, Portland I, LT, and PO) that had been isolated from patients who had acquired their infections in different geographical areas, identi-fied 26 protein bands with molecular weights ranging from 10,000 to 140,000. Two main groups were recognized with molecular weights between 12,000 and 20,000 and between 28,000 and 38,000. The electrophoretic patterns of the strains were similar. By crossed-immunoelectrophoresis using rabbit antiserum raised against one of the four strains tested, there was overall similarity. There were, however, minor antigenic differences between the strains. These differences were also found when each strain was tested against 10 human antisera in ELISA tests run in parallel.

Cultured *G. intestinalis* releases excretory-secretory (ES) materials into the culture medium (Nash et al., 1983). By PAGE the predominant ES product is polydisperse with a molecular weight that varies between 94,000 and 225,000; ES material of lower molecular weight (16,500-21,000) is also found. Although the precise nature of these ES products is unknown, their hydrophobic properties, their sensitivity to protease and periodate, and their failure to bond to lectins suggest that they are a proteolipid. As PAGE analysis of the radiolabeled antigen in the ES products shows that they are identical to the labeled material found on the trophozoites of *Giardia* spp., it is reasonable to assume that ES material is derived from the surface of the parasite.

An analysis of the surface antigens of *G. intestinalis* was undertaken by Einfeld and Stibbs (1984). When rabbit antiserum against the P-1 strain was absorbed with live or formaldehyde-treated trophozoites, it failed to precipitate a major surface antigen that had been detected by crossed-immunoelectrophoresis of a sonicate of the organism. In immunoblotting experiments, monospecific rabbit antisera against this antigen identified a single antigenic component of molecular weight 82,000. Further, SDS-PAGE analysis of radiolabeled P-1 trophozoites showed a prominent band of identical molecular weight that could be precipitated, together with other components of molecular weights 105,000, 30,000, and 24,000, by the monospecific antiserum. Virtually identical results were obtained when these experiments were repeated using three other strains of *G. intestinalis*. Although there were some differences between the results obtained by Einfeld and Stibbs (1984) and Nash et al. (1983), there were important similarities: an antigenic component of molecular weight 82,000 was visible in some autoradiographs shown by the latter authors. Both groups identified antigens with molecular weights of about 21,000-24,000 and 30,000, and the 105,000 molecular weight components in Einfeld's study fell within the range of Nash's polydisperse antigen.

Results from a variety of methods used by Nash et al. (1983) indicated that the ES material of strain P-1 differed antigenically from that of strain WB. In an extension of this study (Nash and Keister, 1985), the ES products and surface antigens of 19 isolates of giardia were compared by reactivity with homologous and heterologous antisera and by acrylamide slab gel electrophoresis. Although recovered from patients and animals in different geographical areas, some isolates appeared similar. Other human isolates showed marked differences of the surface antigens. There was partial correlation between the DNA-binding patterns after endonuclease restriction analysis and the characteristics of the ES products or surface antigens.

Although the surface antigens are likely to be most important in eliciting a humoral immune response to *Giardia* sp. in the host, MAbs may be reactive with other cellular components (Sect. III.e). By use of detergents, the cytoskeleton (flagellar axonemes and striated disk) of giardia can be extracted and analyzed

(Crossley and Holberton, 1983). Fractionation of SDS-solubilized cytoskeleton yields two important protein fractions: one containing tubulin and the other containing a protein of molecular weight 30,000 (giardin). By comparison with other tubulins the giardia tubulin is markedly heterogeneous, but its amino acid composition is very similar to that of rat brain tubulin. Giardin also appears heterogeneous by isoelectric focusing, but its amino acid composition is considerably different from that of tubulin. As an integral protein of the disk microribbons, giardin is associated in vivo with tubulin.

E. Development of Monoclonal Antibodies Against *Giardia intestinalis*

The development of MAbs against *G. intestinalis* was first described by Torian et al. (1984).

1. Organisms

The Portland 1 strain of *G. intestinalis* was cultured in Diamond's modified TY1-S-33 medium (Diamond et al., 1978). After washing three times in phosphate-buffered saline (PBS) (ph 7.0; 0.01 M) the protozoa were suspended in PBS to a concentration of 3.2×10^7 cells per milliliter.

2. Immunization

BALB/c mice were immunized by the intraperitoneal injection of 8×10^5 live *G. intestinalis* suspended in 0.25 ml PBS. Adjuvant was not used. Mice were re-inoculated intravenously 41 days later with 8×10^5 trophozoites, and after a further 21 days, they were injected intravenously with 8×10^5 organism. Three days later, they were humanely killed.

3. Hybridization Procedure

The myeloma cell line BALB/c MOPC 21 NS1/1 (NS/1) was cultivated in RPM1 1640 containing heat-inactivated fetal calf serum. Using polyethylene glycol at a concentration of 40%, NS/1 cells and splenic lymphocytes from immunized mice were fused at a ratio of 1:7. Selection for hybrid cells was undertaken using HAT medium (see Chap. 1).

4. Detection of Giardia intestinalis *Antibodies in Culture Supernatants*

An ELISA method was used for the detection of antibodies in the supernatant of the hybrid culture, and cells that produced giardia antibody were cloned by endpoint dilution on thymocyte feeder layers in microtiter plates. Seventeen phenotypically stable cloned cell lines that produced MAbs against *G. intestinalis* were produced; nine MAbs (four were of the IgM class, two were of the IgG class, and the antibody class of the other three was not determined) were chosen for further analysis. By immunofluorescence it was found that each antibody reacted

against the four strains of formalin-fixed giardia tested; unfixed trophozoites
did not stain, suggesting that the antigen determinants are not located on the
surface of the membrane. Four antibodies reacted with only the body of the organism (3-7, 3-11, 3-15, 3-16), two with only the flagella (3-5, 3-14), one with
only the attachment disk (3-12), and two with the body and flagella with equal
intensity (3-4, 3-17). By immunoblotting, it was found that the MAbs that reacted in the immunofluorescent test with the trophozoite body and body/flagella
reacted with two pronase-sensitive, heat-stable antigenic components of molecular weight 170,000 and 155,000 from all four strains of giardia. Antigens prepared
from whole trophozoites or isolated cytoskeletons gave identical results. Monoclonal antibodies that identified flagella and attachment disk, however, reacted
principally with two components of lower molecular weight 53,000 and 55,000:
at lower dilutions five additional polypeptides of molecular weight 160,000,
116,000, 110,000, 38,000, and 31,000 were identified by the flagellum-specific
MAbs. As these flagellum- and disk-specific antibodies reacted strongly with a
purified bovine brain tubulin preparation, and as the polypeptides that reacted
with them comigrated with bovine brain tubulin, it was concluded that these
MAbs identify giardia tubulin. The different immunofluorescent-staining patterns
obtained by MAbs 3-5/3-14 (flagellum-specific) and 3-12 (disk-specific) may be
explained by differences in the antigen determinants in the flagellar and disk microtubules. Because the MAbs to tubulin show extensive cross-reactivity, for example with *Candida albicans*, it is unlikely that they will be useful for diagnostic
purposes.

F. Immunological Tests

As the detection of giardial trophozoites and/or cysts in the feces or duodenojejunal contents can be difficult, often necessitating the examination of multiple
stool samples and duodenal intubation is unpleasant for the patients, immunological tests that have proved so useful in other protozoal infections have been
evaluated.

1. Serological Tests

a. Indirect Immunofluorescence. Ridley and Ridley (1976) were the first to
describe a fluorescent antibody method (IFA test) for the detection of serum
antibodies to *G. intestinalis*. As antigen in the test they used washed cysts, preliminary experiments having shown that trophozoites in aspirates and frozen sections of jejunal mucosa were unsuitable because they were lost in washing and
were too scant, respectively. Antibodies at a titer of $\geqslant 10$ were detected in the
sera of 89% of infected symptomatic patients but in none of the 17 control subjects (Table 3). The high sensitivity of the test was shown by other workers but
Visvesvara and Healy (1978) found that antibodies were not detectable in 33%
of sera from infected patients.

Table 3 Results of the Immunofluorescence Method for the Detection of Serum Antibodies Against *G. intestinalis*

No. of patients whose sera gave positive results/no. of patients with giardiasis tested		No. of individuals whose sera gave positive results/no. of noninfected individuals tested	Antigen used	Ref.
Symptomatic patients	Asymptomatic patients			
32/36	0/2	0/17	Cysts	Ridley and Ridley (1976)
44/68	28/40	0/53	Trophozoites	Visvesvara and Healy (1978)
29/30	—	0/19	Trophozoites	Visvesvara et al. (1980)
29/29	25/30	—	Trophozoites	Wittner et al. (1983)

The antibody detected by the IFA test is preponderantly of the IgG class (Ridley and Ridley, 1976); specific IgM and IgA has been only rarely detected. After successful treatment, the antibody titer decreases only slowly (Visvesvara et al., 1980; Wittner et al., 1983), making the serological diagnosis of repeated infection difficult.

b. Enzyme-Linked Immunosorbent Assay. The use of whole trophozoites of *G. intestinalis* as antigen, detected serum antibodies of the IgG class in 81% of 59 patients with symptomatic giardiasis and 12% of 17 apparently noninfected control subjects (Smith et al., 1981). The specificity of the antibody was confirmed by absorption with *G. intestinalis* trophozoites but not by *E. histolytica* or *Trichomonas vaginalis*. These antibodies persist for many months after successful treatment; in five of seven patients who were reinfected, high-titered serum antibody was produced.

Wittner et al. (1983) found that the IFA and ELISA titers within the groups of infected and noninfected patients studied were similar, but more false-positive results were obtained in the ELISA. This, however, may reflect IgG antibody from a previous undiagnosed infection.

Although possibly of some value in seroepidemiological studies, a lack of sensitivity of the serological tests and the persistence of antibody after successful treatment, limits their diagnostic value.

As *G. intestinalis* is a luminal parasite that excretes/secretes antigenic material into the contents of the intestine, methods for the detection of such antigens have been developed.

2. Detection of Giardia Antigen in Feces

By using repeated washed cysts recovered from the feces of patients with symptomatic giardiasis as an antigen, Craft and Nelson (1982) raised antibodies in rabbits for use in the detection of giardia antigen by counterimmunoelectrophoresis. Two parallel precipitin lines which represented reactivity of antigen with specific IgG and IgM and which were equidistant from the antigen and antiserum-containing wells were obtained. All 62 fecal samples which by microscopy contained giardia cysts, and each of three jejunal aspirates containing trophozoites gave positive results; a positive reaction was noted in only one of the 162 apparently noninfected (by microscopy) individuals. Within 2 weeks of successful treatment fecal antigen was not detectable, but positive results were still obtained in patients whose therapy had failed. Preliminary experiments had shown that the antibodies produced against the trophozoites used for immunization did not produce precipitin lines in the test.

An ELISA method for the detection of giardia antigen was described by Ungar et al. (1984) who used goat and rabbit antisera against cultured trophozoites of two human isolates. This method, which in a model system detected between 37 and 375 trophozoites and 12 and 125 cysts, gave positive results in 36 of 39 fresh unpreserved stool samples from patients with proven infection. Only three of 128 specimens from apparently noninfected individuals were positive; two, however, probably had giardiasis. The overall sensitivity and specificity of the test were then 92 and 98%, respectively, and the predictive values of a positive and negative ELISA were 92 and 98%, respectively. After successful treatment, the ELISA optical density readings declined. Although ELISA is unsuitable for use with preserved fecal specimens, repeated freezing and thawing of unpreserved specimens and storage at 4°C for up to 100 days did not interfere with the sensitivity of the test.

A simplified ELISA method involving only three manipulative stages was described by Green et al. (1985). Affinity-purified rabbit antibody against giardia was used in the test, which on a model system could detect 40 ng/ml and 25 ng/ml trophozoite and cyst protein, respectively, and 75/76 samples that were positive by microscopy gave positive results; all 27 reference-negative specimens were negative by ELISA.

The sensitivity and specificity were, therefore, 98.7 and 100%, respectively, with predictive values for positive and negative samples of 100 and 96.4%, respectively. Within 5 days of treatment with a single oral dose of tinidazole, the test became negative—2 days after the disappearance of cysts from the stool. An advantage of this test system is that as the results of direct visual inspection agree with optical density readings with a threshold of 3 SD above the reference negative mean, the use of colorimeters in field studies can be obviated.

IV. CONCLUSIONS

From the foregoing discussion it is clear that methods currently used for the detection of trophozoites or cysts of protozoa in feces, intestinal secretions, or tissues are unsatisfactory. Tests based on the detection of specific antigens in such mterial should be more reliable and indeed preliminary data suggests that this is so (Sects. II.F.4. and II.F.2.). Because the protozoa are antigenically complex and the parasite preparations often contaminated with the protein components of the culture medium, diagnostic methods that employ polyclonal antisera lack sensitivity and specificity. As the need for antigen purification is obviated, many of these difficulties are circumvented by the use of MAbs, and it is anticipated that their use as diagnostic reagents will become routine. Antigen detection tests based on the inhibition by antigen of the interaction between an MAb and its anti-idiotype should be explored. Such a method has proved useful in the detection of malarial sporozoite antigen in mosquitoes (Potocnjak et al., 1982). The use of polyclonal antibodies for serological differentiation between pathogenic and nonpathogenic strains of *E. histolytica* has not proved effective. The production and use of MAbs against a variety of epytopes, however, may be helpful and deserves further attention.

REFERENCES

Albach, R. A. and Booden, T. (1978). Amoebae. In *Parasitic Protozoa* (J. P. Kreier, ed.), Vol. 2. Academic Press, New York, pp. 455-506.

Aley, S. B., Scott, W. A., and Cohn, Z. A. (1980). Plasma membrane of *Entamoeba histolytica*. *J. Exp. Med. 152*:391-404.

Ambroise-Thomas, P. (1974). Sero diagnostic de l'amibiase par un test rapide d'agglutination de particules de latex sesibelisees. Resultats de 462 examens et comparaison a la reaction d'immuno-gluorescence indirecte. *Bull. Soc. Pathol. Exot. 67*:156-166.

Ambroise-Thomas, P. (1976). Immunofluorescence in diagnosis, posttherapeutic control and seroepidemiology of amoebiasis. In *Proceedings of the International Conference on Amoebiasis* (B. Sepulveda and L. S. Diamond, eds.). Instituto Mexicano del Seguro Social. Mexico City, pp. 594-498.

Ambroise-Thomas, P., Desgeorges, P. T., and Monget, D. (1978). Diagnostic immunoenzymologique (ELISA) des maladies parasitaires par une micromethode modifiee. 2. Resultats pour la toxoplasmase, l'amibiase, la trichinose, l'hydatidose et l'aspergillose. *Bull. WHO 56*:797-804.

Arroyo-Begovich, A. (1978). Induccion de immunidad protectora antiambiana con "neuvos" antigenos en el hamster lactante. B Material antigenico. *Arch. Invest. Med. 9*(Suppl. 1):311-314.

Bertram, M. A., Meyer, E. A., Lile, J. D., and Morse, S. A. (1983). A comparison of isozymes of five axenic *Giardia* isolates. *J. Parasitol. 69*:793-801.

Ghatia, V. N. and Warhurst, D. C. (1981). Hatching and subsequent cultivation of cysts of *Giardia intestinalis* in Diamond's medium. *Trans. R. Soc. Trop. Med. Hyg. 84*:45.

Boonpucknavig, S. and Nairn, R. C. (1967). Serological diagnosis of amoebiasis by immunofluorescence. *J. Clin. Pathol. 20*:875-878.

Bos, H. J. (1978). Fractionation and serological characterization of *Entamoeba histolytica* antigen. *Acta Leiden. 45*:105-116.

Bos, H. J. and Eijk, A. A., Van den (1976). Enzyme-linked immunosorbent assay (ELISA) in the serodiagnosis of amoebiasis. In *Proceedings of the International Conference on Amoebiasis* (B. Sepulveda and L. S. Diamond, eds.). Instituto Mexicano del Securo Social, Mexico City, pp. 721-727.

Bos, H. J., Schonten, W. J., Noordpool, H., Makbin, M., and Oostburg, B. F. J. (1980). A seroepidemiological study of amoebiasis in Surinam by the enzyme linked immunosorbent assay (ELISA). *Am. J. Trop. Med. Hyg. 29*: 358-363.

Brandt, H. and Tamayo, R. P. (1970). Pathology of human amoebiasis. *Hum. Pathol. 1*:351-385.

Brooke, M. M. and Goldman, M. (1949). Polyvinyl alcohol-fixative as a preservative and adhesive for protozoa in dysenteric stools and other liquid materials. *J. Lab. Clin. Med. 34*:1554-1560.

Burnham, W. R., Reeve, R. S., and Finch, R. (1980). *Entamoeba histolytica* infection in male homosexuals. *Gut 21* :1097-1099.

Calderon, J., Munoz, M. L., and Acosta, H. M. (1980). Surface redistribution and release of antibody in induced caps in *Entamoebae. J. Exp. Med. 151*:184-193.

Chang, S. M., Lin, C. M., Dusanic, D. G., and Cross, J. H. (1979). Antigenic analyses of two axenized strains of *Entamoeba histolytica* by two dimensional immunoelectrophoresis. *Am. J. Trop. Med. Hyg. 28*:845-853.

Chin, A. T. L. and Gerken, A. (1984). Carriage of intestinal protozoal cysts in homosexuals. *Br. J. Vener. Dis. 60*:193-195.

Craft, J. C. and Nelson, J. D. (1982). Detection of giardiasis by counterimmunoelectrophoresis of feces. *J. Infect. Dis. 145*:499-504.

Crossley, R. and Holberton, D. V. (1983). Characterization of proteins from the cytoskeleton of *Giardia lamblia. J. Cell Sci. 59*:81-103.

Danciger, M. and Loqez, M. (1975). Numbers of *Giardia* in the feces of infected children. *Am. J. Trop. Med. Hyg. 24*:237-242.

Diamond, L. S. (1968). Techniques of axenic cultivation of *Entamoeba histolytica* Schaudinn 1903 and *Entamoeba histolytica*-like samoebae. *J. Parasitol. 54*:1047-1056.

Diamond, L. S., Harlow, D. R., and Cunnick, C. C. (1978). A new medium for the axenic cultivation of *Entamoeba histolytica* and other *Entameoba. Trans. R. Soc. Trop. Med. Hyg. 72*:431-432.

Editorial (1982). Battles against *Giardia* in gut mucosa. *Lancet 2*:527-528.

Editorial (1985). Is that amoeba harmful or not? *Lancet 1*:732-734.

Einfeld, D. A. and Stibbs, H. H. (1984). Identification and characterization of a major surface antigen of *Giardia lamblia. Infect. Immun. 46*:377-383.

Garcia, L. S., Bruckner, D. A., Brewer, T. C., and Shimizu, R. Y. (1982). Comparison of indirect fluorescent antibody amoebic serology with counterimmunoelectrophoresis and indirect hemagglutination amoebic serologies. *J. Clin. Microbiol. 15*:603-605.

Goldman, M. (1953). Cytochemical differentiation of *Entamoeba histolytica* and *Endamoeba coli* by means of fluorescent antibody. *Am. J. Hyg. 58*: 319-328.

Goldman, M. (1966). Evaluation of a fluorescent antibody test for amoebiasis using two widely differing amoeba strains as antigen. *Am. J. Trop. Med. Hyg. 15*:694-700.

Goldmeier, D., Sargeaunt, P. G., Price, A. S. et al. (1986). Is *Entamoeba histolytica* in homosexual men a pathogen? *Lancet 1*:641-644.

Gordts, B., Hemelhof, W., Retore, P., Rahman, M., Cadranel, S., and Butzler, J. P. (1984). Routine culture of *Giardia lamblia* trophozoites from human duodenal aspirates. *Lancet 2*:137.

Green, E. L., Miles, M. A., and Warhurst, D. C. (1985). Immunodiagnostic detection of giardia antigen in feces by a rapid visual enzyme-linked immunosorbent assay. *Lancet 2*:691-693.

Grundy, M. S. (1982). Preliminary observations using a multilayer ELISA method for the detection of *Entamoeba histolytica* trophozoite antigens in stool samples. *Trans. R. Soc. Trop. Med. Hyg. 76*:396-400.

Ishaq, M. and Pudma, M. C. (1980). Antigenic variation among strains of *Entamoeba histolytica. Ann. Trop. Med. Parasitol. 74*:373-375.

Izar, G. (1914). Studien ueber Amoebenenteritis. Mitteilung IV, Ueber das Vorkommen spezifischer Antikoerper im serum von Amoebenruhr kranken. *Arch. Schiffs Trop. Hyg. 18* (suppl.):45-79.

Jackson, T. F. H. G., Gathiram, V., and Simjee, A. E. (1985). Seroepidemiological study of antibody responses to the syndromes of *Entamoeba histolytica. Lancet 1*:716-718.

Jeanes, A. L. (1969). Evaluation in clinical practice of the fluorescent amoebic antibody test. *J. Clin. Pathol. 22*:427-429.

Juniper, K., Worrell, C. L., Miushew, M. C., Roth, L. S., Cypert, H., and Lloyd, R. E. (1972). Serologic diagnosis of amoebiasis. *Am. J. Trop. Med. Hyg. 21*: 157-168.

Kamath, K. R. and Murugasu, R. A. (1974). A comparative study of four methods for detecting *Giardia lamblia* in children with diarrheal disease and malabsorption. *Gastroenterology 66*:16-24.

Kessel, J. F., Lewis, W. P., Ma, S., and Kem, H. (1961). Preliminary report on a hemagglutination test for entamoebae. *Proc. Soc. Exp. Biol. Med. 106*: 409-413.

Kessel, J. F., Lewis, W. P., Pasquel, E. M., and Turner, J. A. (1965). Indirect hemagglutination and complement fixation tests in amoebiasis. *Am. J. Trop. Med. Hyg. 14*:540-550.

Kettis, A. A., Thorstensson, R., and Utter, G. (1983). Antigenicity of *Entamoeba histolytica* strain NIH 200: A survey of clinically relevant antigenic components. *Am. J. Trop. Med. Hyg. 32*:512-522.

Keystone, J. S., Keystone, D. L., and Proctor, E. M. (1980). Intestinal parasitic infection in homosexual men; prevalence, symptoms and factors in transmission. *Can. Med. Assoc. J. 123*:512-514.

Knoblock, J. and Mannweiler, E. (1983). Development and persistence of antibodies to *Entamoeba histolytica* in patients with amoebic liver abscess. *Am. J. Trop. Med. Hyg. 32*:727-732.

Kobayashi, T. K., Koretoh, O., Kamachi, M., Watanabe, S., Ishigooka, S., Matsushita, I., and Sawaragi, I. (1985). Cytologic demonstration of *Entamoeba histolytica* using immunoperoxidase technique. Report of two cases. *Acta Cytol. 29*:414-418.

Krupp, I. M. (1974). Comparison of counterimmunoelectrophoresis with other serologic tests in the diagnosis of amoebiasis. *Am. J. Trop. Med. Hyg. 23*: 27-30.

Krupp, I. M. (1977). Definition of the antigenic pattern of *Entamoeba histolytica* and immunoelectrophoretic analysis of the variations of patient response to amoebic disease. *Am. J. Trop. Med. Hyg. 26*:387-392.

Krupp, I. M. and Powell, S. J. (1971). Comparative study of the antibody response in amoebiasis. Persistence after successful treatment. *Am. J. Trop. Med. Hyg. 20*:421-424.

Kulda, J. and Nohynkova, E. (1978). Flagellates of the human intestine and of intestines of other species. In *Parasitic Protozoa* (J. P. Kreier, ed.), Vol. 2. Academic Press, New York, pp. 1-138.

Lumsden, W. H. R. and McMillan, A. (1987). Protozoa. In *Mackie and McCartney's Medical Microbiology* (J. P. Duguid, B. P. Marmion, and J. G. Collee, eds.), Vol. 2. Churchill Livingston, Edinburgh.

McGowan, K., Deneke, C. F., Thorne, G. M., and Gorback, S. L. (1982). *Entamoeba histolytica* cytotoxin: Purification, characterization strain virulence and protease activity. *J. Infect. Dis. 146*:616-625.

McMillan, A. (1980). Intestinal parasites in homosexual men. *Scot. Med. J. 25*: 33-35.

McMillan, A., Gilmour, H. M., McNeillage, G., and Scott, G. R. (1984). Amoebiasis in homosexual men. *Gut 25*:356-360.

McMillan, A. and McNeillage, G. J. C. (1984). Comparison of the sensitivity of microscopy and culture in the laboratory diagnosis of intestinal protozoal infection. *J. Clin. Pathol. 37*:809-811.

Maddison, S. E., Powell, S. J., and Elsdon-Dew, R. (1965). Application of serology to the epidemiology of amoebiasis. *Am. J. Trop. Med. Hyg. 17*:554-557.

Mattern, C. F. T. and Keister, D. B. (1977). Experimental amoebiasis. II. Hepatic amoebiasis in the newborn hamster. *Am. J. Trop. Med. Hyg. 26*:402-411.

Markell, E. K., Havens, R. F., Kuritsubo, R. A., and Wingerd, J. (1984). Intestinal protozoa in homosexual men of the San Francisco Bay area: Prevalence and correlates of infection. *Am. J. Trop. Med. Hyg. 33*:239-245.

Meyers, J. D., Kuharic, H. A., and Holmes, K. K. (1977). *Giardia lamblia* infection in homosexual men. *Br. J. Vener. Dis. 53*:54-55.

Milgram, E. A., Healy, G. R., and Kagan, I. G. (1966). Studies on the use of the indirect hemagglutination test in the diagnosis of amoebiasis. *Gastroenterology 50*:645-649.

Morris, M. N. and Powell, S. J. (1970). Latex agglutination test for invasive amoebiasis. *Lancet 1*:1362-1363.

Nash, T. E., Gillin, F. D., and Smith, P. D. (1983). Excretory-secretory products of *Giardia lamblia. J. Immunol. 131*:2004-2010.

Nash, T. E. and Keister, D. B. (1985). Differences in excretory-secretory products and surface antigens among 19 isolates of *Giardia. J. Infect. Dis. 152*:1166-1171.

Nash, T. E., McCutchan, T., Keister, D., Dame, J. B., Conrad, J. D., and Gillin, E. D. (1985). Restriction-endonuclease analysis of DNA from 15 *Giardia* isolates obtained from humans and animals. *J. Infect. Dis. 152*:64-73.

O'Shea, M. S. and Feria-Velasco, A. (1974). Demonstracion ultramicroscopica de antigenos de superficie en tropozoitos de *E. histolytica* por immunofluorescencias con IgG humana especifica. *Arch. Invest. Med. 5* (Suppl. 2):307-314.

Ortega, H. B., Borchardt, K. A., Hamilton, R., Ortega, P., and Mahood, J. (1984). Enteric pathogenic protozoa in homosexual men from San Francisco. *Sex. Transm. Dis. 11*:59-63.

Owen, R. L. (1980). The ultrastructural basis of *Giardia* function. *Trans. R. Soc. Trop. Med. Hyg. 74*:429-433.

Palacios, O., de la Hoz, R., and Sosa, H. (1978). Determinacion del antigenos amibiano enheces por el metodo ELISA (enzyme-linked immunosorbent assay) para la identificacion de *Entambe histolytica*. *Arch. Invest. Med. 9* (Suppl. 1):339-348.

Parelkar, S. N., Stamm, W. P., and Hill, K. R. (1971). Indirect immunofluorescent staining of *Entamoeba histolytica*. *Trans. R. Soc. Trop. Med. Hyg. 67*: 659-662.

Phillips, S. C., Mildvan, D., Williams, D. C., Gelb, A. M., and White, M. C. (1981). Sexual transmission of enteric protozoa and helminths in a venereal disease clinic population. *N. Engl. J. Med. 305*:603-606.

Pillai, S. and Mohimen, A. (1982). A solid phase sandwich radioimmunoassay for *Entamoeba histolytica* proteins and in the detection of circulating antigens in amoebiasis. *Gastroenterology 83*:1210-1216.

Pittman, F. E. and Hennigar, G. R. (1974). Sigmoidoscopic and colonic mucosal biopsy findings in amoebic colitis. *Arch. Pathol. 97*:155-158.

Potocnjak, P., Zavala, F., Nussenzweig, R., and Nussenzweig, V. (1982). Inhibition of idiotype-anti-idiotype interaction for detection of a parasite antigen: A new immunoassay. *Science 215*:1637-1639.

Prathap, K. and Gilman, R. (1970). The histopathology of acute intestinal amoebiasis. A rectal biopsy study. *Am. J. Pathol. 60*:229-239.

Randall, G. P., Goldsmith, R. S., Shek, J., Mehalko, S., and Heyneman, D. (1984). Use of the enzyme-linked immunosorbent assay (ELISA) for detection of *Entamoeba histolytica* antigen in faecal samples. *Trans. R. Soc. Trop. Med. Hyg. 78*:593-595.

Rendtorff, R. C. (1954). The experimental transmission of human intestinal protozoan parasites. II. *Giardia lamblia* cysts given in capsules. *Am. J. Hyg. 59*: 209-220.

Ridley, D. S. and Hagwood, B. C. (1956). The value of formol-ether concentration of faecal cysts and ova. *J. Clin. Pathol. 9*:74-76.

Ridley, M. J. and Ridley, D. S. (1976). Serum antibodies and jejunal histology in giardiasis associated with malabsorption. *J. Clin. Pathol. 29*:30-34.

Robinson, G. L. (1968). The laboratory diagnosis of human parasitic amoebae. *Trans. R. Soc. Trop. Med. Hyg. 62*:285-294.

Root, D. M., Cole, F. X., and Williamson, J. A. (1978). The development and standardization of an ELISA method for the detection of *Entamoeba histolytica* antigens in fecal samples. *Arch. Invest. Med. 9*(Suppl. 1):203-210.

Saha, T. K. and Ghosh, T. K. (1977). Invasion of small intestinal mucosa by *Giardia lamblia* in man. *Gastroenterology 72*:402-405.

Sargeaunt, P. G. and Williams, J. E. (1978). Electrophoretic isoenzyme patterns of *Entamoeba histolytica* and *Entamoeba coli*. *Trans. R. Soc. Trop. Med. Hyg. 72*:164-166.

Sargeaunt, P. G., Oates, J. K., MacLennan, I., Oriel, J. D., and Goldmeier, D. (1983). *Entamoeba histolytica* in male homosexuals. *Br. J. Vener. Dis. 59*: 193-195.

Savanat, T. and Chaicumpa, W. (1969). Immunoelectrophoresis test for amoebiasis. *Bull. WHO 40*:343-353.

Sawhney, S., Chakravarti, R. N., Jain, P., and Vinayak, V. K. (1980). Immunogenicity of axenic *Entamoeba histolytica* antigen and its fractions. *Trans. R. Soc. Trop. Med. Hyg. 74*:26-29.

Sawitz, W. G. and Faust, E. C. (1942). The probability of detecting intestinal protozoa by successive stool examinations. *Am. J. Trop. Med. Hyg. 22*:131-136.

Scalas, L. (1921). Contributo allo studio della deviazione del complemento nella dissenteria amebica. *Reforma Med. 37*:103-104.

Sheehan, D. J., Bottone, E. J., Pavletick, K., and Heath, M. C. (1979). *Entamoeba histolytica* efficacy of microscopic cultural and serological techniques for laboratory diagnosis. *J. Clin. Microbiol. 10*:128-133.

Smith, P. D., Gillin, F. D., Brown, W. R., and Nash, T. E. (1981). IgG antibody to *Giardia lamblia* detected by enzyme-linked immunosorbent assay. *Gastroenterology 80*:1476-1480.

Smith, P. D., Gillin, F. D., Kaushal, N. A., and Nash, T. E. (1982). Antigenic analysis of *Giardia lemblia* from Afghanistan, Puerto Rico, Ecuador and Oregon. *Infect. Immun. 36*:714-719.

Speiser, F. (1980). Anwendung einer Enzym-Immunmethode (Elisa) fur die serologie der Amobiase. *Schweiz. Med. Wochenschr. 110*:404-407.

Stamm, W. P., Ashley, M. J., and Parelkar, S. N. (1973). Evaluation of latex agglutination test for amoebiasis. *Trans. R. Soc. Trop. Med. Hyg. 67*:211-213.

Stamm, W. P., Ashley, M. J., and Bell, K. (1976). The value of amoebic serology in an area of low endemicity. *Trans. R. Soc. Trop. Med. Hyg. 70*:49-53.

Stamm, W. P. and Phillips, E. A. (1977). A cellulose acetate membrane precipitin (CAP) test for amoebiasis. *Trans. R. Soc. Trop. Med. Hyg. 71*:490-492.

Thompson, J. E., Freischlag, J., and Thomas, D. S. (1983). Amoebic liver abscess in a homosexual man. *Sex. Transm. Dis. 10*:153-155.

Thompson, P. E., Graedel, S. K., Schneider, C. R., Stucki, W. P., and Gordon, R. M. (1968). Preparation and evaluation of standardized amoebic antigen from axenic cultures of *Entamoeba histolytica*. *Bull. WHO 39*:349-365.

Torian, B. E., Barnes, R. C., Stephens, R. S., and Stibbs, H. H. (1984). Tubulin and high molecular weight polypeptides as *Giardia lamblia* antigens. *Infect. Immun. 46*:152-158.

Ungar, B. L. P., Yolken, R. H., Nash, T. E., and Quinn, T. C. (1984). Enzyme-linked immunosorbent assay for the detection of *Giardia lamblia* in fecal specimens. *J. Infect. Dis. 149*:90-97.

Ungar, B. L. P., Yolken, R. H., and Quinn, T. C. (1985). Use of a monoclonal antibody in an enzyme immunoassay for the detection of *Entamoeba histolytica* in fecal specimens. *Am. J. Trop. Med. Hyg. 34*:465-472.

Visvesvara, G. S., Healy, G. R., and Brown, W. R. (1980). An immunofluorescence test to detect serum antibody to *Giardia lamblia*. *Ann. Intern. Med. 93*:802-805.

Walls, K. W. and Wilson, M. (1983). The use of the solid phase indirect immunofluorescent assay (FIAX) in the serodiagnosis of amoebiasis. *Ann. N.Y. Acad. Sci. 420*:422-430.

Ward, H. D., Alroy, J., Lev, B. I., Keusch, G. T., and Pereira, M. E. A. (1985). Identification if chitin as a structural component of *Giardia* cysts. *Infect. Immun. 49*:629-634.

William, D. C., Shookhoff, H. B., Felman, Y. M., and DeRamos, S. W. (1978). High rates of enteric protozoal infections in selected homosexual men attending a venereal disease clinic. *Sex. Transm. Dis. 5*:155-157.

Wittner, M., Maayan, S., Farrer, W., and Tanowitz, H. B. (1983). Diagnosis of giardiasis by two methods: Immunofluorescence and enzyme-linked immunosorbent assay. *Arch. Pathol. Lab. Med. 107*:524-527.

Wolfe, M. S. (1978). Managing the patient with giardiasis: Clinical, diagnostic and therapeutic aspects. In *Waterborne Transmission of Giardiasis* (W. Jakubowski and J. C. Hoff, eds.). National Technical Information Service, Springfield, Va., pp. 39-52.

World Health Organization (1969). Amoebiasis. Report of a WHO Expert Committee. Geneva.

Wright, S. G., Tomkins, A. M., and Ridley, D. S. (1977). Giardiasis: Clinical and therapeutic aspects. *Gut 18*:343-350.

Yang, J. and Kennedy, M. T. (1979). Evaluation of enzyme-linked immunosorbent assay for the serodiagnosis of amoebiasis. *J. Clin. Microbiol. 10*:778-985.

Ylvisaker, J. A. and McDonald, G. B. (1980). Sexually acquired amoebic colitis and liver abscess. *West. J. Med. 132*:153-157.

ELEVEN

Development of Monoclonal Antibodies Against Herpes Simplex Virus

Ian W. Halliburton
University of Leeds
Leeds, England

I. INTRODUCTION

The most common herpesvirus infections of man are caused by herpes simplex virus. There are two serotypes, herpes simplex virus type 1 (HSV-1) and herpes simplex virus type 2 (HSV-2) which can be differentiated from each other by biochemical, immunological, and biological tests. Type 1 isolates are commonly obtained from lesions of the lips, mouth, and upper parts of the body, whereas type 2 isolates are associated principally with genital lesions. The two viruses are not, however, mutually exclusive in their site of infection, and about 30% of genital isolates are type 1, and a small number of isolates from nongenital sites are type 2 (Buckmaster et al., 1984; Herrod et al., 1984).

II. MORPHOLOGY OF THE HERPES SIMPLEX VIRUS PARTICLE

The morphology of the herpesvirus particle is the primary means of classification of the virus family. Figure 1 shows the basic appearance of the virus particle. Herpesvirions have four distinct morphological regions: an electron-opaque core, an icosahedral capsid enclosing the core, and electron-dense amorphous region called the tegument (Roizman and Furlong, 1974), and an outer glycoprotein-containing envelope. The nucleoprotein core contains a cylindrical protein structure around

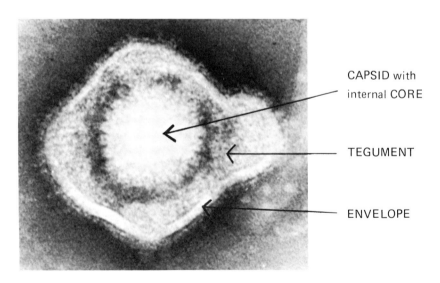

CAPSID with
internal CORE

TEGUMENT

ENVELOPE

Fig. 1 Electron micrograph of the HSV virus particle indicating the four distinct morphological regions.

which the double-stranded DNA of 100×10^6 molecular weight (Becker et al., 1968; Wilkie, 1973) is wound in a toroidal structure (Furlong et al., 1972). Also present within the core is a polyamine, spermine, which may play a role in condensation of the virus DNA (Gibson and Roizman, 1971; McCormick, 1978). Surrounding the core is an icosahedral capsid composed of 150 hexameric and 12 pentameric capsomeres. The diameter of the capsid is approximately 100 nm. Exterior to the capsid is the tegument, a loosely defined structure of highly variable size that has no distinctive structural features in thin sections of virions but that sometimes appears to have components with a fibrous structure in negatively stained particles (Wildy et al., 1960; Morgan et al., 1968; Schwartz and Roizman, 1969). Another polyamine, spermidine, appears to be localized in the tegument (Gibson and Roizman, 1971; McCormick, 1978). Surrounding the tegument is the triple-layered lipid and glycoprotein-containing envelope derived from altered patches of cellular membranes (Morgan et al., 1954; Epstein, 1962). As with most enveloped viruses, there are protrusions or spikes of about 8 nm in length on the surface of the envelope (Watson, 1973).

III. HERPES SIMPLEX VIRUS PROTEINS

The DNA contains about 150,000 nucleotide base pairs, which is enough to code for 5.5×10^6 daltons of protein. In addition, however, there is growing realization of the existence of a number of overlapping genes, hence, the true coding potential of the DNA is greater than this. At least 50 virus-specified polypeptides varying in molecular weight from about 12,000 to 275,000 have now been identified by sodium dodecyl sulfate-polyacrylamide gel electrophoresis (SDS-PAGE) (Honess and Roizman, 1973; Marsden et al., 1976; Powell et al., 1977). Unfortunately there is no general agreement about a system of nomenclature for herpes simplex virus proteins. Some groups refer to polypeptides by their molecular weight while others use one of several numbering systems related largely to the order of polypeptides as seen on SDS-PAGE. In this chapter, a number system based on that of Spear and Roizman (1972) and Honess and Roizman (1973) will essentially be used. This system numbers polypeptides from the largest molecular weight at the top of the gel as ICP 1 (infected cell polypeptide 1) or VP 1 (virion polypeptide 1) to the smallest molecular weight at the bottom of the gel. Glycoproteins will be referred to by a universally accepted nomenclature in which they have been assigned an alphabetical designation preceded by g for the fully processed glycoprotein or by pg for a precursor to the fully processed glycoprotein.

When the polypeptides in virus infected cells are examined by SDS-PAGE at different times postinfection, it is apparent that many of the polypeptides exhibit temporal control in their rates of synthesis (Honess and Roizman, 1973; Powell and Courtney, 1975). Additional studies using inhibitors of protein, RNA, and DNA synthesis have identified three groups of HSV proteins, α, β, and γ, whose synthesis

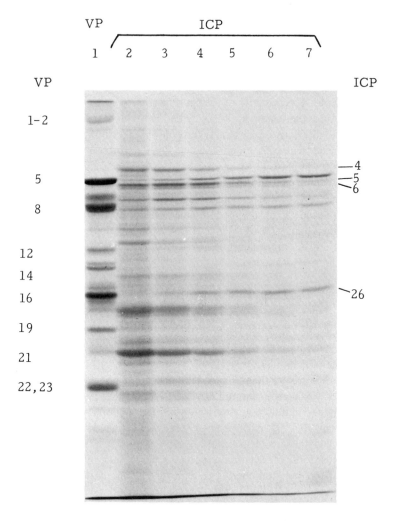

Fig. 2 Structural and nonstructural polypeptides of HSV-1. Lane 1 is an autora-
diogram of the structural polypeptides of HSV-1 strain HFEM. Lanes 2-7 are a
timecourse study of the polypeptides in cells infected with *ts LB2*, a *ts* mutant
of strain HFEM, at 38°C, a temperature slightly below its restrictive temperature.
The polypeptides were labeled with [^{35}S] methionine during successive 90-min
intervals from 1.0-2.5 hr (lane 2) to 8.5-10 hr postinfection (lane 7). The VP
numbers at the left indicate the position of some of the major HSV-1 virion polypeptides and the ICP numbers at the right indicate the corresponding infected cell
polypeptides (cf. Table 1).

is coordinately regulated in a cascade fashion (Honess and Roizman, 1974, 1975a; Powell and Courtney, 1975). The groups α, β, and γ correspond to immediate-early, early, and late-temporal classes of synthesized proteins. Figure 2 illustrates these temporal classes with a timecourse study of the proteins made by *ts LB2* (Halliburton et al., 1977, 1980), a *ts* mutant of HSV-1 strain HFEM at 38°C, a temperature slightly below a completely restrictive temperature (Honess et al., 1980). The α proteins are exemplified by ICP 4, the β proteins by ICP 6 and the γ proteins by ICP 5 or ICP 26. Polypeptides associated with virus replication are of the α or β class, the virion structural proteins tending to be of the γ class.

Specific functions, as yet, have been assigned to only a few of the polypeptides. To review our knowledge of polypeptide function it is convenient to consider two groups, the structural and the nonstructural polypeptides.

A. Structural Polypeptides

The number of structural polypeptides reported has varied from 13 to 33 of which several are glycosylated (Spear and Roizman, 1972; Heine et al., 1974; Powell and Watson, 1975; Strnad and Aurelian, 1976). Differences in the number detected probably arise largely because of differences in the purification methods used, resulting in various degrees of contaminating cellular polypeptides or because of the electrophoretic system employed. Figure 2, lane 1 illustrates the separation of structural polypeptides of HSV-1 strain HFEM in a comparison of the polypeptides in cells infected with a *ts* mutant of the same strain and Table 1 indicates the molecular weight and established location of the major structural polypeptides within the virion.

Of the structural polypeptides, at least seven are present in the virus capsid. Two forms of the capsid (A and B) have been demonstrated, A capsids lacking DNA and B capsids containing DNA (Gibson and Roizman, 1972). The A capsids contain VP 5, VP 19C, VP 23, and VP 24. The B capsids contain in addition VP 21 and VP 22a, a modified form of VP 22 (Gibson and Roizman, 1972; Braun et al., 1984) and a polypeptide of 12,000 molecular weight (Heilman et al., 1979). VP 5 is considered to be the major capsid polypeptide.

The virion's glycoproteins are exposed on the envelope surrounding the capsid as shown by preferential labeling by lactoperoxidase-catalyzed iodination (Olshevsky and Becker, 1972) or by tritiated borohydride reduction of Schiff's bases formed between pyridoxal phosphate and reactive groups on the virion (Roizman and Furlong, 1974). In addition, antibodies to gC, gB (Powell et al., 1974; Eberle and Courtney, 1980), gD (Watson and Wildy, 1969; Cohen et al., 1978), or gE (Para et al., 1982a) have neutralizing activity, indicating the presence of the glycorproteins on the surface of the virions.

Despite many studies on the glycoproteins of HSV, the precise number of glycosylated species is not yet known, and our knowledge of the function of individual glycoproteins is very limited. The subject has been recently reviewed by

Table 1   Identified Function or Site in the Virion of HSV Polypeptides and Availability of Monoclonal Antibodies

ICP[a]	Mol. wt. ($\times\ 10^{-3}$)	VP[b]	Suggested function or site in the virion	MAb available?
1-2	275	1-2	Tegument	–
3	260	3	Tegument	–
4	175	–	Immediate-early[c]	Yes
5	155	5	Major capsid protein	Yes
6	144	–	Ribonucleotide reductase	Yes
7	138	–	DNA polymerase?	–
0	110	–	Immediate-early[c]	Yes
8	135	–	Major DNA-binding protein	Yes
9	130	8	gC, envelope	Yes
10	126	7	gB, envelope	Yes
11	119	8.5	pgB	Yes
12	117	–	–	–
13	116	–	–	–
14	115	9	–	–
15	109	–	–	–
16	105	–	–	–
17	100	10	–	–
18	94	11	–	–
18.5	92	12	Tegument	–
19	90	–	Alkaline nuclease	Yes
20	86	13	gE, envelope	Yes
21	80	14	–	–
22	68	–	Immediate-early[c]	–
23	67	–	–	–
24	66	–	–	–
25	65	15	Tegument	–
26	64	16	Tegument	Yes
27	63	–	Immediate-early[c]	Yes
28	59	17	gD, envelope	Yes
29	58	–	DNA-binding protein	Yes
30	57	18	–	–
31	53	19	Capsid	–
32	50	20	–	–
33	48	–	–	–
34	44	21	Core	–
35	43	–	Thymidine kinase	Yes
36	42	–	–	–

Table 1 *continued*

ICP[a]	Mol. wt. ($\times 10^{-3}$)	VP[b]	Suggested function or site in the virion	MAb available?
37	40	–	–	–
38	37	–	Ribonucleotide reductase?	–
39	36	22	Capsid	Yes
40	33	23	Capsid	–
41	32	–	–	–
42	31	–	–	–
43	30	–	–	–
44	27	–	–	–
45	25	24	Capsid	–
46	23	–	–	–
47	12	–	Immediate-early[c]	–
48	–	–	–	–
49	–	–	–	–

[a]ICP, infected cell polypeptide.
[b]VP, virion polypeptide.
[c]The function of immediate-early polypeptides is discussed in the text.

Spear (1985). To date, six type 1 [gB-1 (VP 7), gC-1 (VP 8), gD-1 (VP 17), gE-1 (VP 13), gG-1, and gH-1] and five type 2 glycoproteins (gB-2, gC-2, gD-2, gE-2 and gG-2) have been identified. The glycoprotein designated gC-2 of molecular weight 75,000 was originally called gF (Balachandran et al., 1981, 1982b) and was renamed on the basis of its antigenic cross-reaction with gC-1 of molecular weight 130,000 (Zezulak and Spear, 1983; Zweig et al., 1983) and on the location of its coding sequence on the genome (Para et al., 1983; Zezulak and Spear, 1984). The glycoprotein previously designated gA (VP 8.5) is now known to be a precursor of gB and has been renamed pgB (Cohen et al., 1981).

Glycoprotein B is essential for the production of infectious virus and *ts* mutants mapping in that gene have been isolated (Manservigi et al., 1977; Little et al., 1981), and the phenotypes of these mutants suggest that gB has multiple functions. Thus, although the mutants adsorb to cells at nonpermissive temperature, they cannot penetrate, indicating that gB is essential for penetration of the virus into cells (Little et al., 1981; Sarmiento et al., 1979). The glycoprotein is also involved in fusion of infected cells because *syn* loci map within the structural gene of gB (Ruyechan et al., 1979; Honess et al., 1980; Little and Schaffer, 1981; DeLuca et al., 1982; Kousoulas et al., 1984).

In addition, gB of wild-type virus exists in a heat-unstable oligomeric form in infected cells and in the virus particle (Sarmiento and Spear, 1979; Snowden et al., 1985). Antiserum to gB of HSV-1 contains type-common and type-specific neutralizing activity and cross-reacts not only with gB-2 but also with glycoproteins in cells infected with bovine mammillitis virus, equine herpesvirus type 1 (Snowden et al., 1985; Snowden and Halliburton, 1985), varicella zoster virus, Epstein-Barr virus, pseudorabies virus, and feline rhinotracheitis virus (I. W. Halliburton and B. W. Snowden, unpublished observations). The gene coding for gB has recently been sequenced, permitting predictions about secondary structure of the glycoprotein (Bzik et al., 1984; Pellett et al., 1985).

Glycoprotein C is not essential for productive infection of HSV in tissue culture because mutants lacking gC are viable (Hoggan and Roizman, 1959; Heine et al., 1974; Holland et al., 1983a, 1984; Zezulak and Spear, 1984). The glycoprotein has also been implicated in syncytial formation in an as yet unknown manner (Honess et al., 1980; Lee et al., 1982) and it binds to the C3b component of complement (Friedman et al., 1984).

Glycoprotein D stimulates the production of high titers of neutralizing antibody, contains both type-common and type-specific antigenic sites, and is likely to play an important role in the initial stages of virus infection (Sim and Watson, 1973; Cohen et al., 1978; Halliburton, 1980). Tryptic peptide analysis (Eisenberg et al., 1980; Balachandran et al., 1982c) and sequencing (Watson et al., 1982; Watson, 1983; Laskey and Dowbenko, 1984) have shown that gD-1 and gD-2 are structurally similar but not identical, sharing 85% homology, which would strongly suggest that they are also functionally similar. No specific functional role for gD has been conclusively identified, but it has been suggested to be a likely candidate for the cellular receptor-binding protein and may, therefore, be important in attachment (Spear, 1980a). It has also been implicated in fusion of infected cells (Noble et al., 1983; Norrild et al., 1983).

Glycoprotein E was originally identified by its ability to bind to the Fc portion of IgG (Baucke and Spear, 1979). The glycoprotein is present in purified virions and binds specifically to IgG, not to Fab fragments (Para et al., 1982b). Antiserum to gE also neutralizes virus infectivity in the presence of complement, but the specific role of gE in virion infectivity is not known, although it has been proposed that it may be involved in virus pathogenesis because the binding of IgG to receptors at the surface of infected cells could interfere with immune cytolysis (Westmoreland and Watkins, 1974; Costa and Robson, 1975).

Glycoprotein H could play a role in cell-to-cell spread of virus (Buckmaster et al., 1985), but no functions have yet been associated with gG.

The location of the remaining structural polypeptides is not really known, but it is generally assumed that they are located in the tegument. Extraction of virions with the nonionic detergent NP 40 results in differential solubilization of the putative tegument polypeptides. Thus, whereas, VP 13, VP 14, and VP 16 are readily extracted by NP 40, VP 1-2, VP 3, and VP 12 are appreciably more resistant to extraction (Spear, 1980b). A protein kinase activity (Rubenstein et al., 1972; Lemaster and Roizman, 1980; Katan et al., 1985) and an ATPase activity (Epstein and Holt, 1963) have been shown to be extractable by NP 40, and therefore, have also been associated with the tegument or envelope.

B. Nonstructural Polypeptides

As with the structural polypeptides, the function of many of the nonstructural polypeptides is not known. However, those to which function has been assigned by inference or by experiment will be discussed and are indicated in Table 1.

The first proteins synthesized in HSV-infected cells have been designated α, or immediate-early, proteins. They are ICP 4, 0, 22, 27, and 47, and their mRNAs are transcribed in the absence of prior viral protein synthesis (Honess and Roizman, 1974, 1975b; Clements et al., 1977). Functional immediate-early polypeptides are required for efficient expression of early (β_1 or β_2) or late (γ_1 or γ_2) viral genes (Honess and Roizman, 1975b).

The most extensively studied immediate-early gene product is ICP 4, largely because a number of temperature-sensitive mutants in the ICP 4 gene exist. These mutants dramatically overproduce all the immediate-early polypeptides at the nonpermissive temperature and it seems that ICP 4 is required for expression of early and late genes and is responsible for controlling its own synthesis and that of the other immediate-early genes (Halliburton et al., 1977; Preston, 1979; Dixon and Schaffer, 1980; Honess et al., 1980). These findings have been confirmed by the isolation and characterization of ICP 4 deletion mutants (De Luca et al., 1985). Transfection experiments with plasmids containing various combinations of immediate-early genes have suggested that ICP 0 may be able to act in *trans* with ICP 4 to stimulate expression from early promoters (DeLuca and Schaffer, 1985; Quinlan and Knipe, 1985). Isolation and characterization of insertion and deletion mutants in the ICP 22 gene established that ICP 22 function was not required for growth of the virus in Vero cells. However, it has subsequently been established that these mutants are host-range mutants that will grow in some cell lines such as Vero, HEp-2, or MRC-5s but not as well in cells such as BHK or Rat-1 cells (Halliburton et al., 1983; Sears et al., 1985). It is probable that the permissive cells can substitute a host function for the ICP 22 function, whereas the nonpermissive cells, to various degrees, cannot do so. The function involved appears to be required remarkably late in the growth cycle for an immediate-early gene function and affects the expression of late (γ_2) genes (Halliburton et al., 1983; Sears et al., 1985). Isolation of *ts* mutants in the ICP 27 gene have established that the ICP 27 protein is required for virus replication and, like ICP 22, affects the expression of late viral genes (Sacks et al., 1985). No function has yet been assigned to ICP 47.

The synthesis of β polypeptides depends upon the presence of functional α polypeptides and reaches peak rates between 5 and 7 hr after infection (Honess and Roizman, 1974, 1975b). Ribonucleotide reductase, which catalyzes the synthesis of deoxyribonucleotides by direct reduction of the four ribonucleotides, has been shown to be essential for virus replication and to be, at least partially, virus coded by the isolation and characterization of a temperature-sensitive mutant affecting this activity (Dutia, 1983). The enzyme activity has been specifically associated with two polypeptides of 144,000 (ICP 6) and 38,000 molecular weight, both of which are phosphorylated (Huszar et al., 1983; Bachetti et al., 1984).

The virus-induced thymidine kinase has also been extensively studied and is associated with a 44,000 molecular weight polypeptide, but higher-molecular-weight complexes of this polypeptide have also been demonstrated (Ogino et al., 1973; Honess and Watson, 1974).

The enzyme is not required for growth of the virus in tissue culture since TK$^-$ mutants grow satisfactorily (Aron et al., 1973), but the enzyme is required for growth of the virus in resting cells (Jamieson and Subak-Sharpe, 1974). Several additional enzyme activities in HSV-infected cells, such as uracil-DNA-glycolase and UTP nucleotidohydrolase (molecular weight 53,000), have been shown to be biochemically distinct from the host cell-coded enzymes (Caradonna and Cheng, 1981).

One group of nonstructural proteins that have been extensively studied are the DNA-binding proteins, as many as 23 of which have been reported (Bayliss et al., 1975; Powell and Purifoy, 1976; Bookout and Levy, 1980; Wilcox et al., 1980). Most of these belong to the β kinetic class, but α proteins have also been shown to have affinity for DNA (Bookout and Levy, 1980; Hay and Hay, 1980), although the binding of ICP 4 has been shown to be indirect and via a component of uninfected cells (Freeman and Powell, 1982). The binding of a protein to a DNA cellulose column clearly does not by itself prove any functional relationship, but the approach has, in general, been used to look principally for proteins involved in DNA synthesis. The function of some of these proteins has, however, been identified.

The most abundant DNA-binding protein is ICP 8 which has a molecular weight of 135,000 and is referred to as the major DNA-binding protein. Antiserum to this protein neutralizes in vitro DNA synthesis in chromatin extracts of HSV-infected cells, suggesting that the polypeptide has a role in DNA synthesis (Powell et al., 1981). It has also been suggested that ICP 8 is involved in the negative regulation of γ_2 genes (Godowski and Knipe, 1985).

Purification of the HSV-specified DNA polymerase has been reported (Weissbach et al., 1973). The enzyme has a molecular weight of 143,000, and a second polypeptide (ICP 29) of molecular weight 54,000 copurifies with it. The polymerase polypeptide has, in addition, a 3',5'-exonuclease activity for which a proofreading role has been proposed (Weissbach et al., 1973; Knopf, 1979). A fourth DNA-binding protein that has been purified is the alkaline nuclease (Banks et al.,

1983). The enzyme (ICP 19) has both endo- and exonucleolytic activity in vitro, but its role in vivo is not known (Hoffman and Cheng, 1979). By use of a mutant that has at least one lesion in the alkaline nuclease gene, it has been established that the enzyme has an essential role in virus replication (Halliburton and Timbury, 1976; Francke and Garrett, 1982; Moss, 1986).

IV. PRODUCTION AND SCREENING OF MONOCLONAL ANTIBODIES

A. Immunization

In our department the general approach that has been used in the production of monoclonal antibodies (MAbs) is as follows: Lysates, sonicates, or the detergent-solubilized membrane fraction (Roberts et al., 1985) of infected cells or purified polypeptides (Banks et al., 1984, 1985; Vaughan et al., 1984) were inoculated twice, along with Freund's incomplete adjuvant, into the footpad of inbred BALB/c mice, with a 14-day interval between injections. Three days before cell fusion the mice were given, in the tail vein, an intravenous boost of the extract or polypeptide.

B. Cell Fusion

The procedure used in cell fusion is essentially as described by Kennett et al. (1978). The mice were bled and the blood screened for antibody. The spleen cells from the immunized mice were mixed with a nonproducing myeloma cell line such as SP2/0-Ag-14 (Shulman et al., 1978) at a ratio of 10:1 and resuspended in culture medium containing hypoxanthine, aminopterin, and thymidine (HAT) to select hybridomas (Killington et al., 1981). Individual colonies of hybrid cells were transferred to Linbro panel wells, and antibody-producing hybrids were detected by, e.g., enzyme-linked immunosorbent assay (ELISA).

C. Production of Ascitic Fluid

Six- to 12-week-old inbred mice were sensitized with pristane 1 week before injection with hybrid cells to produce ascites tumors. Generally, 1×10^7 cells were used per animal. The mice were killed after 10-14 days and ascitic fluid harvested from the peritoneal cavity. The antibody was purified from the ascitic fluid using DEAE-cellulose chromatography as described by Fahey and Horbett (1959).

D. Screening of Monoclonal Antibodies

Monoclonal antibodies can be screened by any of a variety of tests, as illustrated in Sect. V. The tests most commonly used are immunoglobulin classification, ELISA, immunoperoxidase, immunofluorescence, radioimmunoassay, Western

blot analysis, SDS-PAGE of immunoprecipitates, immunoadsorbent chromatography, enzyme neutralization (Banks et al., 1985), reverse passive hemagglutination (Cranage et al., 1983) immune electron microscopy, neutralization, or im-
munocytolysis (Oakes and Lausch, 1984).

V. A REVIEW OF MONOCLONAL ANTIBODIES CURRENTLY AVAILABLE AGAINST HERPES SIMPLEX VIRUS AND THEIR POTENTIAL USES

A. Proteins

Herpes simplex virus type 1 specifies approximately 50 infected cell polypeptides
forming three groups, α, β, and γ, whose synthesis is coordinately regulated and
sequentially ordered in a cascade fashion (Honess and Roizman, 1974, 1975b).
Type 2 HSV appears to specify the same number of infected cell polypeptides
(Powell and Courtney, 1975). Monoclonal antibodies have been isolated to about
a third of these polypeptides as summarized in Table 1 and as indicated in more
detail in this section. Braun et al. (1983) and Showalter et al. (1981) have each
isolated MAbs to a number of infected cell polypeptides. Braun et al. (1983) have
isolated 113 MAbs that reacted specifically with infected cells by immunofluorescence. However, only seven MAbs reacted by immunoprecipitation (with ICP
5, 8, and gB), 12 reacted with electrophoretically separated polypeptides transferred to nitrocellulose strips (ICP 4, 5, 6, 8, 29, and 35-37), but only three reacted by both techniques, all with ICP 8. Ninety-one of the MAbs failed to react
by either technique, either because of denaturation of antigenic sites or because
they failed to form precipitates. It is unlikely that any single assay technique will
allow the identification of all MAbs. The authors also looked at the type specificity of the antibodies, the location of the genes specifying the polypeptides on
the physical map of the DNA, the site of accumulation of the viral polypeptides
in the cell, the nature of posttranslational modification, the electrophoretic mobility, and the oligomeric cr monomeric nature of the viral proteins.

Showalter et al. (1981) isolated 52 MAbs against 10 HSV proteins including
three glycosylated proteins (gB, gC, and gD) and six nonglycosylated proteins
[ICP 4, 5, 6, 8, 9, and an unclassified (uncharacterized) 68,000-molecular-weight
protein] . Glycoprotein D, gA, the 68,000 protein, ICP 9, and ICP 6 express both
type-specific and cross-reactive antigenic determinants. In contrast, nine antibodies against gB all showed cross-reactivity between HSV-1 and HSV-2, whereas eight
antibodies against gC all reacted type specifically. Given these findings, the authors suggested that gB expresses only cross-reactive determinants and gC only
type-specific determinants. Since then, however, it has been established that gB
also possesses type-specific determinants (Snowden et al., 1985) and gC cross-
reactive determinants (Zweig et al., 1983).

1. Immediate Early Polypeptides

For the immediate-early polypeptides, MAbs specific for ICP 4 (Showalter et al., 1981; Braun et al., 1983; Ackermann et al., 1984), ICP 0 and ICP 27 (Ackermann et al., 1984) have been produced. All three polypeptides have been shown to accumulate primarily in the nuclei of infected cells. Monoclonal antibodies specific for ICP 22 and ICP 47 have not yet been produced, but antisera specific for 12 and 16 residue peptides of the essential polypeptide ICP 22 (Sears et al., 1985) have been produced (Ackermann et al., 1985).

2. Enzymes

By use of MAbs to HSV-1 and HSV-2 early antigens Bachetti et al. (1984) have shown that in both serotypes, ribonucleotide reductase activity is associated with phosphoproteins of molecular weight 144,000 and 38,000 encoded between map units 0.566 and 0.602. The major 144,000 antigenic species was identified as ICP 6 in HSV-1 and ICP 10 in HSV-2.

Banks et al. (1983) have purified the alkaline nuclease induced by HSV-1 and HSV-2 and used the HSV-2 nuclease as an immunogen to prime BALB/c mice, which were then used to prepare MAbs. Five MAbs were used in immunoperoxidase tests to demonstrate the nuclear localization of the enzyme and to identify it as an 85,000-molecular-weight phosphoprotein (ICP 19) which was mapped by analysis of intertypic recombinants (Halliburton, 1980) as 0.168 to 0.175 map units on the genome (Banks et al., 1985). Three of the MAbs were directed against HSV type-common epitopes and two against HSV-2-specific epitopes on the enzyme.

Purified HSV thymidine kinase has been used to immunize mice for the production of MAbs to the enzyme. Purified preparations of HSV-2 DNA polymerase contain at least two polypeptides, a major one of about 150,000 molecular weight and a minor one of 54,000 molecular weight (ICP 29). Vaughan et al. (1985) have purified the latter, prepared polyclonal rabbit antiserum and MAbs to it, and used these reagents to characterize the protein, to map it to 0.525 to 0.627 map units, a position quite distinct from that of DNA polymerase itself, and to verify the close association between these two polypeptides. After using these MAbs to the HSV-induced alkaline nuclease, to ICP 29, and to the major DNA-binding protein, ICP 8, Vaughan et al. (1984) suggested that these polypeptides interact as part of an HSV DNA replication complex. Norrild et al. (1985), using a MAb to a 91,000-molecular-weight protein, thought to be the alkaline nuclease, showed that it coprecipitated a 121,000-molecular-weight protein identified as the major DNA-binding protein, ICP 8.

3. DNA-Binding Proteins

The major DNA-binding protein of HSV, ICP 8, is a β or early protein, has a molecular weight of about 130,000, and is essential for DNA replication. Several groups have isolated MAbs to ICP 8 (Showalter et al., 1981; McLean et al., 1982; Braun et al., 1983; La Thangue et al., 1984; Vaughan et al., 1984, 1985) and to at least five other DNA-binding proteins of molecular weight 155,000 (ICP 5), 115,000 (gB), 60,000, and 40,000 (ICP 39), in addition to the MAbs described previously. The expression of ICP 8 in COS-1 cells transfected with an SV40 origin-of-replication plasmid vector containing the Bgl II 0 fragment of HSV-2 has been verified using a MAb to ICP 8 (Sheppard et al., 1985). ICP 8 may also be a major component of the AG-4 antigen of HSV-2 (Evans et al., 1985; Flanders et al., 1985).

4. Structural Polypeptides

Monoclonal antibodies have been produced to at least three nonglycosylated structural proteins: VP 5, 16, and 22a.

The MAbs against VP 5 (ICP 5), the major capsid polypeptide, have been produced by a number of groups (Showalter et al., 1981; McLean et al., 1982; Braun et al., 1983; La Thangue and Chan, 1984). All the MAbs are cross-reacting by PAGE of radioimmunoprecipitates, Western blot analysis, immunofluorescence, or solid phase immunoassay, with the heterologous virus whether produced against HSV-1 (Showalter et al., 1981; Braun et al., 1983; La Thangue and Chan, 1984) or HSV-2 (McLean et al., 1982). An MAb against HSV-2 VP 16 (ICP 26) has been produced and is cross-reactive with HSV-1 (McLean et al., 1982). A 57,000-molecular-weight HSV-1 polypeptide isolated by reversed phase high-performance liquid chromatography (RP-HPLC) also reacted with the same MAb (Welling-Wester et al., 1985).

An MAb reactive with a 40,000-molecular-weight phosphoprotein, designated VP 22a or p40 (ICP 39), has been isolated (Zweig et al., 1979). This polypeptide is present in full, but not in empty, capsids purified from nuclei of infected cells. The MAb immunoprecipitated a cluster of three to four closely spaced polypeptides ranging in molecular weight from 39,000 to 45,000. Another panel of MAbs has also been shown to react with at least six bands of molecular weight 39,000-50,000, designated ICP 35a to 35f (Braun et al., 1983; Braun et al., 1984), whose genes map between 0.32 and 0.36 map units. This family of polypeptides are genetically and immunologically related. ICP 35a to 35d are cytoplasmic precursors to 35e and 35f, which are nuclear products, one of which corresponds to the virion capsid component VP 22a. None of the members of the ICP 35 family have been found in empty capsids, and it has been proposed that ICP 35e and 35f coat the surface of the capsid of full virions (Braun et al., 1984). A *ts* mutant [HSV-1 (17)ts VP 1201] in the gene coding for ICP 35, mapping at about 0.33 map units, has been characterized (Preston et al., 1983) with the aid of the MAb to p40 produced by Zweig et al. (1979). At the nonpermissive temperature the infected cells accumulated the polypeptides forming the slowest migrating forms of ICP 35, and the mutant was defective in encapsidation of viral DNA. The temperature-sensitive lesion, therefore, prevents the processing of the polypeptides and thereby the encapsidation of viral DNA.

5. Glycoproteins

Monoclonal antibodies to the six characterized glycoproteins gB, gC, gD, gE, gG, and gH have been isolated. In addition, by using a combination of immunoprecipitation with MAbs and analysis of the immune precipitates by two-dimensional PAGE, Palfreyman et al. (1983) have identified additional intermediates in the processing of gB, gC, gD, and gE, and possible additional previously unreported glycoproteins. Norrild et al. (1986) have also shown by indirect immunofluorescence using MAbs to gB, gC, and gD that these glycoproteins interact with the cytoskeletal elements actin, myosin, and tubulin during intracellular transport. The MAbs to the six characterized glycoproteins have been used to purify individual glycoproteins by immune affinity chromatography, to study the processing of glycoproteins, to study cross-reactions with heterologous HSV and with glycoproteins of other herpesviruses, to identify antigenic sites, and in several other ways. Each of these will now be illustrated by reference to individual glycoproteins.

a. Glycoprotein B. Pereira et al. (1981) isolated 24 independently derived MAbs reactive with gB and its precursor gA (pgB), 12 of which neutralized virus infectivity. All MAbs precipitated gA and gB. Twenty-three of the MAbs precipitated gA and gB from HEp-2 or Vero cells infected with HSV-1 or HSV-2. One MAb neutralized only HSV-2 and precipitated gA and gB from extracts of HEp-2 but not of Vero-infected cells. Glycoproteins A and B had faster electrophoretic mobilities in Vero cells than in HEp-2 cells and the infected Vero cell lysates contained three relatively small proteins that were also precipitated by 23 of the 24 MAbs (Pereira et al., 1981, 1982b). Showalter et al. (1981) also observed degradation of gB in mouse and Vero cells but not in HEp-2 cells.

Using a panel of MAbs to gB, Kousoulas et al. (1984) have segregated the MAbs into nine groups on the basis of immunological reactivity, a series of spontaneous and mutagen-induced virus mutants nonreactive in at least one immune reaction with two of the MAbs, preliminary mapping of the mutations by marker transfer or marker rescue, and a technique for rapid selection of mutants reactive or nonreactive with specific MAbs. Pellett et al. (1985) have presented the nucleotide sequence of the gB gene of HSV-1 strain F, the specific amino acid substitutions in three of the mutants selective for loss of reactivity with two MAbs, and a model of the structure of gB and the predicted changes in the structure of the gB induced by the mutations was also presented.

The importance of gB has been enhanced by evidence of cross-reactivity between gB of HSV-1 and glycoproteins of other herpesviruses. We have shown that a monoprecipitin antiserum to gB of HSV-1, immunoprecipitates not only gB and pgB from cells infected with HSV-1 or HSV-2 but also precipitates at least three glycoproteins from cells infected with bovine mammillitis virus or equine herpesvirus type 1 (Snowden et al., 1985). The precipitated glycoproteins were digested with trypsin and the resulting peptides separated by two-dimensional thin-layer chromatography or by HPLC. The resulting profiles were almost identical, suggesting considerable structural conservation of the polypeptide backbone of the antigenically related glycoproteins of these four viruses. Cross-reactions between the gB-related glycoproteins of these four viruses have also been shown by Western blot analysis, but use of polyclonal or MAbs to HSV-1 gC or gD did not reveal any such cross-reactions other than between gD of HSV-1 and HSV-2 (Snowden and Halliburton, 1985). We have extended these latter studies to show antigenic relatedness of HSV-1 gB and a glycoprotein of varicella zoster virus, Epstein-Barr virus, pseudorabies virus, and feline rhinotracheitis virus. With MAbs to HSV-1, Edson et al. (1985) and Kitamura et al. (1986) have also shown cross-reaction by immune precipitation and SDS-PAGE between HSV-1 gB and a 63,000 or 64,000-molecular weight varicella zoster virus envelope glycoprotein and have suggested that these two proteins may have similar functions. Such cross-reactions could also have great relevance to vaccine studies.

b. Glycoprotein C. Antisera prepared against individual glycoproteins gB, gD, and gE of HSV-1 have frequently been cross-reactive with HSV-2, whereas antibody to gC was type-specific (Spear, 1976). When MAbs to gC were first obtained, they were also found to be type-specific whether prepared against HSV-1 or against HSV-2 (Pereira et al., 1980; Balachandran et al., 1982c; Pereira et al., 1982a). At that stage, an HSV-2 glycoprotein of molecular weight similar to that of HSV-1 gC had been designated gC solely on the basis of electrophoretic mobility, even though the biochemical and immunological characteristics of the HSV-1 and HSV-2 glycoproteins were quite distinct and the genes specifying them were not colinear. Monoclonal antibodies were then described that precipitated HSV-2 glycoproteins of multiple electrophoretic forms ranging from 50,000 to 80,000 molecular weight (Balachandran et al., 1981; Para et al., 1983). This glycoprotein was designated gF by Balachandran et al. (1981). The MAbs reacted type specifically and the glycoprotein's gene mapped to 0.58 to 0.69 map units on the HSV-2 genome, the same coordinates as HSV-1 gC (Para et al., 1983). Zweig et al. (1983) isolated an MAb that reacted with both the 75,000-molecular-weight HSV-2 gF and the 130,000-molecular-weight HSV-1 gC. The HSV-1 gC and HSV-2 gF, therefore, contain at least one related epitope. The name of HSV-2 gF has, thus, now been changed to gC, even though HSV-1 and HSV-2 gC have considerably different electrophoretic mobilities. The amino acid sequences of gC of HSV-1 and HSV-2 have recently been deduced (Frink et al., 1983; Dowbenko and Laskey, 1984), and antibodies prepared to a synthetic peptide of 12 amino acids, corresponding to that predicted for the amino acids of HSV-1 from positions 128 to 139, reacts with both HSV-1 and HSV-2 gC thus defining a conserved cross-reactive region of HSV-1 gC (Zweig et al., 1984). Marlin et al. (1985) using MAb-resistant mutants (*mar* mutants) with an antigenically altered form of gC and a panel of 22 gC MAbs, have identified a minimum of nine epitopes, which clustered in two distinct antigenic sites.

c. Glycoprotein D. Monoclonal antibodies to gD have confirmed the existence of type-specific and type-common domains within the gD molecule (Pereira et al., 1980; Balachandran et al., 1982c), and an MAb recognizing both gD-1 and gD-2 linked to Sepharose has been used as an immunoadsorbent for the large-scale purification of both glycoproteins (Eisenberg et al., 1982b). Monoclonal antibodies to gD, selected for ability to bind to the surface of purified virions, have been shown to exhibit potent neutralizing activity (Para et al., 1985), to block HSV-induced cell fusion (Noble et al., 1983), and to block the adsorption of virions to cells (Eisenberg et al., 1985).

In attempts to relate the structure of the protein to its biological functions, Eisenberg et al. (1982a) using 17 MAbs have defined eight epitopes within gD based on differences in radioimmunoprecipitation and neutralization assays. Four of these determinants were type-common, three were gD-1-specific, and one was gD-2-specific. One group of antibodies, group VII, was shown to react with a type-common continuous epitope within residues 11-19 of the mature glycoprotein (residues 36 to 44 of the predicted sequence of gD) (Cohen et al., 1984). The site of binding of two additional MAb groups that recognize continuous epitopes has now been established (Eisenberg et al., 1985). Groups II and V (Eisenberg et al., 1982a) bind specifically to residues 268-287 of gD-1 and gD-2 and residues 340-356 of gD-1 (Eisenberg et al., 1985). In addition, competition studies have been carried out to map the relative positions of four discontinuous epitopes corresponding to MAbs in groups I, III, IV, and VI (Eisenberg et al., 1985). In different studies a type 2-specific MAb has been found to bind to amino acid 97 in HSV-2 gD (Rawls et al., 1984).

d. Glycoprotein E. Balachandran et al. (1981) described two type-specific MAbs that precipitated different HSV-2 glycoproteins, the multiple electrophoretic forms of which ranged in molecular weight from 50,000 to 80,000. One they designated gF which, as indicated previously, has now been identified as gC-2, the other they identified as the Fc-binding glycoprotein gE which precipitated a 60,000-molecular-weight polypeptide that chased into a 66,000- and 79,000-molecular-weight polypeptide. Para et al. (1983) isolated MAbs to gE, one of which has tentatively been implicated in adsorption of the virus to infected cells (Fuller and Spear, 1985).

e. Glycoprotein G. As indicated previously, a glycoprotein, initially designated gF, was shown to share antigenic determinants with gC-1 and its gene was shown to comap with that of gC-1. This left uncertain the origin and nature of the glycoprotein of about 124,000 molecular weight originally designated gC-2 (Spear, 1976). This glycoprotein has been renamed gG (Roizman et al., 1984). It reacts with an MAb H966 and its gene has been mapped by analysis of intertypic recombinants to the S component of the genome (Roizman et al., 1984). These results have been confirmed by Marsden et al. (1984) who identified a glycoprotein of 92,000 molecular weight whose gene mapped at 0.846 to 0.924 map units. Although the molecular weight of this glycoprotein is rather lower than that for gG (124,000) the discrepancy is probably a result of the different gel system or virus strain, or both, used by the two groups, because the characteristics and genome map position of the two glycoproteins suggest that they are one and the same.

Recently, Richman et al. (1986) precipitated a type 1 glycoprotein with a molecular weight of 59,000 with MAb LP10 and Ackermann et al. (1986) identified two broad bands of molecular weights 60,000-68,000 and 44,000-48,000 by Western blot analysis with MAb H1379. In both studies the genes coding for the glycoproteins mapped in the U_S region as U_S4 (McGeoch et al., 1985). The exact location (0.892-0.924) was established when the in vitro translation product of the cloned gene U_S4 was precipitated by LP10 (Richman et al., 1986). From a comparison of sequences of the genes and the mapping data of this new glycoprotein with those of gG-2 it was concluded that this was the HSV-1 equivalent of gG-2 (Frame et al., 1986).

Balachandran and Hutt-Fletcher (1985) have also isolated MAbs to gG (molecular weight 108,000) and exchanged reagents with A.C. Minson to confirm that they are dealing with the same glycoprotein. They have also proposed a hypothetical model for the processing of gG involving proteolytic cleavage and addition of *0*- and *N*-linked sugars. Similar observations have been made by H. Su and R. Courtney (personal communication).

f. Glycoprotein H. Glycoprotein H is the most recently named glycoprotein. An MAb, LP 11, was isolated by Buckmaster et al. (1985) which precipitated two glycosylated polypeptides of approximate molecular weight 120,000 from HSV-1-infected cells, and neutralization experiments with intertypic recominants have mapped the glycoprotein gene to within 0.26 to 0.51 map units on the HSV-1 genome. Pulse and pulse-chase experiments have shown that this glycoprotein may be the same as the 110,000-molecular-weight glycoprotein described by Showalter et al. (1981), but experiments with exchanged MAbs have not been performed. Antibody LP11 inhibits plaque formation when added to cell monolayers, suggesting that gH-1 may play a role in cell-to-cell spread of infectious virus (Buckmaster et al., 1985).

B. Monoclonal Antibody-Resistant (*mar*) Mutants

Monoclonal antibodies specific for HSV-1 glycoproteins have been used to demonstrate that HSV undergoes mutagen-induced and spontaneous antigenic variation.

Initially, two neutralizing MAbs, one type-specific for gB and one type-specific for gC, were used to select from untreated or from 5-bromodeoxyuridine- or nitrosoguanidine-treated stocks of HSV-1 strain KOS viral variants resistant to neutralization by MAbs plus complement (Holland et al., 1983a). The *mar* mutants, however, may remain reactive with antibodies that define other antigenic sites. Thus by analyzing the patterns of resistance of neutralization of *mar* mutants with panels of MAbs, discrete antigenic sites on the HSV glycoprotein can be defined and enumerated. Thus, four gC and four gB antigenic variants were isolated. Two of the former failed to express gC, but the other two gC antigenic variants and the four gB variants expressed antigenically altered gC or gB, respectively. Analysis of the *marC* mutants with seven gC specific MAbs provided evidence for at least two antigenic sites on gC (Holland et al., 1983a). In a more extensive study, a panel of 22 MAbs was tested against 22 *marC* mutants. A minimum of nine epitopes were identified that clustered in two distinct antigenic sites, which were shown by MAb-competition studies to be topographically separated on the glycoprotein (Marlin et al., 1985). The mutation in one of the *marB* mutants, *marB1.1* was mapped to a 1.6-kilobase region of the HSV-1 genome (coordinates 0.350 to 0.361) which lies within the structural gene for gB (Holland et al., 1983b).

C. Protection in Mice

Monoclonal antibodies directed against virus glycoproteins have been used successfully to passively protect mice against HSV infection (Dix et al., 1981; Balachandran et al., 1982a; Rector et al., 1982; Sethi, 1983; Kümel et al., 1985; Roberts et al., 1985). Monoclonal antibodies to gB (Balachandran et al., 1982a; Rector et al., 1982; Kümel et al., 1985; Roberts et al., 1985), gC (Dix et al., 1981; Balachandran et al., 1982a; Rector et al., 1982; Sethi, 1983; Kümel et al., 1985; Roberts et al., 1985), gD (Dix et al., 1981; Balachandran et al., 1982a; Rector et al., 1982; Sethi, 1983; Kümel et al., 1985), and gE (Balachandran et al., 1982a; Rector et al., 1982) all protected mice from lethal infection by the virus, although there is no agreement on which antibody provides the best protection; for example, Kümel et al. (1985) found antibodies specific for gB to be less effective than antibodies against gC in providing immunity, and antibodies against gD were the least effective, whereas Balachandran et al. (1982a) found antibodies to gB and to gD equally effective and more so than antibodies to gC or gE. However, Roberts et al. (1985) did not find MAbs to gB or to gC at all effective for the passive immunization of mice, there being no protection when the MAbs were used individually and only a slight increase in mouse survival time when used together. Certainly, the times of virus challenge and the route by which the challenge virus is inoculated varies from study to study, which may well affect the outcome.

There is also no agreement regarding the mechanism by which the antibodies protected the mice. Dix et al. (1981) attributed protection to neutralization of virus in vivo, whereas the antibodies used by Balachandran et al. (1982a) did not neutralize virus infectivity, but a good correlation was found between protection and titers of MAbs assessed by antibody-dependent cellular cytoxicity. Rector et al. (1982), however, found no correlation of the ability of the antibodies to neutralize HSV-1, to promote complement-mediated cell lysis or antibody-dependent cellular cytoxicity, or to protective activity, and Kümel et al. (1985) found no correlation between immune protection and neutralization or antibody isotype. Sethi (1983) found that the passive transfer of MAbs resulted in generation of potent HSV-specific cytotoxic T lymphocytes in the lymph nodes of recipients, provided that the immunization was administered 12-hr postinfection. When the same antibody was injected at 3 hr before HSV infection, no primary cytotoxic T-lymphocyte response was obtained, but the MAbs protected the recipients from death in both cases. Protection, however, is affected by many factors such as the dose of both the protecting antibody and the challenge virus, and antibodies recognizing different epitopes on a single glycoprotein are not equally protective even if the antibody doses are equivalent based on the in vitro neutralization titer (Kümel et al., 1985). It appears, therefore, that the therapeutic effectiveness of MAbs in protecting against HSV infection does not correlate with immunological reactivity in vitro.

Following inoculation of athymic nude mice in the ear pinna with HSV-1 followed by passive transfer of neutralizing MAb or polyclonal HSV antiserum, Kapoor et al. (1982) suggested that neutralizing antibodies play an important role in restricting the movement of virus to the nervous system but that cell-mediated immune mechanisms are essential for the elimination of virus from the pinna. Studying virus growth in the trigeminal ganglia of HSV-1-infected mice, Oakes and Lausch (1984) found that inoculation of infected ganglia in the presence of a pool of nonneutralizing MAbs specific for gB and gE suppressed virus growth by more than 90%. Removal of antibody was followed by a rapid rise in virus production. Use of a pool of MAbs was appreciably more effective in suppressing growth than was any of the antibodies used individually, hence, suppression was strongest when multiple epitopes on the infected cell surface were bound by antibody. Thus the critical functional role for antibody may be simply to slow the rate of virus replication to give time for the cell to develop and mediate reactions capable of destroying virus-infected cells (Oakes and Lausch, 1984).

Active immunization using purified glycoproteins has also been used to protect mice. Roberts et al. (1985) used glycoproteins, purified by immunoadsorption chromatography with MAbs to gB or gC to protect mice successfully against a lethal HSV-1 challenge. Purification of gD by immunoadsorption chromatography using an MAb and its use as a successful vaccine in mice has also been described (Eisenberg et al., 1982b; Long et al., 1984).

D. Detection and Typing of Herpes Simplex Virus

Because type 1 and type 2 HSV share a number of common antigens, typing of isolates with hyperimmune animal antisera is not specific unless the antiserum is first adsorbed with an excess of heterologous antigen to remove cross-reacting antigens. Such type-specific (adsorbed) antisera has been useful in a number of studies such as typing of isolates (Herrod et al., 1984) or enumeration of type-specific antigenic sites (Halliburton, 1980). This adsorbed antiserum is very effective but time-consuming to prepare and variable from batch to batch. Monoclonal antibodies offer a considerable practical advantage in providing a continuous supply of material of defined epitope specificity. They have been used to type isolates by direct immunofluorescence (Volpi et al., 1983; Swierkosz et al., 1985), indirect immunofluorescence (Balachandran et al., 1982b; Pereira et al., 1982a; Goldstein et al., 1983; Legacé-Simard et al., 1983; Peterson et al., 1983; Teh and Sacks, 1983; Docherty et al., 1984; Gleaves et al., 1985; Swierkosz et al., 1985; Zimmerman et al., 1985), ELISA (Nilheden et al., 1983; Frame et al., 1984; Clayton et al., 1985), enzyme immunofiltration technique (Richman et al., 1982) or reverse passive hemagglutination (Buckmaster et al., 1984). Typing of isolates or of specimens that have previously been shown to be virus-positive by tissue culture by all of these tests is very reliable as illustrated in Table 2. Of over 2000 isolates typed with a variety of MAbs, eight type 1 and 22 type 2 isolates behaved anomalously, i.e., about 1.5% of the total. Attempts made to type the virus specimen from lesions without having first verified the presence of virus by tissue culture are less satisfactory (Chap. 12).

It has frequently been suggested that the very restricted specificity of MAbs might limit their application in the detection and typing of viruses and, in addition, because of intratypic antigenic variation, it might be that a number of strains would escape recognition. From the results in Table 2 it would seem that even though examples of nonreactive antigenic variants have been detected (Balachandran et al., 1982b; Pereira et al., 1982a; Lagacé-Simard et al., 1983; Buckmaster et al., 1984; Swierkosz et al., 1985), nevertheless antigenic changes in HSV and nonrecognition by MAbs is not as serious a problem as first suggested. With clinical specimens the rate of HSV detection relative to that obtained in tissue culture is often lower, but the major reason for this is simply the low concentration of virus present in some specimens.

One of the weaknesses of several of these studies, however, has been that the authors often typed the isolates using the MAbs without also typing by some other method, or alternatively, another immunological method using the same MAbs was used as a comparison. In many studies, therefore, it is stated that the isolates were successfully typed using the MAbs without the assurance that none of the results were false-positive. Often a proportion of the isolates (but sometimes

Table 2 Typing of HSV Isolates[a] Using MAbs

MAb	Reactive with	Test	No. positive/No. tested HSV-1	No. positive/No. tested HSV-2	Ref.
Commercial	HSV-1 TS[b]	Direct IF	49/49	38/39	Swierkosz et al. (1985)
	HSV-2 TS				
HD1	HSV TC gD	Indirect IF	56/56	55/55	Pereira et al. (1982a)
HC1	HSV-1 gC	Indirect IF	63/63	2/67	
H222	HSV-2 gE	Indirect IF	0/30	62/64	
H368	HSV-2 gB	Indirect IF	0/30	44/52	
Commercial	HSV-1 TC[c]	Indirect IF	10/14	16/16	Swierkosz et al. (1985)
	HSV-2 TS				
3G11	HSV-1 gC		34/34		
6-A6	HSV-2 140 kd	Indirect IF		83/83	Peterson et al. (1983)
6-E12	HSV-2 55 kd				
6-H11	HSV-2 38 kd				
18βB3	HSV gD	Indirect IF	98/99	48/48	Balachandran et al. (1982b)
17αA2	HSV-2 gC				
17βA3	HSV-2 gD	Indirect IF	101/101		Lagacé-Simard et al. (1983)
Various	HSV-1 TS				
G3	HSV-2 TS		—	97/97	
E6	HSV-2 TS		—	86/97	

Clone	Antigen	Method			Reference
HC-1	HSV-1 gC		22/22		
H222	HSV-2 gE				
H368	HSV-2 gB	Indirect IF		22/22	Teh and Sachs (1983)
H379	?				
3-G11	HSV-1 gC		76/76		
6-A6	HSV-2 140 kd	Indirect IF		187/187	Goldstein et al. (1983)
6A12	HSV-2 55 kd				
6-H11	HSV-2 38 kd				
S-200	HSV-TC	Indirect IF	4/4	11/11	Docherty et al. (1984)
S-141	HSV TS				
S-200	HSV 105-130 kd	Indirect IF	95/95		Zimmerman et al. (1985)
S-141	HSV 110-130 kd	Indirect IF		78/78	
18βB3	HSV gD	ELISA	45/45	30/30	Frame et al. (1984)
17αA2	HSV-2 gF				
17βA3	HSV-2 gD				
G11	HSV-1 gC	Enzyme immunofiltration	131/131		
A6					Richman et al. (1982)
E12, H11	HSV-2 TS			374/374	
LP2	HSV gD				
LP11	HSV-1 gB	Passive hemagglutination			Buckmaster et al. (1984)
LP10	HSV-1 gG		62/63	37/37	
LP4	HSV-2 DNA BP				

[a] Virus stocks or specimens identified as virus positive by tissue culture.
[b] TS, type-specific.
[c] TC, type-common.

a very small proportion) was typed by an unequivocal typing method such as restriction endonuclease analysis of DNA or by SDS-PAGE of polypeptides (Herrod et al., 1984). However, this is no assurance that the isolates not so checked have been correctly typed.

Clearly, no single MAb should ever be used to differentiate type 1 and type 2. Many, however, appear to be directed against sufficiently conserved sites that a combination of one type 1 and one type 2 MAb should never lead to an incorrect diagnosis, even though rare isolates might give ambiguous results by reacting with neither antibody. Several of the studies mentioned earlier employed a combination of a type-common and type-specific MAb; therefore, identification of one type is by reaction with the type-common but failure to react with the type-specific. It may be that use of two type-specific antibodies, such that positive reactions are always detected, could be advantageous. Certainly rapid and accurate typing of HSV isolates is going to assume greater importance if additional selective antiviral drugs such as bromovinyl deoxyuridine (De Clerq et al., 1979) are developed. In addition, an accurate, simple method of typing large numbers of isolates is currently needed simply to establish a picture of the epidemiology of HSV-1 and HSV-2. The use of MAbs by methods such as those discussed present rapid, sensitive, highly specific, and relatively inexpensive methods of diagnosis which can be performed in any clinical laboratory.

ACKNOWLEDGMENTS

I would like to thank the Medical Research Council for Project Grants toward my research incorporated into this chapter, Mrs. S.D. Smith for her excellent technical assistance and Mrs. C.I. Moorhouse for typing this chapter.

REFERENCES

Ackermann, M., Braun, D. K., Pereira, L., and Roizman, B. (1984). Characterisation of herpes simplex virus 1α proteins, 0, 4, and 27 with monoclonal antibodies. *J. Virol. 52*:108-118.

Ackermann, M., Longnecker, R., Roizman, B., and Pereira, L. (1986). Identification, properties and gene location of a novel glycoprotein specified by herpes simplex virus 1. *Virology 150*:207-220.

Ackermann, M., Sarmiento, M., and Roizman, B. (1985). Application of antibody to synthetic peptides for characterisation of the intact and truncated α22 protein specified by herpes simplex virus 1 and the R325 α22⁻ deletion mutant. *J. Virol. 56*:207-215.

Aron, G. M., Schaffer, P. A., Courtney, R. J., Benyesh-Melnick, M., and Kit, S. (1973). Thymidine kinase activity of herpes simplex virus temperature sensitive mutants. *Intervirology 1*:96-109.

Bachetti, S., Evelegh, M. J., Muirhead, B., Sartori, C. S., and Huszar, D. (1984). Immunological characterization of herpes simplex virus type 1 and 2 polypeptide(s) involved in viral ribonucleotide reductase activity. *J. Virol. 49*: 591-593.

Balachandran, N., Bachetti, S., and Rawls, W. E. (1982a). Protection against lethal challenge of BALB/c mice by passive transfer of monoclonal antibodies to five glycoproteins of herpes simplex virus type 2. *Infect. Immun. 37*:1132-1137.

Balachandran, N., Frame, B., Chernesky, M., Kraiselburd, E., Louri, Y., Garcia, D., Lavery, C., and Rawls, W. E. (1982b). Identification and typing of herpes simplex viruses with monoclonal antibodies. *J. Clin. Microbiol. 16*:205-208.

Balachandran, N., Harnish, D., Killington, R. A., Bachetti, S., and Rawls, W. E. (1981). Monoclonal antibodies to two glycoproteins of herpes simplex virus type 2. *J. Virol. 39*:438-446.

Balachandran, N., Harnish, D., Rawls, W. E., and Bachetti, S. (1982c). Glycoproteins of herpes simplex virus type 2 as defined by monoclonal antibodies. *J. Virol. 44*:344-355.

Balachandran, N. and Hutt-Fletcher, L. M. (1985). Synthesis and processing of glycoprotein gG of herpes simplex virus type 2. *J. Virol. 54*:825-832.

Banks, L., Halliburton, I. W., Purifoy, D. J. M., Killington, R. A., and Powell, K. L. (1985). Studies on the herpres simplex virus alkaline nuclease: Detection of type-common and type-specific epitopes on the enzyme. *J. Gen. Virol. 66*:1-14.

Banks, L., Purifoy, D. J. M., Hurst, P.-F., Killington, R. A., and Powell, K. L. (1983). Herpes simplex virus non-structural proteins. IV. Purification of the virus-induced deoxyribonuclease and characterization of the enzyme using monoclonal antibodies. *J. Gen. Virol. 64*:2249-2260.

Banks, L. M., Vaughan, P. J., Meredith, D., and Powell, K. L. (1984). Monoclonal antibodies to herpes simplex virus thymidine kinase. *J. Gen. Virol. 65*:1625-1630.

Baucke, R. B. and Spear, P. G. (1979). Membrane proteins specified by herpes simplex viruses. V. Identification of an Fc-binding glycoprotein. *J. Virol. 32*:779-789.

Bayliss, G. J., Marsden, H. S., and Hay, J. (1975). Herpes simplex virus proteins: DNA binding proteins in infected cells and in the virus structure. *Virology 68*:124-134.

Becker, Y., Dym, H., and Sarov, I. (1968). Herpes simplex virus DNA. *Virology 36*:184-192.

Bookout, J. B. and Levy, C. C. (1980). Comparative examination of the polypeptides of herpes simplex virus: Types 1 and 2. *Virology 101*:198-216.

Braun, D. K., Pereira, L., Norrild, B., and Roizman, B. (1983). Application of denatured, electrophoretically separated, and immobilized lysates of herpes simplex virus-infected cells for detection of monoclonal antibodies and for studies of the properties of viral proteins. *J. Virol. 46*:103-112.

Braun, D., Roizman, B., and Pereira, L. (1984). Characterization of post-translational products of herpes simplex virus gene 35 proteins binding to the surfaces of full capsids but not empty capsids. *J. Virol.* 49:142-153.

Buckmaster, E. A., Cranage, M. P., McLean, C. S., Coombs, R. R. A., and Minson, A. (1984). The use of monoclonal antibodies to differentiate isolates of herpes simplex types 1 and 2 by neutralization and reverse passive haemagglutination tests. *J. Med. Virol.* 13:193-202.

Buckmaster, A., Gompels, U., and Minson, A. (1985). Characterization and physical mapping of an HSV-1 glycoprotein of approximately 115 X 10³ molecular weight. *Virology* 139:408-413.

Bzik, D. J., Fox, B. A., DeLuca, N. A., and Person, S. (1984). Nucleotide sequence specifying the glycoprotein gene, *gB*, of herpes simplex virus type 1. *Virology* 133:301-314.

Caradonna, S. J. and Cheng, Y.-C. (1981). Induction of uracil-DNA glycosylase and dUTP nucleotidohydrolase activity in herpes simplex virus infected human cells. *J. Biol. Chem.* 256:9834-9837.

Clayton, A.-L., Beckford, U., Roberts, C., Sutherland, S., Druce, A., Best, J., and Chantler, S. (1985). Factors influencing the sensitivity of herpes simplex virus detection in clinical specimens in a simultaneous enzyme-linked immunosorbent assay using monoclonal antibodies. *J. Med. Virol.* 17:275-282.

Clements, J. B., Watson, R. J., and Wilkie, N. M. (1977). Temporal regulation of herpes simplex virus type 1 transcription: Location of transcripts on the viral genome. *Cell* 12:275-285.

Cohen, G. H., Dietzschold, B., Ponce de Leon, M., Long, D., Golub, E., Varrichio, A., Pereira, L., and Eisenberg, R. J. (1984). Localization and synthesis of an antigenic determinant of herpes simplex virus glycoprotein D that stimulates the production of neutralizing antibody. *J. Virol.* 49:102-108.

Cohen, G. H., Halliburton, I. W., and Eisenberg, R. J. (1981). Glycoproteins of herpesviruses. In *Human Herpesviruses* (A. J. Nahmias, W. R. Dowdle, and R. G. Schinazi, eds.). Elsevier, New York, pp. 549-554.

Cohen, G. H., Katze, M., Hydrean-Stern, C., and Eisenberg, R. J. (1978). Type-common CP-1 antigen of herpes simplex virus is associated with a 59,000 molecular-weight envelope glycoprotein. *J. Virol.* 27:172-181.

Costa, J. C. and Robson, A. S. (1975). Role of Fc receptors in herpes simplex virus infection. *Lancet* 1:77-78.

Cranage, M. P., McLean, C. S., Buckmaster, E. A., Minson, A. C., Wildy, P., and Coombs, R. R. A. (1983). The use of monoclonal antibodies in (reverse) passive haemagglutination tests for herpes simplex virus antigens and antibodies. *J. Med. Virol.* 11:295-306.

DeClerq, E., Descamps, V., DeSomer, P., Barr, P. J., Jones, A. S., and Walker, R. T. (1979). E-5-(2-bromovinyl)-2'-deoxyuridine: A potent and selective anti-herpes agent. *Proc. Natl. Acad. Sci. USA* 76:2947-2951.

DeLuca, N., Bzik, D. J., Bond, V. C., Person, S., and Snipes, W. (1982). Nucleotide sequences of herpes simplex virus type 1 (HSV-1) affecting virus entry, cell fusion and production of glycoprotein B (VP 7). *Virology* 122:411-423.

DeLuca, N. A., McCarthy, A. M., and Schaffer, P. A. (1985). Isolation and characterization of deletion mutants of herpes simplex virus type 1 in the gene encoding immediate-early regulatory protein ICP 4. *J. Virol.* 56:558-570.

DeLuca, N. A. and Schaffer, P. A. (1985). Activation of immediate-early, early, and late promoters by temperature-sensitive and wild-type forms of herpes simplex virus type 1 protein ICP4. *Mol. Cell. Biol.* 5:1997-2008.

Dix, R. D., Pereira, L., and Baringer, J. R. (1981). Use of monoclonal antibody directed against herpes simplex virus glycoproteins to protect mice against acute virus-induced neurological disease. *Infect. Immun.* 34:192-199.

Dixon, R. A. F. and Schaffer, P. A. (1980). Fine-structure mapping and functional analysis of temperature-sensitive mutants in the gene encoding the herpes simplex virus type 1 immediate early protein VP 175. *J. Virol. 36:* 189-203.

Docherty, J. J., Lohse, M. A., Dellaria, M. F., Naugle, F. P., Mason, C. W., Knerr, R. A., McDermott, H. M., Mundon, F. K., and Zimmerman, D. H. (1984). Incidence of herpes simplex virus types 1 and 2 in penile lesions of college men. *J. Med. Virol. 13:*163-170.

Dowbenko, D. J. and Laskey, L. A. (1984). Extensive homology between the herpes simplex virus type 2 glycoprotein g*F* gene and the herpes simplex virus type 1 glycoprotein *C* gene. *J. Virol. 52:*154-163.

Dutia, B. M. (1983). Ribonucleotide reductase induced by herpes simplex virus has a virus-specified constituent. *J. Gen. Virol. 64:*513-521.

Eberle, R. and Courtney, R. J. (1980). Preparation and characterization of specific antisera to individual glycoprotein antigens comprising the major glycoprotein region of herpes simplex virus type 1. *J. Virol. 35:*902-917.

Edson, C. M., Hosler, B. A., Respess, R. A., Waters, D. J., and Thorley-Lawson, D. A. (1985). Cross-reactivity between herpes simplex virus glycoprotein B and a 63,000-dalton varicella-zoster virus envelope glycoprotein. *J. Virol. 56:*333-336.

Eisenberg, R. J., Long, D., Pereira, L., Hampar, B., Zweig, M., and Cohen, G. H. (1982a). Effect of monoclonal antibodies on limited proteolysis of native glycoprotein gD of herpes simplex virus type 1. *J. Virol. 41:*478-488.

Eisenberg, R. J., Long, D., Ponce de Leon, M., Matthews, J. T., Spear, P. G., Gibson, M. G., Lasky, L. A., Berman, P., Golub, E., and Cohen, G. H. (1985). Localization of epitopes of herpes simplex virus type 1 glycoprotein D. *J. Virol. 53:*634-644.

Eisenberg, R. J., Ponce de Leon, M., and Cohen, G. H. (1980). Comparative structural analysis of glycoprotein gD of herpes simplex virus types 1 and 2. *J. Virol. 35:*428-435.

Eisenberg, R. J., Ponce de Leon, M., Pereira, L., Long, D., and Cohen, G. H. (1982b). Purification of glycoprotein gD of herpes simplex virus types 1 and 2 by use of monoclonal antibody. *J. Virol. 41:*1099-1104.

Epstein, M. A. (1962). Observations of the fine structure of mature herpes virus and on the composition of its nucleoid. *J. Exp. Med. 115:*1-11.

Epstein, M. A. and Holt, S. J. (1963). Adenosine triphosphatase activity at the surface of mature extracellular herpes virus. *Nature 198:*509-510.

Evans, L. A., Sheppard, M., and May, J. T. (1985). Analysis of the HSV-2 early AG-4 antigen. *Arch. Virol.* 85:13-23.

Fahey, J. L. and Horbett, A. P. (1959). Human gamma globulin fractionation on anion exchange cellulose columns. *J. Biol. Chem.* 234:2645-2651.

Flanders, R. T., Kucera, L. S., Raben, M., and Ricardo, M. J. (1985). Immunologic characterization of herpes simplex virus type 2 antigens ICP10 and ICSP11/12. *Virus Res.* 2:245-260.

Frame, B., Mahony, J. B., Balachandran, N., Rawls, W. E., and Chernesky, M. A. (1984). Identification and typing of herpes simplex virus by enzyme immunoassay with monoclonal antibodies. *J. Clin. Microbiol.* 20:163-166.

Frame, M. C., Marsden, H. S., and McGeoch, D. J. (1986). Novel herpes simplex virus type 1 glycoproteins identified by antiserum against a synthetic oligonucleotide from the predicted product of U_S4. *J. Gen. Virol.* 67:745-751.

Francke, B. and Garrett, B. (1982). The effect of a temperature sensitive lesion in the alkaline DNAse of herpes simplex virus type 2 on the synthesis of viral DNA. *Virology* 116:116-127.

Freeman, M. J. and Powell, K. L. (1982). DNA-binding properties of a herpes simplex virus immediate early protein. *J. Virol.* 44:1084-1087.

Friedman, H. M., Cohen, G. H., Eisenberg, R. J., Seidel, C. A., and Cines, D. B. (1984). Glycoprotein C of herpes simplex virus 1 acts as a receptor for the C3b complement component of infected cells. *Nature* 309:633-635.

Frink, R. J. R., Eisenberg, R., Cohen, G., and Wagner, E. K. (1983). Detailed analysis of the portion of the herpes simplex virus type 1 genome encoding glycoprotein C. *J. Virol.* 45:634-647.

Fuller, A. O. and Spear, P. G. (1985). Specificities of monoclonal and polyclonal antibodies that inhibit adsorption of herpes simplex virus to cells and lack of inhibition by potent neutralizing antibodies. *J. Virol.* 55:475-482.

Furlong, D., Swift, J., and Roizman, B. (1972). Arrangement of herpesvirus deoxyribonucleic acid in the core. *J. Virol.* 10:1071-1074.

Gibson, W. and Roizman, B. (1971). Compartmentalization of spermine and spermidine in the herpes simplex virion. *Proc. Natl. Acad. Sci. USA* 68: 2818-2821.

Gibson, W. and Roizman, B. (1972). Proteins specified by herpes simplex virus VIII. Characterization and composition of multiple capsid forms of subtypes 1 and 2. *J. Virol.* 10:1044-1052.

Gleaves, C. A., Wilson, D. J., Wold, A. D., and Smith, T. F. (1985). Detection and serotyping of herpes simplex virus in MRC-5 cells by use of centrifugation and monoclonal antibodies 16 h postinoculation. *J. Clin. Microbiol.* 21:29-32.

Godowski, P. J. and Knipe, D. M. (1985). Identification of a herpes simplex virus function that represses late gene expression from parental viral genomes. *J. Virol.* 55:357-365.

Goldstein, L. C., Corey, L., McDougall, J. K., Tolentino, E., and Nowinski, R. C. (1983). Monoclonal antibodies to herpes simplex viruses: Use in antigenic typing and rapid diagnosis. *J. Infect. Dis.* 147:829-837.

Halliburton, I. W. (1980). Intertypic recombinants of herpes simplex virus. *J. Gen. Virol.* 48:1-23.

Halliburton, I. W., Morse, L. S., Roizman, B., and Quinn, K. E. (1980). Mapping of the thymidine kinase genes of type 1 and type 2 herpes simplex viruses using intertypic recombinants. *J. Gen. Virol.* 49:235-253.

Halliburton, I. W., Post, L. E., and Roizman, B. (1983). Analysis of the function of a gene 22 of HSV type 1 using host range mutants. In *Abstracts 8th International Herpesvirus Workshop*, Oxford, England, p. 119.

Halliburton, I. W., Randall, R. E., Killington, R. A., and Watson, D. H. (1977). Some properties of recombinants between type 1 and type 2 herpes simplex viruses. *J. Gen. Virol.* 36:471-484.

Halliburton, I. W. and Timbury, M. C. (1976). Temperature sensitive mutants of herpes simplex virus type 2: Description of three new complementation groups and studies on the inhibition of host cell DNA synthesis. *J. Gen. Virol.* 30:207-221.

Hay, R. T. and Hay, J. (1980). Properties of herpesvirus-induced 'immediate early' polypeptides. *Virology* 104:230-234.

Heilman, Jr. C. J., Zweig, M., Stephenson, J. R., and Hampar, B. (1979). Isolation of a nucleocapsid polypeptide of herpes simplex viruses types 1 and 2 possessing immunologically type-specific and cross-reactive determinants. *J. Virol.* 29:39-42.

Heine, J. W., Honess, R. W., Cassai, E., and Roizman, B. (1974). Proteins specified by herpes simplex virus. XII. The virion polypeptides of type 1 strains. *J. Virol.* 14:640-651.

Herrod, H. A., McLean, B., Hambling, M. H., and Halliburton, I. W. (1984). Efficiency of the use of pock size on the chorioallantoic membrane of fertile hen's eggs as a method of typing herpes simplex viruses. *J. Hyg.* 93:95-103.

Hoffman, P. J. and Cheng, Y. C. (1979). DNase induced after infection of KB cells by herpes simplex virus type 1 or type 2. II. Characterisation of an associated endonuclease activity. *J. Virol.* 32:449-457.

Hoggan, M. D. and Roizman, B. (1959). The isolation and properties of a variant of herpes simplex producing multinucleated giant cells in monolayer cultures in the presence of antibody. *Am. J. Hyg.* 70:208-219.

Holland, T. C., Homa, F. L., Marlin, S. D., Levine, M., and Glorioso, J. C. (1984). Herpes simplex virus type 1 glycoprotein C-negative mutants exhibit multiple phenotypes including secretion of truncated glycoproteins. *J. Virol.* 52:566-574.

Holland, T. C., Marlin, S. D., Levine, M., and Glorioso, J. (1983a). Antigenic variants of herpes simplex virus selected with glycoprotein-specific monoclonal antibodies. *J. Virol.* 45:672-682.

Holland, T. C., Sandri-Goldin, R. M., Holland, L. E., Marlin, S. D., Levine, M., and Glorioso, J. C. (1983b). Physical mapping of the mutation in an antigenic variant of herpes simplex virus type 1 by use of an immunoreactive plaque assay. *J. Virol.* 46:649-652.

Honess, R. W., Buchan, A., Halliburton, I. W., and Watson, D. H. (1980). Recombination and linkage between structural and regulatory genes of herpes simplex virus type 1: A study of the functional organisation of the genome. *J. Virol.* 34:716-742.

Honess, R. W. and Roizman, B. (1973). Proteins specified by herpes simplex virus. XI. Identification and relative molar rates of synthesis of structural and nonstructural herpesvirus polypeptides in the infected cell. *J. Virol. 12*:1347-1365.

Honess, R. W. and Roizman, B. (1974). Regulation of herpesvirus macromolecular synthesis. I. Cascade regulation of the synthesis of three groups of viral proteins. *J. Virol. 14*:8-19.

Honess, R. W. and Roizman, B. (1975a). Proteins specified by herpes simplex. VIII. Glycosylation of viral polypeptides. *J. Virol. 16*:1308-1326.

Honess, R. W. and Roizman, B. (1975b). Regulation of herpesvirus macromolecular synthesis: Sequential transition of polypeptide synthesis requires functional viral polypeptides. *Proc. Natl. Acad. Sci. USA 72*:1276-1280.

Honess, R. W. and Watson, D. H. (1974). Absence of a requirement for host polypeptides in the herpes virus thymidine kinase. *J. Gen. Virol. 24*:215-220.

Huszar, D., Beharry, S., and Bachetti, S. (1983). Herpes simplex virus-induced ribonucleotide reductase: Development of antibodies specific for the enzyme. *J. Gen. Virol. 64*:1327-1335.

Jamieson, A. T. and Subak-Sharpe, J. H. (1974). Biochemical studies on the herpes simplex virus-specified deoxypyrimidine kinase activity. *J. Gen. Virol. 24*:481-492.

Kapoor, A. K., Nash, A. A., Wildy, P., Phelan, J., McLean, C. S., and Field, H. J. (1982). Pathogenesis of herpes simplex virus in congenitally athymic mice: The relative roles of cell-mediated and humoral immunity. *J. Gen. Virol. 60*:225-233.

Katan, M., Stevely, W. S., and Leader, D. P. (1985). Partial purification and characterization of a new phosphoprotein kinase from cells infected with pseudorabies virus. *Eur. J. Biochem. 152*:57-65.

Kennett, R. H., Denis, K. A., Tung, A. S., and Klinman, N. R. (1978). Hybrid plasmacytoma production: Fusions with adult spleen cells, monoclonal spleen fragments, neonatal spleen cells and human spleen cells. *Curr. Top. Microbiol. Immunol. 81*:77-91.

Killington, R. A., Newhook, L., Balachandran, N., Rawls, W. E., and Bachetti, S. (1981). Production of hybrid cell lines secreting antibodies to herpes simplex virus type 2. *J. Virol. Methods 2*:223-236.

Kitamura, K., Namazue, J., Campo-Vera, H., Ogino, T., and Yamanishi, K. (1986). Induction of neutralizing antibody against varicella-zoster virus (VZV) by VZV gp3 and cross-reactivity between VZV gp3 and herpes simplex viruses gB. *Virology 149*:74-82.

Knopf, K. W. (1979). Properties of herpes simplex virus DNA polymerase and characterisation of its associated exonuclease activity. *Eur. J. Biochem. 98*:231-244.

Kousoulas, K. G., Pellett, P. E., Pereira, L., and Roizman, B. (1984). Mutations affecting conformation or sequence of neutralizing epitopes identified by reactivity of viable plaques segregate from *syn* and *ts* domains of HSV-1 (F) *gB* gene. *Virology 135*:379-394.

Kumel, G., Kaerner, H. C., Levine, M., Schröder, C. H., and Glorioso, J. C. (1985). Passive immune protection by herpes simplex virus-specific monoclonal antibodies and monoclonal antibody-resistant mutants altered in pathogenicity. *J. Virol. 56*:930-937.

Lagacé-Simard, J., Fauvel, M., and Lecomte, J. (1983). Analysis and selection of hybridoma antibodies for typing isolates of herpes simplex virus. *J. Infect. Dis. 147*:593.

Laskey, L. A. and Dowbenko, D. J. (1984). Sequence analysis of the type-common glycoprotein-D genes of herpes simplex virus types 1 and 2. *DNA 2*: 23-29.

LaThangue, N. B. and Chan, W. L. (1984). The characterization and purification of DNA binding proteins present within herpes simplex virus infected cells using monoclonal antibodies. *Arch. Virol. 79*:13-33.

LaThangue, N. B., Shriver, K., Dawson, C., and Chan, W. L. (1984). Herpes simplex virus infection causes the accumulation of a heat-shock protein. *EMBO J. 3*:267-277.

Lee, G. T., Pogue-Geile, K. L., Pereira, L., and Spear, P. G. (1982). Expression of herpes simplex virus glycoprotein C from a DNA fragment inserted into the *tk* gene of this virus. *Proc. Natl. Acad. Sci. USA 79*:6612-6616.

Lemaster, S. L. and Roizman, B. (1980). Characterization of the virion protein kinase of proteins phosphorylated in the virion. *J. Virol. 35*:798-811.

Little, S. P., Jofre, J. T., Courtney, R. J., and Schaffer, P. A. (1981). A virion-associated glycoprotein essential for infectivity of herpes simplex virus type 1. *Virology 115*:149-160.

Little, S. P. and Schaffer, P. A. (1981). Expression of the syncytial (syn) phenotype in HSV-1, strain KOS: Genetic and phenotypic studies of mutants in two *syn* loci. *Virology 112*:686-702.

Long, D., Madara, T. J., Ponce de Leon, M., Cohen, G. H., Montgomery, P. C., and Eisenberg, R. J. (1984). Glycoprotein D protects mice against lethal challenge with herpes simplex virus types 1 and 2. *Infect. Immun. 37*:761-764.

McCormick, F. (1978). Polyamine turnover and leakage during infection of HeLa and L cells with herpes simplex virus type 1. *Virology 91*:496-503.

McGeoch, D. J., Dolan, A., Donald, S., and Rixon, F. J. (1985). Sequence determination and genetic content of the short unique region in the genome of herpes simplex virus type 1. *J. Mol. Biol. 181*:1-13.

McLean, C., Buckmaster, A., Hancock, D., Buchan, A., Fuller, A., and Minson, A. (1982). Monoclonal antibodies to three nonglycosylated antigens of herpes simplex virus type 2. *J. Gen. Virol. 63*:297-305.

Manservigi, R., Spear, P. G., and Buchan, A. (1979). Cell fusion induced by herpes simplex virus is promoted and suppressed by different viral glycoproteins. *Proc. Natl. Acad. Sci. USA 74*:3913-3917.

Marlin, S. D., Holland, T. C., Levine, M., and Glorioso, J. C. (1985). Epitopes of herpes simplex virus type 1 glycoprotein gC are clustered in two distinct antigenic sites. *J. Virol. 53*:128-136.

Marsden, H. S., Buckmaster, A., Palfreyman, J. W., Hope, R. G., and Minson, A. C. (1984). Characterization of the 92,000-dalton glycoprotein induced by herpes simplex virus type 2. *J. Virol. 50*:547-554.

Marsden, H. S., Crombie, I. K., and Subak-Sharpe, J. H. (1976). Control of protein synthesis in herpesvirus infected cells: Analysis of the polypeptides induced by wild-type and sixteen temperature-sensitive mutants of HSV strain 17. *J. Gen. Virol. 31*:347-372.

Morgan, C., Ellison, S. A., Rose, H. M., and Moore, D. H. (1954). Structure and development of viruses as observed in the electron microscope. I. Herpes simplex virus. *J. Exp. Med. 100*:195-202.

Morgan, C., Rose, H. M., and Mednis, B. (1968). Electron microscopy of herpes simplex virus 1. Entry. *J. Virol. 2*:507-516.

Moss, H. (1986). The herpes simplex virus type 2 alkaline exonuclease activity is essential for replication and growth. *J. Gen. Virol. 67*:1173-1178.

Nilheden, E., Jeansson, S., and Vahlne, A. (1983). Typing of herpes simplex virus by an enzyme-linked immunosorbent assay with monoclonal antibodies. *J. Clin. Microbiol. 17*:677-680.

Noble, A. G., Lee, G. T.-Y., Sprague, R., Parish, M. L., and Spear, P. G. (1983). Anti-gD monoclonal antibodies inhibit cell fusion induced by herpes simplex virus type 1. *Virology 129*:218-224.

Norrild, B., Anderson, A. B., and Feldborg, R. (1985). Crossed immunoelectrophoretic analysis of herpes simplex virus type 2 proteins. Characterization of antigen-5. *Arch. Virol. 85*:95-108.

Norrild, B., Lehto, V.-P., and Virtanen, I. (1986). Organization of cytoskeleton elements during herpes simplex virus type 1 infection of human fibroblasts: An immunofluorescence study. *J. Gen. Virol. 67*:97-105.

Norrild, B., Virtanen, I., Lehto, V. P., and Pederson, B. (1983). Accumulation of herpes simplex virus type 1 glycoprotein D in adhesion areas of infected cells. *J. Gen. Virol. 64*:2499-2503.

Oakes, J. E. and Lausch, R. N. (1984). Monoclonal antibodies suppress replication of herpes simplex virus type 1 in trigeminal ganglia. *J. Virol. 51*:656-661.

Olshevsky, U. and Becker, Y. (1972). Surface glycopeptides in the envelope of herpes simplex virions. *Virology 50*:277-279.

Ogino, T., Shiman, R., and Rapp, F. (1973). Deoxythymidine kinase from rabbit kidney cells infected with herpes simplex virus types 1 and 2. *Intervirology 1*:80-95.

Palfreyman, J. W., Haarr, L., Cross, A., Hope, R. G., and Marsden, H. S. (1983). Processing of herpes simplex virus type 1 glycoproteins: Two-dimensional gel analysis using monoclonal antibodies. *J. Gen. Virol. 64*:873-886.

Para, M. F., Baucke, R. B., and Spear, P. G. (1982a). Glycoprotein gE of herpes simplex virus type 1: Effects of anti-gE on virion infectivity and on virus-induced Fc-binding receptors. *J. Virol. 41*:129-136.

Para, M. F., Goldstein, L., and Spear, P. G. (1982b). Similarities and differences in the Fc-binding glycoprotein (gE) of herpes simplex virus types 1 and 2 and tentative mapping of the viral gene for this glycoprotein. *J. Virol. 41*:137-144.

Para, M. F., Parish, M. L., Noble, A. G., and Spear, P. G. (1985). Potent neutralizing activity associated with anti-glycoprotein D specificity among monoclonal antibodies selected for binding to herpes simplex virions. *J. Virol. 55*: 483-488.

Para, M. F., Zezulak, K. M., Conley, A. J., Weinberger, M., Snitzer, K., and Spear, P. G. (1983). Use of monoclonal antibodies against two 75,000-molecular-weight glycoproteins specified by herpes simplex virus type 2 in glycoprotein identification and mapping. *J. Virol. 45*:1223-1227.

Pellett, P. E., Kousoulas, K. G., Pereira, L., and Roizman, B. (1985). Anatomy of the herpes simplex virus 1 strain F glycoprotein B gene: Primary sequence and predicted protein structure of the wild type and of monoclonal antibody-resistant mutants. *J. Virol. 53*:243-253.

Pereira, L., Dondero, D. V., Gallo, D., Devlin, V., and Woodie, J. D. (1982a). Serological analysis of herpes simplex virus types 1 and 2 with monoclonal antibodies. *Infect. Immun. 35*:363-367.

Pereira, L., Dondero, D., Norrild, B., and Roizman, B. (1981). Differential immunologic reactivity and processing of glycoproteins gA and gB of herpes simplex virus types 1 and 2 made in Vero and HEp-2 cells. *Proc. Natl. Acad. Sci. USA 78*:5202-5206.

Pereira, L., Dondero, D., and Roizman, B. (1982b). Herpes simplex virus glycoprotein gA/B: Evidence that the infected Vero cell products comap and arise by proteolysis. *J. Virol. 44*:88-97.

Pereira, L., Klassen, T., and Baringer, J. R. (1980). Type-common and type-specific monoclonal antibody to herpes simplex virus type 1. *Infect. Immun. 29*:724-732.

Peterson, E., Schmidt, O. W., Goldstein, L. C., Nowinski, R. C., and Corey, L. (1983). Typing of herpes simplex virus isolates with mouse monoclonal antibodies to herpes simplex virus types 1 and 2: Comparison with type-specific rabbit antisera and restriction endonuclease analysis of viral DNA. *J. Clin. Microbiol. 17*:92-96.

Powell, K. L., Buchan, A., Sim, C., and Watson, D. H. (1974). Type-specific protein in herpes simplex virus envelope reacts with neutralizing antibody. *Nature 249*:360-361.

Powell, K. L. and Courtney, R. J. (1975). Polypeptides synthesised in herpes simplex virus type 2 infected HEp2 cells. *Virology 66*:217-228.

Powell, K. L., Littler, E., and Purifoy, D. J. M. (1981). Nonstructural proteins of herpes simplex virus II. Major virus-specific DNA-binding protein. *J. Virol. 39*:894-902.

Powell, K. L., Mirkovic, R., and Courtney, R. (1977). Comparative analysis of polypeptides induced by type 1 and type 2 strains of herpes simplex virus. *Intervirology 8*:18-29.

Powell, K. L. and Purifoy, D. J. M. (1976). DNA-binding proteins of cells infected by herpes simplex virus type 1 and type 2. *Intervirology 7*:225-239.

Powell, K. L. and Watson, D. H. (1975). Some structural antigens of herpes simplex virus type 1. *J. Gen. Virol. 29*:167-178.

Preston, C. M. (1979). Control of herpes simplex virus type 1 mRNA synthesis in cells infected with wild-type virus or the temperature sensitive mutant *tsK*. *J. Virol. 29*:275-284.

Preston, V. G., Coates, J. A. V., and Rixon, F. J. (1983). Identification and characterization of a herpes simplex virus gene product required for encapsidation of virus DNA. *J. Virol. 45*:1056-1064.

Quinlan, M. P. and Knipe, D. M. (1985). Stimulation of a herpes simplex virus DNA-binding protein by two viral functions. *Mol. Cell. Biol. 5*:957-963.

Rawls, W. E., Balachandran, N., Sisson, G., and Watson, R. J. (1984). Localization of a type-specific antigenic site on herpes simplex virus type 2 glycoprotein D. *J. Virol. 51*:263-265.

Rector, J. T., Lausch, R. N., and Oakes, J. E. (1982). Use of monoclonal antibodies for analysis of antibody-dependent immunity to ocular herpes simplex virus type 1 infection. *Infect. Immun. 38*:168-174.

Richman, D. D., Buckmaster, A., Bell, S., Hodgman, C., and Minson, A. C. (1986). Identification of a new glycoprotein of herpes simplex virus type 1 and genetic mapping of the gene that codes for it. *J. Virol. 57*:647-655.

Richman, D. D., Cleveland, P. H., and Oxman, M. N. (1982). A rapid enzyme immunofiltration technique using monoclonal antibodies to serotype herpes simplex virus. *J. Med. Virol. 9*:299-305.

Roberts, P. L., Duncan, B. E., Raybould, T. J. G., and Watson, D. H. (1985). Purification of herpes simplex virus glycoproteins B and C using monoclonal antibodies and their ability to protect mice against lethal challenge. *J. Gen. Virol. 66*:1073-1085.

Roizman, B. and Furlong, D. (1974). The replication of herpesviruses. In *Comprehensive Virology 3* (H. Fraenkel-Conrat and R. R. Wagner, eds.). Plenum Press, New York, pp. 229-403.

Roizman, B., Norrild, B., Chan, C., and Pereira, L. (1984). Identification and preliminary mapping with monoclonal antibodies of a herpes simplex virus 2 glycoprotein lacking a known type 1 counterpart. *Virology 133*:242-247.

Rubenstein, A. S., Gravell, M., and Darlington, R. (1972). Protein kinase in enveloped herpes simplex virions. *Virology 50*:287-290.

Ruyechan, W. T., Morse, L. S., Knipe, D. M., and Roizman, B. (1979). Molecular genetics of herpes simplex virus. II. Mapping of the major viral glycoproteins and of the genetic loci specifying the social behaviour of infected cells. *J. Virol. 29*:677-697.

Sacks, W. R., Greene, C. C., Aschman, D. P., and Schaffer, P. A. (1985). Herpes simplex virus type-1 ICP27 is an essential regulatory protein. *J. Virol. 55*: 796-805.

Sarmiento, M., Haffey, M., and Spear, P. G. (1979). Membrane proteins specified by herpes simplex viruses. III. Role of glycoprotein VP7 (B$_2$) in virion infectivity. *J. Virol. 29*:1149-1158.

Sarmiento, M. and Spear, P. G. (1979). Membrane proteins specified by herpes simplex viruses. IV. Conformation of the virion glycoprotein designated VP7 (B$_2$). *J. Virol. 29*:1159-1167.

Schwartz, J. and Roizman, B. (1969). Concerning the egress of herpes simplex virus from infected cells: Electron and light microscope observations. *Virology 38*:42-49.

Sears, A., Halliburton, I. W., Meignier, B., Silver, S., and Roizman, B. (1985). Herpes simplex virus 1 mutant deleted in the *a22* gene: Growth and gene expression in permissive and restrictive cells and establishment of latency in mice. *J. Virol. 55*:338-346.

Sethi, K. (1983). Effects of monoclonal antibodies directed against herpes simplex virus-specified glycoproteins on the generation of virus-specific and H-2-restricted cytotoxic T-lymphocytes. *J. Gen. Virol. 64*:2033-2037.

Sheppard, M., Evans, L., and May, J. T. (1985). Expression of the herpes simplex virus type-2 major DNA-binding protein (ICP 8) gene in COS-1 cells. *Virus Res. 3*:287-292.

Showalter, S. D., Zweig, M., and Hampar, B. (1981). Monoclonal antibodies to herpes simplex virus type 1 proteins, including the immediate-early protein ICP 4. *Infect. Immun. 34*:684-692.

Shulman, M., Wilde, C. D., and Köhler, G. (1978). A better cell line for making hybridomas secreting specific antibodies. *Nature 276*:269-270.

Sim, C. and Watson, D. H. (1973). The role of type specific and cross reacting structural antigens in the neutralization of herpes simplex virus types 1 and 2. *J. Gen. Virol. 19*:217-233.

Snowden, B. W. and Halliburton, I. W. (1985). Identification of cross-reacting glycoproteins of four herpesviruses by Western blotting. *J. Gen. Virol. 66*: 2039-2044.

Snowden, B. W., Kinchington, P. R., Powell, K. L., and Halliburton, I. W. (1985). Antigenic and biochemical analysis of gB of herpes simplex virus type 1 and type 2 and of cross-reacting glycoproteins induced by bovine mammillitis virus and equine herpesvirus type 1. *J. Gen. Virol. 66*:231-247.

Spear, P. G. (1976). Membrane proteins specified by herpes simplex viruses. I. Identification of four glycoprotein precursors and their products in type-1 infected cells. *J. Virol. 17*:991-1008.

Spear, P. G. (1980a). In *Cell Membranes and Viral Envelopes* (H. A. Blough and J. M. Tiffany, eds.). Academic Press, New York, pp. 709-750.

Spear, P. G. (1980b). Composition and organization of herpesvirus virions and properties of some of the structural proteins. In *Oncogenic Herpesviruses* (F. Rapp, ed.) Vol. 1, CRC Press, Boca Raton, pp. 53-84.

Spear, P. G. (1985). Glycoproteins specified by herpes simplex viruses. In *The Herpesviruses 3* (B. Roizman, ed.). Plenum Press, New York and London, pp. 315-356.

Spear, P. G. and Roizman, B. (1972). Proteins specified by herpes simplex virus. V. Purification and structural proteins of the herpesvirion. *J. Virol. 9*:143-159.

Strnad, B. C. and Aurelian, L. (1976). Proteins of herpesvirus type 2: 1. Virion, non-virion and antigenic polypeptides in infected cells. *Virology 69*:438-452.

Swierkosz, E. M., Arens, M. Q., Schmidt, R. R., and Armstrong, T. (1985). Evaluation of two immunofluorescence assays with monoclonal antibodies for typing of herpes simplex virus. *J. Clin. Microbiol.* 21:643-644.

Teh, C.-Z. and Sacks, S. L. (1983). Susceptibility of recent clinical isolates of herpes simplex virus to 5-ethyl-2'-deoxyuridine: Preferential inhibition of herpes simplex virus type 2. *Antimicrob. Agents Chemother.* 23:637-640.

Vaughan, P. J., Banks, L. M., Purifoy, D. J. M., and Powell, K. L. (1984). Interactions between herpes simplex virus DNA-binding proteins. *J. Gen. Virol.* 65:2033-2041.

Vaughan, P. J., Purifoy, D. J. M., and Powell, K. L. (1985). DNA-binding protein associated with herpes simplex virus DNA polymerase. *J. Virol.* 53: 501-508.

Volpi, A., Lakeman, A. D., Pereira, L., and Stagno, S. (1983). Monoclonal antibodies for rapid diagnosis and typing of genital herpes infections during pregnancy. *Am. J. Obstet. Gynecol.* 146:813-815.

Watson, D. H. (1973). Morphology. In *The Herpes Viruses* (A. S. Kaplan, ed.). Academic Press, New York and London, pp. 27-43.

Watson, D. H. and Wildy, P. (1969). The preparation of "monoprecipitin" antisera to herpes virus specific antigens. *J. Gen. Virol.* 4:163-168.

Watson, R. J. (1983). DNA sequence of the herpes simplex virus type 2 glycoprotein D gene. *Gene 26*:307-312.

Watson, R. J., Weis, J. H., Salstrom, J. S., and Enquist, L. W. (1982). Herpes simplex virus type-1 glycoprotein D gene: Nucleotide sequence and expression in *E. coli. Science 218*:381-384.

Weissbach, A., Hong, S.-C. L., Aucker, J., and Muller, R. (1973). Characterisation of herpes simplex virus-induced deoxyribonucleic acid polymerase. *J. Biol. Chem. 248*:6270-6277.

Welling-Wester, S., Popken-Boer, T., Wilterding, J. B., van Beeumen, J., and Welling, G. W. (1985). Isolation by high performance liquid chromatography and partial characterization of a 57,000-dalton herpes simplex virus type 1 polypeptide. *J. Virol.* 54:265-270.

Westmoreland, D. and Watkins, J. F. (1974). The IgG receptor induced by herpes simplex virus; studies using radio-iodinated IgG. *J. Gen. Virol.* 24:167-178.

Wilcox, K. W., Kohn, A., Sklyanskaya, E., and Roizman, B. (1980). Herpes simplex virus phosphoproteins. I. Phosphate cycles on and off some viral polypeptides and can alter their affinity for DNA. *J. Virol. 33*:167-182.

Wildy, P., Russell, W. C., and Horne, R. W. (1960). The morphology of herpes virus. *Virology 12*:204-222.

Wilkie, N. M. (1973). The synthesis and substructure of herpesvirus DNA: The distribution of alkali labile single stranded interruptions in HSV-1 DNA. *J. Gen. Virol. 21*:453-467.

Zezulak, K. M. and Spear, P. G. (1983). Characterization of a herpes simplex virus type 2 75,000 molecular weight glycoprotein antigenically related to herpes simplex virus type 1 glycoprotein C. *J. Virol.* 47:553-562.

Zezulak, K. M. and Spear, P. G. (1984). Mapping of the structural gene for herpes simplex virus type 2 counterpart of herpes simplex virus type 1 glycoprotein C and identification of a type 2 mutant which does not express this glycoprotein. *J. Virol. 49*:741-747.

Zimmerman, D. H., Mundon, F. K., Croson, S. E., Henchal, L. S., Docherty, J. J., and O'Neill, S. P. (1985). Identification and typing of herpes simplex virus types 1 and 2 by monoclonal antibodies, sensitivity to the drug (E)-5-(2-bromovinyl)-2'-deoxyuridine, and restriction endonuclease analysis of viral DNA. *J. Med. Virol. 15*:215-222.

Zweig, M., Heilman, C. J., Rabin, H., Hopkins, R. F., Neubauer, R. H., and Hampar, B. (1979). Production of monoclonal antibodies against nucleocapsid proteins of herpes simplex virus types 1 and 2. *J. Virol. 32*:676-678.

Zweig, M., Showalter, S. D., Bladen, S. V., Heilman, C. J., and Hampar, B. (1983). Herpes simplex virus type 2 glycoprotein gF and type 1 glycoprotein gC have related antigenic determinants. *J. Virol. 47*:185-192.

Zweig, M., Showalter, S. D., Simms, D. J., and Hampar, B. (1984). Antibodies to a synthetic oligopeptide that react with herpes simplex virus type 1 and 2 glycoprotein C. *J. Virol. 51*:430-436.

TWELVE

Immunological Diagnosis of Herpes Simplex Virus

Isabel W. Smith and John F. Peutherer

Edinburgh University
Medical School
Edinburgh, Scotland

I. INTRODUCTION

Herpes simplex viruses, types 1 and 2 (HSV-1 and HSV-2) can infect many different sites on the skin and mucous membranes. Less frequently, the central nervous system (CNS) may be involved and disseminated infections occur in the newborn. Herpes simplex infections can be divided by clinical and serological features into primary and recrudescent infections. Primary infections occur in the absence of a prior immune response and may be accompanied by fever and adenitis. After the primary infection, virus persists and may be reactivated to cause recrudescent lesions: these are usually less extensive and of shorter duration than the primary infection. Reactivation of the virus occurs in the presence of high levels of neutralizing antibody (Douglas and Couch, 1970).

Exogenous reinfection with a second virus can occur despite previous infection with the heterologous virus or with the homologous type (Buchman et al., 1979; Gerson et al., 1984; Kit et al., 1983; Maitland et al., 1982; Schmidt et al., 1984). Clinically, the first infection with the heterologous type is known as an initial infection and is intermediate in severity between primary and recrudescent disease.

II. CLINICAL PRESENTATION AND EPIDEMIOLOGY OF HERPES SIMPLEX INFECTIONS

A. Persistence of Virus

The site of viral persistence is within the sensory root ganglia of the appropriate areas; for oral and facial infections, this is the trigeminal ganglion and for anogenital infections the sacral ganglia. The viral genome can remain in a latent state within the neuron with little or no evidence of virus expression. The block may be at the transcriptional level, and virus cannot be isolated directly from ganglionic extracts. Virus expression can be detected only after the neurons have been cultured for some time, often in the presence of permissive cells. Most patients with humoral antibody carry the virus in the ganglion (Baringer and Swoveland, 1973; Bastian et al.,1972), although only about one-half suffer from recrudescent disease, e.g., herpes labialis. Local effects on Langerhans cells in the skin are important in producing localized disease (Toews et al., 1980). The frequency and severity of recrudescences decrease with age (Grout et al., 1976) but are markedly affected by the immune competence of the host. Immune depression that results from malignant disease and its therapy or that is induced for organ transplantation (Rand et al., 1977) or that resulting from a congenital defect, leads to a high rate of recrudescence and extensive clinical disease. A similar picture occurs in the acquired immune-deficiency syndrome (AIDS).

B. Epidemiology and Clinical Features

The two virus types are associated with infections at different clinical sites. Thus, HSV-1 causes oral, facial, eye, and skin infections above the waist, whereas HSV-2 is found in the genital tract (Nahmias and Dowdle, 1968).

Genital herpes is an increasing problem both in the United States and the United Kingdom (Fig. 1). There was a steady increase in the number of notifications of genital herpetic infections over the period 1968-1980, and it is of interest that the rate per 100,000 population in both countries is similar.

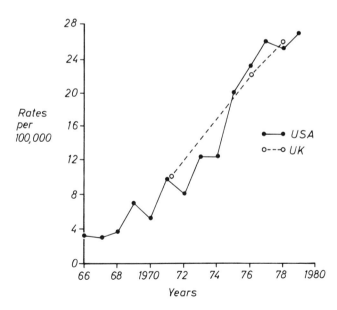

Fig. 1 Rates per 100,000 of patients with clinically diagnosed genital herpetic infection in the United States and the United Kingdom (*Source*: adapted from Becker and Nahmias, 1985).

Primary infection with HSV-1 is most often manifested in children as an acute gingivostomatitis with vesicular and ulcerative lesions in the mouth and on the lips. Pharyngitis is also seen in some patients. Social and economic factors have long been recognized as of great importance in determining the age of infection and the proportion of the population who are infected (Smith et al., 1967). Genital infections occur in the sexually active individual and appear as vesicular and ulcerative lesions of the penis, vulva, vagina, cervix, rectum and perineum, and nearby skin areas. Urethral infection and dysuria occur: aseptic meningitis is a further complication (Corey et al., 1983). Clinical features are more severe in primary genital infections, and are more marked in the female, than are recrudescent episodes, which are less severe and are not accompanied by systemic features. Initial genital infections with HSV-2 in patients with a history of previous HSV-1 infection are intermediate in severity.

C. Association of Virus Type with Clinical Site

It is now clear that the association of virus type with clinical site is not absolute. This is well established for HSV-1 infection of the genital tract, although there are marked differences in the proportion of genital HSV-1 isolates in different reports. In the United States some studies have found only a small proportion of HSV-1 isolates (Corey et al., 1983; Dowdle et al., 1967; Nahmias and Roizman, 1973). We reported in 1973 that 17% of genital isolates from a study of Edinburgh patients were HSV-1 (Smith et al., 1973). This was confirmed in a larger study (Peutherer et al., 1981; Smith et al., 1976). A high prevalence of HSV-1 has also been reported by other groups, e.g., 33-40% in the United States (Kalinyak et al., 1977); 35% in Japan (Kawana et al., 1976); 16.7% in Sweden (Wolontis and Jeansson, 1977); and 50% in Sheffield (Barton et al., 1982).

Our observations are given in Table 1 from which it is seen that the proportion of HSV-1 infections of the genital tract has remained at approximately 30% in female patients, whereas the rate in male patients has risen from 5.7% in the first period to approximately 16%. Among isolates from female patients aged less than 20 years, 50% were HSV-1. This is in definite agreement with both the Sheffield and Japanese findings.

One-third to one-quarter of all genital herpes infections are primary, and most HSV-1 genital infections are primary (Smith et al., 1981). Clinically, primary HSV-1 cervical infections are less severe than those with HSV-2. Indeed, the severity of such HSV-1 infections was comparable with recrudescent HSV-2 disease (Smith et al., 1981). Conversely, recrudescent genital HSV-1 disease is much less frequent than is HSV-2 (Corey et al., 1983; Peutherer et al., 1982; Reeves et al., 1981).

Herpes simplex virus type 2 can be isolated from extragenital sites (Kaufman and Rawls, 1972; Wolontis and Jeansson, 1977). Isolation from the pharynx at

Table 1 Number (and Percentage) of Male and Female Patients with Genital Infections from Whom HSV-1 and HSV-2 Were Isolated in Three Cohorts (Edinburgh, 1966-1985)

Study period	Male patients		Female patients	
	Type 1 (%)	Type 2 (%)	Type 1 (%)	Type 2 (%)
1966-1971	2 (6)	33 (94)	9 (30)	21 (70)
1971-1979	13 (16)	68 (84)	22 (32)	48 (68)
1980-1985	83 (15)	464 (85)	169 (29)	376 (71)

the time of genital infection has been reported from 13% of female and 7% of male patients (Corey et al., 1983). In a small study in Edinburgh, 10 patients with concurrent oral and genital infection were examined. Herpes simplex virus was isolated from both sites in all cases and four of the 10 patients yielded HSV-2 while undergoing primary or initial infections.

Excretion of virus in oral secretions in the absence of clinical disease has been often described (Buddingh et al., 1953). Sequential sampling of the oral secretions of a group of patients has shown that 27% of those with antibody excrete virus at some time in the absence of symptoms (Douglas and Couch, 1970). Comparable studies of genital secretions have shown that the virus could be isolated from 0.3% of college students in the United States with some gynecological problem (Kalinyak et al., 1977). McCaughtry et al. (1982), however, concluded that four of the five patients from whom they isolated HSV did have other infections, e.g., candidal, at the time of isolation. Excretion of the virus persists in women after clinical recovery from herpes genitalis (Adam et al., 1979). Isolation of virus from the urethra of asymptomatic male patients has been reported.

D. Infection in Pregnancy

The newborn baby is at risk of infection with HSV-1 from oral lesions (Light, 1979) and epidemics have been described in nurseries (Buchman et al., 1978; Linneman et al., 1978). The genital tract of the mother, however, can also present a serious risk to the baby. During vaginal delivery, a 50% incidence of infection has been reported in babies born during primary maternal genital infection, compared with a 5% risk during reactivated disease (Nahmias and Visintine, 1976). Interestingly, most infants are reported to acquire the virus from asymptomatic mothers (Corey et al., 1983; Whitley et al., 1980). Recent reports from Birmingham (Woodman and Weaver, 1986) and Sheffield (Woolley et al., 1986) present a different picture. In a study of 29 "at-risk" women in Birmingham, the virus was never isolated in the absence of lesions during the later stages of pregnancy.

The Sheffield study showed that 22 of the 49 women studied had a recurrence of herpetic infection during pregnancy. Nineteen of these occurred in the third trimester, but isolations were made only from vaginal swabs. There was no evidence of cervical infection from smears or culture. Harger et al. (1983) reported that 3% of the cervical cultures they collected late in pregnancy contained HSV in the absence of clinical disease. A comparable isolation rate was reported by Yaeger (1984) in samples collected at delivery. The potentially serious risk to the baby and the possible absence of clinical features in the mother underline the importance of screening for virus throughout the later stages of pregnancy as a means of deciding on the need for delivery by ceserean section. Such screening should be available during the last 4-8 weeks (Light and Linneman, 1974), and isolation should be repeated weekly and as close as possible to the beginning of labor. Women with a history of genital herpes, those with antibodies to HSV-2, and those whose sexual partners have herpes genitalis, should all be monitored. Proper management of the pregnancy requires both the use of rapid diagnostic techniques to detect the virus and the ability to measure specific antibody to HSV-2. Similar considerations apply to the diagnosis of infection in the baby.

E. Conclusions

The management of patients with genital ulcers would be aided by rapid diagnosis. The two most important causes of painful ulceration of the perianal region or anal canal are trauma and HSV-1 infection (McMillan and Smith, 1984). Rapid diagnosis would allow prompt treatment of the infected group with specific antiviral therapy. The diagnosis of infection at other sites is not usually required as urgently, although direct methods would be suitable for the examination of specimens from high-risk patients, e.g., those with hepatitis B and AIDS. The rapid diagnosis of herpetic encephalitis is also important, but it is difficult to detect virus in the cerebrospinal fluid (CSF), although it should be attempted along with serological studies to detect specific antibody in the CSF and blood. Aseptic meningitis caused by HSV-2 can be confirmed by virus isolation from the CSF or the buffy coat.

III. LABORATORY DIAGNOSIS OF HERPETIC INFECTIONS

A. Tissue Culture

Isolation of the virus in tissue culture is considered to be the most sensitive method of detecting virus. It has the advantage that by continuing incubation of the culture, low titers of virus can replicate and produce a cytopathic effect (CPE) up to a week or more after inoculation. This time interval can, however, be a disadvantage when dealing with specimens from a pregnant woman as results are required quickly. The speed at which the CPE develops depends not only upon the inoculum size but also upon the sensitivity of the cell cultures. Various cell strains (primary rabbit kidney, PRK), semicontinuous cell strains (human embryo fibroblasts, HEF; MRC-5; W1-38; human foreskin fibroblasts, HFF), and cell lines (Hep-2; Vero cells) have been used. Some authors (Rubin and Rogers, 1984) consider that PRK cells are more sensitive than human diploid fibroblasts, and as fewer other virus groups produce a CPE in PRK cells, the CPE is easier to identify. Other authors (Callihan and Menegus, 1984; Moore, 1984) did not find any significant difference between PRK and human fibroblasts. They reported that variation in sensitivity can occur between batches of commercial PRK cells. Moore (1984) established a semicontinuous HFF cell stain that was less variable in sensitivity, whereas Callihan and Menegus (1984) used both MRC-5 and W1-38 cells from commercial sources.

Once a CPE develops, the virus must be identified. Previously, this was done by neutralization with antiserum and could take another 3 days.

Various combinations of tissue culture and immunological tracing of HSV using polyclonal and monoclonal antibodies (MAbs) have been tried to speed up the laboratory diagnosis of HSV infections. Unfortunately, this would preclude the isolation and identification of other viruses such as cytomegalovirus (CMV) (Hughes et al., 1986).

1. Detection by Polyclonal Antibody

a. Cultureset.   A coverslip in a Leighton tube is seeded with Vero cells. The resultant monolayer is inoculated with the specimen and incubated for 24 or 48 hr. After fixing with formalin, the cells are stained using rabbit antiherpes antibody and an indirect peroxidase-antiperoxidase (PAP) reagent. The manufacturers recommend that three stained foci should be visible before the test is considered positive. Phillips et al. (1985) achieved a sensitivity of over 90% in 48 hr, whereas the sensitivities in other studies ranged from 65-79% at 48 hr and 56-73% at 24 hr (Table 2). These results fall below the manufacturer's claim of 95% sensitivity after 24 hr incubation. These authors point out that some of the groups, e.g., Fayram et al. (1983) inoculated up to six tissue culture tubes and used these results to compare with two Cultureset observations. It is, therefore, difficult to evaluate the Cultureset results in an unbiased manner.

The importance of the type of specimen on the sensitivity was commented upon by Hayden et al. (1983) who noted that most discrepant results were found in specimens from the female genital tract. It was suggested that this could be a reflection of varying amounts of virus present at this site.

Both Hayden et al. (1983) and Sewell et al. (1984) reported that a number of specimens that were Cultureset-negative did not produce a CPE in tissue culture until after 2-5 days incubation. This indicated that when the specimens contained a low titer of virus the amount of viral antigen was below the level of detection by Cultureset at 24-48 hr.

Table 2 Sensitivity of HSV Detection by Conventional Culture and Cultureset

Conventional culture			Cultureset		Ref.
Number (%) of specimens positive by					
24 hr	48 hr	>48 hr	24 hr	48 hr	
—	—	54[a] (100)	—	35 (64.8)	Fayram et al. (1983)
31 (49.2)	55 (87.3)	63[b] (100)	46 (73)	—	Hayden et al. (1983)
—	—	58[c] (100)	—	53 (91.4)	Phillips et al. (1985)
25 (45.5)	46 (83.6)	55[d] (100)	31 (56.4)	43 (78.2)	Rubin and Roger (1984)
—	25 (34.7)	72[e] (100)	—	57 (79.2)	Sewell et al. (1984)

[a]5 days
[b]≥4 days
[c]7 days
[d]>48 hr
[e]≥5 days

Despite the manufacturer's recommendation that three stained foci should be visible before a specimen is classed as positive, Hayden et al. (1983) noted that nine of 46 specimens that were tissue culture-positive had only one to three densely staining cells in the Cultureset. Likewise, Rubin and Rogers (1984) considered a single focus as positive. These workers noted that epithelial cells in the inoculum could stain a pale red, possibly because of the endogenous cellular peroxidase reacting with the substrate. It was, therefore, recommended that specimens should be centrifuged before inoculation to remove these epithelial cells.

Balkovic and Hsiung (1985) reported the use of Cultureset mouse Mabs for typing (Sect. IV.B.1). These reagents have now replaced the polyclonal rabbit antiserum for diagnostic use.

b. Scott Selecticult. The Scott Selecticult method is similar to Cultureset, except that it uses a horseradish peroxidase as the enzyme. The polyclonal antibody detects both HSV-1 and HSV-2 and can confirm the presence of HSV more quickly than tissue culture (Johnson et al., 1985). However, three of the specimens had to be incubated for 5 days before detection by Scott Selecticult was possible. By this time all but one of the specimens were positive by tissue culture.

c. Indirect Peroxidase-Antiperoxidase in Multiwell Plates. Mayo et al. (1985) inoculated 4261 specimens into multiwell plates. At 24 hr, 696 were positive by PAP compared with 237 by tissue culture. By 72 hr a further 311 were positive by PAP and 490 by tissue culture. However, when the tissue cultures were incubated for a total of 11 days the final number producing CPE was 1019—12 more than that by PAP. Thus, the sensitivity of PAP at 72 hr was 98.7%.

d. Direct Immunoperoxidase Test. Sewell et al. (1984) tested the cultures after 48 hr incubation and found the test easier to carry out than the indirect PAP but the sensitivity was only 79% compared with tissue culture. Johnson et al. (1985) had to continue their observations up to 5 days to obtain a sensitivity equal to tissue culture, but in addition, they reported one false-positive reaction.

e. Lab-Lock Chamber Slides and Immunological Staining. Lab-lock chamber slides were seeded with HFF, inoculated, and incubated for 24 hr, after which the monolayers were stained with a rabbit anti-HSV-2 antibody in conjunction with fluorescent reagents (Nerurkar et al., 1984b). Compared with the tissue culture results, the sensitivity and specificity of biotin-avidin-fluorescent antibody (BA-FA) (Nerurkar et al., 1983) were 100% at 24 hr compared with CPE at 7 days. Direct fluorescent-conjugated antibody was less sensitive (68%) but 100% specific: an indirect fluorescent antibody test, although more sensitive (88%), was less specific (88%).

f. Enzyme-Linked Immunosorbent Assay Detection of Antigen. Morgan and Smith (1984) used "Removawell" Ortho strips and a horseradish peroxidase-labeled serum (Ortho) to detect HSV antigens by the enzyme-linked immunosorbent assay (ELISA) method. A sensitivity of 63% was found in a direct test. After two days of incubation in tissue culture, however, the sensitivity was 79-87%, at 4 days it was 96-98%, and by 7 days it reached 98-100%, depending upon the cells in which the virus was grown. The sensitivity of herpes antigen detection by ELISA was increased when the inoculum was centrifuged onto the tissue culture cells (one RK and one MRC-5) at 2500 g for 30 min. After a subsequent 44 hr incubation 80% of each culture was pooled, lysed with lysing agent (Ortho Diagnostics), and assayed by Ortho Diagnostics HSV ELISA-spin amplification technique (SAT) (Michalski et al., 1986). The sensitivity of tissue culture isolation was 95.2% and that of ELISA-SAT 97.6% both being 100% specific. The time to reporting a positive ELISA-SAT was 48 hr, at which time only 69% of the cultures were positive.

g. Conclusions. It can be seen that only Nerurkar et al. (1984b) and Michalski et al. (1986) have succeeded in shortening the time for detection without sacrificing sensitivity.

2. Monoclonal Antibody Detection

a. Centrifugation of the Inoculum Followed by Direct Immunofluorescence. A series of 98 specimens were inoculated into MRC-5 tissue cultures, and over a period of 6 days 22 produced a CPE. When the inoculum was centrifuged onto coverslip monolayers of MRC-5 cells, however, 23 specimens were positive at 16 hr when stained with mouse monoclonal antibodies (MAbs) (Syva-type 1 and 2 to unspecified antigens) conjugated with fluorescein (compared with 8 showing CPE at 16 hr) (Gleaves et al., 1985). Twenty-one known positive specimens that had been stored were also examined by this method. All 21 were positive 16 hr after centrifugation, but 3 days were required for all to develop CPE in tissue culture. The value of centrifugation was also examined. With both the fresh and the stored specimens, two fewer coverslips were positive if the culture was not centrifuged. In addition there were apparently more fluorescent foci in the centrifuged specimens.

b. Microcarrier Cultures and Enzyme-Linked Immunosorbent Assay Detection. Microcarrier cultures were used by Rossier et al. (1985) to support the growth of HSV. At various intervals a sample of the beads can be removed, the antigen harvested, and detected by ELISA using a mouse MAb H3-30-1-B-3 which reacted with the 100,000-molecular-weight protein of HSV-1 and HSV-2. This latter technique has the advantage that one culture can be tested over a number of days and allows a low titer of virus to replicate and give sufficient amount of antigen for detection.

c. Conclusions. Gleaves et al. (1985) have succeeded in shortening the time for detection of the virus without sacrificing sensitivity.

B. Direct Antigen Detection

The detection methods discussed so far have all required the use of tissue culture to amplify the virus, but attempts have also been made to use immunofluorescence and the ELISA method to detect HSV antigen in clinical specimens (Table 3).

1. Polyclonal Antibody Detection

a. Immunofluorescence in Direct Smears. Three groups used direct smears from the lesions. Adam et al. (1980) detected HSV antigen more easily with an indirect horseradish peroxidase (HRP) test using polyclonal rabbit antibody to HSV-1 or HSV-2 than in tissue culture. Schmidt et al. (1983) stored their slides at −70°C. After acetone fixation, staining was carried out using direct immunofluorescence with hamster antiherpes serum or direct immunoperoxidase with Dako rabbit antiherpes serum. About 19% of the smears examined were unsatisfactory because they did not contain five to ten basal cells. The sensitivity with the satisfactory smears as compared with tissue culture was 75-76% for both methods, although

Table 3 Noncultural Detection of HSV Antigens in Clinical Specimens

Method	Ag+/TC+[a]	Ag+/TC−[b]	Comment	Ref.
Polyclonal antibodies				
Direct IF[c]	60/78	2/31	25 other smears unsatisfactory	Schmidt et al. (1983)
Direct IP[d]	59/77	2/34	23 other smears unsatisfactory	
Indirect BA/FA[e]	32/36	23/42	Some smears of poor quality	Nerurkar et al. (1984a)
ELISA	74/79	25/327	Specimens concentrated before testing	Land et al. (1984)
ELISA	94/186	4/427	Specimens collected in 3 ml	Lawrence et al. (1984)
ELISA	155/295	26/836	Cervical specimens had insufficient antigen	Warford et al. (1984)
ELISA	38/45	0/58	Specimens collected in 0.5 ml	Alexander et al. (1985)
Monoclonal antibodies				
Indirect IF	12/13	2/7	Good cell preparations from fresh lesions required	Balachandran et al. (1982)
Direct IF	48/54	6/50	Require at least 20 cells/well of Hendley-Essex slide	Goldstein et al. (1983)
Direct IF	14/18	1/48	81 other cell preparations unsatisfactory	Volpi et al. (1983)
Direct IF	27/35	0/127		Fung et al. (1985)
ELISA biotin IgM	69/140	122/281	Specimens extracted in 400 ml	Adler-Storthz et al. (1983)
ELISA amplified	48/50	5/98		Clayton et al. (1986)

[a]Antigen-positive: tissue culture-positive.
[b]Antigen-positive: tissue culture-negative.
[c]IF, immunofluorescence.
[d]IP, immunoperoxidase.
[e]BA/FA, biotin-avidin fluorescence.

positive results were not always obtained by both methods on the same specimens. Both methods demonstrated positivity in two specimens from which HSV
was not isolated. The authors noted that endogenous cellular peroxidase must be
differentiated from the true viral reaction. Nerurkar et al. (1984b) used the same
rabbit anti-HSV BA-FA reagent that had shown 100% sensitivity with tissue culture to stain direct smears. They found 37.7% false-positives but noted that the
results were very dependent upon the quality of the cells in the preparation.

b. Immunofluorescence in Cellular Deposits.   Other workers did not use smears
made directly from lesion swabs but made preparations of the cellular deposit
from the specimen transport medium after the inoculation to tissue cultures.
Lawrence et al. (1984) who used a human anti-HSV serum had a very low sensitivity with this method, detecting only 1% of the positive tissue cultures.

c. Enzyme-Linked Immunosorbent Assay of Clinical Specimens.   When compared
with tissue culture techniques Warford et al. (1984) reported an overall sensitivity
of 52.5% and a specificity of 96.9% with Ortho reagents. However, they comment on the low correlation of ELISA results from cervical specimens compared
with tissue culture (cf. Hayden et al., 1983) and also on false-positive reactions.
Lawrence et al. (1984) reported a 50.5% sensitivity using a human antiherpes
serum for detection. They found four of 427 culture-negative specimens were
positive by ELISA but showed by a specific blocking test that these four specimens contained nonviable HSV antigen. A sensitivity of 69.6% and a specificity
of 93.3% were reported by Sewell and Horn (1985) using an Ortho ELISA reagent. One of their ELISA-positive, tissue culture-negative specimens, came from
a patient who had yielded HSV 10 days earlier in tissue culture. The reason for
the other "false-positive" results is unknown. Alexander et al. (1985) used an
ELISA method based on that of Vestigaard and Jensen marketed by Mercia. They
found a sensitivity of 84.4% and no false-positive results with a purified rabbit
antiherpes serum. When they compared their method and results with those of
Lawrence et al. (1984) they suggested that their increased sensitivity may have
been due to the small volume in which the specimen was collected. Land et al.
(1984) also concentrated the specimen by centrifuging the cells out of the transport medium and lysing them in a small volume. They used rabbit anti HSV-1
(RIgα1, Dako) and anti HSV-2 (RIgα2, Dako) to capture and detect antigen. Of
457 specimens, 79 were positive in tissue culture and 94% of these were also ELISA
positive. Five of the specimens that were tissue culture-positive had very few cells,
so these may have been below the detection level of the ELISA test. The ELISA
detection rate could, however, be increased to 100% if the specimens were tested
within 24 hr of sampling or up to 14 days if stored at $-20°C$.

*d. Biotin Streptavidin Amplification of Enzyme-Linked Immunosorbent Assay
Test.*   Nerurkar et al. (1984a) reported a sensitivity of 95.6% and specificity of

91.4% using the same rabbit serum as they used for the immunofluorescent test (Nerurkar et al., 1983). Similarly to Lawrence et al. (1984) these authors found that the antigen in the ELISA-positive, tissue culture-negative specimens could be blocked with specific antibody. It was also noted by Nerurkar et al. (1984a) that the presence of *Candida albicans* or *Staphylococcus aureus* in the specimens did not substantially affect the ELISA result.

e. Enzyme-Linked Fluorescence Assay. Shekarchi et al. (1985) used 4-methylumbelliferyl phosphate as the substrate and measured the resulting fluorescence in a Micro-Fluor reader. This substrate gave a quicker reaction, thus, the test time was reduced.

2. Detection by Monoclonal Antibody

a. Immunofluorescence on Direct Smears. In 1982 Balanchandran et al. examined scrapes from the base of lesions by indirect IF (using MAbs specified in Chap. 11, Table 2) and found that if the specimen was from a primary infection or from a vesicle of less than 4 days duration in a recurrence, 80% of the specimens were positive compared with 93% by virus isolation. Specimens taken from vesicles older than 4 days did not yield virus in culture, but two of seven specimens were shown to contain HSV antigen by IF. The authors comment that good preparations are required for this test. Goldstein et al. (1983) also noted that the lack of cells in six of 106 specimens accounted for the loss of sensitivity in their indirect IF test (using MAbs specified in Chap. 11, Table 2). They required at least 20 cells per well of a Hendley-Essex slide and found a 90% sensitivity by both tissue culture and indirect IF. In both assays, six specimens reacted in only one of the tests. Volpi et al. (1983) reported a 77% sensitivity with one possible false-positive result.

b. Immunofluorescence on Cellular Deposits. Fung et al. (1985), using Electronucleonics mouse IgM MAbs (HSV type-common and HSV-2 type-specific) in an indirect test, detected herpes antigen in 27 of the 35 positive tissue culture specimens. this is a sensitivity of 77.1% compared with 62-86% with polyclonal antibodies, but the specificity with MAbs was 100%. These authors found that they had fewer than the manufacturer's recommended two or more intact cells per high-power field in one-third of their preparations and even with freshly prepared smears, 23% of the specimens had insufficient cells. This shows that for either prepared smears or those from transport medium, taking the sample is a very critical part of the test.

c. Enzyme-Linked Immunosorbent Assay. A biotin-avidin amplification step has been introduced into the ELISA test by Adler-Storthz et al. (1983) who conjugated biotin to IgM MAbs (18b.2 reacts with both HSV-1- and HSV-2-infected cells) and found a 49% sensitivity. They detected antigen, however, in 122 specimens that were tissue culture-negative. They claim that a high proportion of these results were specific; if an IgM MAb (E19.2) which did not react with HSV, was substituted in the test, 100 of these positive results became negative. Six specimens were subjected to serological blocking which invariably reduced the positivity. Although this test is claimed to detect 90 plaque-forming units or 6 X 10^3 particles of HSV-1 or HSV-2, its sensitivity for tissue culture is only 49%. As antigen is apparently detected in a high proportion of culture-negative specimens, further work is required to establish the specificity of the reaction.

A type-common MAb to viral glycoprotein was used to capture the HSV antigen which was subsequently detected by another type-common MAb. The sensitivity of this reaction was 55.5% (Clayton et al., 1985). When Clayton et al. (1986) used an amplified detection system the sensitivity obtained with swab specimens sent to the laboratory in 3 ml of transport medium was 78%. However, when swabs were sent to the laboratory in plastic sleeves and antigen extracted in 400 µl of diluent prior to testing by the amplified ELISA method the sensitivity increased to 92%. A number (eight) of the specimens that did not yield virus in culture were shown to contain nonviable herpes antigen by specific naturalization of the ELISA reaction.

3. Conclusions

The detection sensitivity of herpes antigen by immunofluorescence using either polyclonal antibodies or MAbs is dependent upon the quality of the smears or cellular deposits examined. Monoclonal antibodies should have the potential to be useful in such a test, but there are no well-documented studies using commercially available MAbs.

The ELISA tests also have a low sensitivity, again dependent upon the amount of viral material in the specimen. Concentration of the specimen improves sensitivity but there can also be a problem with false-positive readings. A proportion of these are possibly true-positive results where no viable virus is present in the specimen. If the amplified ELISA system of Clayton et al. (1986) performs well in other centers, this test will be useful for the detection of HSV antigen in specimens that cannot be transported quickly to the laboratory and that have lost part or all of their viability.

C. Detection of Herpes Simplex Virus Nucleic Acid

As well as examining the cellular deposit from the transport medium for the presence of viral antigen, Fung et al. (1985) attempted to detect HSV DNA by hybridization. Single-stranded HSV DNA labeled with either radioactive nucleotides or biotin (a probe) is allowed to interact with the denatured DNA in the cells. If there is any HSV DNA in the cells the probe will anneal to it. Fung et al. (1985) used Patho-Gene Kit (Enzo Biochem) to probe for HSV DNA. This commercial product was made from cloned fragments of HSV-1 and HSV-2 DNA labeled with biotin, and the test was developed with streptavidin, horseradish peroxidase, and substrate. Again at least two intact cells should be present per high-power field and staining should be in the nucleus of the cell. Of the 35 specimens that were positive by tissue culture 25, or 71.4% were also positive by hybridization. However, 12 of the tissue culture-negative specimens gave a positive hybridization, reducing the specificity to 90.6%. The authors discuss the possibility of detecting latent virus. Although more rapid, hybridization should be used as an adjunct to tissue culture and not as a replacement.

D. Detection of Antibody to Herpes Simplex Virus

The complement fixation test, which has been used for many years, is capable of demonstrating primary infections with either HSV-1 or HSV-2, but it cannot detect initial infections, e.g., a first infection with HSV-2 in the presence of HSV-1 antibody.

IV. TYPING AND SUBTYPING OF HERPES SIMPLEX VIRUS ISOLATES

The typing of isolates is useful for epidemiological studies, but as the association between HSV-2 and cervical cancer becomes more tenuous, it does not seem to be so imperative to type the virus. Some clinicians, however, still feel that the information is useful for the management of pregnant women or to assess the possible recurrence rate.

Typing has been performed by estimating the size of the pock produced on the chorioallantoic membrane of the developing chick embryo (Parker and Banatvala, 1967); by the electron microscopic detection of filaments in the nucleus of the host cell (Couch and Nahmias, 1969); by microneutralization (Peutherer, 1970); by the limitation of growth in chick embryo fibroblasts (Balkovic and Hsiung, 1985; Zheng et al., 1983); and by inhibition of growth of virus by E-5-(2-bromovinyl)-2'-deoxyuridine (BVDU) (Balkovic and Hsiung, 1985; Swierkosz et al., 1985a; Zheng et al., 1983; Zimmerman et al., 1985). This last method can be unreliable: Balkovic and Hsiung (1985) and Swierkosz et al. (1985a) both reported that one HSV isolate was incorrectly typed by BVDU. One was acycloguanosine (ACG)-resistant and the other was from an immunocompromised patient. Growth of herpes virus in vitro in the presence of ACG produced six more ACG^r strains. With the increasing use of antiviral agents, care will be required with the method of typing because ACG^r isolates of HSV-1 will also be resistant to BVDU and so be typed as HSV-2.

A. Typing with Polyclonal Antibodies

1. Microneutralization

Pauls and Dowdle (1967) introduced the microneutralization test. It was modified by Peutherer (1970) and when compared with the size of pocks produced on the chorioallanoic membrane of developing chick embryos it had a sensitivity of 98% and a 100% specificity (Smith et al., 1973). Zheng et al. (1983) also used a microneutralization test based on commercial sera. They found that the sera were cross-reactive and, hence, could not type the HSV-1 strains. Two-thirds of the HSV-2 isolates were identifiable, giving an overall sensitivity of 32% when compared with BVDU resistance.

2. Immunofluorescence

Maitland et al. (1982), using polyclonal rabbit anti HSV-1 serum with and without absorption with HSV-2 infected cells, found 100% sensitivity and specificity compared with restriction enzyme analysis. Zheng et al. (1983), using commercial reagents, found that there was a sensitivity of only 17%, although the specificity was 100%.

B. Typing with Monoclonal Antibodies

1. Immunofluorescence

Balkovic and Hsiung (1985) used both Micro Trak (Syva) (see earlier discussion) and Ortho MAbs to type HSV isolates. When compared with culture in chick embryo fibroblasts and inhibition with BVDU, both tests were 100% specific. The inclusion of a counterstain in the Syva reagent made it easier to read, and as it was a direct method, it was quicker to perform than the indirect method of Ortho. When Zimmerman et al. (1985) compared MAb typing with inhibition of BVDU and restriction enzyme analysis, they also found 100% agreement. Also, in 1983 Peterson et al. showed that MAbs were superior to polyclonal antibodies for typing HSV. Five isolates could not be typed by MAbs and were subsequently shown to be a mixture of HSV-1 and HSV-2 by plaque purification and restriction enzyme analysis.

Swierkosz et al. (1985b) compared an indirect (Electronucleonic) and a direct (Kallestad Lab Inc.) IF test for typing HSV. The isolates were all typed by restriction enzyme analysis. The indirect test used a type-common MAb and a type-specific HSV-2 MAb. The HSV-2 MAb gave 100% agreement but four of the 14 HSV-1 isolates could not be typed by this method. These workers commented on the amount of background fluorescence with the Electronucleonic reagents—a problem that did not arise with those from Kallestad Lab Inc. whose MAbs were type-specific. All the HSV-1 strains could be correctly typed, but one of the 38 HSV-2 isolates failed to react with the specific HSV-2 MAb. This particular strain of HSV-2 may have lacked the epitope detected by this MAb.

Fung et al. (1985) inoculated tissue cultures and subsequently typed 11 viruses using the Syva type-specific MAbs. Following inoculation, the viral transport medium was centrifuged and smears prepared from the resultant cell deposit. Upon typing of the cell deposits by the indirect method with Electronucleonic reagents, one specimen did not react with either MAb. Six smears and isolates correlated, one being HSV-1 the rest HSV-2, but the remaining four, which on isolation were shown to be HSV-2, were incorrectly typed in the deposit smears. As the intensity of staining with the type-specific HSV-2 MAb was less than that of the type-common MAb, this could have caused the mistyping in the smears. Thus, careful evaluation of the MAb used in typing is essential, especially if one of a pair is type-common.

2. Enzyme-Linked Immunosorbent Assays

The ELISA method for typing employed an antigen-capture step followed by detection with MAb (Frame et al., 1984) or indirect and antibody sandwich techniques (Gerna et al., 1983). Another approach was to inoculate monolayers on multiwell plates and to use these as the antigen which was detected by mouse MAbs—one HSV-1-specific and the other type-common—followed by an antimouse enzyme conjugate serum and substrate (Nilheden et al., 1983). All these tests gave satisfactory results when compared with restriction enzyme analysis of the HSV genome.

3. Reverse Passive Hemagglutination Test

Monoclonal antibody was precipitated by ammonium sulfate, redissolved in water, and dialyzed before being linked to trypsin-treated red blood cells by chromic chloride. The antigen was diluted, mixed with the antibody-linked red blood cells, and after incubation, hemagglutination was recorded. The MAbs LP10 and LP4 (see Chap. 11, Table 2) that are type-specific for HSV-1 and HSV-2, respectively, gave 100% agreement with typing by BVDU (Buckmaster et al., 1984).

4. Enzyme Immunofiltration Technique

The infected cell lysate was applied to a disk (934 AH Whatman) in a multiwell suction plate (V & P Enterprises, San Diego, California). This was followed by MAbs G11 (HSV-1) or A6, E12, and H11 (HSV-2) (see Chap. 11, Table 2). After removal of the unbound antibodies, either HRP staphylococcal protein A (SPA) or HRP goat antimouse IgG was added and the color reaction developed by the addition of substrate. The HRP goat antimouse serum gave little or no background, but the HRP-SPA was more versatile as it could be used for both mouse MAbs and antibodies from other species. The sensitivity and specificity of this method was 100% (Richman et al., 1982).

C. Immunological Subtyping

Subtyping is useful in studying the microepidemiology of infection. In 1963 Ashe and Scherp raised polyclonal antibodies to a number of HSV-1 isolates and by neutralization kinetics grouped their isolates; unfortunately, two isolates from one patient fell into different groups.

Pereira et al. (1982) used 18 MAbs (two to gC-1; eight to gD-1 and gD-2; one to gD-2; three to pgB/gB-1 and pgB/gB-2; one to pgB/gB-2; two to gE-2; and one of unknown specificity) to type 36 HSV isolates (18 HSV-1 and 18 HSV-2). Seven of the MAbs were useful: three divided the 18 HSV-1 into four subgroups, and four MAbs divided the HSV-2 isolates into six subgroups. In the HSV-2 isolates, three were epidemiologically related and all fell into the same subgroup. In 1986 Sutherland et al. reported a study of 64 isolates from 18 patients. Six of the patients were infected with HSV-1 and did not suffer from recurrences during the period of study. Five of the six patients had the same subtype of HSV-1 (no information is given on the relationship or otherwise of these patients). Of the 12 patients from whom HSV-2 was isolated, all but one had at least one recurrence, and viruses were isolated from different sites during one episode. In only one instance was there a difference in the subtype of a virus from two different sites during the same episode. Four of the 12 patients had different subtypes in successive recurrences. The subtypes did not appear to correlate with the BamHI restriction enzyme (RE) profile in that isolates with the same profiles exhibited different epitopes and vice versa. In only one instance a patient yielded a virus at the second recurrence that had a different RE profile and a different epitope thus, presumably, this was a reinfection rather than a recrudescence. The inclusion of additional MAbs in the panel further subdivided the isolates, but the epidemiological value of this is not yet clear.

Theoretically it should be possible to raise MAbs to epitopes on every antigen expressed by HSV, but whether or not such reagents would give a true picture of the spread of infection remains to be assessed.

D. Restriction Enzyme Analysis

The alternative approach is to analyze the genome of HSV by restriction enzymes (RE), which recognize certain, usually palindromic, sequences in double-stranded DNA, e.g., the enzyme from *Escherichia coli* designated *EcoRI* recognizes the sequences and cleaves the strands at the points indicated in Fig. 2. Each time the sequence occurs in the viral DNA, the enzyme cleaves the DNA to give a number of fragments that can be separated electrophoretically in agarose.

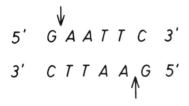

Fig. 2   The recognition and cleavage site for the restriction endonuclease *EcoRI*.

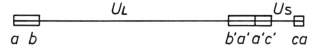

Fig. 3   The organization of the genome of HSV.

The genome of HSV consists of two covalently linked pieces of double-stranded DNA. The unique long (U_L) and unique short (U_S) regions are flanked by inverted terminal repeat sequences, ab, a'b', ac, and a'c' (Fig. 3). The genome exists in four possible isomeric forms as both the U_L and U_S regions may invert. All four isomers are thought to occur equally in isolates.

The RE pattern of HSV can vary in two ways: (1) major variations that involve the loss or acquisition of a recognition site and would be recognized by finding a new high-molecular-weight fragment or two lower-molecular-weight fragments (Fig. 4) and (2) minor variations that are reflected by alterations in the mobilities of fragments from the terminal regions (see Fig. 4).

1. Typing of Herpes Simplex Virus DNA

Restriction enzyme analysis is a powerful tool in the distinction of HSV-1 and HSV-2 (see Fig. 4). The genomes have the same organization but because of differences in their nucleotide sequences give rise to different profiles in gels after treatment with restriction enzymes. The technique is, therefore, very reliable for typing HSV. Both Lonsdale (1979) and Darville (1983) used virus labeled with ^{32}P and detected the resultant fragments by autoradiography. While these results are clear, it is not always possible to use radioactivity in a diagnostic laboratory, and in addition, the half-life of ^{32}P is short so that either frequent supplies of the nucleotide are required or the isolates can be typed only in batches. Arens and Swierkosz (1983) used unlabeled virus. They attempted to remove the cellular DNA from the sample by separating the nuclear and cytoplasmic fractions. Thus, they examined only DNA that had been packaged in virus particles. After the DNA had been digested, separated on agarose, and stained with ethidium bromide, they were able to type all but one isolate. When the results of this simplified technique were compared with those of sodium iodide gradient-purified DNA, the major bands agreed. This simple method using unlabeled virus is more suited to a diagnostic laboratory. However, problems may result from lack of stability of the total cytoplasmic DNA and contamination of the digests with RNA.

2. Subtyping of Herpes Simplex Virus DNA

In addition to typing HSV isolates, it has been shown that the RE profiles of the DNA from different HSV-1 isolates could be distinguished on the basis of the major variations. This technique was applied to tracing the spread of HSV-1 in

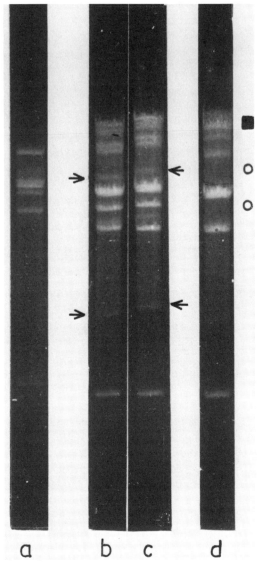

Fig. 4 Agarose gel separation of the fragments generated by *EcoRI* digestion of HSV DNA stained by ethidium bromide. Lane a HSV-1; lanes b-d HSV-2. A major difference shown by the loss (open circle) of two bands and gain of a larger band (closed square) is illustrated in lane d compared with c. Minor variations due to mobility differences (arrows) are shown in lanes b and c.

nurseries (Buchman et al., 1978) and in a dental practice (Manzella et al., 1984). In our series of 49 unrelated genital HSV-1 isolates, it was again possible to distinguish them on the basis of major variations, as all unrelated HSV-1 isolates have their own unique profile. When isolates from five consorts of these patients were examined it was shown that both partners yielded identical viruses, but all five couples had their own HSV-1 substrain. Thus, RE analysis can be used to trace genital infections with HSV-1. Previously published work on a very few strains of HSV-2 used both major and minor variations to distinguish isolates (Barton et al., 1985; Buchman et al., 1979; Chaney et al., 1983). We have shown that although the major variations are constant in sequential isolates from the same patients, mobility differences in the joint and terminal region occur (Maitland et al., 1982). Also, different DNA preparations from the same isolate can show mobility differences. These results corroborate Roizman and Tognon (1983) who state that mobility differences should not be used to distinguish strains of HSV-2. We examined 198 HSV-2 isolates from unrelated patients with genital herpetic infections using five enzymes: *EcoRI, BglII, HindIII, Kpn,* and *BamHI* (for all of which there are published maps). It was impossible to distinguish all of these viruses on the basis of major variations. Again we were able to compare the isolates from nine of the consorts of the unrelated patients. Fewer than nine RE patterns were found in the 18 isolates, so despite both members of each couple yielding identical viruses, other couples were apparently infected with the same substrain of HSV-2. Thus, it was impossible to trace person-to-person spread of HSV-2 using the currently mapped restriction enzymes.

E. Conclusions

Although the ultimate in typing is RE analysis, this procedure is possibly not suited to routine diagnostic virology laboratories. Monoclonal antibodies, therefore, would appear to be a more practical approach, especially if two type-specific MAbs reacting with the appropriate epitopes are used. A counterstain is useful for fluorescence but both fluorescence and ELISA tests appear to be satisfactory.

V. MEASUREMENT OF TYPE-SPECIFIC ANTIBODY

A number of tests have been developed in an attempt to distinguish HSV-1 and HSV-2 antibody. These include microneutralization tests expressed as the potency of neutralization (pN) value (Nahmias et al., 1969; 1970) or as the II/I index (Rawls et al., 1970); neutralization kinetic studies (Skinner et al., 1971); fluorescent antibody studies (Smith et al., 1972b); and antibody complement cytolysis (Smith et al., 1972a). None of these tests measured solely type-specific antibodies, so both type-common and type-specific antibodies were measured together.

In an attempt to measure type-specific antibody Hampar et al. (1985) prepared MAb affinity-purified antigens: gC and gD from HSV-1 and gD and gC from

HSV-2. In addition, the sera under test were absorbed with either Vero cells or cells infected with HSV-1 or HSV-2. The residual antibody was then measured by ELISA and results compared with those of microneutralization. A 91% agreement was found with HSV-2 antibody and 99% with HSV-1 antibody.

A. Radioimmune Precipitation Tests

Both Eberle and Courtney (1981) and Ashley et al. (1985) have looked at the antibody response to different polypeptides during acute recrudescent infections. Eberle and Courtney (1981) reported that they could distinguish by radioimmune precipitation (RIP) assay a type-1 from a type-2 response on the basis of the reaction with gC-1 and some low-molecular-weight HSV-2 glycoproteins. However, Ashley et al. (1985) performed both homologous and heterologous reactions and found that although the homologous antibody could be detected earlier, cross-reacting antibody very soon developed to pgB/gB, gC, gD, and nonglycosylated proteins, (they did not, however, report an antibody production to gG-2).

B. Western Blot Analysis

Eberle et al. (1984, 1985) used the Western blot method and found that different polypeptides were detected by this technique. The earliest antibody to be detected was to the p40 complex, which has been shown to be the intracellular form of the capsid protein. Antibody to p40 appears early in both HSV-1 and HSV-2 infections: this is followed by antibodies to gG-2 and the 80,000-molecular-weight protein in HSV-2 infection; and possibly by antibodies to gB and p80 in HSV-1 infection.

C. Glycoprotein G

Roizman et al. (1984) had indicated that gG-2 was type-specific. By an immuno-blot assay Eberle et al. (1984) detected gG-2 antibody in patients' sera following either a primary HSV-2 infection or a recurrence of such an infection. Ashley et al. (1985) did not report on gG-2 reactivity in their RIP assay because they found that gG-2 was not efficiently labeled with [^{35}S]methionine. However, Teglbjaerg et al. (1986) who used a [^{14}C]amino acid label suggested the strong band at a relative molecular weight of 127,000 may have been partly due to gG-2g (see Chap. 11).

The gG-1 and gG-2 antigens were purified in affinity columns. For gG-2 MAbs, H966 or H1206 were used, although H1206 gave the better yield. Glycoprotein G-1 was prepared by the sequential removal of all other HSV-1 glycoproteins (Lee et al., 1985a,b). Recently Olofsson et al. (1986) have shown that gG-2 will attach to gel-bound *Helix pomatia* lectin, thus, this is an alternative method for the purification of gG-2. As previous work has shown that gC-1 binds to the same lectin, this method is not suitable for the purification of gG-1.

The specificity of gG-1 and gG-2 was examined by using the purified antigens in an immunodot blot test (Lee et al., 1985a,b). It was found that patients had detectable antibody to gG in sera taken more than 10 days postinfection and that there was no cross-reactivity of gG-1 antibody with gG-2 antigen and vice versa. Thus, it appears that gG-1 and gG-2 are type-specific antigens and could be used for screening patients' sera for the presence of antibody to either, or both, types of HSV.

D. Conclusions

Although both RIP and the Western blot techniques have been useful in determining the various antigens to which antibody is produced during the course of an herpetic infection, the immunodot blot test (Lee et al., 1985a,b) is the most straightforward type-specific assay yet developed, provided the results are substantiated by other laboratories. It does not require specialized facilities or containment, thus it could be carried out in routine diagnostic laboratories, especially if gG-1 and gG-2 were to become available commercially.

VI. CONCLUSIONS

The case for rapid diagnosis or simple detection methods for specimens from high-risk patients has been made. The obvious tests that should be useful are either IF or ELISA tests performed directly on the patients' specimens. Unfortunately, even with the advent of MAbs, IF tests are not sufficiently sensitive to give reliable results. The problem appears to be insufficient virus in certain specimens which, on occasions, may be due to the poor quality of the material sampled from clinical lesions. ELISA tests are more encouraging.

Tissue culture has long been considered to be the most sensitive method for detection of HSV. It does, however, suffer from the disadvantage that it may take 5-10 days for the CPE to appear. Recently, two groups of workers have succeeded in speeding up the detection of HSV while retaining the sensitivity and specificity. Both methods involve centrifuging the inoculum onto the monolayers. After 16 hr Gleaves et al. (1985) were able to detect HSV antigen by a direct IF with MAbs. The interpretation of IF slides requires some technical expertise, so the report of Michalski et al. (1986) of an ELISA-SAT test giving almost 100% sensitivity at 48 hr may well be more acceptable. This test gives an objective result and, certainly, amplification of the amount of virus in the specimen is necessary, as Clayton et al. (1985) point out. In their experience the amount of virus in the specimens submitted can vary considerably from week to week and this variation was reflected in the direct ELISA tests.

The typing of isolates is considered useful by some clinicians either to forecast the probability of recurrence of genital herpes or possibly in the choice of antiviral agent. A number of methods are available, but MAbs, either singly or in pools, give quick reliable results. The MAbs are commercially available, and the most common technique used is immunofluorescence, preferably with two type-specific antibodies.

When there is a problem with herpes in pregnancy, it is considered wise to try to establish whether or not the woman has antibodies to HSV-2. Previously, this has been both time-consuming and complex, but with the report that gG-2 is specific for HSV-2 it should be possible to determine the level of HSV-2 antibody present. This will detect women who have suffered from asymptomatic genital infection with HSV-2. These patients, along with any known to suffer from genital herpes or to be at risk from an infected partner, should be screened during the last 4-8 weeks of pregnancy, possibly by an accelerated isolation technique (Gleaves et al., 1985; Michalski et al., 1986), and any woman who has no HSV-2 antibody should be screened as near to delivery as possible to attempt to identify any primary asymptomatic infection. Such information should be useful in deciding if it is necessary to carry out a ceseren section.

REFERENCES

Adam, E., Dreesman, G., Kaufman, R., and Melnick, J. (1980). Asymptomic virus shedding after herpes genitalis. *Am. J. Obstet. Gynecol. 137*:827-830.

Adam, E., Kaufman, R. H., Mirkovic, R. R., and Melnick, J. L. (1979). Persistence of virus shedding in asymptomatic women after recovery from herpes genitalis. *Obstet. Gynecol. 54*:171-173.

Adler-Storthz, K., Kendall, C., Kennedy, R. C., Henkel, R. D., and Dreesman, G. R. (1983). Biotin-avidin-amplified enzyme immunoassay for detection of herpes simplex virus antigen in clinical specimens. *J. Clin. Microbiol. 18*: 1329-1334.

Alexander, I., Ashley, C. R., Smith, K. J., Harbour, J., Roome, A. P. C. H., and Darville, J. M. (1985). Comparison of ELISA with virus isolation for the diagnosis of genital herpes. *J. Clin. Pathol. 38*:554-557.

Arens, M. Q. and Swierkosz, E. M. (1983). Simplified method for typing herpes simplex virus by restriction enzyme analysis. *J. Clin. Microbiol. 17*:548-551.

Ashe, W. K. and Scherp, H. W. (1963). Antigenic analysis of herpes simplex virus by neutralization kinetics. *J. Immunol. 91*:658-665.

Ashley, R., Benedetti, J., and Corey, L. (1985). Humoral immune response to HSV-1 and HSV-2 viral proteins in patients with primary genital herpes. *J. Med. Virol. 17*:153-166.

Balachandran, N., Frame, B., Chernesky, M., Kraiselburd, E., Kouri, Y., Garcia, D., Lavery, C., and Rawls, W. E. (1982). Identification and typing of herpes simplex viruses with monoclonal antibodies. *J. Clin. Microbiol. 16*:205-208.

Balkovic, E. S. and Hsiung, G. D. (1985). Comparison of immunofluorescence with commercial monoclonal antibodies to biochemical and biological techniques for typing clinical herpes simplex virus isolates. *J. Clin. Microbiol.* *22*:870-872.

Baringer, J. R. and Swoveland, P. (1973). Recovery of herpes simplex virus from human trigeminal ganglions. *N. Engl. J. Med.* *288*:648-650.

Barton, I. G., Kinghorn, G. R., Najem, S., Al-Omar, L. S., and Potter, C. W. (1982). Incidence of herpes simplex virus types 1 and 2 isolated in patients with herpes genitalis in Sheffield. *Br. J. Vener. Dis.* *58*:44-47.

Barton, S. E., Munday, P. E., Davis, J. M., Tyms, A. S. (1985). Restriction enzyme analysis and herpes simplex infections. *Lancet 1*:1448-1449.

Bastian, F. O., Rabson, A. S., Yee, C. L., and Tralka, T. S. (1972). *Herpesvirus hominis* isolation from human trigeminal ganglia. *Science 178*:306-307.

Becker, T. M. and Nahmias, A. J. (1985). Genital herpes—yesterday, today, tomorrow. *Ann. Rev. Med. 36*:185-193.

Buchman, T. G., Roizman, B., Adams, G., and Stover, B. H. (1978). Restriction endonuclease fingerprinting of herpes simplex virus DNA. A novel epidemiological tool applied to a nosocomial outbreak. *J. Infect. Dis. 138*:488-498.

Buchman, T. C., Roizman, B., and Nahmias, A. J. (1979). Demonstration of exogenous genital reinfection with herpes simplex virus type 2 by restriction endonuclease fingerprinting of viral DNA. *J. Infect. Dis. 140*:295-304.

Buckmaster, E. A., Cranage, M. P., McLean, C. S., Combs, R. R. A., and Minson, A. (1984). The use of monoclonal antibodies to differentiate isolates of herpes simplex types 1 and 2 by neutralisation and reverse passive haemagglutination tests. *J. Med. Virol. 13*:193-202.

Buddingh, G. J., Schrum, D. I., Lanier, J. C., and Guidry, D. J. (1953). Studies of the natural history of herpes simplex infections. *Pediatrics 11*:595-610.

Callihan, D. R. and Menegus, M. A. (1984). Rapid detection of herpes simplex virus in clinical specimens with human embryonic lung fibroblasts and primary rabbit kidney cell cultures. *J. Clin. Microbiol. 19*:563-565.

Chaney, S. M. J., Warren, K. G., Kettyls, J., Zbitnue, A., and Subak-Sharpe, J. H. (1983). A comparative analysis of restriction endonuclease digests of the DNA of herpes simplex virus isolated from genital and facial lesions. *J. Gen. Virol. 64*:357-371.

Clayton, A.-L., Beckford, U., Roberts, C., Sutherland, S., Druce, A., Best, J., and Chantler, S. (1985). Factors influencing the sensitivity of herpes simplex virus detection in clinical specimens in a simultaneous enzyme-linked immunosorbent assay using monoclonal antibodies. *J. Med. Virol. 17*:275-282.

Clayton, A. L., Roberts, C., Godley, M., Best, J. M., and Chantler, S. M. (1986). Herpes simplex virus detection by ELISA: Effect of enzyme amplification, nature of lesion sampled and specimen treatment. *J. Med. Virol. 20*:89-97.

Corey, L., Adams, H. G., Brown, Z. A., and Holmes, K. K. (1983). Genital herpes simplex virus infections: Clinical manifestation, course and complications. *Ann. Intern. Med. 98*:958-972.

Couch, E. F. and Nahmias, A. J. (1969). Filamentous structures of type 2 herpesvirus hominis infection of the chorioallantoic membrane. *J. Virol. 3*:228-232.

Darville, J. M. (1983). A miniaturised and simplified technique for typing and subtyping herpes simplex virus. *J. Clin. Pathol. 36*:929-934.

Douglas, R. G. and Couch, R. B. (1970). A prospective study of chronic herpes simplex virus infection and recurrent herpes labialis in humans. *J. Immunol. 104*:289-295.

Dowdle, W. R., Nahmias, A. J., Harwell, R. W., and Pauls, F. P. (1967). Association of antigenic type of *Herpesvirus hominis* with site of viral recovery. *J. Immunol. 99*:974-980.

Eberle, R. and Courtney, R. J. (1981). Assay of type-specific and type-common antibodies to herpes simplex virus types 1 and 2 in human serum. *Infect. Immun. 31*:1062-1070.

Eberle, R., Mou, S.-W., and Zaia, J. A. (1984). Polypeptide specificity of the early antibody response following primary and recurrent herpes simplex virus type 2 infections. *J. Gen. Virol. 65*:1839-1843.

Eberle, R., Mou, S.-W., and Zaia, J. A. (1985). The immune response to herpes simplex virus: Comparison of the specificity and relative titres of serum antibodies directed against viral polypeptides following primary herpes simplex virus type 1 infections. *J. Med. Virol. 16*:147-162.

Fayram, S. L., Aarnaes, S., and de la Maza, L. M. (1983). Comparison of Culture-set to a conventional tissue culture-fluorescent-antibody technique for isolation and identification of herpes simplex virus. *J. Clin. Microbiol. 18*:215-216.

Frame, B., Mahony, J. B., Balachandran, N., Rawls, W. E., and Chernesky, M. A. (1984). Identification and typing of herpes simplex virus by enzyme immunoassay and monoclonal antibodies. *J. Clin. Microbiol. 20*:162-166.

Fung, J. C., Shanley, J., and Tilton, R. C. (1985). Comparison of the detection of herpes simplex virus in direct clinical specimens with herpes simplex virus specific DNA probes and monoclonal antibodies. *J. Clin. Microbiol. 22*:748-753.

Gerna, G., Battaglia, M., Revello, M. G., and Gerna, M. T. (1983). Typing of herpes simplex virus isolates by enzyme-linked immunosorbent assay: Comparison between indirect and double antibody sandwich techniques. *J. Clin. Microbiol. 17*:942-944.

Gerson, M., Portnoy, J., and Hamelin, C. (1984). Consecutive infections with herpes simplex virus types 1 and 2 within a three-week period. *J. Infect. Dis. 149*:655.

Gleaves, C. A., Wilson, D. J., Wold, A. D., and Smith, T. F. (1985). Detection and serotyping of herpes simplex virus in MRC-5 cells by use of centrifugation and monoclonal antibodies 16 hours postinoculation. *J. Clin. Microbiol. 21*:29-32.

Goldstein, L. C., Corey, L., McDougall, J. K., Tolentino, E., and Nowinski, R. C. (1983). Monoclonal antibodies to herpes simplex viruses: Use in antigenic typing and rapid diagnosis. *J. Infect. Dis. 147*:829-837.

Grout, P. and Barber, V. E. (1976). Cold sores—an epidemiological survey. *J. R. Coll. Gen. Pract. 26*:428-434.

Hampar, B., Zweig, M., Showalter, S. D., Bladen, S. V., and Riggs, C. W. (1985). Enzyme-linked immunosorbent assay for determination of antibodies against herpes simplex virus types 1 and 2 in human serum. *J. Clin. Microbiol. 21*: 496-500.

Harger, J. H., Pazia, G. J., Armstrong, J. A., Breinig, M. C., and Ho, M. (1983). Characteristics and management of pregnancy in women with genital herpes simplex virus infections. *Am. J. Obstet. Gynecol. 145*:784-791.

Hayden, F. G., Sorensen, A. S., and Bateman, J. A. (1983). Comparison of the Immunolok Cultureset Kit and virus isolation for detection of herpes simplex virus in clinical specimens. *J. Clin. Microbiol. 18*:222-224.

Hughes, J. H., Mann, D. R., and Hamparian, V. V. (1986). Viral isolation versus immune staining of infected cell cultures for the laboratory diagnosis of herpes simplex virus infections. *J. Clin. Microbiol. 24*:487-489.

Johnson, F. B., Leavitt, R. W., and Richards, D. F. (1985). Comparison of Scott Selecticult-HSV Kit with conventional culture and direct immunoperoxidase staining for detection of herpes simplex virus in cultures of clinical specimens. *J. Clin. Microbiol. 21*:438-441.

Kalinyak, J. E., Fleagle, G. E., and Docherty, J. J. (1977). Incidence and distribution of herpes simplex virus types 1 and 2 from genital lesions in college women. *J. Med. Virol. 1*:175-181.

Kaufman, R. H. and Rawls, W. H. (1972). Extragenital type 2 herpesvirus infection. *Am. J. Obstet. Gynecol. 112*:866-867.

Kawana, T., Kawaguchi, T., and Sakamoto, S. (1976). Clinical and virological studies on genital herpes. *Lancet 2*:964.

Kit, S., Trkula, D., Qavi, H., Dreesman, G., Kennedy, R. C., Adler-Storthz, K., Kaufman, R., and Adam, E. (1983). Sequential genital infections by herpes simplex viruses types 1 and 2: Restriction endonuclease analysis of viruses from recurrent infections. *Sex. Transm. Dis. 10*:67-71.

Land, S.-A., Skurrie, I. J., and Gilbert, G. L. (1984). Rapid diagnosis of herpes simplex virus infections by enzyme-linked immunosorbent assay. *J. Clin. Microbiol. 19*:865-869.

Lawrence, T. G., Budzko, D. B., and Wilcke, B. W., Jr. (1984). Detection of herpes simplex virus in clinical specimens by an enzyme-linked immunosorbent assay. *Am. J. Clin. Pathol. 81*:339-341.

Lee, F. K., Coleman, R. M., Pereira, L., Bailey, P. D., Tatsuno, M., and Nahmias, A. J. (1985a). Detection of herpes simplex virus type 2-specific antibody with glycoprotein G. *J. Clin. Microbiol. 22*:641-644.

Lee, F., Pereira, L., Coleman, R. M., Bailey, P., Tatsuno, M., Griffin, C., and Nahmias, A. (1985b). New type-specific antigens for detecting antibodies to herpes simplex viruses type 1 (HSV-1) and type 2 (HSV-2). 6th International Meeting International Society for STD Research. Brighton.

Light, I. J. (1979). Postnatal acquisition of herpes simplex virus by the newborn infant: A review of the literature. *Pediatrics 63*:480-482.

Light, I. J. and Linnemann, C. C. (1974). Neonatal herpes simplex infection following delivery by cesarean section. *Obstet. Gynecol. 44*:496-499.

Linnemann, C. C., Buchman, T. G., Light, I. J., and Ballard, J. L. (1978). Transmission of herpes simplex virus type 1 in a nursery for the newborn. Identification of viral isolates by DNA "fingerprinting." *Lancet 1*:964-966.

Lonsdale, D. M. (1979). A rapid method for distinguishing herpes simplex virus type 1 from type 2 by restriction enzyme technology. *Lancet 1*:849-852.

McCaughtry, M. L., Fleagle, G. S., and Docherty, J. J. (1982). Inapparent genital herpes simplex virus infection in college women. *J. Med. Virol. 10*:283-290.

McMillan, A. and Smith, I. W. (1984). Painful anal ulceration in homosexual men. *Br. J. Surg. 71*:215-216.

Maitland, N. J., Smith, I. W., Peutherer, J. F., Robertson, D. H. H., and Jones, K. W. (1982). Restriction enzyme analysis of DNA from genital isolates of herpes simplex virus type 2. *Infect. Immun. 38*:834-842.

Manzella, J. P., McConville, J. H., Valenti, W., Menegus, M. A. Swierkosz, E. M., and Arens, M. (1984). An outbreak of herpes simplex virus type 1 gingivostomatitis in a dental hygiene practice. *J. Am. Med. Assoc. 252*:2019-2022.

Mayo, D. R., Brennan, T., Egbertson, S. H., and Moore, D. J. (1985). Rapid herpes simplex virus detection in clinical samples submitted to a state virology laboratory. *J. Clin. Microbiol. 21*:768-771.

Michalski, F., Shaikh, M., Sahraie, F., Desai, S., Verano, L., and Vallabhaneni, J. (1986). Enzyme linked immunosorbent assay spin amplification technique for herpes virus antigen detection. *J. Clin. Microbiol. 24*:310-311.

Moore, D. F. (1984). Comparison of human fibroblast cells and primary rabbit kidney cells for the isolation of herpes simplex virus. *J. Clin. Microbiol. 19*: 548-549.

Morgan, M. A. and Smith, T. F. (1984). Evaluation of enzyme-linked immunosorbent assay for the detection of herpes simplex virus antigen. *J. Clin. Microbiol. 19*:730-732.

Nahmias, A. J. and Dowdle, W. R. (1968). Antigenic and biologic differences in *Herpesvirus hominis*. *Prog. Med. Virol. 10*:110-159.

Nahmias, A. J., Dowdle, W. R., Kramer, J. L., Luce, C. F., and Mansour, S. C. (1969). Antibodies to *Herpesvirus hominis* types 1 and 2 in the rabbit. *J. Immunol. 102*:956-962.

Nahmias, A. J., Josey, W. E., Naib, Z. M., Luce, C., and Duffey, A. (1970). Antibodies to *Herpesvirus hominis* types 1 and 2 in humans. 1. Patients with genital herpetic infections. *Am. J. Epidemiol. 91*:539-546.

Nahmias, A. J. and Roizman, B. (1973). Infection with herpes simplex viruses 1 and 2. *N. Engl. J. Med. 289*:781-789.

Nahmias, A. J. and Visintine, M. (1976). Herpes simplex virus. In *Infectious Diseases of the Fetus and Newborn* (J. S. Remington and J. D. Kilin, eds.). W. B. Saunders, Philadelphia, pp. 156-190.

Nerurkar, L. S., Jacob, A. J., Madden, D. L., and Sever, J. L. (1983). Detection of genital herpes simplex infections by a tissue culture-fluorescent-antibody technique with biotin avidin. *J. Clin. Microbiol. 17*:149-154.

Nerurkar, L. S., Namba, M., Brashears, G., Jacob, A. J., Lee, Y. J., and Sever, J. L. (1984a). Rapid detection of herpes simplex virus in clinical specimens by use of a capture biotin-streptavidin enzyme linked immunosorbent assay. *J. Clin. Microbiol. 20*:109-114.

Nerurkar, L. S., Namba, M. A., Sever, J. L. (1984b). Comparison of standard tissue culture, tissue culture plus staining and direct staining for detection of genital herpes simplex virus infection. *J. Clin. Microbiol. 19*:631-633.

Nilheden, E., Jeansson, S., and Vahlne, A. (1983). Typing of herpes simplex virus by enzyme-linked immunosorbent assay with monoclonal antibodies. *J. Clin. Microbiol. 17*:677-680.

Olofsson, S., Lundström, M., Marsden, H., Jeansson, S., and Vahlne, A. (1986). Characterisation of a herpes simplex virus type 2-specified glycoprotein and affinity for *N*-acetyl-galactosamine-specific lectins and its identification as 92K or gG. *J. Gen. Virol. 67*:737-744.

Parker, J. and Banatvala, J. (1967). Herpes genitalis—clinical and virological studies. *Br. J. Vener. Dis. 43*:212-216.

Pauls, F. P. and Dowdle, W. R. (1967). A serologic study of *Herpesvirus hominis* strains by microneutralization tests. *J. Immunol. 98*:941-947.

Pereira, L., Dondero, D. V., Gallo, D., Devlin, V., and Woodie, J. D. (1982). Serological analysis of herpes simplex virus types 1 and 2 with monoclonal antibodies. *Infect. Immun. 35*:363-367.

Peterson, E., Schimdt, O. W., Goldstein, L. C., Nowinski, R. C., and Corey, L. (1983). Typing of clinical herpes simplex virus isolates with mouse monoclonal antibodies to herpes simplex virus types 1 and 2: Comparison with the type specific rabbit sera and restriction endonuclease analysis of viral DNA. *J. Clin. Microbiol. 17*:92-96.

Peutherer, J. F. (1970). The specificity of rabbit antisera to *Herpesvirus hominis* and its dependence on the dose of virus inoculated. *J. Med. Microbiol. 3*: 267-272.

Peutherer, J. F., Smith, I. W., and Robertson, D. H. H. (1981). Association of herpes simplex virus types 1 and 2 with clinical sites of infection. In *The Human Herpesviruses* (A. J. Nahmias, W. R. Dowdle, and R. F. Schinazi, eds.). Elsevier, New York, p. 595.

Peutherer, J. F., Smith, I. W., and Robertson, D. H. H. (1982). Genital infection with herpes simplex virus type 1. *J. Infect. 4*:33-35.

Phillips, L. E., Magliolo, R. A., Stehlik, M. L., Whiteman, P. A., Faro, S., and Rogers, T. E. (1985). Retrospective evaluation of the isolation and identification of herpes simplex virus with Cultureset and human fibroblasts. *J. Clin. Microbiol. 22*:255-258.

Rand, K. H., Rasmussen, L. E., Pollard, R. B., Arvin, A., and Merigan, T. C. (1977). Cellular immunity and herpesvirus infection in cardiac-transplant patients. *N. Engl. J. Med. 296*:1372-1377.

Rawls, W. E., Iwamoto, K., Adam, E., Melnick, J. L. (1970). Measurement of antibodies to herpesvirus types 1 and 2 in human sera. *J. Immunol. 104*:599-606.

Reeves, W. C., Corey, L., Adams, H. G., Vontver, L. A., and Holmes, K. K. (1981). Risk of recurrence after first episodes of genital herpes; relation to HSV type and antibody response. *N. Engl. J. Med. 305*:315-319.

Richman, D. D., Cleveland, P. H., and Oxman, M. N. (1982). A rapid enzyme immunofiltration technique using monoclonal antibodies to serotype herpes
simplex virus. *J. Med. Virol.* 9:299-305.

Roizman, B., Norrild, B., Chan, C., and Pereira, L. (1984). Identification and preliminary mapping with monoclonal antibodies of a herpes simplex virus type
2 glycoprotein lacking a known type 1 counterpart. *Virology* 133:242-247.

Roizman, B. and Tognon, M. (1983). Restriction endonuclease patterns of herpes
simplex virus DNA: Application to diagnosis and molecular epidemiology.
Curr. Top. Microbiol. Immunol. 104:273-286.

Rossier, E., Scalia, V., Phipps, P. H., Kennedy, D. A., and Brodeur, B. (1985).
Microcarriers in combination with enzyme immunofiltration and immuno-
fluorescence for detection of herpes simplex virus antigens in culture. *J.
Clin. Microbiol.* 21:335-339.

Rubin, S. J. and Rogers, S. (1984). Comparison of Cultureset and primary rabbit kidney cell culture for the detection of herpes simplex virus. *J. Clin.
Microbiol.* 19:920-922.

Schmidt, N. T., Dennis, J., Devlin, V., Gallo, D., and Mills, J. (1983). Comparison of direct immunofluorescence and direct immunoperoxidase for detection of herpes simplex virus antigen in lesion specimens. *J. Clin. Microbiol.*
18:445-448.

Schmidt, O. W., Fife, K. H., and Corey, L. (1984). Reinfection is an uncommon
occurrence in patients with symptomatic recurrent genital herpes. *J. Infect.
Dis.* 149:645-646.

Sewell, D. L. and Horn, S. A. (1985). Evaluation of a commercial enzyme-linked
immunosorbent assay for the detection of herpes simplex virus. *J. Clin. Microbiol.* 21:457-458.

Sewell, D. L., Horn, S. A., and Dilbeck, P. W. (1984). Comparison of Cultureset
and Bartels immunodiagnostics with conventional tissue culture for isolation
and identification of herpes simplex virus. *J. Clin. Microbiol.* 19:705-706.

Shekarchi, I. C., Sever, J. L., Nerurkar, L., and Fuccillo, D. (1985). Comparison
of enzyme-linked immunosorbent assay with enzyme-linked fluorescence
assay with automated readers for the detection of rubella virus antibody and
herpes simplex virus. *J. Clin. Microbiol.* 21:92-96.

Skinner, G. R. B., Thouless, M. E., and Jordan, J. A. (1971). Antibodies to type
1 and type 2 herpesvirus in women with abnormal cervical cytology. *Br. J.
Obstet. Gynaecol.* 78:1031-1038.

Smith, J. W., Adam, E., Melnick, J. L., and Rawls, W. E. (1972a). Use of the [51]Cr
release test to demonstrate antibody responses to herpes simplex types 1
and 2. *J. Immunol.* 109:554-564.

Smith, J. W., Lowry, S. P., Melnick, J. L., and Rawls, W. E. (1972b). Antibodies
to surface antigens of herpesvirus type 1 and type 2 infected cells among
women with cervical cancer and control women. *Infect. Immun.* 5:305-310.

Smith, I. W., Peutherer, J. F., and MacCallum, F. O. (1967). The incidence of
Herpesvirus hominis antibody in the population. *J. Hyg. (Lond.)* 65:395-
408.

Smith, I. W., Peutherer, J. F., and Robertson, D. H. H. (1973). Characterization
of genital strains of *Herpesvirus hominis. Br. J. Vener. Dis.* 49:385-390.

Smith, I. W., Peutherer, J. F., and Robertson, D. H. H. (1976). Virological studies in genital herpes. *Lancet 2*:1089-1090.

Smith, I. W., Peutherer, J. F., and Hunter, J. M. (1981). Cervical infection with herpes simplex virus. *Lancet 1*:1051.

Sutherland, S., Morgan, B., Mindel, A., and Chan, W. L. (1986). Typing and subtyping of herpes simplex isolates by monoclonal fluorescence. *J. Med. Virol. 18*:235-245.

Swierkosz, E. M., Arens, M. Q., and Rivetna, K. A. (1985a). Problems associated with the use of (*E*)-5-(2-bromovinyl)-2'-deoxyuridine for typing herpes simplex virus. *J. Clin. Microbiol. 21*:459-461.

Swierkosz, E. M., Arens, M. Q., Schmidt, R. R., and Armstrong, T. (1985b). Evaluation of two immunofluorescence assays with monoclonal antibodies for typing herpes simplex virus. *J. Clin. Microbiol. 21*:643-644.

Teglbjaerg, C. C., Feldborg, R., and Norrild, B. (1986). Immunological reactivity of human sera with individual herpes simplex proteins. A comparative study of sera from patients with preinvasive or invasive cervical cancer and controls. *J. Med. Virol. 18*:169-180.

Toews, G. D., Bergstresser, P. R., and Streilein, J. W. (1980). Epidermal Langerhans cell density determines whether contact hypersensitivity or unresponsiveness follows skin painting with DNFB. *J. Immunol. 124*:445-453.

Volpi, A., Lakeman, A. D., Pereira, L., and Stagno, S. (1983). Monoclonal antibodies for rapid diagnosis and typing of genital herpes infections during pregnancy. *Am. J. Obstet. Gynecol. 146*:813-815.

Warford, A. L., Levy, R. A., and Rekrut, K. A. (1984). Evaluation of a commercial enzyme-linked immunosorbent assay for detection of herpes simplex virus antigen. *J. Clin. Microbiol. 20*:490-493.

Whitley, R. J., Nahmias, A. J., Visintine, A. M., Fleming, C. L., and Alford, C. A. (1980). The natural history of herpes simplex virus infection of mother and newborn. *Pediatrics 66*:489-494.

Wolontis, S. and Jeansson, S. (1977). Correlation of herpes simplex virus types 1 and 2 with clinical features of infection. *J. Infect. Dis. 135*:28-33.

Woodman, C. B. J. and Weaver, J. B. (1986). Virological screening for herpes simplex virus (HSV) in late pregnancy. *Lancet 1*:744.

Woolley, P. D., Monteiro, E., Wilson, J., and Kinghorn, G. R. (1986). Virological screening in late pregnancy in recurrent genital herpes. *Lancet 1*:1336.

Yaeger, A. (1984). Genital herpes simplex infections: Effects of asymptomatic shedding and latency on management of infections in pregnant women and neonates. *J. Invest. Dermatol. 83*:53S-56S.

Zheng, Z. M., Mayo, D. R., and Hsiung, G. D. (1983). Comparison of biological, biochemical, immunological and immunochemical techniques for typing herpes simplex virus isolates. *J. Clin. Microbiol. 17*:396-399.

Zimmerman, D. H., Mundon, F. R., Croson, S. E., Henchal, L. S., Docherty, J. J., and O'Neill, S. P. (1985). Identification and typing of herpes simplex virus types 1 and 2 by monoclonal antibodies, sensitivity to the drug (*E*)-5-(2-bromovinyl)-2'-deoxyuridine and restriction enzyme endonuclease analysis of the viral DNA. *J. Med. Virol. 15*:215-222.

THIRTEEN

Detection of Human Papilloma Viruses of the Genital Tract

Mary Norval
Edinburgh University
Medical School
Edinburgh, Scotland

I. INTRODUCTION

Papilloma viruses are known to infect a variety of species including man, dogs, horses, rabbits, deer, sheep, cattle, mice, and birds, and to induce papillomatosis (warts) in these animals (Lancaster and Olson, 1982). Warts have been recognized for centuries and were transmitted experimentally almost 80 years ago (Ciuffo, 1907). Traditionally warts were thought of as benign or even hyperplastic lesions of cutaneous or mucosal tissues, but gradually their potential for transformation to carcinomas was recognized. In particular, in recent years an association between human papilloma viruses (HPV) and the development of genital neoplasias has been found, which has fostered interest in the papilloma viruses and their detection. Concomitantly, major advances in the molecular cloning of papilloma viruses have partly compensated for our inability to culture the viruses in vitro and have made possible some studies on their behavior.

This chapter outlines the biology of HPV types and reviews genital warts and the association of HPV with genital carcinomas. Methods for the detection of HPV in genital lesions are assessed, including the relevance of monoclonal antibodies (MAbs) and polyclonal antibodies.

II. HUMAN PAPILLOMA VIRUSES

A. Papilloma Virus Types

Papilloma viruses belong to the genus A of the family *Papovaviridae*. The virions are naked, about 50 nm in diameter, with icosahedral symmetry and contain 72 capsomeres. Particles of HPV prepared from plantar warts by grinding skin scrapings followed by equilibrium centrifugation in CsC1 are shown in Fig. 1.

In the past few years it has become clear that there are many types of papilloma viruses that infect particular species in preferential sites and with typical clinical manifestations. In man, the number of types has risen to 45, and more are still being discovered. Types 1-18 and their associated clinical lesions are outlined in Table 1.

A new type is designated if it shares less than 50% sequence homology with other papilloma viruses as tested by reassociation kinetics under stringent conditions of nucleic acid hybridization (Coggin and zur Hausen, 1979) (see Sect. VI.E for an explanation of hybridization conditions). There should also be significant antigenic variation from any other type, although this is often not possible to test if virus particles are either not present or are present in low numbers. Furthermore, viral protein products are not now well defined either in terms of molecular weight or function. In practice, typing is based on molecular cloning of viral DNA, followed by blot hybridization with known human types under different stringency conditions. A subtype has less than 100%, but more than 50%, sequence

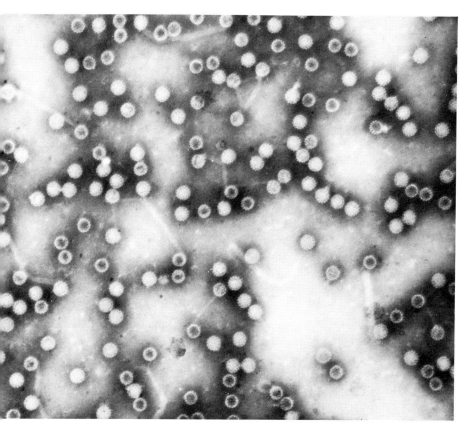

Fig. 1 Negative stain of HPV-1 particles prepared by grinding plantar warts and purifying by CsC1 gradient centrifugation. Particles are about 55 nm in diameter.

homology with known types. Perhaps it is surprising that typing without characterization of viral mRNA and viral proteins should lead to such good concordance with clinical lesions. Recombination between different types has been suggested (Gissmann, 1984).

B. Genomic Organization

The genome of HPV types consists of a double-stranded, covalently closed, circular DNA molecule containing about 7900 base pairs. As papilloma viruses cannot be cultured in vitro it is important to ascertain their genomic organization from nucleotide sequence analysis so that predictions can be made about their possible protein products, control elements, and associations with different types of cells.

Table 1 Types of HPV and Their Predominant Clinical Lesions

HPV type	Lesion
1	Plantar wart
2	Common wart (mosaic type)
3	Plane wart
4	Palmar and plantar warts
5, 8, 9, 12, 14, 15, 17	Epidermodysplasia verruciformis (EV)
6	Condyloma acuminatum, flat condyloma, CIN 1 and 2
7	Butchers' hand wart
10	Plane wart
11	Condyloma acuminatum, flat condyloma, laryngeal papilloma, CIN 1 and 2
13	Focal epithelial hyperplasia
16, 18	Carcinoma of uterine cervix, vulva, and penis, bowenoid papulosis, vulval intraepithelial neoplasia grade 3, CIN 3

Some HPV types are found in small numbers only in wart lesions, as in genital warts, and some are present only in the form of viral DNA, not as mature virus particles, as in cervical carcinomas. Thus, sequencing here depends upon successful molecular cloning of papilloma virus DNA. Where possible, the cloning methods depend upon the isolation and purification of viral DNA, followed by linearization, either at the single *BamHI* or *EcoRI* site; making recombinant plasmids, often with (pBR322); and cloning in suitable bacterial strains. When viral particles are not found, a genomic library of the appropriate tissue is made by cleaving cellular DNA with a restriction endonuclease using bacteriophage as vector. Recombinant phages containing viral DNA are then cloned. These strategies are reviewed by Gissmann and Schwarz (1985).

Initial studies led to the elucidation of the nucleotide sequence of bovine papilloma virus type 1 (BPV 1) (Chen et al., 1982), and subsequently the sequence of HPV-1a (Clad et al., 1982; Danos et al., 1982), HPV-6b (Schwarz et al., 1983), and HPV-16 (Seedorf et al., 1985) have been found. The general organization is very similar in all these types and is illustrated in Fig. 2 for HPV-6b and HPV-16.

Intracellular replication of DNA viruses is often split into three phases: first, early proteins are synthesized which are preponderantly nonstructural in function, then viral DNA is replicated, and finally late proteins are synthesized which are mostly structural, making up the capsomere subunits of the virus particle. The proteins are coded for by open-reading frames on the viral DNA. All major open-reading frames (ORFs) are on one DNA strand. Potentially, these encode polypeptides larger than 90 amino acids. There are several presumptive early ORFs,

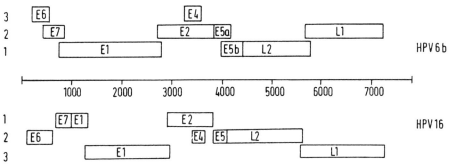

Fig. 2 Open-reading frames of HPV-6b and HPV-16 genomes (*Source*: data from Schwarz et al., 1983 and Seedorf et al., 1985).

designated *E1* to *E7*, on the basis of size, and two late ORFs, *L1* and *L2*. Between *L1* and *E6* is a noncoding region of about 1000 base pairs that is thought to contain the origin of DNA replication and the promoter for early gene transcription. Transcriptional enhancer elements functioning in a position-independent and orientation-independent manner have been mapped within this region and also in the other region between the *E* and *L* parts of the genome (Lusky et al., 1983; Spalholz et al., 1985).

An in vitro transforming system is available for BPV-1 and has yielded interesting results on genomic organization. A segment containing 69% of the viral genome was found to be necessary for transformation of certain mouse cells to focus formation, growth in soft agar, and tumorigenicity in athymic nude mice (Lowy et al., 1980); furthermore, the genetic information encoded by *E2, E3, E4,* and *E5* was sufficient to induce transformation (Lusky and Botchan, 1985; Yang et al., 1985a). *E1* function is involved in extrachromosomal viral DNA maintenance in transformed cells (Lusky and Botchan, 1984). *E2* is responsible for the transactivation of the enhancer located in the noncoding region (Yang et al., 1985b). This could lead to a direct effect on transformation as well as increased expression of other ORFs including *E6, E7,* and *E1. E5* may be involved in inducing proliferation of dermal fibroblasts in fibropapillomas. It will be interesting to see if the early ORFs of HPV have similar functions, despite their lack of homology with BPV-1 and their biological differences in inducing epithelial proliferation rather than fibropapillomas.

Differences in coding potential between different HPV types may be of functional importance. For example, HPV-16, which is associated mainly with genital carcinomas, is not like HPV-1a and HPV-6b in some respects. The ORFs for *E1* of HPV-16 are split into two reading frames, and *E4* and *E5* do not have a translation initiation codon (Seedorf et al., 1985). The importance of these changes is not known at the present time. By studying the sequences of HPV-16 and HPV-18

in various cervical cell lines derived from carcinomas, the presence of *E1* but probably not *E2* was thought to be necessary for expression of the malignant phenotype (Pater and Pater, 1985).

Viral mRNA synthesis has been examined mainly in BPV-1 and cottontail
rabbit papilloma virus (CRPV) systems (Pfister, 1984). Some interesting results
with CRPV show that transcription differs in virus-producing benign tumors from
malignant nonproductive tumors (Phelps et al., 1985). The regions of the genome
containing the ORFs, once transcribed to RNA, probably undergo excision and
splicing to make the mRNAs. Work has begun on analyzing viral mRNAs in cervical cell lines to find out which regions of the genome are transcribed, whether
or not splicing occurs, and whether cotranscribed host sequences are important
(Schwarz et al., 1985). In one report, HPV-16 mRNA was found only rarely in
cervical carcinoma biopsies containing HPV-16 DNA (Lehn et al., 1985). Thus,
continuous expression of HPV may not be necessary for the maintenance of a
transformed state. The implications for detection methods, such as assaying for
HPV protein products, are obvious.

C. Viral Protein Products

None of the early gene products of HPV types have yet been identified in in vitro
transforming systems or in warts, and no specific tumor antigens are characterized
in vivo. It is likely that such proteins are, in fact, synthesized as shown by the
conservation of the amino acid sequences coded for by the early regions of different papilloma virus genomes. They may be present, however, only in small
quantities or be weakly antigenic so that new methods may have to be developed
to detect them. One approach may be to translate viral mRNAs in vitro. Another
may be to take segments of ORFs, especially the early ORFs, and to insert these
into bacterial expression vectors under the control of inducible promoters, in the
hope of getting translation of viral products.

L1 and *L2* are expected to code for the viral structural polypeptides. Major
polypeptides of molecular weight 57,000, 54,000, and 44,000 have been described
in purified HPV-1, HPV-2, and HPV-3, in association with other minor polypeptides of smaller molecular weights, which varied among isolates (Gissmann et al.,
1977). Such work has been dogged by difficulties in the preparation of adequately
purified virus particles, in sufficient quantity for analysis, from pooled clinical
material. It should be possible, however, to obtain a sufficient quantity for the
preparation of monoclonal antibodies (MAbs). In BPV-2, *L1* codes for the major
polypeptide of the capsid, which has a molecular weight 55,000; *L2* probably
codes for a polypeptide of molecular weight 50,000 (Potter and Meinke, 1985).

Antisera have been prepared against purified HPV, where it is possible to prepare sufficient quantities of purified virions, i.e., types 1, 2, 3, 5, 8, and 9 (Gissmann et al., 1977; Jablonska et al., 1982). These are type-specific and detect viral

capsid antigens in the nuclei of infected cells. If the antisera are prepared using virus particles disrupted with sodium dodecyl sulfate (SDS), the type specificity is then lost and the antisera cross-react, not only with the capsid antigens of other HPV types but also with papilloma viruses from other species, such as cattle, dogs, horses, and deer (Jenson et al., 1980). Again the antigen is located in the nuclei of infected cells. Probably there are genus-specific amino acid sequences, shared among all papilloma viruses, which lie in a part of the capsid protein not normally exposed on the surface of virions. As outlined in Sect. VI.D, both the genus-specific and type-specific antisera to the capsid antigens are of use in screening tissues for evidence of papilloma virus infection.

III. HUMAN WARTS

Wart lesions induced by HPV infection are primarily epithelial proliferations of the skin or mucosa. This results in overgrowth of subepithelial capillaries (papillomatosis) and in thickening of the stratum spinosum (acanthosis) and stratum corneum (hyperkeratosis). Eventually, probably to accommodate the epithelial proliferation on a limited base, the basement membrane and the overlying strata corrugate, creating strands or outgrowths whose vessels (which grow correspondingly) nourish the epithelium. The lesion is thus essentially fibroepithelial with, usually, some (limited) branching of the processes or "asperities."

Warts are ordinarily benign, showing limited growth and generally regress spontaneously after several weeks or months. They can persist, however, and can recur. Abrasion of the skin is probably required before the virus is able to infect a new host, and the incubation period is thought to be between 3 and 18 months (Rowson and Mahy, 1967). It is not known what happens during this period, how infective HPV types are, or if subclinical infections occur.

A few cells of the basal layer contain HPV DNA in their nuclei (Beckmann et al., 1985) and many more in the first or second suprabasal layer of the stratum spinosum (Grussendorf and zur Hausen, 1979). The viral DNA may be integrated or extrachromosomal, although the latter is the more commonly found state with most, but not all, types. The parabasal cells probably represent the first target for the virus. The structural proteins begin to appear in the cells of the upper layers of the stratum spinosum, and virus particles, when present, appear in this layer and the stratum granulosum. The virions can sometimes be seen in paracrystalline arrays in the nuclei and enmeshed in keratin in the stratum corneum. Figure 3 shows a diagram of the epidermis infected with HPV, and Fig. 4 an array of HPV-1 in the stratum granulosum of a plantar wart.

The cells of the basal and suprabasal layers may be nonpermissive for HPV and the association with virus a transforming one (Fletcher and Norval, 1983). In vitro, HPV fails to replicate productively, even in cultures of keratinocytes that

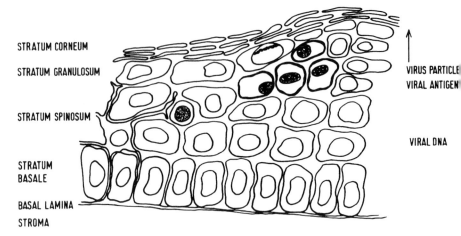

STRATUM CORNEUM

STRATUM GRANULOSUM

STRATUM SPINOSUM

STRATUM
BASALE

BASAL LAMINA

STROMA

VIRUS PARTICLE
VIRAL ANTIGEN

VIRAL DNA

Fig. 3   Diagram of the epidermis showing an area where papilloma virus is replicating.

are forming a granular layer, and it is found only as viral DNA, 50-250 copies per cell, present as stable nonintegrated genomes (Taichman et al., 1983). As the keratinocytes become more differentiated in the stratum spinosum, the association with virus probably becomes permissive. The productive infection in the superficial cells is marked by the presence of koilocytic cells, first noted by Koss and Durfee (1956). In brief, these can be described as having densely staining irregular indented or folded nuclei and a ballooned cytoplasm with a clear, glycogen-free perinuclear halo. Sometimes, there are basophilic nuclear inclusions that consist of arrays of virus particles. The koilocytes are considered pathognomonic of HPV infection. Different types of koilocytes have been described by their histopathological appearance (Crum et al., 1985), but whether these represent separate clinical entities, infection with different HPV types, or stages of permissiveness for HPV replication is not known.

There is increasing evidence that HPV can become latent and may be present in the epidermis without clinical lesions and morphological signs. The cervix, in particular, may be subject to latency which may be important for the diagnosis and management of patients (Ferenczy et al., 1985; Syrjanen et al., 1985).

IV. GENITAL WARTS

It has become increasingly evident that papilloma viruses associated with infections of the male and female genital areas are spread preponderantly by sexual transmission. There is probably no correlation between genital and skin warts.

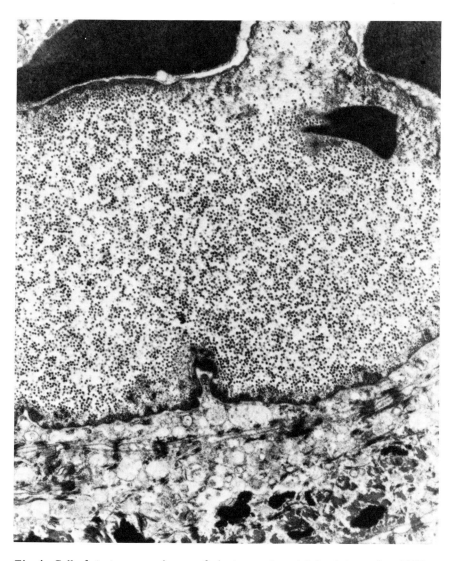

Fig. 4   Cell of stratum granulosum of plantar wart containing intranuclear HPV particles, an osmiophilic intranuclear inclusion, and cytoplasmic keratin masses (X15,000).

Genital warts are found in populations of high promiscuity (Waugh, 1972), in age groups of sexual maturity, and where sexual activity is highest (zur Hausen, 1977). The sites of genital warts are commonly those of frequent contact during coitus. Horizontal spread can be traced from subjects with the disease (Oriel, 1971). The incidence of genital HPV infection increased during the last decade and, in Britain, now represents at least 6% of all cases seen in departments of genitourinary medicine (Adler, 1984). During 1984, 13% of 5013 men and 13% of 3230 women who attended the Department of Genitourinary Medicine in Edinburgh had genital warts (A. McMillan, personal communication).

In men, genital warts are found on the glans and shaft of the penis, prepuce, frenum, and coronal sulcus, urethral meatus, scrotum, and anus. In women, they are present on the introitus, vulva, vagina, cervix, perineum, and anus. Until 1976, condyloma acuminatum was the only known manifestation of genital HPV infection. With the introduction of colposcopy into clinical practice and the use of DNA hybridization methods, other clinical features of genital infection, particularly the flat condyloma and bowenoid papulosis have been recognized.

A. Condyloma Acuminatum

The classic exophytic genital wart or condyloma acuminatum is characterized by papillomatosis, acanthosis, elongation and thickening of the rete pegs, and koilocytosis (Woodruff and Peterson, 1958): its growth pattern is illustrated in Fig. 5A. It is found on the penis, anus, vulva, perineum, and cervix (zur Hausen, 1977). Virus particles are seen in some lesions, around 50% in most surveys, although not normally in high numbers. Viral antigens have also been detected and viral DNA, preponderantly types 6 and 11 (Gissmann et al., 1983). Malignant conversion into carcinomas of the penis and vulva is rare (zur Hausen, 1977).

Giant condylomata located on the penis were described by Buschke and Lowenstein in 1931. They have invasive growth properties after long periods but without metastases. They are associated with HPV-6 and HPV-11 (Zachow et al., 1982).

B. Flat Condyloma (Flat Koilocytosis)

In the cervix, predominantly, HPV infections assume a less exophytic form and flat lesions are found. Often they appear as white epithelium in the transformation zone of cervical ectropion where subcolumnar reserve cells are proliferating and redifferentiating into squamous epithelium. It is not known why there should be a preferential site for this type of wart, but perhaps the rate of cell or tumor production is highest here, or the keratin pattern may be unusual. Flat condylomata were not recognized as wart lesions until 1976 (Meisels and Fortin, 1976) and, on colposcopy, are often very difficult to distinguish from lesions of cervical

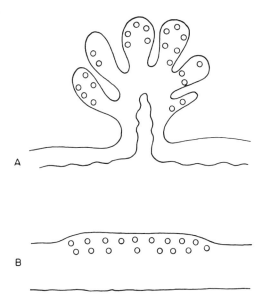

Fig. 5   Diagram of growth pattern of (A) condyloma acuminatum and (B) flat condyloma. Koilocytes denoted by o.

intraepithelial neoplasia (CIN), being classified traditionally as CIN grade 1 (mild dysplasia). They are also found on the vulva and penile glans (Gross et al., 1985b). The growth pattern of flat condyloma is shown in Fig. 5B. The nomenclature of this type of wart is confusing as it has been called variously a flat wart, a non-condylomatous cervical wart, subclinical HPV, flat koilocytic lesion, and atypical condyloma, but the term flat condyloma is being used increasingly despite the inherent contradiction in this description (condyloma is derived from the Greek *kondylos*: knuckle) (see Fletcher, 1983, for a critical review of nomenclature and classification).

   In this decade, flat condylomata of the uterine cervix have become recognized as common infections. It has been estimated that 1.3% of unselected women show cytological changes consistent with HPV infections on routine Papanicolaou smears and 25% of colposcopically directed punch biopsies also show similar changes (Reid et al., 1980). There is evidence to suggest that the prevalence of flat condylomata of the cervix is increasing, although there is more awareness of this condition and better detection methods than formerly (Oriel, 1983). Histologically, as with condylomata acuminata, flat condylomata show koilocytic cells; genus-specific viral antigen is present in about half the cases, although its distribution is often patchy and sparse compared with exophytic genital warts (Woodruff et al., 1980). The DNAs of HPV-6 and HPV-11 are found in 50-60% flat condylomata (Gissmann et al., 1982; Gross et al., 1985b).

In addition to the flat condyloma, an endophytic or inverted condyloma has been described (Meisels et al., 1977). Here squamous epithelium has proliferated in the necks of the endocervical glands with superficial koilocytosis. It is possible that this is merely a papilloma virus infection of a branching epidermized gland, and Fletcher (1983) has suggested that it should not be considered as different from flat condyloma.

C. Bowenoid Papulosis

First noted in 1970 (Lloyd, 1970), bowenoid papulosis consists of flat, multifocal, slightly pigmented papules, often verrucoid, on the shaft of the penis, and affects young adults. Although appearing to be benign macroscopically and often regressing spontaneously, these papules show microscopic tissue changes of squamous cell carcinoma in situ. They assume a flat, papillary endophytic or papillomatous exophytic form (Gross et al., 1985a). Only 5% of lesions show the genus-specific antigen of HPV, but over 50% contain HPV-16 DNA (Braun et al., 1983; Gross et al., 1985a; Ikenberg et al., 1983). This is taken to indicate low productive infection with HPV-16 in epithelial cells primarily nonpermissive for the virus and transformed to some extent by the presence of viral DNA. Bowenoid papulosis of men may represent an important reservoir of HPV-16.

Histologically genital Bowen's disease is very similar to bowenoid papulosis, except lesions are not multifocal and they occur on the glans of the penis (Wade, 1978). The average age of patients is 50, and HPV-16 is found in 80% of the patients (Ikenberg et al., 1983).

V. ASSOCIATION OF HUMAN PAPILLOMA VIRUS WITH GENITAL CARCINOMAS

Almost 150 years ago Rigoni-Stern (1842) observed that uterine cancers were more prevalent in married than in unmarried women, and were almost absent in certain orders of nuns. Confirmation of these findings, indicating that sexual behavior and cervical cancer were associated, was published in 1973 (Rotkin), and since then a sexually transmitted agent has been sought. In addition, based on epidemiological data, a progression from a premalignant change in the cervix to a truly malignant state is suggested (Meisels et al., 1982). These stages are recorded histologically as CIN 1 (mild dysplasia), CIN 2 (moderate dysplasia), CIN 3 (severe dysplasia/carcinoma in situ), and invasive carcinoma. Various viruses, such as herpes simplex type 2 and cytomegalovirus, have been implicated as possible agents in this neoplastic process, whereas HPV was suggested only a few years ago (zur Hausen, 1976). The association between HPV and abnormalities

Table 2 The Association of HPV with Neoplastic Changes in the Uterine Cervix

	% with koilocytes on cytology	% with koilocytes on histopathology	HPV antigen-positive		DNA content		HPV type by DNA hybridization
					% diploid	% aneuploid	
CIN 1	80.6	95	28	43	33	8	HPV-6 or 11 (42%) HPV-16 or 18 (18%)
CIN 2	72	77	22	15	12	65	HPV-6 or 11 (8%)
CIN 3	58.1	54	9	15[a]	0	82	HPV-6 or 11 (1%)
Cervical carcinoma							HPV-16 or 18 (51%)
Ref.	Baird (1985)	Kurman et al. (1983)	Reid et al. (1982)	Kurman et al. (1983)	Reid et al. (1984)		Reviewed in Gissmann (1984)

[a]In epithelium adjacent to lesion.

of the uterine cervix rapidly gained ground, however, after it was realized that CIN often occurred in conjunction with koilocytosis (Meisels et al., 1982).

Various groups soon added data in support of HPV infections being important in CIN: their studies, some of which are summarized in Table 2, included histopathology, looking for features of papilloma virus infection, screening for HPV antigen using an antiserum against the genus-specific papilloma antigen, and detection of HPV DNA by nucleic acid hybridization. In addition to these data, HPV-16 is found in CIN lesions where there are abnormal mitotic figures and nuclear atypia in all layers of the squamous epithelium. These lesions have an aneuploid nuclear DNA content and a high risk of progression to malignancy (Crum et al., 1984; Crum et al., 1985).

Similar results to those found in the cervix have been obtained for vulval condylomata and vulval intraepithelial neoplasia (VIN) (Boshart et al., 1984, Ferenczy et al., 1985; Gissmann, 1984).

Although the viral DNA in HPV-6 and HPV-11 lesions is in the same state as in other papilloma virus infections, i.e., nonintegrated and circular (Lehn et al., 1984), that of HPV types 16 and 18 in carcinomas may be different. There is evidence for head-to-tail tandem genomic repeats persisting in a nonintegrated and circular form, and for some integrated genomes persisting as head-to-tail repeated oligomers of up to 20 per integration site or as monomers (Boshart et al., 1984; Durst et al., 1985). In another study, HPV-16 DNA was found as a single copy covalently linked to tumor cell DNA in a cervical carcinoma (Lehn et al., 1985). Integration of HPV-16 and HPV-18 also occurs in some cervical cell lines (Pater and Pater, 1985; Schwarz et al., 1985; Yee et al., 1985). In contrast, Fukushima et al. (1985) failed to find HPV DNA sequences in the majority of invasive squamous cell carcinomas of the cervix. The sensitivity of the assay system used was estimated at one copy of viral genome per 20 cells with a homologous HPV probe and one copy per three cells with a heterologous DNA probe.

The consensus is that HPV-6 and HPV-11 are found in a nonintegrated form most commonly in genital warts and in CIN and VIN of low grades and that this association is one of low malignant potential; on the other hand, HPV-16 and HPV-18 are found most commonly in genital carcinomas in an integrated form and have high malignant potential (Crawford, 1984). Various cofactors such as infection with a second virus or bacteria, or even smoking, are undoubtedly important (zur Hausen, 1982). It has not yet been possible to document if HPV plays a casual or causal role in genital neoplasias (Singer et al., 1984) and more data are required, particularly on what happens during progression of the lesions.

VI. DETECTION OF GENITAL HUMAN PAPILLOMA VIRUS INFECTIONS

These methods are wide-ranging and include gross appearance, colposcopy, cervical cytological and histopathological studies of cervical biopsies, electron microscopy, detection of HPV antigens, detection of HPV DNA, and immune responses. Each test gives valuable information, although the only reliable method of typing HPV at the present time is by DNA hybridization. Most reports combine more than one technique, which is prudent until the position becomes clearer and definitive reagents are available.

A. Gross Appearance and Colposcopy

There is little problem in identifying the classic condyloma acuminatum by its gross appearance, and a good description is given in Woodruff et al. (1958). On colposcopic examination of the vagina and cervix, there is often a thick white epithelial focus with surface projections containing capillary loops. Early lesions are more difficult to define and have only small surface projections (asperities) (Meisels et al., 1979; Reid et al., 1980).

Flat condylomata have a smooth or irregular surface, only slightly raised from the surrounding epithelium. They exist in both dysplastic and nondysplastic forms. Recently, the colposcopic appearances of HPV lesions in the cervix have been classified as normal, mosaic, warty, leukoplakial (thickened white epithelium), or a combination (Vayrynen et al., 1985). Colposcopic approaches, however, do not reliably detect and separate the types, and in practice, clinicians are more concerned about dysplastic zones, whether koilocytic or not, and tend to direct their attention and their biopsies to them. Distinguishing patches of dysplasia from nondysplastic flat condylomata or coincident dysplasia and koilocytosis is unreliable colposcopically and requires histological examination (Kirkup et al., 1982). Condylomata can be suspected if the lesions are multiple, if they are present outside the transformation zone, and if there are dilated capillaries in the surrounding native squamous epithelium (Meisels et al., 1977).

B. Cytology and Histopathology

There are characteristic cellular changes in Papanicolaou smears of women with condylomata (Meisels et al., 1984; Syrjanen, 1984). Normally, inflammatory cells are absent, whereas koilocytes and dyskeratotic cells are present, although not invariably so. The koilocyte is considered pathognomonic for HPV infection. It is an intermediate or superficial squamous cell with enlarged hyperchromatic nucleus and an area of perinuclear clearing. The rest of the cytoplasm is thickened, often with an amphophilic-staining pattern. It may be binucleated or multinucleated. Dyskeratocytes are often shed singly or in clusters. They are small keratinized squamous cells with orangeophilic cytoplasm and large homogeneous nuclei. Sometimes the nuclei are atypical and it is difficult to distinguish papilloma virus infections from CIN or carcinoma. Neoplastic cells have a well-reserved chromatin structure, defined nuclear membranes, and abnormal nucleocytoplasmic ratios but these features are hard to define and sometimes characteristic cells are not shed

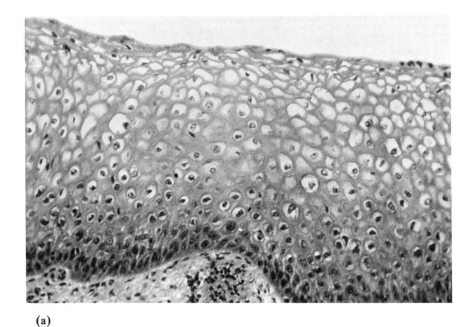

(a)

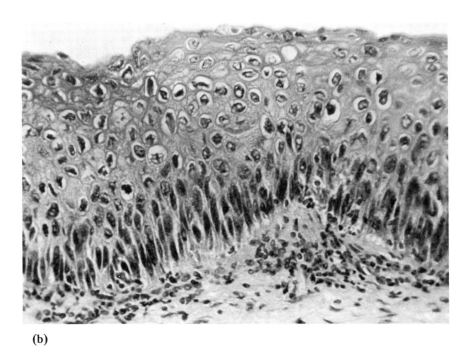

(b)

Fig. 6 Histopathology of cervical biopsies showing (a) normal epithelium with koilocytosis and (b) CIN 2 (moderate dysplasia) with concurrent koilocytosis (hematoxylin-eosin; ×160).

from the condyloma. Colposcopically directed cervical biopsies should be taken when there is an abnormal Papanicolaou smear.

Some features of the histopathology of genital warts have already been covered in Sect. IV. Condyloma acuminatum is distinguished by papillomatous growth with acanthosis. There is elongation and thickening of rete pegs, and koilocytes are prominent, often in the tips of the papillary projections. In the flat condyloma, the most striking feature is the presence of koilocytes in the middle and upper epithelial layers.

The flat condylomata are sometimes found in association with CIN, either within the premalignant lesion or adjacent to it (Fig. 6). This makes the detection of HPV infection and the grading of the dysplasia particularly difficult. A simplified and helpful scheme for reporting the histopathology of cervical biopsies is to grade the dysplasia with and without koilocytosis and, if desired, to note whether the koilocytes are adjacent to, remote from, or coincident with the dysplasia (Fletcher, 1983).

Recently an attempt has been made to forecast more accurately which lesions might progress by reporting on the ploidy pattern of biopsies (Fu et al., 1983). While diploidy represents a normal cellular pattern, polyploidy is indicative of hyperplasia and benign neoplasms, and aneuploidy of a malignancy (Bohm and Sandritter, 1975). It is possible to quantitate nuclear DNA in smears or tissue sections by microspectrophotometry or computerized image analysis after Feulgen staining. In condylomata, diploid or polyploid DNA is found, while in CIN, persisting for a year or more, aneuploid DNA is detected; in CIN that has regressed, most nuclei are diploid or polyploid. This technique is demanding and time-consuming, perhaps not likely to be useful in a routine laboratory, but automated fluorescent flow cytometry may be developed in the near future to give similar information.

Measurement of DNA content of cells has been complemented by observations of abnormal mitotic figures and diffuse nuclear atypia in VIN lesions (Crum et al., 1982). In vulval condylomata, nuclear atypia is seen only in the mature epithelial cells and abnormal mitoses are absent. Furthermore, Crum et al. (1985) have shown that a distinction between HPV types in CIN might be made histologically. In condylomatous lesions containing koilocytic atypia and nuclear atypia in the upper epithelial layers, 61% were infected with HPV-6 or HPV-11. In CIN lesions in association with condylomata showing nuclear atypia in all the epithelial layers, or abnormal mitoses plus koilocytic atypia, or both, 82% were infected with HPV-16. In CIN lesions with minimal epithelial layer maturation and nuclear atypia in all epithelial layers, or with abnormal mitoses, or with both, 33% had evidence of HPV-16 DNA and 22% had untypable viral DNA. This analysis shows that careful histopathological assessment may be able to pinpoint those lesions containing HPV-16 that may have a tendency to progress. However, the CIN lesions of grades 1 and 2 in association with HPV infections may be difficult to fit into this histological categorization. Furthermore, in contrast to the results of Crum et al. (1985) another study of HPV infections of condylomatous and condylomatalike lesions of the male and female genital tract, perianal skin, and anal mucosa, concluded that the structural abnormality of a lesion was not sufficient to predict HPV type, even taking details of the koilocytic features into account (Gross et al., 1985b). The only correlation found between severe epithelial atypia without koilocytosis and HPV-16 DNA was in bowenoid papulosis.

Therefore, it currently seems wise to substantiate the microscopically abnormal appearance of condylomatous or dysplastic lesions with detection of HPV by additional methods. However, from the viewpoint of the patient, a useful grading of cervical dysplasias can be made using quick-frozen sections which avoids the inevitable delay with paraffin sections. The patient can, therefore, be advised at the time of colposcopy and treated immediately after diagnosis (Fletcher et al., 1985).

C. Electron Microscopy

Condylomata acuminata prepared for electron microscopy by standard procedures were first shown to contain HPV virions in 1968 in Edinburgh (Dunn and Ogilvie, 1968). The virus particles have a characteristic size and shape which makes them relatively easy to detect in cells, even at low densities. Since then, several groups have undertaken surveys of flat condylomata and reported HPV in approximately half the biopsies screened (Ferenczy et al., 1981; Pilotti et al., 1981; Reid et al., 1980). The particles are always found within the nuclei of koilocytic cells and sometimes in the superficial dyskeratotic cells, but in all types of genital warts, they are present in only low numbers. The HPV particles have never been reported in malignant squamous cell tumors (Kurman et al., 1981; Syrjanen and Pyrohonen, 1982).

It is possible to reprocess cells for electron microscopy from Papanicolaou smears using the methods outlined in Smith and Coleman (1983). Virus particles are seen in koilocytes and dyskeratocytes in about half the smears showing overall cytological evidence of HPV infection (Meisels et al., 1984).

Although electron microscopy has provided valuable information about productive HPV infections in genital condylomata, it is a painstaking technique given the paucity of virus particles. It will not distinguish different types of HPV and obviously cannot be used to detect HPV DNA in malignant tumors. Apart from research purposes, it has been largely superseded by detection of HPV antigens (see Sect. VI.D). However recently, by use of electron microscopy, interesting results have been obtained related to the possible latency of HPV in the cervix. In a prospective follow-up study of women who had had abnormal smears, Syrjanen et al. (1985) screened punch biopsies by electron microscopy and found HPV particles in tissues that were colposcopically and histologically normal. Although these studies could be undertaken by DNA hybridization methods

(Ferenczy et al., 1985), information on the structure and numbers of virions and on the cell types infected can be obtained only from electron microscopy.

D. Detection of Viral Antigens

1. Polyclonal Antibodies

The method commonly employed for the detection of HPV antigens in genital condylomata is the peroxidase-antiperoxidase technique, as outlined by Sternberger, 1979 (reviewed in Leisels et al., 1984). This procedure has a great advantage in that sections of formalin-fixed, paraffin-embedded material can be used. A genus-specific papilloma virus antiserum is made by injecting rabbits with purified disrupted HPV-1 from pooled plantar warts or BPV-1 from bovine fibropapillomas. This antiserum binds to viral antigens and is detected by adding a secondary antiserum followed by a soluble complex of peroxidase-antiperoxidase which binds to the free site of the secondary antibody. A substrate of peroxidase and H_2O_2 are added; in a positive test, a dark brown staining results.

In essence, HPV antigen is detected in the nuclei of some koilocytes and occasionally in dyskeratocytes. In some surveys it is found more often in flat condylomata than in exophytic lesions (Ferenczy et al., 1981; Morin et al., 1981), whereas in others, the reverse is found (Syrjanen et al., 1983). The degree of positive staining is always variable, although it is most marked where the koilocytosis is most extensive, and it ranges from abundant, patchy, and sparse, to negative. Even examining adjacent epithelial asperities in condylomata acuminata showed great variation in staining for no known reasons (Woodruff et al., 1980). Syrjanen et al. (1985) found no correlation between the presence of HPV particles seen on electron microscopy and the presence of viral antigens, and surmised that the genus-specific antigen may not necessarily be expressed or exposed at the same time as virus particles are found.

With CIN and VIN, positive staining is inversely related to the degree of dysplasia and is not found, generally, in carcinomas (Crum et al., 1982; Kurman et al., 1983; Reid et al., 1982).

Variations of the peroxidase-antiperoxidase method include using biotinylated secondary antibodies with a detection system of avidin and biotinylated horseradish peroxidase. In a study by Gupta et al. (1983), this method was employed to compare positive staining for HPV antigens in Papanicolaou smears with cervical biopsies; HPV antigens were detected in 67% of smears and 62% of biopsies. Thus, cervical smears may be just as effective a starting material for detection of HPV antigens as biopsies are.

2. Monoclonal Antibodies

Antibodies that can differentiate the genital HPV types are not now available. It would be extremely useful to develop such antibodies, especially directed against early viral products. Attempts are being made in this direction and, now that the nucleotide sequences of HPV-1a, HPV-6b, and HPV-16 are known, it may be possible to create artificial oligopeptides with type-specificity against which antibodies could be produced.

Recently, Gorra et al. (1985) characterized several MAbs to BPV-1 that could distinguish lesions induced by BPV-1 from those of BPV-2 and HPV-1, as tested by avidin-biotin immunoperoxidase staining. The BPV-1 was purified from bovine fibropapilloma, disrupted with SDS, and used to immunize mice. Sera from the mice were tested for antibodies to papilloma virus by immunofluorescence on acetone-fixed sections of bovine fibropapillomas. Mice with high antibody titers were killed and their spleen cells fused with a nonimmunoglobulin-secreting myeloma cell line. Hybridomas were screened for immunoglobulin production, then by immunofluorescence for anti-BPV antibodies. Positive cultures were cloned and further tested for type specificity. Three antibodies, all of the IgG2a subclass, were found with type specificity for BPV-1. It should be possible to make similar MAbs against the HPV types present in large numbers in skin warts, but it would be difficult to collect sufficient purified particles from genital warts. As there is no expression of the genus-specific antigen in malignant genital tumors, MAbs with type specificity for early viral proteins may be necessary to detect and type any HPV present in such a lesion.

Thus, screening for HPV antigens using existing antibody preparations are of use in detecting HPV-productive infections, but great advances would be made if antibodies were available of either type specificity or directed against antigens expressed in transformed cells.

E. Detection of Viral DNA by Hybridization

This approach is the only one that now leads to typing of HPV. Furthermore, the state of viral DNA (whether integrated or not, whether a single copy, or whether repeated and in what manner) within the infected cell or tumor can be ascertained. Hybridization depends upon single-stranded nucleic acids forming stable duplexes under appropriate conditions if their base sequences are sufficiently complementary. If double-stranded nucleic acid is heated, it denatures to single strands. The temperature at which half the double strands become single-stranded is called the T_m.

The optimal temperature for duplex formation is 25°C below T_m. At this point (high stringency) only single strands with a high degree of complementarity remain as stable duplexes; if the hybridization temperature is lower (low stringency), then fewer well-matched duplexes remain together. These differential hybridization conditions have proved very useful in HPV studies. Thus, it is possible, first, to screen DNA from a lesion at low stringency with an HPV DNA as probe to look for any evidence of HPV DNA; then, if present, the conditions of stringency can be increased with use of different types of HPV DNA as probes, and this will specifically type the HPV DNA in the lesion (Bornkamm et al., 1983). A T_m of $-18°C$ has been used for stringent hybridization, and a T_m of $-40°C$ for nonstringent (Boshart et al., 1984; Ikenberg et al., 1983).

Methods of hybridization include Southern blotting, adaptations of dot blotting, and in situ hybridization. An analysis of condylomata acuminata for HPV-6 DNA by Southern blotting is outlined in Gissman et al. (1982) and the detection of HPV-18 in cervical carcinomas in Boshart et al. (1984). Methods used to determine the state of the viral genome are illustrated in Durst et al. (1985).

Dot blotting has recently been tried by several groups, mostly in attempts to use cervical scrapes for typing HPV without the need for cervical biopsies. The clinical procedure is no more demanding than collecting routine Papanicolaou smears. In one study (Schneider et al., 1985), smears were taken with swabs from the vagina, vulva, endocervix and ectocervix, and the cells suspended by mixing in buffer before filtering directly onto nitrocellulose membranes for hybridization, without first extracting cellular DNA as is necessary for Southern blotting. Results obtained with dot blotting showed good correlation with Southern blotting. Sometimes infection with more than one type of HPV was detected which may reflect the relative cell populations obtained from smears and biopsies and the relative sensitivities of dot blotting and Southern blotting. The HPV DNA was largely confined to the tissue seen to be colposcopically and cytologically abnormal, but occasionally it was found in normal tissue. It is not known if this result is due to latent HPV infections or to "false-positive" hybridizations. Follow-up studies are required.

Wickenden et al. (1985) also used cervical scrapes, but here the cellular DNA was extracted, put on gels, and transferred to robust Zetaprobe nylon filters which can be stored before hybridization. These filters can be stored and are rehybridizable. A check was made on the quantity of DNA extracted from the scrape by hybridization with an *alu*-repeat sequence probe. This particular sequence is found 5×10^5 times in human genomes, and 16% of samples had insufficient DNA. Only HPV-6 DNA was used as a probe in this study, and it will be interesting to obtain data using a wider range of HPV DNA types.

Dot blotting must be carefully controlled to ensure that the probe does not bind nonspecifically to the filter. The probes are usually labeled with ^{32}P. This makes the procedure fairly slow (autoradiography requires 1-6 days for adequate exposure) and labor-intensive. Efforts are being made to label the probe with a substance other than a radioactive isotope, such as a fluorochrome or biotin (see later discussion). This would eliminate the need for radioactive substances, enable batches of probes to be synthesized that would be stable, and reduce the time needed to detect duplex formation.

In situ hybridization has proved a powerful tool in locating viral DNA or mRNA in specific cells from tumors and other tissues. It has the advantage over other hybridization methods of locating specific cells that contain viral information within a lesion. In addition, paraffin sections prepared for routine histopathological examination can be used. Grussendorf and zur Hausen (1979) were the first to show which cells in plantar and finger warts contained HPV DNA. A similar study recently located HPV-16 DNA in nuclei of tumour cells from cervical carcinomas (Grussendorf-Conen et al., 1985).

The HPV DNA has been labeled with biotin in vitro instead of with a radioactive substance. Condylomata acuminata were then screened by in situ hybridization (Beckmann et al., 1985). Hybridization was carried out under stringent and nonstringent conditions using HPV-1, HPV-6, HPV-11, and HPV-16 DNAs as probes. After hybridization, avidin was added, followed by goat antiavidin, biotinylated rabbit antigoat IgG, avidin-biotinylated peroxidase, and finally a substrate for peroxidase. Each of these steps amplifies the sensitivity of the method, which was estimated at 50-100 viral copies per cell genome using a reconstruction dot blotting experiment on nitrocellulose membranes.

At the moment, the sensitivity of hybridization using biotinylated probes is about 100 times less than using radioactive probes. However, the method is attractive, and it is hoped that further improvements will include synthesizing more suitable biotinylated nucleotides.

F. Immune Response

There is little information available on the immune response to HPV infections, although it is generally agreed that circulating antibody titer is not a major factor in predicting regression or persistence of warts or reinfection (Cubie, 1972; Pfister and zur Hausen, 1978). However, more sensitive methods for measuring antibodies, such as enzyme-linked immunosorbent assay (ELISA), have been developed in the past few years. One study with disrupted BPV-1 as antigen and an ELISA test has shown that IgG antibodies to papilloma antigens were present in 95% of patients with anogenital warts, 60% with CIN, and 93% with cervical carcinomas. Immunoglobulin M antibodies were present in 54% of patients with anogenital warts, 29% with CIN, and 95% with cervical carcinomas. Control groups of children and adults without cervical lesions were never positive (Baird, 1985). It is difficult to understand the implications of these data, both for the IgM and the IgG results. Some corroboration is required before such a test would be of use as a detection method for cervical abnormalities.

Cell-mediated immune responses are thought to play a role in regression of warts, with inflammatory cell exudates being characteristically found (Tagami et al., 1977). It has been suggested that the initial cells of the wart may not be recognized by immune effector cells, perhaps because the products of the virally infected cells are locally immunosuppressive (Kirchner, 1984). Recently, it has proved possible to examine wart and CIN lesions from the cervix for the distribution of such effector cells. Specific MAbs were used that differentiate B lymphocytes, T cells of the helper and cytotoxic/suppressor subsets, and Langerhans cells. Langerhans cells and T lymphocytes were much depleted in wart epithelium compared with normal epithelium, whereas there was an increase in Langerhans cells and T-cytotoxic/suppressor cells, together with increased stromal lymphocytes in CIN 3 (Morris et al., 1983). The Langerhans cells of the epidermis are important in recognition and processing of exogenous antigens within local sites, presenting antigens to the T lymphocytes and thus playing a crucial role during viral infection of the skin and in tumor induction (Wolff and Stingl, 1983).

Another study has characterized mononuclear cell infiltrates in cervical biopsies of women followed for at least 12 months (Syrjanen et al., 1984). No differences were found in the percentage of T-cell subsets, B cells, or mononuclear phagocytes between lesions that remained stationary, regressed, or progressed. Progression was related only to the degree of CIN, although there was a marked reduction in Langerhans cells in lesions that progressed compared with those that regressed or remained stationary. The significance of this finding is not known. The presentation of HPV to the immune system in the epidermis and the local immune response is a topic of utmost interest, and information of diagnostic or prognostic importance may well be forthcoming from its study.

VII. CONCLUSIONS AND FUTURE PROSPECTS

As may be seen from the previous section, no one method is now readily available for the detection of genital HPV infections, although nucleic acid hybridization, if well controlled, gives the most information about the virus. From the patient's viewpoint, assessments made at the time of colposcopic and other examinations are most valuable, especially if treatment is then immediate. A pathologist, working in conjunction with a clinician, can provide information rapidly using frozen sections of tissue. It remains to be seen if most HPV infections can be typed correctly on the distribution of nuclear atypia in sections. Much more information is required about the induction of dysplasia and what governs its progression, stationary phase, or regression. It is important to ascertain the transmission of HPV types, especially of types 16 and 18. Whether or not these viruses can be latent in the genital tract of men and women remains to be determined.

Nucleic acid hybridization by Southern blot analysis of DNA from biopsies is a technique requiring expertise and is expensive and time-consuming. However, recent advances using cervical scrapes in place of biopsies, probes labeled with biotin instead of a radioactive isotope, and dot blotting, have almost brought hybridization into the realm of diagnostic virology. More information should be available in the near future from laboratories around the world about the association of HPV-6, HPV-11, HPV-16, and HPV-18 with CIN, VIN, and other neoplasms of the genital tract, which should give a clearer indication of their putative role in genital carcinomas.

Antibodies against HPV that are now available do not provide all of the information required. Antibodies that are type-specific and/or that can detect early viral proteins are necessary, and it should be feasible to produce such reagents. The only MAbs used thus far in HPV infections are ones that distinguish mononuclear cells in sections of tissues. This type of study is important, not so much in the context of detection of HPV, but in understanding the local immune response in lesions that progress, regress, or remain stationary.

ACKNOWLEDGMENTS

I wish to thank Dr. S. Fletcher and Mrs. H. Cubie for their critical readings of the manuscript, and my colleagues for many helpful discussions. Mrs. H. Cubie kindly provided Figs. 1 and 4, and Dr. S. Fletcher Fig. 6.

REFERENCES

Adler, M. W. (1984). Genital warts and molluscum contagiosum. *Br. Med. J.* *288*:213-215.

Baird, P. J. (1985). The role of human papilloma and other virus. *Clin. Obstet. Gynecol.* *12*:19-32.

Beckmann, A. M., Myerson, D., Daling, J. R., Kiviat, N., Fenoglio, C. M., and McDougall, J. K. (1985). Detection and localisation of human papillomavirus DNA in human genital condylomas by in situ hybridisation with biotinylated probes. *J. Med. Virol.* *16*:265-273.

Bohm, N. and Sandritter, W. (1975). DNA in human tumours: A cytophotometric study. *Curr. Top. Pathol.* *60*:151-219.

Bornkamm, G. W., Desgranges, C., and Gissmann, L. (1983). Nucleic acid hybridisation for the detection of viral genomes. *Curr. Top. Microbiol. Immunol.* *104*:287-298.

Boshart, M., Gissmann, L., Ikenberg, H., Kleinheinz, A., Scheurlen, W., and zur Hausen, H. (1984). A new type of papillomavirus DNA, its presence in genital cancer biopsies and in cell lines derived from cervical cancer. *EMBO J.* *3*:1151-1157.

Braun, L., Farmer, E. R., and Shah, K. V. (1983). Immunoperoxidase localization of papillomavirus antigen in cutaneous warts and bowenoid papulosis. *J. Med. Virol.* *12*:187-193.

Buschke, A. and Lowenstein, L. (1931). Uber carcinomahnliche Condylomata acuminata des Penis. *Arch. Dermatol. Syphilol.* *163*:30-46.

Chen, E. Y., Howley, P. M., Levinson, A. D., and Seeburg, P. H. (1982). The primary structure and genetic organization of the bovine papillomavirus type 1 genome. *Nature 299*:529-534.

Ciuffo, G. (1907). Innesto positivo con filtrato di verrucae volgare. *G. Ital. Mal. Venerol.* *48*:12-17.

Clad, A., Gissmann, L., Meier, B., Freese, U. K., and Schwarz, E. (1982). Molecular cloning and partial nucleotide sequence of human papillomavirus type 1a DNA. *Virology 118*:254-259.

Coggin, J. R. and zur Hausen, H. (1979). Workshop on papillomavirus and cancer. *Cancer Res. 39*:545-546.

Crawford, L. (1984). Papillomavirus and cervical tumours. *Nature 310*:16.

Crum, C. P., Fu, Y. S., Levine, R. U., Richart, R. M., Townsend, D. E., and Fenoglio, C. M. (1982). Intraepithelial squamous lesions of the vulva: Biologic and histologic criteria for the distinction of condylomas from vulvar intraepithelial neoplasia. *Am. J. Obstet. Gynecol. 144*:77-83.

Crum, C. P., Ikenberg, H., Richart, R. M., and Gissmann, L. (1984). Human papillomavirus type 16 and early cervical neoplasia. *N. Engl. J. Med. 310*:880-883.

Crum, C. P., Mitao, M., Levine, R. U., and Silverstein, S. (1985). Cervical papillomaviruses segregate within morphologically distinct precancerous lesions. *J. Virol. 54*:675-681.

Cubie, H. A. (1972). Serological studies in a student population prone to infection with human papilloma virus. *J. Hyg. 70*:677-690.

Danos, O., Katinka, M., and Yaniv, M. (1982). Human papillomavirus 1a complete DNA sequence: A novel type of genomic organization among *Papovaviridae. EMBO J. 1*:231-236.

Dunn, A. E. and Ogilvie, M. M. (1968). Intranuclear virus particles in human genital wart tissue: Observations on the ultrastructure of epidermal layer. *J. Ultrastruct. Res. 22*:282-295.

Durst, M., Kleinheinz, A., Hotz, M., and Gissmann, L. (1985). The physical state of human papillomavirus type 16 DNA in benign and malignant genital tumours. *J. Gen. Virol. 66*:1515-1522.

Ferenczy, A., Braun, L., and Shah, K. V. (1981). Human papillomavirus (HPV) in condylomatous lesions of cervix. *Am. J. Surg. Pathol. 5*:661-670.

Ferenczy, A., Mitao, M., Nobutka, N., Silverstein, S., and Crum, C. (1985). Latent papillomaviruses and recurring genital warts. *N. Engl. J. Med. 313*: 784-788.

Fletcher, S. (1983). Histopathology of papilloma virus infection of the cervix uteri: The history, taxonomy, nomenclature and reporting of koilocytic dysplasias. *J. Clin. Pathol. 36*:616-624.

Fletcher, S. and Norval, M. (1983). On the nature of the deep cellular disturbances in human-papilloma virus infection of the squamous cervical epithelium. *Lancet 2*:546-549.

Fletcher, S., Smart, G. E., and Livingstone, J. J. (1985). Grading of cervical dysplasias by frozen section. *Lancet 2*:599-600.

Fu, Y. S., Reagan, J. W., and Richart, R. M. (1983). Precursors of cervical cancer. *Cancer Surveys 2*:359-382.

Fukushima, M., Okagaki, T., Twiggs, L. B., Clark, B. A., Zachow, K. R., Ostrow, R. S., and Faras, A. J. (1985). Histological types of carcinoma of the uterine cervix and the detectability of human papillomavirus DNA. *Cancer Res. 45*: 3252-3255.

Gissmann, L. (1984). Papillomaviruses and their association with cancer in animals and in man. *Cancer Surveys 3*:161-181.

Gissmann, L., De Villiers, E. M., and zur Hausen, H. (1982). Analysis of human genital warts (condylomata acuminata) and other genital tumours for human papillomavirus type 6 DNA. *Int. J. Cancer. 29*:143-146.

Gissman, L., Pfister, H., and zur Hausen, H. (1977). Human papilloma virus (HPV): Characterization of 4 different isolates. *Virology 76*:569-580.

Gissmann, L. and Schwarz, E. (1985). Cloning of papillomavirus DNA. In *Recombinant DNA Research and Viruses* (Y. Becker, ed.). Martinus Nijhoff, Boston, pp. 173-197.

Gissmann, K., Wolnik, L., Ikenberg, H., Koldovsky, U., Schnurch, H. G., and zur Hausen, H. (1983). Human papillomavirus type 6 and 11 DNA sequences in genital and laryngeal papillomas and in some cervical cancers. *Proc. Natl. Acad. Sci. USA 80*:560-563.

Gorra, J. B., Lancaster, W. D., Kurman, R. J., and Jenson, A. D. (1985). Bovine papillomavirus type 1 monoclonal antibodies. *J. Natl. Cancer Inst. 75*:121-125.

Gross, G., Hagedorn, M., Ikenberg, H., Rufli, T., Dahlet, C., Grosshans, E., and Gissmann, L. (1985a). Bowenoid papulosis. Presence of human papillomavirus (HPV) structural antigens and of HPV 16-related DNA sequences. *Arch. Dermatol. 121*:858-863.

Gross, G., Ikenberg, H., Gissmann, L., and Hagedorn, M. (1985b). Papillomavirus infection of the anogenital region: Correlation between histology, clinical picture, and virus type. Proposal of a new nomenclature. *J. Invest. Dermatol. 85*:147-152.

Grussendorf, E.-I. and zur Hausen, H. (1979). Localization of viral DNA-replication in sections of human warts by nucleic acid hybridization with complementary RNA of human papillomavirus type 1. *Arch. Dermatol. Res. 264*: 55-63.

Grussendorf-Conen, E.-I., Ikenberg, H., and Gissmann, L. (1985). Demonstration of HPV-16 genomes in the nuclei of cervix carcinoma cells. *Dermatologica 170*:199-201.

Gupta, J. W., Gupta, P. K., Shah, K. V., and Kelly, D. P. (1983). Distribution of human papillomavirus antigen in cervico-vaginal smears and cervical tissues. *Int. J. Gynecol. Pathol. 2*:160-170.

Ikenberg, H., Gissmann, L., Gross, G., Grussendorf-Cohen, E.-I., and zur Hausen, H. (1983). Human papillomavirus type 16 related DNA in genital Bowen's disease and in bowenoid papulosis. *Int. J. Cancer 32*:563-565.

Jablonska, S., Orth, G., and Lutzner, M. A. (1982). Immunopathology of papillomavirus-induced tumors in different tissues. *Springer Semin. Immunopathol. 5*:33-62.

Jenson, A. B., Rosenthal, J. R., Olson, C., Pass, F., Lancaster, W. D., and Shah, K. (1980). Immunological relatedness of papillomaviruses from different species. *J. Natl. Cancer Inst. 64*:495-500.

Kirchner, H. (1984). Immunologic surveillance and human papillomaviruses. *Immunol. Today 5*:272-276.

Kirkup, W., Evans, A. S., Brough, A. K., Davis, J. A., O'Loughlin, T., Wilkinson, G., and Monaghan, J. M. (1982). Cervical intraepithelial neoplasia and 'warty' atypia: A study of colposcopic, histological and cytological characteristics. *Br. J. Obstet. Gynaecol.* *89*:571-577.

Koss, L. G. and Durfee, G. R. (1956). Unusual patterns of squamous epithelium of the uterine cervix: Cytologic and pathologic study of koilocytic atypia. *Ann. N.Y. Acad. Sci.* *63*:1245-1261.

Kurman, R. J., Jenson, A. B., and Lancaster, W. D. (1983). Papillomavirus infection of the cervix. II. Relationship to intraepithelial neoplasia based on the presence of specific viral structural proteins. *Am. J. Surg. Pathol.* *7*:39-52.

Kurman, R. J., Shah, K. H., Lancaster, W. D., and Jenson, A. B. (1981). Immunoperoxidase localization of papillomavirus antigens in cervical dysplasia and vulvar condylomas. *Am. J. Obstet. Gynecol.* *140*:931-935.

Lancaster, W. D. and Olson, C. (1982). Animal papillomavirus. *Microbiol. Rev.* *46*:191-207.

Lehn, H., Ernst, T.-M., and Sauer, G. (1984). Transcription of episomal papillomavirus DNA in human condylomata acuminata and Buschke-Lowenstein tumours. *J. Gen. Virol.* *65*:2003-2010.

Lehn, H., Krieg, P., and Sauer, G. (1985). Papillomavirus genomes in human cervical tumors: Analysis of their transcriptional activity. *Proc. Natl. Acad. Sci. USA* *82*:5540-5544.

Lloyd, K. M. (1970). Multicentric pigmented Bowen's disease of the groin. *Arch. Dermatol.* *101*:48-51.

Lowy, D. R., Dvoretzky, I., Shober, R., Law, M.-F., Engel, L., and Howley, P. M. (1980). In vivo tumorigenic transformation by a defined subgenomic fragment of bovine papilloma virus DNA. *Nature 287*:72-74.

Lusky, M., Berg, L., Weiher, H., and Botchan, M. (1983). The bovine papillomavirus contains an activator of gene expression at the distal end of the transcriptional unit. *Mol. Cell. Biol.* *3*:1108-1122.

Lusky, M. and Botchan, M. R. (1984). Characterization of the bovine papillomavirus plasmid maintenance sequences. *Cell 36*:391-401.

Lusky, M. and Botchan, M. R. (1985). Genetic analysis of bovine papillomavirus type 1 *trans*-acting replication factors. *J. Virol.* *53*:955-965.

Meisels, A. and Fortin, R. (1976). Condylomatous lesions of the cervix and vagina. I. Cytologic patterns. *Acta Cytol.* *20*:505-509.

Meisels, A., Fortin, R., and Roy, M. (1977). Condylomatous lesions of the cervix. II. Cytologic, colposcopic and histopathologic study. *Acta Cytol.* *21*: 373-390.

Meisels, A., Morin, C., and Cases-Codero, M. (1982). Human papillomavirus infection of the uterine cervix. *Int. J. Gynecol. Pathol.* *1*:75-94.

Meisels, A., Morin, C., and Casas-Codero, M. (1984). Lesions of the uterine cervix associated with papillomavirus and their clinical consequences. *Adv. Clin. Cytol.* *2*:1-31.

Meisels, A., Roy, M., Fortier, M., and Morin, C. (1979). Condylomatous lesions of the cervix. Morphologic and colposcopic diagnosis. *Am. J. Diagnos. Gynecol. Obstet.* *1*:109-116.

Morin, C., Braun, L., Casas-Cordero, M., Shah, K. V., Roy, M., Fortier, M., and Meisels, A. (1981). Confirmation of the papillomavirus etiology of condylomatous cervix lesions by the peroxidase antiperoxidase technique. *J. Natl. Cancer Inst.* 66:831-835.

Morris, H., Gatter, K., Sykes, G., Caesmore, V., and Maron, D. (1983). Langerhans cells in human cervical epithelium: Effects of wart virus infection and intraepithelial neoplasia. *Br. J. Obstet. Gynaecol.* 90:412-420.

Oriel, J. d. (1971). Natural history of genital warts. *Br. J. Vener. Dis.* 47:1-8.

Oriel, J. D (1983). Condylomata acuminata as a sexually transmitted disease. *Dermatol. Clin.* 1:93-102.

Pater, M. M. and Pater, A. (1985). Human papillomavirus types 16 and 18 sequences in carcinoma cell lines of the cervix. *Virology* 145:313-318.

Pfister, H. (1984). Biology and biochemistry of papillomaviruses. *Rev. Physiol. Biochem. Pharmacol.* 99:111-181.

Pfister, H. and zur Hausen, H. (1978). Seroepidemiological studies of human papillomavirus (HPV-1) infections. *Int. J. Cancer.* 21:161-165.

Phelps, W. C., Leary, S. L., and Faras, A. J. (1985). Shope papillomavirus transcription in benign and malignant rabbit tumours. *Virology* 146:120-129.

Pilotti, S., Rolke, F., De Palo, G., Della Torre, C., and Alasio, L. 91981). Condylomata of the uterine cervix and koilocytosis of cervical intraepithelial neoplasia. *J. Clin. Pathol.* 34:532-541.

Potter, H. L. and Meinke, W. J. (1985). Nucleotide sequence of bovine papillomavirus type 2 late region. *J. Gen. Virol.* 66:187-193.

Reid, R., Crum, C. P., Herschman, B. R., Fu, Y. S., Braun, L., Shah, K. V., Agronow, S., and Stanhope, C. R. (1984). Genital warts and cervical cancer. III. Subclinical papillomaviral infection and cervical neoplasia are linked by a spectrum of continuous morphologic and biologic change. *Cancer* 53:943-953.

Reid, R., Laverty, C. R., Coppleson, M., Isarangkul, W., and Hills, E. (1980). Noncondylomatous cervical wart virus infection. *Obstet. Gynecol.* 55:476-483.

Reid, R., Stanhope, C. R., Herschman, B. R., Booth, E., Phibbs, G. D., and Smith, J. P. (1982). Genital warts and cervical cancer. I. Evidence of an association between subclinical papillomavirus infection and cervical malignancy. *Cancer* 50:377-387.

Rigoni-Stern, D. (1842). Fatti statistici relativi alle mallattic cancrose che servirono de base alle poche cose dette dal dott. *G. Servire Prog. Patol. Terap.* 2:507-517.

Rotkin, I. D. (1973). A comparison review of key epidemiological studies in cervical cancer related to current searches for transmissible agents. *Cancer Res.* 33:1353-1367.

Rowson, K. E. and Mahy, B. W. (1967). Human papova (wart) virus. *Bacteriol. Rev.* 31:110-131.

Schneider, A., Kraus, H., Schuhmann, R., and Gissmann, L. (1985). Papillomavirus infection of the lower genital tract: Detection of viral DNA in gynaecological swabs. *Int. J. Cancer* 35:443-448.

Schwarz, E., Durst, M., Demankowski, C., Lattermann, O., Zech, R., Wolfsperger, E., Suhai, S., and zur Hausen, H. (1983). DNA sequence and genome organization of human papillomavirus type 6b. *EMBO J. 2*:2341-2348.

Schwarz, E., Freese, U. K., Gissmann, L., Mayer, W., Roggenbuck, B., Stremlau, A., and zur Hausen, H. (1985). Structure and transcription of human papillomavirus sequences in cervical carcinoma cells. *Nature 314*:111-114.

Seedorf, K., Krammer, G., Durst, M., Suhai, S., and Rowekamp, W. G. (1985). Human papillomavirus type 16 DNA sequence. *Virology 145*:181-185.

Singer, A., Walker, P. G., and McCance, D. J. (1984). Genital wart virus infections: Nuisance or potentially lethal? *Br. Med. J. 288*:735-736.

Smith, J. and Coleman, D. V. (1983). Electron microscopy of cells showing viral cytopathic effects in Papanicolaou smears. *Acta Cytol. 27*:605-613.

Spalholz, B. A., Yang, Y.-C., and Howley, P. M. (1985). Transactivation of a bovine papilloma virus transcriptional regulatory element by the E2 gene product. *Cell 42*:183-191.

Sternberger, L. A. (1979). *Immunocytochemistry*, 2nd ed. John Wiley & Sons, New York, pp. 104-169.

Syrjanen, K. J. (1984). Current concepts of human papillomavirus infections in the genital tract and their relationship to intraepithelial neoplasia and squamous cell carcinoma. *Obstet. Gynecol. Surv. 39*:252-265.

Syrjanen, K. J. and Pyrhonen, S. (1982). Immunoperoxidase demonstration of human papilloma virus (HPV) in dysplastic lesions of the uterine cervix. *Arch. Gynecol. 233*:53-61.

Syrjanen, K. J., Vayrynen, M., Castren, O., Mantyjarvi, R., and Yliskoski, M. (1984). The relation between the type of immunoreactive cells found in human papillomavirus (HPV) lesions of the uterine cervix and the subsequent behaviour of these lesions. *Arch. Gynecol. 234*:189-196.

Syrjanen, K. J., Vayrynen, M., Hippelainen, M., Castren, O., Saarikoski, S., and Mantyjarvi, R. (1985). Electron microscopic assessment of cervical punch biopsies in women followed-up for human papillomavirus (HPV) lesions. *Arch. Geschwulstforsch. 55*:131-138.

Tagami, H., Takigawa, M., Ogino, A., Imamura, S., and Ofugi, S. (1977). Spontaneous regression of plane warts after inflammation. *Arch. Dermatol. 113*: 1209-1213.

Taichman, L. B., Reilly, S. S., and La Porta, R. F. (1983). The role of keratinocyte differentiation in the expression of epitheliotropic viruses. *J. Invest. Dermatol. 81*:137S-140S.

Vayrynen, M., Syrjanen, K., Castren, O., Saarikoski, I. S., and Mantyjarvi, R. (1985). Colposcopy in women with papillomavirus lesions of the uterine cervix. *Obstet. Gynecol. 65*:409-415.

Wade, T. R., Kopf, A. W., and Ackerman, A. B. (1978). Bowenoid papulosis of the penis. *Cancer 42*:1890-1903.

Waugh, M. (1972). Condylomata acuminata. *Br. Med. J. 2*:527-528.

Wickenden, C., Steele, A., Malcolm, A. D., and Coleman, D. V. (1985). Screening for wart virus infection in normal and abnormal cervices by DNA hybridisation of cervical scrapes. *Lancet 1*:65-67.

Wolff, K. and Stingl, G. (1983). The Langerhans cell. *J. Invest. Dermatol. 80*: 17S-21S.

Woodruff, J. D. and Peterson, W. F. (1958). Condylomata acuminata of the cervix. *Am. J. Obstet. Gynecol. 75*:1354-1362.

Woodruff, J. D., Braun, L., Cavallieri, R., Gupta, P., Pass, F., and Shah, K. V. (1980). Immunological identification of papillomavirus antigen in paraffin-processed condyloma tissues from the female genital tract. *Obstet. Gynecol. 56*:727-732.

Yang, Y.-C., Okayama, H., and Howley, P. M. (1985a). Bovine papillomavirus contains multiple transforming genes. *Proc. Natl. Acad. Sci. USA 82*:1030-1034.

Yang, Y.-C., Spalholz, B. A., Rabson, M. S., and Howley, P. M. (1985b). Dissociation of transforming and *trans*-activation functions for bovine papillomavirus type 1. *Nature 318*:575-577.

Yee, C., Krishnan-Hewlett, I., Baker, C. C., Schlegel, R., and Howley, P. M. (1985). Presence and expression of human papillomavirus sequences in human cervical carcinoma cell lines. *Am. J. Pathol. 119*:361-366.

Zachow, K. R., Ostrow, R. S., Bender, M., Watts, S., Okagaki, T., Pass, F., and Faras, A. J. (1982). Detection of human papillomavirus DNA in anogenital neoplasias. *Nature 300*:771-773.

zur Hausen, H. (1976). Condylomata acuminata and human genital cancer. *Cancer Res. 36*:794.

zur Hausen, H. (1977). Human papillomaviruses and their possible role in squamous cell carcinomas. *Curr. Top. Microbiol. Immunol. 78*:1-30.

zur Hausen, H. (1982). Human genital cancer—synergism between two virus infections or synergism between a virus infection and initiating events. *Lancet 2*:1370-1372.

FOURTEEN

Diagnosis of Hepatitis B Infection

Edward A. C. Follett
Hepatitis Reference Laboratory
Regional Virus Laboratory
Ruchill Hospital
Glasgow, Scotland

I. THE DISEASE

Hepatitis B infection is normally a self-limiting infection in that over 90% of those infected clear all markers of infectious virus from their blood and become immune to further infection. Acute illness is associated with abnormal liver function and jaundice and, although usually mild, can be prolonged. The disease is not usually life-threatening and acute clinical cases recover without chronic sequelae. A proportion of those infected do not eliminate the virus, remain chronically infected, and become long-term carriers who may have the virus, its specific antigens, or both, circulating in their blood for many years. Persisting infection is more likely to develop following a mild or asymptomatic infection (Sherlock, 1981). Very few blood donors who are found to be long-term carriers give any history of jaundice/hepatitis that would account for their chronic infection (Crawford et al., 1979). Long-term carriage is more likely to be associated with chronic liver disease. There is increasing evidence of a link between hepatocellular carcinoma and hepatitis B infection, especially when the hepatitis B infection has resulted in long-term carriage (Beasley, 1982).

II. EPIDEMIOLOGY OF HEPATITIS B

A. Geographical Distribution

Hepatitis B infection is a global problem. It has been estimated that there are around 200 million asymptomatic carriers of hepatitis B surface antigen (HBsAg) in the world's population (Gust, 1981). The distribution of these carriers worldwide is very uneven, with prevalence rates ranging from 0.1% in Western Europe and North America, through 5-10% in southern and Eastern Europe, to about 20% in parts of Asia (Sobeslavsky, 1980) and, on the Pacific island of Rapa, 50% (Deinhardt and Gust, 1982). In addition, even in countries with a low prevalence, evidence of widespread infection can be found in specific population groups, e.g., intravenous drug abusers and homosexual men, to an extent approaching that found in areas of Southeast Asia where hepatitis B is endemic and most prevalent. Even in countries with a low prevalence, there are groups in the population in whom the infection is becoming endemic and who represent a continuing and increasing reservoir of infection.

B. Patterns of Infection

Two patterns of infection can be distinguished depending upon the local prevalence of HBsAg carriage. In countries with a high carriage rate, infection occurs perinatally or in early childhood, and the highest rates of infection are seen in children and young adults. In countries with a low carrier rate, hepatitis B infection in children is uncommon and the peak age for infection is between 16 and

Table 1 Analysis of Acute Hepatitis B Cases in Western Scotland According to Age

Year	0-15 (yr)	16-20 (yr)	21-30 (yr)	31-40 (yr)	41-50 (yr)	51-60 (yr)	61+ (yr)
1982	0	53	54	13	10	3	1
1983	4	97	83	15	7	6	4
1984	9	159	129	18	17	3	1

Cases were only included if positive for both HBsAg and anti-HBc IgM.

30 years (Table 1) and is associated with drug abuse and sexual promiscuity. Substantially more infections are seen in males.

C. Transmission

1. Vehicle of Transmission

Blood contains the highest titer of HBsAg and hepatitis B virus (HBV) of any body fluid and is the most effective vehicle for transmitting infection. The HBsAg has also been demonstrated in saliva (Bancroft et al., 1977), semen (Alter et al., 1977), urine (Villarejos et al., 1974), tears (Darrell and Jacob, 1978), menstrual blood, and vaginal secretions (Darani and Gerber, 1974). Apart from blood, only semen and saliva have been demonstrated to transmit infection to chimpanzees, and saliva only when administered subcutaneously (Scott et al., 1980). Transmission of HBV infection by saliva administered orally has not been accomplished. Neither HBsAg nor HBV can normally be demonstrated in feces.

2. Modes of Transmission

Before the introduction of screening of all blood donations for HBsAg, cases of posttransfusion hepatitis B infection formed a large proportion of the reported annual total of acute cases. This route of transmission has been virtually eliminated, but blood products such as factor VIII and factor IX prepared from plasma pooled from several thousand donations still present some slight risk to recipients. Transfusion of small amounts of infected blood can occur during any procedure where the skin is broken by an instrument previously used on an infected person. Procedures, such as tattooing, acupuncture, ear-piercing, and hair electrolysis, have been implicated in the transmission of hepatitis B. Health care personnel, particularly those using invasive procedures involving breakage of the skin or mucous membranes, are at risk of infection. The group at greatest risk from this particular route of transmission are intravenous drug abusers. Sharing of contaminated needles and syringes is commonplace among abusers, and the extent of hepatitis B infection in abusers (Table 2) illustrates the effectiveness of needle inoculation as a method of transmission. Regular abusers of long-standing in the

Table 2   Markers of Prior HBV Infection in Blood Donors and Risk Groups in Western Scotland

Category	No. tested	No. positive for anti-HBc + anti-HBs	% positive
Blood donor[a]	2400	31	1.3
Male homosexuals[b]	217	56	25.8
Drug abusers[c]	606	356	58.7

Sources: data from [a]Follett et al., 1980; [b]Follett and McMillan, 1980; [c]Follett et al., 1986.

west of Scotland have markers of hepatitis B infection equivalent to those found in a population with a carrier rate of 20%. The carrier rate in the blood donor population of western Scotland averages 0.129% (Barr et al., 1981).

It was apparent many years ago that not all cases of hepatitis B could be attributed to a suitable percutaneous incident at an appropriate time in the past. That hepatitis B might be spread by the sexual route was originally suggested by Mirick and Shank (1959) to explain the observation of secondary cases in the wives of servicemen inoculated with a contaminated batch of yellow fever vaccine. Various studies of spouses of acute cases and carriers, female prostitutes, and patients attending venereal disease clinics have demonstrated much greater evidence of hepatitis B infection than in control groups. Male-to-female, female-to-male, and male-to-male transmission occur. Homosexual men are at particular risk of hepatitis B infection (Szmuness et al., 1975). Infection is significantly related to the duration of homosexual activity, the number of casual partners, and anal intercourse (Schreeder et al., 1982). Within the homosexual population of a given area, the prevalence of markers of hepatitis B infection can be many times that found in a heterosexual group (see Table 2). Although clinical hepatitis does occur in this group, most infections are subclinical (Coleman et al., 1977).

Not all carriers of HBsAg are equally infectious, and it may be that some carriers are totally noninfectious, although this can be proved absolutely only by testing for infectivity in chimpanzees. Babies born to mothers who are HBsAg carriers provide the clearest example of this differing infectivity. Most carrier mothers do not transmit infecton to their babies who show no evidence of infection, either HBsAg or any other marker, at any time. A few do become infected, HBsAg appearing at 2-3 months of age usually without symptoms, the child thereafter becoming a long-term carrier. The timing of the appearance of HBsAg indicates infection at or around the time of birth, and this form of HBV transmission is referred to as perinatal transmission.

The discovery of hepatitis B e antigen (HBeAg) (Magnius and Espmark, 1972) and the subsequent development of tests for the antigen and its antibody, anti-HBe (Sect. III.D.4) provided an explanation for this difference in infectivity. Early studies in Japan (Okada et al., 1976) demonstrated that infants who became carriers had mothers with circulating HBeAg; infants who were not infected had mothers with anti-HBe. Many studies have confirmed the general truth of this finding, but sufficient exceptions have been noted to signify that there is no absolute correlation between HBeAg and infectivity and anti-HBe and noninfectivity. In general terms, mothers with circulating HBeAg are very likely to transmit infection to their offspring (85%, Beasley et al., 1977; 83%, Boxall, 1982), those with anti-HBe are much less likely.

In countries with a high carrier rate, perinatal transmission is one of the principal routes whereby HBV is transmitted from generation to generation. A means is now available to eliminate this route of transmission by treatment of the newborn with a combination of hepatitis B immunoglobulin and hepatitis B vaccine. A 95% success rate has been reported from an extensive study in Taiwan (Beasley et al., 1983). Increasing drug abuse has resulted in many more such cases being seen in countries with low carrier rates, and any antenatal patients giving a history of drug abuse or association with drug abusers should be screened for HBsAg. A baby born to any HBsAg carrier, irrespective of HBeAg status, should be given a course of hepatitis B immunoglobulin and hepatitis B vaccine to ensure, as far as possible, that HBV infection is not transmitted.

The observation that carriers with circulating HBeAg are much more likely to transmit infection also applies to sexual transmission, both homosexual and heterosexual. Semen from HBeAg carriers has produced infection when inoculated into chimpanzees (Alter et al., 1977). Molecular hybridization techniques have provided evidence of virus in semen of HBeAg carriers but not in semen of those with anti-HBe (Karayiannis et al., 1985). There is no doubt that carriers with circulating HBeAg are much more likely to infect their sexual partners, but carriers with anti-HBe cannot be considered risk-free. The most recent evidence compelling caution in interpreting the infectivity of carriers with anti-HBe is the observation of fulminant hepatitis in successive female sexual partners of two anti-HBe-positive males (Fagan et al., 1986).

D. Incubation Period

The average incubation period for hepatitis B infection given in standard textbooks is 3 months, a figure based on well-documented exposures, e.g., from a blood transfusion. With the decline in posttransfusion cases, the study of incubation periods has become difficult as it is almost impossible to date the infection-causing event in cases seen in drug abusers and promiscuous homosexuals. There is, however, an awareness that incubation periods can be shorter than 3 months and can also be prolonged to even 6 months (Zuckerman and Howard, 1979). Differences in the dose of virus received and in the host's response to the dose would explain this wide divergence.

E. Control by Vaccines

Hepatitis B virus cannot be grown readily in cell culture, and thus, the normal methods of preparation of a virus vaccine are not available to developers of a hepatitis B vaccine. Fortunately, long-term carriers have high titers of HBsAg ($> 10^{10}$ particles/ml of serum) and it is this HBsAg that stimulates anti-HBs, the protective antibody in an HBV infection. The HBsAg particles contain neither DNA nor RNA and are noninfectious, but when purified and inoculated into a human host, they stimulate the production of protective anti-HBs (Hilleman et al., 1978). A vaccine prepared in this way from the plasma of human carriers has been produced, thoroughly investigated by many groups and is now available commercially and licensed worldwide (HB Vax; Merck Sharp + Dohme). An extensive trial in New York homosexuals demonstrated the efficacy and safety of this plasma-derived vaccine (Szmuness et al., 1980). The techniques of modern molecular biology have allowed the development of another vaccine based on the HBsAg particle. The complete nucleotide sequence of the HBV genome is known, and the segment of DNA coding for HBsAg can be excised and inserted into the genome of a yeast vector. When cultured, the yeast produces large quantities of HBsAg in the same particulate form found in human serum. Two such yeast-derived, HBsAg subunit vaccines produced by Merck Sharp + Dohme and Smith-Kline Biologicals have been licensed in several countries. Both vaccines show responses that are as good as those shown by the plasma-derived vaccine in clinical trials, but they have the additional benefit that there is no risk of contamination by any infectious agent or toxic component from the plasma of the human donors used for the plasma-derived vaccine.

At the time of writing over 3 million doses of Merck's plasma-derived vaccine have been used worldwide. Side effects are minimal and a protective response is achieved in 96-97% of vaccinees. The titer of protective antibody declines with time, and it is clear that, although protection will last for 5 years in many vaccinees, in a substantial proportion a booster dose will be required earlier, and in some individuals even after a year, to maintain the antibody titer above 10 IU/L, the generally accepted minimum level for protection. In the original trial of the vaccine in New York homosexuals, it was shown that nonresponders were susceptible to subsequent infection with HBV. It is essential, therefore, that a post-vaccination check on antibody response be made on all recipients of vaccine so that nonresponders can be alerted and protected with hepatitis B immunoglobulin after any inoculation accident. Responders to the vaccine should be informed and an estimate given of the length of protection.

Apart from a small number of doses used to prevent perinatal transmission, most of the doses of vaccine administered so far have been given to health care staff working in environments where they may be at risk of HBV infection. While this is understandable, the policy has done nothing to control or prevent the spread of infection in the population groups in whom the infection is endemic—drug abusers, homosexuals, patients in institutes for the mentally handicapped. Cost remains the biggest obstacle to widespread use of the vaccine in these groups. It is to be hoped that competition will result in a reduction in cost and allow the vaccines to be used to their full potential in controlling what is now a preventable disease.

III. DIAGNOSIS OF HEPATITIS B INFECTION

A. Introduction

Diagnosis of a viral infection can be a lengthy procedure and many clinicians are deterred from sending suitable specimens to a diagnostic laboratory because by the time the result is returned to them, it may have no effect on their management or care of the patient. The diagnosis of hepatitis B infection is an outstanding example of what a diagnostic laboratory can accomplish using modern technology. Evidence of infection can be obtained within 1 hr of receipt of a clotted blood specimen; an assessment of infectivity, an indication of whether the patient is a new acute infection or a long-term carrier, and a measurement of immunity, can all be provided within 24 hr on a single serum specimen. Many factors have contributed to this unusual situation. Hepatitis B virus is a unique human virus producing large quantities of virus and viral components that circulate in the blood of the infected host and, more importantly, in the blood of long-term carriers. A source of viral antigens is thus available, and these can be purified and used to obtain highly specific polyclonal antibodies. The worldwide problem of hepatitis B has stimulated extensive research at the molecular level. The complete sequence of the HBV genome is known (Galibert et al., 1979), and the relevant parts of the genome have been incorporated into *Escherichia coli* and yeast vectors using recombinant DNA techniques to provide hepatitis B core antigen (HBcAg) for use in diagnostic tests and HBsAg for use as a vaccine (McAleer et al., 1984).

Probably the most important diagnostic stimulus has been the requirement of blood transfusion services worldwide for a quick, sensitive test for HBsAg to screen every blood donation. The financial rewards to pharmaceutical companies able to provide such a test revolutionized the methods of testing for HBsAg in the mid 1970s. Such is the sensitivity and specificity of current tests for HBV markers in serum that the availability of monoclonal antibodies (MAbs) has not had such an impact on testing methodology as in other areas. Some extra degree of sensitivity is claimed for tests incorporating MAb, but the most obvious impact of MAbs on testing to date has been on improving convenience and speed.

B. Markers of Hepatitis B Virus Infection

Three distinct antigen-antibody systems specific for HBV infection have been recognized; the surface antigen (Australia antigen), HBsAg, and its antibody, anti-

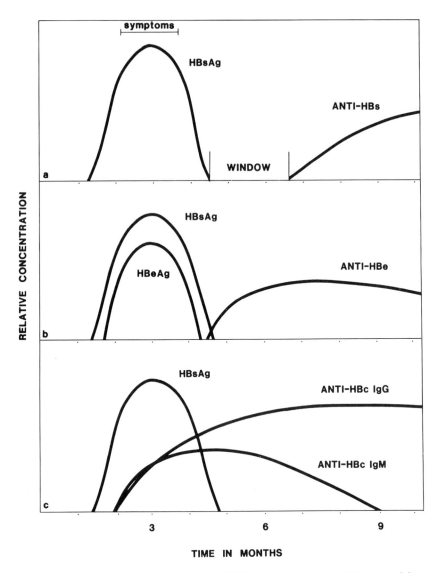

Fig. 1 Time sequence of appearance of HBV markers in acute infection: (a) HBsAg/anti-HBs; (b) HBsAg/HBeAg/anti-HBe; (c) HBsAg/anti-HBc.

HBs; the core antigen, HBcAg, and its antibody, anti-HBc; and the e antigen, HBeAg, and its antibody, anti-HBe. The time of appearance of these markers and the order of their appearance in a typical infection are shown in Fig. 1 together with an indication of the time of acute clinical illness. It is noteworthy that HBsAg can be detected many weeks before clinical illness is apparent and for some time after the patient has recovered clinically. There is often a time interval between the loss of HBeAg and the appearance of anti-HBe. With present test systems there is always a substantial time interval between the loss of HBsAg and the appearance of anti-HBs.

All markers of HBV infection can have clinical importance and, apart from HBcAg, all can be detected in serum at some time during infection. A variety of diagnostic tests have been devised to detect these markers, and their use allows the clinician to follow the course of infection.

C. Design of Test Systems

Three basic types of assay have been utilized for the laboratory detection of HBV markers in serum: the sandwich assay, the competitive assay, and the IgM-antibody capture assay. The sandwich assay produces high specificity as the antigen is first captured by specific antibody, usually attached to a solid phase, and then a second labeled antibody is used to detect any bound antigen. A similar assay can be used to detect antibody with bound and labeled purified antigen as the outer layers of the sandwich. A simpler single-step test is provided by the competitive assay in which labeled antibody and antibody in the specimen compete for antigen bound to a solid phase. The IgM antibody capture assay is used to detect specific IgM, the specificity being introduced by the viral antigen added in the second stage. First, all IgMs present in the serum are captured on a solid phase coated with antihuman IgM. Virus or viral antigen is then added and this binds only to any virus-specific IgM antibody already bound. The bound virus is detected by labeled specific antibody. This type of test is used for the detection of IgM antibody to HBcAg and also for detection of IgM antibody to hepatitis A and rubella viruses.

The most sensitive present test systems use a labeled antigen or antibody in the final stage. This label can be a radioisotope, e.g., ^{125}I, or an enzyme, e.g., horseradish peroxidase. Increasing restrictions placed on the use of radioactive material in the laboratory are making the enzyme label more attractive to many users, but it should be remembered that this label requires one extra step, the demonstration of the presence of enzyme by its reaction on a substrate. Not only does this require further time, but one extra step is one extra opportunity for error. The regulations governing the use of radioactive substances are becoming more stringent, but in the long run, all other factors in the assay being equal, a radioimmunoassay should produce fewer errors than an enzyme immunoassay.

The increasing sophistication of present test methodologies requires sophisticated and expensive equipment such as multiwell gamma counters for radioimmunoassays and automatic plate readers for enzyme immunoassays. Where expense, space, or delivery and storage present problems then consideration should
be given to the simple, unsophisticated, inexpensive test, the reversed passive hemagglutination assay. In this assay, red cells are coated with antibody, and a mixture of the cells and the diluted serum under test are mixed and allowed to settle
at room temperature. Any antigen present binds to the red cells and causes agglutination, usually within 30 min. This test is not as sensitive as the best, enzyme
and radioimmunoassays but it will detect HBsAg in all but the most unusual cases
of clinically apparent acute infection. Tests for other HBV markers are also marketed. These, too, are satisfactory, provided it is remembered that there is some
loss of sensitivity with this system.

D. Test Systems Using Polyclonal Antibodies

1. Hepatitis B Surface Antigen

The best marker of an acute or chronic HBV infection is the presence of HBsAg.
The most sensitive assays can detect HBsAg consistently at concentrations of 0.5
ng/ml (Table 3), at least 6 weeks before clinical illness, and it has been claimed
that surface antigen can be detected as early as 6 days after exposure (Krugman
et al., 1979). The duration of surface antigen in a resolving acute case is highly
variable. In western Scotland, clearing of antigen has been noted within 1 week
in young drug abusers but has taken 1 year in an older patient with systemic lupus
erythematosus. When following up an acute infection, it is useful to ask the testing laboratory to run the current specimen along with a previous specimen. Any
fall in antigen level will then be noticed.

Table 3 Sensitivity of Various Commercial Tests for the Detection of HBsAg

Test	Type	Manufacturer	Sensitivity (ng/ml)
Polyclonal			
Ausria II	RIA	Abbott Laboratories	0.63
Auszyme	EIA	Abbott Laboratories	0.45
Hepanostika HBsAg	EIA	Organon Teknika	0.7
Hepatest	RPHA	Wellcome Diagnostics	5.0
Monoclonal			
Auszyme	EIA	Abbott Laboratories	0.31
Wellcozyme HBsAg	EIA	Wellcome Diagnostics	0.16

Until recently it was believed that the best tests for HBsAg had a sensitivity far in excess of that required for diagnostic purposes and that no benefit would accrue to diagnostic laboratories by further increases in sensitivity. This view has had to be modified following the observations of Kryger et al. (1982) who were able to demonstrate evidence of acute hepatitis B infection (anti-HBc of IgM class) in a group of patients with clinical hepatitis, but who had no detectable HBsAg and who had been classified as cases of non-A, non-B hepatitis. Antigen can be cleared very rapidly by some patients, and if such a patient delays seeking medical advice until the peak of infection is past, then a laboratory test for HBsAg can be misleading. In any case of hepatitis in a high-risk group patient, it is worthwhile testing for anti-HBc of IgM class if HBsAg is not detected. Clearly, a more sensitive test, capable of reducing the time interval or "convalescent window" between loss of HBsAg and development of anti-HBs would be likely to detect antigen in many of these patients. An even more sensitive test for HBsAg could therefore have diagnostic uses.

The blood transfusion services have always sought maximum sensitivity in their tests for HBsAg and have always been concerned that donors with a recent hepatitis B infection, but who are now in the convalescent window, would show no evidence of HBsAg by present tests. If the hepatitis B infection was subclinical then no warning would be noted on questioning the donor, and the donation would be accepted. The simplest method of overcoming this problem would be a more sensitive test capable of eliminating the time interval or convalescent window.

2. Antibody to Hepatitis B Core Antigen

Anti-HBc is normally detected by a single-step competitive assay. After an HBV infection, anti-HBc persists at high titer for many years and is the best marker to assay in epidemiological studies when seeking evidence of prior exposure to HBV. Some current tests use HBcAg prepared by recombinant DNA technology as the solid phase antigen (Peutherer et al., 1981), thus, obviating the necessity of purifying HBcAg from virus particles derived from serum or directly from infected liver tissue.

Diagnostically, evidence of circulating anti-HBc is of limited value, but when the class of the antibody can be determined, clinically useful information is obtained. In most acute cases with clinical hepatitis, anti-HBc is of the IgM class and is normally found at a high titer. In most long-term carriers, especially of more than 1 year duration, tests for anti-HBc IgM are totally negative and the anti-HBc is of the IgG class. Care is needed in interpreting some results, and there are exceptions to the general rule. In early infection, HBsAg and HBeAg may be detected but not anti-HBc IgM. The data could be interpreted to indicate long-term carriage, but a test for total anti-HBc will show very little if any antibody and a further specimen 1-2 weeks later will show rising anti-HBc and the presence of anti-HBc IgM. Some tests for anti-HBc IgM show a prozone effect at high titers.

The specimen will appear negative at low dilution but becomes increasingly positive as dilution increases. If the clinical picture and the anti-HBc IgM result are at variance, then further tests at two dilutions are worthwhile. In some carriers of HBV infection, anti-HBc IgM persists at high titer for many years. Such cases are associated with chronic liver disease and present the diagnostic laboratory with a difficult problem if no evidence of chronic liver disease is reported or suspected. There is evidence from a Japanese group that further differentiation of the IgM antibody into low-molecular-weight (7S) and high-molecular-weight (19S) fractions allows differentiation of acute from persistent infections, the 7S activity being higher in the persistent infections, the 19S being higher in the true acute infections (Tsuda et al., 1984).

As noted in the previous section, a test for anti-HBc IgM can show evidence of acute HBV infection in cases where HBsAg has been rapidly cleared from the serum: a simple negative result for HBsAg may be misleading if a test for anti-HBc IgM is not carried out, as such cases may be labeled non-A, non-B hepatitis. Kryger and colleagues (1982) identified 20% of their non-A, non-B patients as cases of actual HBV infection using this test.

3. Antibody to Hepatitis B Surface Antigen

Anti-HBs is the marker of immunity in HBV infection, and its presence after an acute infection indicates total elimination of HBsAg. Present tests lack specificity at low antibody levels and it is unwise to use anti-HBs as a sole marker or prior hepatitis B infection in epidemiological studies. Anti-HBc is a superior marker of prior infection.

The introduction of hepatitis B vaccine has increased demands for anti-HBs tests both before and after vaccination. Prevaccination checks for immunity to HBV must test for anti-HBs, but immunity can only be assured if anti-HBc is also present. Weakly positive reactions for only anti-HBs (< 5 IU/L) may be unrelated to HBV infection (Tedder et al., 1980), and such patients should not be considered immune. Prevaccination checks may not be essential or cost-effective in low-risk groups but a postvaccination check for development of antibody should be recommended. Some vaccinees do not respond to the present plasma-derived vaccine, and it is essential that they are aware of this failure, particularly if working in a high-risk environment. The present tests for anti-HBs are time-consuming and expensive, particularly if a measured titer of antibody is required. The increasing use of the plasma-derived vaccine and the early introduction of the new yeast-derived vaccines require the development of a simple, rapid test for anti-HBs that can be widely used to determine immunity in vaccinees.

4. Hepatitis B "e" Antigen and Its Antibody

Hepatitis B virus cannot be grown in any cell culture system and hence, there is no simple virological test for infectivity of blood, body fluids, or tissue extracts.

Some indication of infectivity can be obtained by searching for hepatitis B virions or Dane particles by electron microscopy or by assaying for DNA polymerase activity. Both techniques are complex and not readily available on a routine basis. The HBeAg is a soluble protein whose occurrence during infection correlates with the presence of Dane particles and high levels of DNA polymerase activity. It is a component of HBcAg and can be produced by degradation of purified core particles (Takahashi et al., 1979) or from core antigen synthesized in *E. coli* (MacKay et al., 1981).

In the laboratory HBeAg is assayed using the sandwich principle with polyclonal human anti-HBe on the solid phase and a labeled polyclonal antibody as final stage. The test for anti-HBe is a modified HBeAg test in that a precise amount of HBeAg is incubated with the test specimen and residual HBeAg remaining after neutralization with any anti-HBe present is assayed. Most specimens from acute cases and long-term carriers give clear unequivocal results, but a substantial proportion show presence of neither HBeAg nor anti-HBe. Little of relevance to a clinician is gained from such a result, and an improvement in the sensitivity of HBeAg tests is necessary.

5. Conclusions

Any microbiology laboratory considering providing a hepatitis diagnostic service for its local hospital is faced with a bewildering array of possible tests from an ever-increasing number of companies. The single most useful test is for HBsAg, and a test should be chosen that can consistently detect 1.0 ng/ml under standard conditions. This will probably be an enzyme or radioimmunoassay. It is also useful to stock a rapid, reversed passive hemagglutination assay (RPHA) for use in confirming positive test results. Most clinically apparent hepatitis B cases test positive by RPHA, and its use saves the time and expense of confirming all HBsAg positive results by neutralization with specific antibody. The next most useful test for a laboratory is the test for anti-HBc IgM, which will allow differentiation of acute from carrier cases and also permit some investigation of atypical cases when there is suggestion that the patient may be in the convalescent window. The tests for HBeAg/anti-HBe are expensive and may be required infrequently if the local carrier rate is low. It would seem sensible to have these and tests for anti-HBc/anti-HBs centralized. In any laboratory catering to a large population, more extensive use of tests for immunity should be considered. Many individuals in high-risk groups, e.g., drug addicts and homosexuals, appear repeatedly at hospital outpatient clinics or accident/emergency departments. A knowledge of the immune status of such patients can be extremely useful and can often avoid an emergency out-of-hours test for HBsAg. Tests for anti-HBc/anti-HBs on such selected groups are worthy of consideration, especially if there is continual demand for emergency HBsAg tests on these patients.

E. Diagnostic Tests Using Monoclonal Antibodies

1. Hepatitis B Surface Antigen

Monoclonal antibodies (MAbs) can offer high specificity, high affinity, and a constant source of supply. Such is the worldwide demand for HBsAg tests that it would have been expected that tests incorporating MAb would have been available many years ago. However, it is only in the last 2 years that tests have been marketed on a commercial scale. This "failure" has been a result of the high specificity and sensitivity of present polyclonal assays and the unexpected antigenic heterogeneity of HBsAg. Present evidence indicates that the MAb tests are more sensitive because they can detect antigen for a longer period in a patient in the recovery phase of infection, thus reducing the time interval of the convalescent window, and they can also detect antigen at an earlier stage of infection (Wands et al., 1984) (see Table 3).

An additional benefit gained from using MAb technology is that the traditional two-step sandwich assay for HBsAg can be reduced to a one-step procedure. In this system, an antibody to one epitope is used as solid phase antibody and antibody to another epitope is used as labeled antibody. Instead of two incubation steps, as required in the polyclonal sandwich assay, only one is required. Such a system is extremely convenient, especially if a radioimmunoassay system is used, and is ideal for the emergency and out-of-hours tests that are increasingly demanded of a diagnostic laboratory. Before discarding any polyclonal-based assay, however, it should be remembered that sensitivity can be improved by extending incubation times, by increasing incubation temperature, or by reducing the cutoff level. In addition, the only certain method to decide if a patient or donor is in the convalescent window is to test for anti-HBc as well as HBsAg. A combined test able to detect HBsAg by radioimmunoassay and anti-HBc by enzyme immunoassay in a single assay has been developed and found satisfactory (Wylie et al., 1983).

2. Subtyping of Hepatitis B Surface Antigen

It was recognized in the early 1970s, by use of the simple technique of immunodiffusion, that HBsAg was antigenically extremely complex. A common group-specific antigen, a, was identified and further mutually exclusive subdeterminants d or y and w or r. Eight distinct subtypes were recognized and two mixed subtypes containing both d and y. Analysis of surface antigen for the minor subdeterminants was difficult, and very few laboratories tested for other than the ad or ay subtypes. The availability of a variety of MAbs of much greater specificity for the minor subdeterminants than any polyclonal antibody has stimulated interest in the antigenic diversity of HBsAg. Previously unknown subdeterminants have been discovered (Wands et al., 1982), new subgroups have been recognized within the original subtypes, and the a domain has been shown to be antigenically complex (Wands et al., 1984). At present, no specific disease pattern is associated with any particular subtype, and thus extensive subtype analysis has limited clinical value. However, MAbs have already demonstrated a greater antigenic diversity in HBsAg than previously recognized and are the only tools available to further unravel these complexities. Precise subtype analysis is a useful tool in epidemiological studies and should provide valuable information on the transmission of infection, the spread of infection worldwide, and the natural history of HBV infection.

IV. CONCLUSIONS

The present polyclonal-based tests available for the detection of HBsAg and the other markers of HBV infection provide reliable, specific, and sensitive methods for the diagnosis of infection. An increase in the sensitivity of HBsAg tests, in the specificity of tests for anti-HBs at low titer, and in the sensitivity of tests for HBe/anti-HBe would improve current diagnostic methods. The incorporation of MAbs into some test systems has improved convenience and speed of testing. There is still concern that the very high specificity of MAbs could result in failure to detect some unusual antigen even when a cocktail of antibodies is used. This very precise specificity of MAbs makes them ideal tools to investigate the antigenic diversity of HBsAg, and it is in this area that the most valuable contribution has been made to our understanding of HBV infection.

REFERENCES

Alter, H. J., Purcell, R. H., Gerin, J. L., London, W. T., Kaplan, P. M., McAuliffe, V. J., Wagner, J., and Holland, P. V. (1977). Transmission of hepatitis B to chimpanzees by hepatitis B surface antigen-positive saliva and semen. *Infect. Immun. 16*:928-933.

Bancroft, W. H., Snitbhan, R., Scott, R. M., Tingpalapong, M., Watson, W. T., Tanticharoenyos, P., Karwacki, J. J., and Srimarut, S. (1977). Transmission of hepatitis B virus to gibbons by exposure to human saliva containing hepatitis B surface antigen. *J. Infect. Dis. 135*:79-85.

Barr, A., Houston, S. R., Macvarish, I. P., Dow, B. C., Mitchell, R., and Crawford, R. J. (1981). Hepatitis B virus markers in blood donors in the west of Scotland. *Med. Lab. Sci. 38*:405-407.

Beasley, R. P. (1982). Hepatitis B virus as the etiologic agent in hepatocellular carcinoma-epidemiologic considerations. *Hepatology 2*:21-26.

Beasley, R. P., Lee, G. C., Roan, C.-H., Hwang, L.-Y., Lan, C.-C., Huang, F.-Y., and Chen, C.-L. (1983). Prevention of perinatally transmitted hepatitis B virus infections with hepatitis B vaccine. *Lancet 2*:1099-1102.

Beasley, R. P., Trepo, C., Stevens, C. E., and Szmuness, W. (1977). The e antigen and vertical transmission of hepatitis B surface antigen. *Am. J. Epidemiol.* 105:94-99.

Boxall, E. H. (1982). Maternal transmission of hepatitis B. *Recent Adv. Clin. Virol.* 2:17-29.

Coleman, J. C., Waugh, M., and Dayton, R. (1977). Hepatitis B antigen and antibody in a male homosexual population. *Br. J. Vener. Dis.* 53:132-134.

Crawford, R. J., Barr, A., Macvarish, I., Dow, B. C., Mitchell, R., and Follett, E. A. C. (1979). Blood-donors with a history of jaundice. *Lancet* 2:155.

Darani, M. and Gerber, M. (1974). Hepatitis B antigen in vaginal secretions. *Lancet* 2:1008.

Darrell, R. W. and Jacob, G. B. (1978). Hepatitis B surface antigen in human tears. *Arch. Ophthalmol.* 96:674-676.

Deinhardt, R. and Gust, I. D. (1982). *Bull. WHO* 60:661-691.

Fagan, E. A., Davison, F., Smith, P. M., and Williams, R. (1986). Fulminant hepatitis B in successive female sexual partners of two anti-HBe-positive males. *Lancet* 2:538-540.

Follett, E. A. C., Barr, A., Crawford, R. J., and Mitchell, R. (1980). Viral hepatitis markers in blood donors and patients with a history of jaundice. *Lancet* 1:246-249.

Follett, E. A. C., McIntyre, A., O'Donnell, B., Clements, G. B., and Desselberger, U. (1986). HTLV III antibody in drug abusers in the west of Scotland: The Edinburgh connection. *Lancet* 1:446-447.

Follett, E. A. C. and McMillan, A. (1980). Homosexuals—a true "high risk" group for hepatitis B infection. *Commun. Dis. Scot.* (Glasgow) 14:7-8.

Galibert, F., Mandart, E., Fitoussi, F., Tiollais, P., and Charnay, P. (1979). Nucleotide sequence of the hepatitis B virus genome (subtype *ayw*) cloned in *E. coli. Nature* 281:646-650.

Gust, I. D. (1981). Comparison of the epidemiology of hepatitis A and B. In *Viral Hepatitis* (W. Szmuness, H. J. Alter, and J. E. Maynard, eds.). Franklin Institute Press, Philadelphia, pp. 129-143.

Hilleman, M. R., Bertland, A. U., Buynak, E. B., Lampson, G. P., McAleer, W. J., McLean, A. A., Roehn, R. R., and Tytell, A. A. (1978). Clinical and laboratory studies of HBsAg vaccine. In *Viral Hepatitis* (W. Szmuness, H. J. Alter, and J. E. Maynard, eds.). Franklin Institute Press, Philadelphia, pp. 525-537.

Karayiannis, P., Novick, D. M., Lok, A. S. F., Fowler, M. J. F., Monjardino, J., and Thomas, H. C. (1985). Hepatitis B virus DNA in saliva, urine, and seminal fluid of carriers of hepatitis B e antigen. *Br. Med. J.* 290:1853-1855.

Krugman, S., Overby, L. R., Mushahwar, I. K., Ling, C.-M., Frosner, G. G., and Deinhardt, F. (1979). Viral hepatitis, type B. *N. Engl. J. Med.* 300:101-106.

Kryger, P., Aldershvile, J., Mathiesen, L. R., and Nielsen, J. O. (1982). Acute type B hepatitis among HBsAg negative patients detected by anti-HBc IgM. *Hepatology* 2:50-53.

McAleer, W. J., Buynak, E. B., Maigetter, R. Z., Wampler, D. E., Miller, W. J., and Hilleman, M. R. (1984). Human hepatitis B vaccine from recombinant yeast. *Nature 307*:178-180.

MacKay, P., Lees, J., and Murray, K. (1981). The conversion of hepatitis B core antigen synthesized in *E. coli* into e antigen. *J. Med. Virol. 8*:237-243.

Magnius, L. O. and Espmark, J. A. (1972). New specificities in Australia antigen positive sera distinct from the Le Bouvier determinants. *J. Immunol. 109*: 1017-1021.

Mirick, G. S. and Shank, R. E. (1959). An epidemic of serum hepatitis under controlled conditions. *Trans. Am. Clin. Chem. Assoc. 71*:176-180.

Okada, K., Kamiyama, I., Inomata, M., Imai, M., Miyakawa, Y., and Mayumi, M. (1976). e Antigen and anti-e in the serum of asymptomatic carrier mothers as indicators of positive and negative transmission of hepatitis B virus to their infants. *N. Engl. J. Med. 294*:746-749.

Peutherer, J. F., MacKay, P., Ross, R., Stahl, S., and Murray, K. (1981). Use of hepatitis B core antigen produced in *E. coli* in an assay for anti-HBc. *Med. Lab. Sci. 38*:355-358.

Schreeder, M. T., Thompson, S. E., Hadler, S. C., Berquist, K. R., Zaidi, A., Maynard, J. E., Ostrow, D., Judson, F. N., Braff, E. H., Nylund, T., Moore, J. N., Gardner, P., Doto, I. L., and Reynolds, G. (1982). Hepatitis B in homosexual men: Prevalence of infection and factors related to transmission. *J. Infect. Dis. 146*:7-15.

Scott, R. M., Snitbhan, R., Bancroft, W. H., Alter, H. J., and Tingpalapong, M. (1980). Experimental transmission of hepatitis B virus by semen and saliva. *J. Infect. Dis. 142*:67-71.

Sherlock, S. (1981). Virus hepatitis. In *Diseases of the Liver and Biliary System*. Blackwell Scientific, Oxford, pp. 244-269.

Sobeslavsky, O. (1980). Prevalence of markers of hepatitis B virus infection in various countries: A WHO collaborative study. *Bull. WHO 58*:621-628.

Szmuness, W., Much, M. I., Prince, A. M., Hoofnagle, J. H., Cherubin, C. E., Harley, E. J., and Block, G. H. (1975). On the role of sexual behaviour in the spread of hepatitis B infection. *Ann. Intern. Med. 83*:489-495.

Szmuness, W., Stevens, C. E., Harley, E. J., Zang, E. A., Oleszko, W. R., William, D. C., Sadovsky, R., Morrison, J. M., and Kellner, A. (1980). Hepatitis B vaccine. Demonstration of efficacy in a controlled clinical trial in a high-risk population in the United States. *N. Engl. J. Med. 303*:833-841.

Takahashi, K., Akahane, Y., Gotanda, T., Mishiro, T., Imai, M., Miyakawa, Y., and Mayumi, M. (1979). Demonstration of hepatitis B e antigen in the core of Dane particles. *J. Immunol. 122*:275-279.

Tedder, R. S., Cameron, C. H., Wilson-Croome, R., Howell, D. R., Colgrove, A., and Barbara, J. A. J. (1980). Contrasting patterns and frequency of antibodies to the surface, core, and e antigens of hepatitis B virus in blood donors and homosexual patients. *J. Med. Virol. 6*:323-332.

Tsuda, F., Naito, S., Takao, E., Akahane, Y., Furuta, S., Miyakawa, Y., and Mayumi, J. (1984). Low molecular weight (7S) immunoglobulin M antibody against hepatitis B core antigen in the serum for differentiating acute from persistent hepatitis B virus infection. *Gastroenterology 87*:159-164.

Villarejos, V. M., Visona, K. A., Gutierrez, A., and Rodriguez, A. (1974). Role of saliva, urine and faeces in the transmission of type B hepatitis. *N. Engl. J. Med. 291*:1375-1378.

Wands, J. R., Ben-Porath, E., and Wong, M. A. (1984). Monoclonal antibodies and hepatitis B: A new perspective using highly sensitive and specific radio-immunoassays. In *Viral Hepatitis and Liver Disease* (G. W. Vyas, J. L. Dienstag, and J. H. Hoffnagle, eds.). Grune + Stratton, New York, pp. 543-559.

Wands, J. R., Marciniak, R. A., Isselbacher, K. J., Varghese, M., Don, G., Halliday, J. W., and Powell, L. W. (1982). Demonstration of previously undetected hepatitis B viral determinants in an Australian aboriginal population by monoclonal anti-HBs antibody radioimmunoassays. *Lancet 1*:977-980.

Wylie, J. S., Mankikar, S. D., Buchner, B. K., and Moore, B. P. L. (1983). Trial of a combined test for the detection of HBsAg and anti-HBc. *Transfusion 23*:523-525.

Zuckerman, A. J. and Howard, C. R. (1979). *Hepatitis Viruses of Man.* Academic Press, London.

FIFTEEN

Development of Monoclonal Antibodies to Hepatitis B Virus

Hiroshi Takahashi
Jack R. Wands
Massachusetts General Hospital
Boston, Massachusetts

I. INTRODUCTION

This chapter reviews the strategies for production of highly specific monoclonal antibodies (MAbs) to epitopes or antigenic determinants that reside on hepatitis B surface antigen (HBsAg). This viral protein is the specific serological marker for hepatitis B virus (HBV) infection. The importance of immunization schedules as well as the purity of the immunizing antigen preparation are emphasized. Techniques that are useful in characterizing the physical properties of the MAbs are also examined. Another crucial aspect of this research includes studies that focus on the epitope specificity of the MAbs because HBV has far more antigenic heterogeneity than previously recognized with polyclonal antibodies. These considerations become important in selecting appropriate antibodies for use as immunodiagnostic reagents. Appropriate combinations of MAbs to HBsAg (anti-HBs) can be used to construct multisite radioimmunoassays (RIAS). Clinical studies that illustrate the value of such assays are presented. These investigations illustrate the sensitivity and specificity of a first- and second-generation RIA. The development of anti-HBs MAbs has enabled us to extend our diagnostic capabilities and has provided novel information on the importance of HBV as a causitive agent in various acute and chronic liver diseases that show negative results by conventional polyclonal RIA.

II. HEPATITIS B VIRUS ANTIGENS AND ANTIBODIES

In the last decade, considerable progress has been made in identifying and characterizing hepatitis B virus (HBV), in spite of the narrow host range of viral specificity. Only humans and chimpanzees may be infected, and only recently has the virus been propagated in tissue culture (Sureau et al., 1986). The serum of infected individuals usually contains three particulate structures with distinct viral antigenic activity. These include a 22-nm spherical particle that contains HBsAg (the specific serological marker for HBV infection), 22-nm tubular structures also containing HBsAg, and 42-nm spherical Dane particles that represent the infectious HBV. The inner lipid shell of the virus contains hepatitis B core antigen (HBcAg), partially double-stranded viral DNA, a viral DNA polymerase, and hepatitis B e antigen (HBeAg). The presence of HBeAg suggests active viral replication and generally indicates highly infectious material. During HBV infection and recovery, the host produces antibodies to all three antigens—namely, anti-HBs, anti-HBc, and anti-HBe. Thus, the presence of anti-HBs and anti-HBc usually (but not always) signifies past exposure and immunity to HBV.

The hepatitis B surface antigen has three major antigenic domains: the group-specific *a* domain, and the subtype-specific *d* or *y* and *r* or *w* domains. Thus, HBV was originally classified into four major subtypes *adr, adw, ayw,* and *ayr.* However, additional subtype specificities have been described and the classification of HBsAg now include nine main subtypes—ayw_1, ayw_2, ayw_3, ayw_4, and the rare ayr found exclusively in the Far East all belong to the y type, whereas adw_2, adw_4, $adrq^+$, $adrq^-$, belong to the d type as measured by polyvalent anti-HBs antibodies. Therefore, most of the subtyping of HBV strains, to date, has been accomplished by polyclonal monospecific antiserum prepared by immunoabsorption of antisera to one subtype with HBsAg representing another subtype. Anti-HBs Mabs generated to native antigen potentially represents a much more precise method for investigating the diversity in antigenic structure of HBsAg subtypes.

III. PRODUCTION OF ANTI-HEPATITIS B SURFACE MONOCLONAL ANTIBODIES

High affinity IgG and IgM Mabs have been produced in our laboratory by the fusion of NS1 myeloma cells and HBsAg-primed splenocytes (Wands and Zurawski, 1981; Wands et al., 1981). There are several essential criteria for the development of high-affinity antibodies to HBsAg. It is important to have highly pure preparations of HBsAg to ascertain the optimal antigen concentration for production of high affinity antibodies. In addition, a pure HBsAg immunogen will help ensure that all the resulting Mabs will react specifically with only HBsAg-associated epitopes. In our studies HBsAg was isolated by density gradient sedimentation from several units of HBsAg-positive plasma containing both ad and ay HBsAg subtypes. The HBsAg preparation contained only 22-nm, small, spherical forms as judged by electron microscopy. No Dane particles were present, thus excluding other structural proteins of HBV from the immunizing preparation. The optimal route and interval of immunization and the antigen concentration were established for the production of stable anti-HBs-secreting hybrids.

We explored several immunization schedules that varied the route of antigen administration, the concentration of antigen, and the interval between primary and secondary immunizations. Primary immunization was always performed by the intraperitoneal (IP) route at one of three different concentrations of HBsAg (1, 10, or 20 µg/mouse) in a complete Freund's adjuvant (CFA) emulsion. The secondary immunization was either by the IP or intravenous (IV) route. We tested antigen concentrations of 0.1, 1, 10, 50, and 100 µg of viral protein per mouse. The interval between the primary and secondary immunization was either 2, 3, 5, or 10 weeks.

In a study involving ten mice, attempts to establish somatic cell hybrids secreting anti-HBs were unsuccessful when secondary immunizing antigen concentrations of 1, 10, or 20 µg HBsAg in CFA were administered IP. Similarly we were unable to establish stable hybrids secreting anti-HBs if the primary IP immunization with 1, 10, or 20 µg HBsAg was followed by an IV boost of 0.1, 1, 50, or 100 µg HBsAg. In addition, serum titers of anti-HBs were relatively low when any of these immunization schedules were used. Results of immunization with 10 µg of antigen IP

Table 1   Effect of Immunization Schedule on the Anti-HBs Serum Titer and Production of Hybrids Secreting Anti-HBs

Mouse serum dilution	Serum anti-HBs activity with various[a] intervals between immunization			
	2 wk[b]	3 wk	5 wk	10 wk
1:10^1	1.60 (16%)[c]	16.0 (28%)	51.67 (33%)	79.29 (68%)
1:10^2	0.70 (7%)	8.43 (14%)	10.74 (15%)	43.61 (40%)
1:10^3	0.20	0.46	1.61 (1.1%)	12.94 (12%)
1:10^4	0.19	0.18	0.33	0.77 (0.71%)
Disposition of microwells	Fraction of wells positive			
	2 wk[b]	3 wk	5 wk	10 wk
Wells containing hybrids (%)[d]	62	80	73	100
Hybrids secreting anti-HBs (%)	0	1	16	100

[a]Serum anti-HBs activity was measured 72 hr after the last antigen boost using a solid phase radio-immunoassay with ^{125}I-labeled HBsAg.
[b]Time between IV secondary immunization (10 μg HBsAg) and the primary IP immunization (10 μg HBsAg in CFA).
[c]^{125}I-labeled HBsAg bound (cpm $\times$ 10^3). The number in parentheses represents the percentage of counts bound, calculated from the total number of ^{125}I-labeled HBsAg counts added in 200 μl.
[d]Cells from individual fusions were seeded into 300 microwells.

followed by an IV boost of 10 μg at 1, 2, 3, 5, or 10 weeks later are shown in Table 1. There were four animals studied at 1 week, three at 2 weeks, four at 3 weeks, and two at 5 and 10 weeks. As might be expected, serum titers of anti-HBs increased progressively as a function of the length of time between the primary immunization and the secondary antigen boost.

More importantly, although hybrids were established when the second antigen boost was at 2 and 3 weeks, these cells produced relatively small amounts of anti-HBs as measured by the solid phase assays. Moreover, these low levels of culture supernatant activity were often lost as the hybrids were serially passed in tissue culture. If, however, a longer maturation time was allowed between the primary and secondary immunizations, there was not only an increase in the percentage of cell lines secreting anti-HBs, but it was also possible to establish a number of stable hybrids, which have retained very high anti-HBs secretory activity. Therefore, the importance of the route and time of immunization and the antigen concentration should not be underestimated in establishing optimal conditions for the production of anti-HBs synthesizing hybrids.

One positive anti-HBs-secreting hybrids have been identified by solid phase radioimmunoassay (RIA) (Ausab, Abbott Laboratories, North Chicago, Illinois) and their stability established, such hybrids were cloned twice at or beyond limiting dilutions. Subsequently, ascites fluid was collected after malignant growth of cloned hybrids in syngeneic mice.

IV. CHARACTERIZATION OF MONOCLONAL ANTIBODIES

Anti-HBs MAbs were characterized as to specificity for determinants of HBsAg, ability to agglutinate erythrocytes coated with HBsAg (subtypes *adw* and *ayw*), antibody class and subclass, and affinity for HBsAg-associated epitopes. The properties of some representative double-cloned anti-HBs MAbs are shown in Table 2.

By competitive-binding studies we determined whether the anti-HBs MAbs recognize the same, closely related, or separate antigenic determinants on HBsAg (Wands et al., 1982) (Fig. 1). In brief, HBsAg was coated on a solid phase support and was incubated with a constant concentration of one ^{125}I-labeled anti-HBs MAb, such as 5D3, in the presence of purified unlabeled 5D3 or 3D4, 5C3, and 2C6 MAbs. It would be expected that high concentration of unlabeled 5D3 would completely inhibit binding of radiolabeled 5D3 to its epitope on HBsAg. If there is no inhibition of 5D3 binding to HBsAg when other anti-HBs MAbs such as 5C3, 2C6, and 3D4 are incubated with radiolabeled 5D3, we may conclude that 5D3 recognizes a different epitope than the other anti-HBs antibodies. Thus, one can

Table 2   Properties of Representative Examples of Anti-HBs MAbs

Clone	Immunoglobulin class	Affinity constant[a]	Specificity[b] adw	ayw
5D3	IgM	4×10^{11}	++++	++++
1F8	IgM	1.4×10^{10}	++++	++
2F11	IgM	4.8×10^{10}	++++	+++
3D4	IgM	1×10^{11}	++++	++++
1C7	IgG1	3.2×10^{10}	++++	++
4E8	IgG1	9.1×10^{9}	++++	++
5C3	IgG2a	8×10^{10}	++++	++++
5C11	IgG1	4×10^{10}	++++	++++
2C6	IgG2b	2×10^{10}	++++	++++

[a]Expressed as liters per mole per molecule of IgM or IgG.
[b]Capability to agglutinate HBsAg-coated, O-negative erythrocytes (subtypes *adw* and *ayw*). The reaction is graded on an arbitrary scale where ++++ designates strong agglutination and +++, ++, and + are lesser degrees of agglutination.

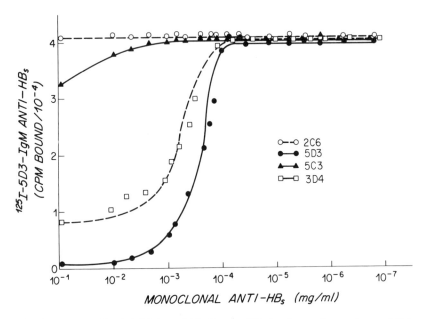

Fig. 1 Competitive inhibition of binding to HBsAg determinants by anti-HBs
MAbs. The four M-RIAs used in the study detect three separate epitopes and one
partial cross-reactive epitope on HBsAg.

establish a matrix of competitive inhibition curves to determine the specificity of
each anti-HBs MAb for separate and distinct epitopes on HBsAg.

Recently, we have demonstrated that at least five noncompeting anti-HBs
MAbs recognize epitopes associated with the a domain of the HBsAg (by definition those antibodies that recognize all subtypes of HBV) (see Table 2). On the
other hand, other MAbs may help distinguish between d and y subtypes (1F8,
2F11, 1C7, and 4E8; Table 2). In brief, RIAs were designed in which one MAb
that recognizes all known HBsAg subtypes was bound to polystyrene beads and
served as capture antibody. Serial 10-fold dilutions of various HBsAg subtypes
were assayed with eight different radiolabeled MAbs. Computer-assisted analysis
of these reactions demonstrated the specificity of these MAbs to epitopes shared

Fig. 2 Signature analysis of 12 HBsAg-positive Ethiopians. They were infected
with two antigenically distinct HBV strains: aligned signature profiles of one
group (six individuals) (top panel); signature profile of the other Ethiopian viral
strain (six individuals) (middle panel); comparison of the signatures (_____)
(_ _ _ _ _), indicating that two distinct variants of HBV are prevalent in this geographical area (bottom panel).

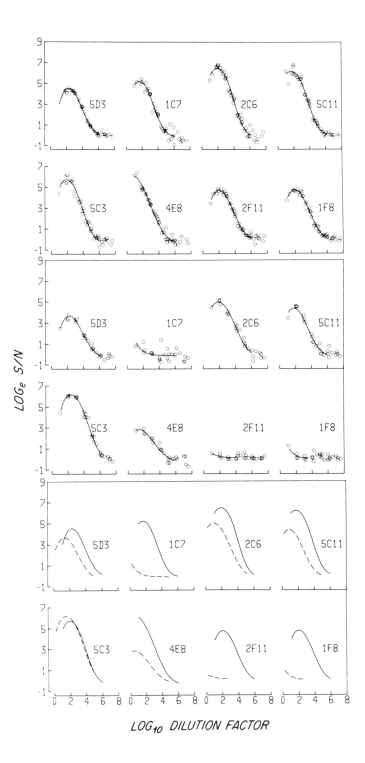

by both *ad* and *ay* subtypes and those more specific to one or the other. We then
began to study HbsAg structure in chronic HBV carriers as shown in Fig. 2. This is
a representative investigation of 12 HBsAg-positive chronic carriers from Ethiopia
as analyzed by the eight monoclonal RIAs. Two distinct binding or viral "signature" profiles representing different HBV strains were observed (Fig. 2, top and
middle). Comparison between the two signatures as depicted in Fig. 2 (bottom)
demonstrates considerable diversity in epitope antigenic structure between the
two Ethiopian HBV strains. Thus, the geographical region from which the Ethiopians originated appeared to harbor two distinct HBV subtypes. It is important
that antibodies 1C7, 4E8, 2F11, and 1F8 showed low-binding activity to one
strain (middle panel) even though the antibodies have high-affinity constants (see
Table 2) for HBsAg-associated epitopes. Herein lies one of the major problems of
the use of MAbs as immunodiagnostic reagents; the antibodies may be too specific,
and as outlined later, one must select antibodies such as 5D3, 5C3, 5C11, 2C6,
and 3D4 that recognized the common *a* domain epitopes so that all HBV strains
are identified with high sensitivity. To select such antibodies, we have had to test
thousands of HBsAg carriers from various regions of the world to assure that all
HBV strains are recognized by the anti-HBs MAbs.

V. CONSTRUCTION OF A FIRST-GENERATION MONOCLONAL RADIOIMMUNOASSAY

Anti-HBs MAbs were isolated and purified from mouse ascites fluid before use in
RIA. The IgM anti-HBs may be effectively purified from ascites fluid using Seph-
arose-4B chromatography. Affinity chromatography on Sepharose-staphylococcal
protein-A columns has proved to be a suitable technique for purification of IgG
isotypes of anti-HBs.

A multiple site monoclonal "simultaneous sandwich" RIA was found to be
a sensitive assay for the detection of HBsAg-associated determinants in serum
(Ben-Porath et al., 1984; 1985). Monoclonal antibodies designated 5D3, 5C3, and
5C11 (IgM, IgG2a, and IgG1, respectively) were selected from a library of anti-
HBs MAbs for use in the monoclonal radioimmunoassay (M-RIA) clinical studies
because of the following special properties: (1) they bind to all known subtypes
of HBsAg (Wands et al., 1984); (2) they recognize distinct and separate determinants on HBsAg by competitive binding studies (Wands et al., 1981); (3) they
possess very high-affinity constants for HBsAg-associated determinants (4×10^{11},
8×10^{10}, and 4×10^{10} L/mol per molecule, respectively). In the simultaneous
sandwich RIA (Fig. 3) polystyrene beads were coated with monoclonal IgM anti-
HBs (5D3) which recognizes all known subtypes of HBsAg, and the other two IgG
MAbs, namely, 5C3 and 5C11 were radiolabeled to a specific activity of 10-12
μCi/μg with the Hunter-Bolton reagent (Bolton and Hunter, 1973). The beads

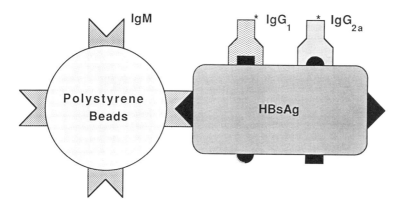

Fig. 3 Diagram demonstrating the immunochemical construction of the first-generation M-RIA. 5D3 an IgM anti-HBs that reacts against repeating determinants within the *a* domain is coupled to a solid phase support (polystyrene beads). The radiolabeled indicator IgG1 (5D3) and IgG2 (5C11) antibodies are also directed against *a* domain-repeating determinants. The assay is performed for 16 hr at 45°C in a simultaneous sandwich mode.

were then incubated with 200 µl of serum sample and 100 µl of radiolabeled probe, consisting of 150,000 cpm of a mixture of 5C3 and 5C11, for 16 hr at 45°C. The beads were washed extensively with distilled water and the radioactivity bound to the beads was measured with a gamma-well counter.

VI. DEVELOPMENT OF A SECOND-GENERATION MONOCLONAL RADIOIMMUNOASSAY

The second-generation, multiple-site M-RIA was developed using the same 5D3-coated beads and radiolabeled indicator antibodies as described in Sect. V. A comparison between the two assays is presented in Table 3. In brief, beads were incubated with 600 µl of serum placed in 2.5-ml plastic tubes with gentle rotary agitation at 45°C for 6-8 hr. Next, the beads were transferred to 25-well plates, 200 µl of fresh serum added to the preincubated beads, and subsequently incubated again with 100 µl of the same 5C3-5C11-radiolabeled indicator antibodies for 16 hr at 45°C; these conditions are identical to the first-generation M-RIA.

To assure the specificity of the antigen-antibody interaction, a neutralization reaction with high-titer polyclonal human anti-HBs antibodies was performed as previously described (Ben-Porath et al., 1985). The neutralization reaction was performed as follows: polyclonal anti-HBs antibodies were obtained from high-titer, anti-HBs-positive plasma by passage of such plasma over an HBsAg-Sepharose-4B affinity column after elution with a glycine HCl buffer, pH 2.6. Polyclonal

Table 3   Comparison of M-RIAs for HBsAg

Measurement	1st-generation M-RIA	2nd-generation M-RIA
Sensitivity	50-100 pg/ml	< 15 pg/ml
Sample volume	200 μl	600 μl
Incubation time	Overnight	6- to 8-hr preincubation and overnight
Method	Simultaneous sandwich RIA at 45°C	Preincubation with rotary agitation at 45°C Simultaneous sandwich RIA at 45°C

anti-HBs thus prepared had a hemagglutination titer of HBsAg-coated O-negative human red blood cells of ~ 1:500,000/20 μl. This reagent provided > 50% neutralization of binding activity in 13 HBsAg-positive human sera in the Ausria II RIA. Concentrated polyclonal anti-HBs (20 μl) was preincubated with 180 μl of M-RIA-reactive serum for 1 hr at 20°C. The binding activity before and after neutralization with anti-HBs was determined. A specific neutralization response of > 50% was considered positive. Finally, as a negative control, 20 μl of anti-HBs-negative plasma prepared in a similar manner was used in parallel experiments.

VII. DATA ANALYSIS

The cutoff values for positive results in the MAb and polyclonal RIAs (P-RIA) were a signal/noise (S/N) ratio of 2.1, defined as the mean counts per minute bound by the experimental serum sample divided by the mean counts per minute of the negative control serum. Such sera were then tested by the first-generation M-RIA. Samples positive only by M-RIA were then retested by Ausria II in the 16-hr incubation protocol according to manufacturer's instructions to reconfirm that they were indeed negative by the polyclonal immunoassay. The remaining first-generation M-RIA nonreactive serum samples were then retested by the second-generation M-RIA as described in Sect. VI. Finally other serological markers indicating recent or past HBV infection, such as anti-HBs and antibodies to hepatitis B core antigen (anti-HBc), were measured in all HBsAg-reactive samples using the Ausab and Corab commercial tests (Abbott Laboratories).

A. Sensitivity of the First- and Second-Generation Monoclonal Radioimmunoassays

The sensitivities of P-RIA and first- and second-generation M-RIAs were evaluated in parallel using a known concentration of HBsAg serially diluted in normal human

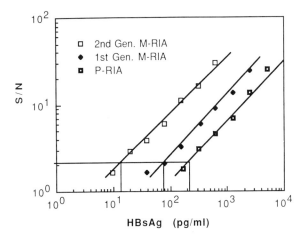

Fig. 4 Comparison of the sensitivity for HBsAg detection in serum by Ausria II, first- and second-generation M-RIAs. Line indicates the cutoff value for positive results.

serum as shown in Fig. 4. The lower limit for HBsAg detection by the P-RIA was about 230 pg/ml. In contrast, the first-generation M-RIA could measure as little as 55 pg/ml, whereas the second-generation M-RIA was found to be very sensitive, with a lower limit of HBsAg detection of about 15 pg/ml. The results demonstrate a four- to fivefold and 16- to 20-fold improvement in sensitivity of the first- and second-generation M-RIAs, respectively, compared with the standard P-RIA.

B. Specificity of the First- and Second-Generation Monoclonal Radioimmunoassays

The specificity of the first-generation (M1-RIA) was assessed (Ben-Porath et al., 1985) using a panel of 2091 serum samples from healthy individuals, patients with liver disease, and controls without liver disease. The results presented in Table 4 indicate that all the serum samples that were reactive by P-RIA were also reactive by the M1-RIA. This information is important because these individuals originated from various regions of the world and were infected with different subtypes of HBV (Courouce-Pauty et al., 1983). Nevertheless, the M1-RIA was capable of detecting all the HBsAg-positive sera, thus recognizing a variety of HBsAg subtypes. Moreover, of the serum samples negative for HBsAg by the P-RIA from patients with liver diseases and from other disease controls, only one was positive by the M1-RIA. This one sample was from a patient with acute hepatitis A who may have been a chronic carrier of HBsAg with a low level of antigen. However, as shown in Sect. VIII that M1-RIA may identify HBsAg-related determinants in patients who are HBsAg-negative by P-RIA.

Table 4   Specificity of First-Generation M-RIA in Healthy Individuals and Control Patients with Liver and Other Diseases

Category	No. tested	M-RIA positive	P-RIA[a] positive
Hepatitis B (acute)[b]	1211	1211	1211
Healthy chronic HBsAg carriers[c]	564	564	564
Alcoholic cirrhosis	50	1	1
Primary biliary cirrhosis	26	0	0
Hemochromatosis	76	0	0
Drug-induced hepatitis	10	0	0
Malignant tumor	76	2	2
Acute hepatitis A[d]	78	1	0
Totals	2091	1779	1778

[a]Ausria II (Abbott Laboratories, North Chicago, Illinois).
[b]Identified initially by P-RIA.
[c]HBsAg was identified in healthy individuals through routine screening by P-RIA and subsequently subtyped as *ayw, adw, ayr,* and *adr* by RIA.
[d]Positive for IgM antihepatitis A antibodies.

Similar, but more limited studies on the specificity of the second-generation (M2-RIA) are presented in Table 5 and Fig. 5. All patients and blood donors positive by P-RIA were also identified as reactive by M2-RIA. Thus, no false-negative results were observed. In addition, low positive patients with chronic active hepatitis by P-RIA (S/N 2.1-10.2) were retested in the M2-RIA. In each instance binding activity was enhanced several-fold presumably because of the greatly increased

Table 5   Specificity of Second-Generation M-RIA in Blood Donors and Disease Controls from Japan

Group	No. tested	M-RIA positive	P-RIA positive
Blood donors	235	14[a]	8
Chronic HBsAg[b] carrier	167	167	167
Hepatitis A[c]	6	0	0
Hepatitis B[b]	7	7	7
Drug-induced hepatitis	2	0	0
Total	417	188	182

[a]Six additional blood donors were positive.
[b]Initially identified as positive by P-RIA (Ausria II).
[c]Positive for IgM antihepatitis A antibodies.

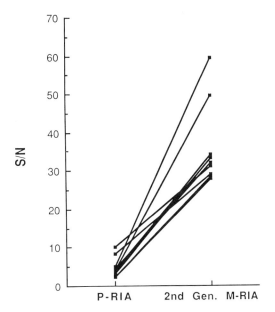

Fig. 5 Analysis of eight patients with chronic active hepatitis as shown by Ausria II and second-generation M-RIA. Note that the low positive values by Ausria II (P-RIA) were substantially higher in the second-generation M-RIA because of the greater sensitivity of the assay.

sensitivity of the M2-RIA as shown by the data depicted in Fig. 5. Finally, there were six blood donors who tested positive only by M2-RIA.

VIII. CLINICAL STUDIES

A. Observations on Patients with Primary Hepatocellular Carcinoma

The development of hepatocellular carcinoma (HCC) occurs in the setting of the HBsAg chronic carrier state. During the last several years, evidence for the association of chronic HBV infection with HCC has become increasingly apparent. By virtue of this association, HCC may now be the most common malignancy in some countries in the world. The epidemiological evidence suggesting that HBV is a causal agent in HCC is most convincing. Such studies have demonstrated a strong geographical correlation between HBsAg prevalence and the prevalence of HCC. Furthermore, case control studies, particularly in Taiwan, shown that HCC patients are almost invariably infected with HBV. The relative risk of developing HCC is approximately 400 times greater for HBsAg carriers than for the general population (Beasley et al., 1981). The risk of developing HCC also correlates well with the duration of the HBsAg carrier state. Thus, if HBV infection occurs in infancy and childhood via vertical transmission from the mother, the risk of manifesting HCC in middle age is highly significant. Furthermore, other epidemiological studies have shown that there is a high prevalence of HBV serological markers (anti-HBs and anti-HBc) in HCC patients who test negatively for HBsAg. This finding suggests, but does not prove, that prior exposure to HBV may have been associated with the pathogenesis of HCC.

We have studied sera from 220 southern African blacks with histologically confirmed HCC (Kew et al., 1986). Both HBsAg-positive and HBsAg-negative (by conventional polyclonal assay) serum samples were sent under code from Johannesburg to Boston for analysis by M1-RIA and M2-RIA. The results of testing for HBsAg by P-RIA, M1-RIA, and M2-RIA in the 220 sera are shown in Fig. 6 and Table 6. All of the patients whose test results were positive for HBsAg by P-RIA

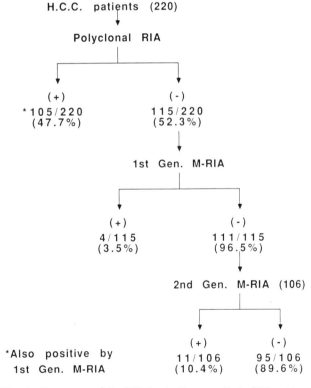

Fig. 6 Summary of the HBsAg-testing results in 220 patients with primary HCC.

Table 6   Summary of Binding Activities and HBV Serological Markers in HBsAg-
Negative Patients Reactive by M1-RIA (Group 1) and M2-RIA (Group 2)

Patient ID no.	Sex	Age	Anti-HBs	Anti-HBc	HBsAg[a] P-RIA	HBsAg[a] M1-RIA	HBsAg[a] M2-RIA
Group 1							
1	M	60	+	+	0.36	3.39	–
2	M	37	+	+	0.45	2.81	–
3	M	17	+	+	0.63	2.62	–
4	M	36	–	+	0.86	2.76	–
Group 2							
5	M	65	+	+	0.48	0.47	10.37
6	M	32	+	+	0.16	1.23	2.25
7	M	50	–	+	0.20	1.06	3.30
8	F	58	–	+	0.12	1.20	2.1
9	F	62	–	+	0.28	1.37	5.45
10	F	60	–	+	0.12	0.44	2.40
11	M	61	–	–	0.48	0.72	10.70
12	F	41	–	–	0.15	0.63	3.70
13	M	63	–	–	0.67	0.54	15.50
14	F	50	–	–	0.14	0.37	2.15
15	M	42	–	–	0.13	1.66	2.90

[a]S/N ratio defined as mean cpm bound in experimental sample divided by mean cpm bound
in the negative control serum. Positive results: S/N > 2.1.

were also positive using M1-RIA. Of the 111 patients whose test results were nega-
tive for HBsAg by both P-RIA and M1-RIA, there was sufficient serum to test for
M2-RIA in only 106. With the 3.5% of patients shown to be HBsAg positive by
M1-RIA and the 10.4% positive with M2-RIA, the number of HCC patients who
tested negative for HBsAg by P-RIA was reduced by 13.9%. The S/N values ranged
from 2.1 to 15.5 for the 11 patients whose test results were positive only by M2-
RIA. As shown in Table 6, of the 11 M2-RIA reactive patients, six had either anti-
HBc and/or anti-HBs (two anti-HBc and anti-HBs; four anti-HBc alone). The remaining five patients had no measurable HBV serological markers in their serum.
Of the 220 patients in the study, 21 demonstrated no virological markers of recent or past HBV infection. However, five of these patients (24%) were reactive
for associated HBsAg epitopes by M2-RIA. Thus, the number of black HCC patients with no apparent serum HBV markers was reduced by one-quarter using
this more sensitive test.

Table 7 Clinical and Serological Profiles on Patients Positive only by First (Group 1)-
and Second (Group 2)-Generation Monoclonal Radioimmunoassays

Patient ID no.	Diagnosis	Anti-HBs	Anti-HBc	HBsAg (S/N) Ausria II	M-RIA
Group 1					
1	Hemodialysis, chronic hepatitis	−	−	< 2.1	6.27
2	Hemodialysis, chronic hepatitis	+	−	< 2.1	20.21
3	Chronic hepatitis, hepatoma	+	+	< 2.1	3.24
4	Chronic active hepatitis	−	−	< 2.1	2.80
5	Cirrhosis	−	+	< 2.1	7.80
6	Cirrhosis	−	+	< 2.1	14.0
7	Acute hepatitis	−	+	< 2.1	9.7
8	Acute hepatitis	+	+	< 2.1	11.8
9	Elevated aminotransferase	−	−	< 2.1	7.4
10	Acute hepatitis	+	+	< 2.1	15.0
Group 2					
1	Hemodialysis, chronic hepatitis	+	+	< 2.1	14.90
2	Hemodialysis, chronic hepatitis	+	+	< 2.1	4.35
3	Chronic hepatitis	−	+	< 2.1	2.35
4	Chronic hepatitis	−	−	< 2.1	14.78
5	Chronic hepatitis	+	+	< 2.1	2.38
6	Cirrhosis	−	−	< 2.1	9.06
7	Cirrhosis	+	−	< 2.1	5.14
8	Cirrhosis	+	+	< 2.1	11.36
9	Cirrhosis	+	+	< 2.1	25.37

B. Observations on Patients with Hepatitis B Surface Antigen-Negative Acute and Chronic Liver Disease

We have begun to investigate patients with chronic liver disease with, and without, recent or past serological markers of HBV infection by M1-RIA and M2-RIA. Table 7 shows some selected patients who were positive only by M1-RIA (group 1) and M2-RIA (group 2). All such patients tested negative by the Ausria II RIA. We also performed a specific viral neutralization test to confirm the positive binding results of the first- and second-generation M-RIAs. In these experiments serum from the M-RIA-positive patients (180 μl) was incubated with 20 μl of high-titer, polyclonal, human-derived anti-HBs antibodies, followed by a repeat measurement of binding activity in the respective M-RIAs. As shown in Fig. 7, binding activity was reduced to undetectable levels by neutralization with polyclonal anti-HBs antibodies, thus confirming the specificity of the antigen-antibody interaction in the M1-RIA and the M2-RIA.

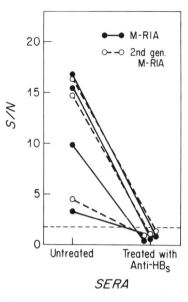

Fig. 7 Representative examples of positive neutralization tests of a serum sample positive only by M-RIA. Results are considered positive if a neutralization result of > 50% is obtained by preincubation with polyclonal human anti-HBs antibodies. The horizontal dotted line is a signal/noise cutoff ratio of 2.1. All samples are completely neutralized in this test.

IX. CONCLUSIONS

Acute and chronic HBV infections present a worldwide problem. For example, it is estimated that worldwide there are now 300 million chronic HBV carriers. There may be a substantial number of patients with acute and chronic hepatitis as well as patients without identifiable liver disease that have HBV infection undetectable by current techniques. Thus, there is a need to improve the sensitivity of present polyclonal HBsAg tests. Given these estimates, we have developed two M-RIAs using the same anti-HBs MAbs, and these RIAs appear to offer certain advantages over current HBsAg immunoassays. The performance of the assays in part depends upon the high-affinity constants of the antibodies for HBsAg-associated epitopes. Furthermore, each antibody recognizes a separate and distinct determinant on HBsAg, and extensive testing with the antibodies revealed that they recognize all known HBV strains. Indeed, in parallel testing of a known concentration of HBsAg in serum, the first- and second-generation M-RIAs improved the detection of HBsAg-associated determinant in serum by four- to fivefold and 16- to 20-fold, respectively. Given the increased sensitivities of the assays, we believe that the M-RIAs would improve the detection of HBV infection.

It was our hypothesis that if a more sensitive assay could be developed, additional HBV-positive patients would be distinguished. Attempts were made, therefore, to develop a second-generation M-RIA. Studies with this M-RIA, which uses a larger sample volume and a longer incubation period to improve the kinetics of the antigen-antibody interaction, resulted in detection of other HBsAg-positive patients reactive to the test. We presume that the improved sensitivity of the second-generation test (about 15 pg/ml) led to the recognition of such patients. Furthermore, these multisite "simultaneous," sandwich M-RIAs have been shown to recognize HBsAg "hidden" in immune complexes formed in anti-HBs excess (Shafritz et al., 1982). Under these circumstances, anti-HBs- and anti-HBc-positive individuals may be reactive in the M-RIAs and not in polyclonal immunoassays (Ben-Porath et al., 1984). It is apparent from the results presented that high-affinity anti-HBs MAbs may be effectively employed in the construction of highly sensitive and specific RIAs and that such assays have improved the diagnostic accuracy of HBV infection.

Finally, it is noteworthy that as the sensitivity of M-RIAs improved for the detection of HBsAg-associated epitopes in serum, a number of patients were recognized without any HBV serological markers such as anti-HBs and anti-HBc. Monoclonal anti-HBs RIA-positive individuals have been associated in recent investigations with the presence of HBV DNA hybridizable sequences in serum and liver (Brechot et al., 1985; Wands et al., 1985). It will be of interest to explore the characteristics of the antigenic and nucleic acid composition of these agents and compare their properties with the known features of HBV.

ACKNOWLEDGMENTS

This research has been supported in part by grants AA-02666, CA-35711, and HD-20469 from the National Institutes of Health. JRW is the recipient of Research Career Development Award AA-00048 from the National Institutes of Health.

REFERENCES

Beasley, R. P., Hwang, L.-U., Lin, C.-C., and Chien, C.-S. (1982). Hepatocellular carcinoma and hepatitis B virus: A prospective study of 22,707 men in Taiwan. *Lancet 2*:1129-1133.

Ben-Porath, E., Wands, J. R., Bar-Shany, S., Huggins, C., and Isselbacher, K. (1985). Improved detection of hepatitis B surface antigen (HBsAg) in blood donors by monoclonal radioimmunoassay. *Transfusion 25*:10-14.

Ben-Porath, E. J., Wands, J., Gruia, M., and Isselbacher, K. J. (1984). Clinical significance of enhanced detection of HBsAg by monoclonal radioimmunoassay. *Hepatology 4*:1269-1273.

Bolton, A. E. and Hunter, W. M. (1973). The labelling of proteins to high specific radioactivities by conjugation to a ^{125}I-containing acetylating agent. *Biochem. J. 133*:529-529.

Brechot, C., Degos, F., Lugassy, C., Thiers, V., Zafrani, S., Franco, C., Bismuth, H., Trépo, C., Benhamou, J.-P., Wands, J., Isselbacher, K., Tiollais, P., and Berthelot, P. (1985). Hepatitis B virus DNA in patients with chronic liver disease and negative tests for hepatitis B surface antigen. *N. Engl. J. Med. 312*:270-276.

Courouce-Pauty, A. M., Plancoz, A., and Soulier, J. D. (1983). Distribution of HBsAg subtypes in the world. *Vox Sang. 44*:197-211.

Kew, M. C., Fujita, Y., Takahashi, H., Coppins, A., and Wands, J. R. (1986). Comparison between polyclonal and first and second generation monoclonal radioimmunoassays in the detection of hepatitis B surface antigen in patients with hepatocellular carcinoma. *Hepatology 6*:636-639.

Shafritz, D. A., Lieberman, H. M., Isselbacher, K. J., and Wands, J. R. (1982). Monoclonal radioimmunoassay for hepatitis B surface antigen: Demonstration of hepatitis B virus DNA or related sequences in serum and viral epitopes in immune complexes. *Proc. Natl. Acad. Sci. USA 79*:5675-5679.

Sureau, C., Romet-Lemonne, J.-L., Mullins, J. I., and Essex, M. (1986). Production of hepatitis B virus by a differentiated human hepatoma cell line after transfection with cloned circular HBV-DNA. *Cell 47*:37-47.

Wands, J. R., Carlson, R. I., Schoemaker, H., Isselbacher, K. J., and Zurawski, V. R. (1981). Immunodiagnosis of hepatitis B with high-affinity IgM monoclonal antibodies. *Proc. Natl. Acad. Sci. USA 78*:1214-1218.

Wands, J. R., Isselbacher, K. J., Brechot, C., and Tiollais, P. (1985). Monoclonal RIAs and HBV-DNA in hepatocellular carcinoma. *Lancet 1*:455.

Wands, J. R., Marciniak, R. A., Isselbacher, K. J., Varghese, M., Don, G., Halliday, J. W., and Powell, L. W. (1982). Demonstration of previously undetected hepatitis B viral determinants in an Australian aboriginal population by monoclonal anti-HBs antibody radioimmunoassay. *Lancet 1*:9777-9780.

Wands, J. R., Wong, M. A., Shorey, J., Brown, R. D., Marciniak, R. A., and Isselbacher, K. J. (1984). Hepatitis B viral antigenic structure: Signature analysis by monoclonal radioimmunoassays. *Proc. Natl. Acad. Sci. USA 81*:2237-2241.

Wands, J. R. and Zurawski, Jr., V. R. (1981). High affinity monoclonal antibodies to hepatitis B surface antigen (HBsAg) produced by somatic cell hybrids. *Gastroenterology 30*:225-232.

SIXTEEN

Diagnosis of Cytomegalovirus Infection

Elizabeth E. Edmond[†]
Edinburgh University
Medical School
Edinburgh, Scotland

Helena F. Hart
Bioscot Ltd.
Edinburgh, Scotland

[†]Deceased.

I. INTRODUCTION

Human cytomegalovirus (HCMV) is an ubiquitous herpesvirus, evidence of infection being present in every population studied. As with other herpesviruses, primary infection with HCMV is followed by lifelong persistence of virus in a manner that is not yet clearly understood, but from which, under certain circumstances, the virus may emerge even after years of quiescence to give a reactivated infection. This virus infrequently causes recognizable disease in normal children or adults, but certain groups of patients, particularly those who are immunocompromised, are at risk of serious and even lethal disease from HCMV infection. Primary infection is most likely to lead to serious illness, but both endogenous reactivation of latent virus and exogenous infection with a genetically different strain of virus may cause severe disease. Primary infection in the immunologically normal individual is associated with the production of IgG and IgM, but only IgG persists as a lifelong marker of previous experience with the virus.

II. CLINICAL PRESENTATION

Community spread of HCMV is mainly subclinical but may manifest as a mononucleosis (Klemona and Kaariainen, 1965). Pyrexia, lymphocytosis, and hepatitis are characteristic features, but pneumonitis and involvement of the central nervous system are rare complications. The Paul-Bunnell type of heterophil antibody does not develop, thus, differentiating the condition from the true infectious mononucleosis caused by Epstein-Barr virus. Headache and myalgia are common presenting symptoms, and the patient may be unwell for 4-6 weeks. Virus is often, but not always, detectable in the saliva and the urine during the acute phase. Viruria may persist for long periods. Virus has also been shown to persist in semen for more than a year following primary infection (Lang et al., 1974).

III. EPIDEMIOLOGY AND TRANSMISSION

A. Community Transmission

Because nearly all infections in the general community are subclinical, assessing the prevalence of infection depends upon demonstrating the presence of IgG antibody in individual sera or upon isolation of virus from secretions of members of a community. Serological surveys have shown that, although the virus is endemic in all communities, the age-related acquisition of IgG antibody varies considerably among countries and among communities within countries. In some communities, more than 90% of the childhood population are seropositive by the age of 4 years, whereas in others, less than 10% of children of the same age have evidence of previous infection. The high frequency of exposure during infancy and early childhood is particularly obvious in communities in which low socioeconomic conditions prevail. Evidence is now accumulating to incriminate close human contact as the most important factor in the spread of infection in these age groups. In communities where a high percentage of individuals escape infection in early life, a significant increase in the rate of infection begins in the adolescent years and continues into adult life. Considerable circumstantial evidence links this rise to the onset of intimate salivary and sexual contact. Virus may be shed in saliva, urine, secretions of the cervix uteri, and breast milk, from individuals who are experiencing active infection with the virus. Prolonged virus shedding in saliva and urine follows primary infection, particularly in childhood. Infection spreads among children grouped together in preschool playgrounds, regardless of the socioeconomic background of the family. Children in residential school are more likely to be infected with HCMV than are children of similar age at day school.

Human cytomegalovirus has been isolated from the cervical secretions of from 1-28% of seropositive pregnant women. Several studies conclude that the proportion of women shedding virus increases with the stage of pregnancy at which virus isolation is attempted, but this may be due to a reduction in shedding in early pregnancy when compared with the infection rate in nonpregnant women (Stagno et al., 1975). Shedding of virus from the cervix in pregnant women is an important source of intrapartum transmission to their offspring. Cervical shedding of virus may also be an important source for venereal spread of infection.

B. Sexual Transmission

Evidence for this route of transmission has mainly been circumstantial. The rise in seropositivity described in the young adult population is not so evident in celibate women of the same age. The prevalence of HCMV positivity and virus shedding are higher in women attending sexually transmitted disease (STD) clinics than other clinics and, moreover, correlate with the prevalence of sexually transmitted disease (Jordan et al., 1973). This virus has been isolated from semen following clinically apparent infection (Lang and Kummer, 1972). The same workers demonstrated virus in the semen of patients attending infertility and STD clinics, as well as from healthy students and blood donors.

Further circumstantial evidence for the sexual spread of HCMV was provided by Chretien et al. (1977), who described the occurrence of HCMV mononucleosis in two male students following intercourse with a female student who had had febrile illness lasting about 1 month before contact with either man. She was seropositive, and HCMV was isolated from her cervix. Another female sexual contact of one of the male students also became ill, whereas roommates remained well and seronegative. More direct evidence for sexual transmission has recently been presented (Handsfield et al., 1985).

Serological tests were carried out on 58 male sex partners of women attending an STD clinic. The serological statuses of the women were known, and each had also been investigated for virus shedding from the cervix and in the urine. A significantly higher proportion of partners of seropositive women had antibody compared with partners of women without antibody. In addition, virus was isolated from serum or urine of four partners of 18 women who shed virus and from no male partners of 42 culture-negative women. The restriction enzyme patterns of pairs of isolates from sex partners were identical in two instances, although a third pair displayed significant differences from each other. Human cytomegalovirus infection is highly prevalent in homosexual men who, in general, have more sexual partners than do heterosexual men. The prevalence of antibody in homosexual men varies from 76-94% compared with approximately 50% in heterosexuals; up to 80% of seropositive homosexual men may be viruric at any time (Drew et al., 1981; Goldmeier et al., 1983; Mindel and Sutherland, 1984; Mintz et al., 1983).

C. Congenital Infection

The major health problem arising from community-acquired infection is that of congenital infection with the virus. Maternal infection resulting in congenital infection may be primary or reactivated. Virus is secreted in 0.3-2.5% of all liveborn infants, maternal reactivation accounting for most cases in highly seropositive communities (Stagno et al., 1977), whereas primary maternal infection precedes most fetal infections when maternal seropositivity is low (Peckham et al., 1983). Fortunately, not all infected infants suffer abnormality or disease; indeed, 90% appear normal at birth, 2% exhibit severe disease with neuronal involvement, and 8% develop perinatal extraneural disease. A proportion of this latter group may demonstrate signs of CNS damage later in childhood in the form of neuromuscular disturbance or auditory defect. Primary maternal infection is more dangerous to the fetus than reactivated infection which occurs in the presence of preexisting maternal antibody, but deafness has been reported following maternal reactivation (Ahlfors et al., 1981). During pregnancy, 1-2% of seronegative women become seropositive.

Prospective studies indicate that between 25 and 75% transmit the infection to their offspring and that transmission may occur at any time during gestation. The control of congenitally acquired HCMV infection currently presents a major challenge to the medical profession.

D. Infection in the Immunocompromised

Infections with HCMV are a major cause of morbidity and mortality in patients who are immunocompromised for any reason, but this is particularly so in organ transplant recipients. Infections may be primary, reactivated, or reinfections from an infectious source. In organ or cardiac transplant recipients, primary infections or reinfections may result from the transmission of virus in blood transfusion or in the transplanted organ itself (Rubin et al., 1985). The most common presentation of HCMV infection is fever, hepatitis, and pneumonia.

Cytomegalovirus infection may be particularly serious in bone marrow transplant recipients who regularly develop a severe form of viral pneumonitis that is often associated with graft-versus-host disease.

IV. PATHOGENESIS

Although community-acquired HCMV infection is not a major health problem, the detailed study of the infection in previously healthy individuals has produced information that has been of crucial value in understanding the pathogenesis of disease caused by the virus, both in this setting and others. During the acute phase of HCMV mononucleosis, virus is readily isolated from buffy coat cultures (Lang and Noren, 1968). Evidence points to the polymorphonuclear or the macrophage monocyte cell type as the main reservoir of virus in the blood during viremia (Carney and Hirsch, 1981; Rinaldo et al., 1977; Rinaldo and DeBiaso, 1983). The disturbance of monocyte function resulting from virus infection has been postulated to be one of the major contributing factors in the excessive production of T-suppressor cells, which is the immunological hallmark of HCMV infection and which, in turn, results in a generalized state of reduced immunocompetence demonstrable in vitro (Carney et al., 1981; Carney et al., 1983).

In vitro lymphocyte proliferative responses from healthy individuals are suppressed when cultured with autologous monocytes infected with HCMV (Carney and Hirsch, 1981). Recently isolated strains of HCMV disturb monocyte function in a similar manner, even though the infection is abortive and only early antigens are expressed (Rice et al., 1984). It appears that the infected monocyte facilitates the proliferation of CD8+ cells while inhibiting the response of the CD4+ cells. This may be due to interference with the antigen-presenting function of monocytes to CD4+ cells, to stimulation of the release of prostaglandins or other substances resulting in the recruitment of suppressor cells, or to other undefined effects on monocyte function. Monocytes with enhanced suppressor function have been observed in other infections (Ellner et al., 1978; Katz et al., 1979).

Lymphocytosis and hypergammaglobulinemia disappear early in convalescence, but the number of CD8+ cells remain elevated for some time (Carney et al., 1981), and lymphocyte responses remain below average for over 2 years in some patients (TenNapel and The, 1980). Usually, during the second week after the onset of symptoms, a humoral response becomes detectable. Specific IgM is always produced in previously immunocompetent individuals; maximum titers are found 3-6 weeks after onset, decline during convalescence, and are generally undetectable after 3-4 months. The IgG response appears at the same time or slightly after the IgM. Specific IgG consists mainly of IgG1 and IgG3 subclasses directed against various structural and nonstructural antigens. Indefinite, probably lifelong, persistence of IgG, at least to some antigens, is usual, although not at the high titers observed during acute infection Specific IgA of both subclasses is also produced against early and late antigens (Riggs and Cremer, 1980). The period during which IgA is detectable varies considerably from one individual to another.

In contrast to the humoral response, the development of specific delayed-type hypersensitivity is markedly delayed (TenNapel and The, 1980) and does not reach levels comparable with those of healthy, previously infected individuals until after the third month. Other proliferative responses begin to recover about this time but, as mentioned previously, may not attain levels comparable with controls for many months.

Cytotoxic responses to HCMV infection have not been studied in depth in previously healthy individuals. In bone marrow transplant patients, however, it has been shown that specific cytotoxic responses develop relatively quickly in those who survive the infection, despite the general immunosuppressed state, and often precede the rise in antibody titer (Quinnan et al., 1981; Rook et al., 1984).

V. STRUCTURE AND REPLICATION

A. Structure

1. Virions

Similarly to other members of the herpesvirus family, CMV produces a complex multilayered virion of approximately 180 nm in diameter. Examined by electron microscopy, these sectioned virus particles have an inner DNA-containing core surrounded by an icosahedral capsid, an opposed tegument layer, and an outer bilaminar envelope (Kanich and Craighead, 1972). Two other types of particles have been recovered from the supernate of human fibroblast cultures infected with HCMV; dense bodies and noninfective enveloped particles.

2. Dense Bodies

Dense bodies are homogeneous electron-dense structures 250-600 nm in diameter, bounded by an outer membrane. These structures accumulate in cytoplasmic inclusions along with structurally typical virions. Originally thought to be lysosomes (Ruebner et al., 1965), dense bodies were difficult to separate from virions until glycerol-tartrate gradients were shown to be especially effective in separating the two (Talbot and Almeida, 1977). Dense bodies contain no DNA, and a large proportion of their protein mass consists of one species of matrix protein found in mature virions (see Sect. V.B.3). The outer envelope, however, is thought to contain a normal complement of virion glycoproteins.

3. Noninfectious Enveloped Particles

A third type of virus structure was described by Irmiere and Gibson (1983, 1985) and was referred to as "noninfectious enveloped particles" (NIEPs). Similar to dense bodies, these particles are noninfectious, lack DNA, but their protein composition is more complex, being similar to, although not identical with, virion protein composition. The NIEPs are produced by all HCMV strains examined and are particularly abundant in preparations of laboratory strain AD169.

The production of these two types of noninfectious particle has complicated the clear recognition and characterization of virion proteins.

B. Replication

The large size (molecular weight approximately 1.55×10^8) and complex nature of the HCMV genome has rendered analysis of viral transcription and protein production difficult. Analysis of the chemical events in infected cells is further complicated because HCMV infection does not shut down cellular protein synthesis. In the early phase of infection, it has been estimated that 70-90% of total protein synthesized are host cell proteins, and even in the late stage after the onset of virus DNA synthesis, approximately 40% of protein synthesis is host-specific (Stinski, 1977). The permissive infection of human fibroblasts by HCMV exhibits three main phases of gene expression.

1. The immediate-early events, which occur independently of any preceding viral protein synthesis
2. The early events, which require the transcription of at least one immediate-early gene
3. Late events, which occur after DNA synthesis has begun

1. Immediate-Early Events

It has long been known that virus-specific antigens can be detected as early as 30 min to 1 hr postinfection, by anticomplement immunofluorescence (Geder, 1976; Tanaka et al., 1981), by indirect immunofluorescence (Michelson-Fiske et al., 1977), and by immunoprecipitation (Michelson et al., 1979; Tanaka et al., 1981). Stinski (1978) used cycloheximide to enhance viral proteins relative to cellular products and detected nine to ten early viral proteins ranging in molecular weight from 21-75 X 10^3. Three of these proteins 68-75 X 10^3 were recognized as the earliest produced and designated "immediate-early" proteins. Later, analysis of the mRNA appearing in cells around this time detected a preponderant 1.95 kilobase messenger that was transcribed abundantly relative to other classes. In vitro this mRNA coded for a 75 X 10^3-mol. wt. protein which represents the preponderant immediate-early protein detected in infected cells (Stinski et al., 1983). This protein is presumably modified in infected cells to a 72 X 10^3-mol. wt. protein, the existence of which has been confirmed by Jahn et al. (1984) and by Wilkinson et al. (1984). This preponderant immediate-early antigen has been shown to be capable of autoregulation (Stenberg and Stinski, 1985). It is thought to play a major role in the regulation of immediate-early events and to exert a major influence in the switch from restricted to extensive transcription. Four other mRNA classes have also been identified that code for at least four minor proteins with approximate molecular weights ranging from 56 X 10^3 to 16.5 X 10^3.

2. Early Events

Early proteins appear 4-48 hr after infection. Four to twenty early polypeptides have been described (Blanton and Tevethia, 1981; Michelson et al., 1979; Stinski, 1978). It has been recognized that some immediate-early and early antigens can be synthesized at late times (Blanton and Tevethia, 1981; Kim et al., 1983) and that the multiplicity of infection can affect their expression and detection (Musiani et al., 1979; Sweet et al., 1985). Sweet et al. (1985) have shown that as many as eight early antigens can be extracted from cytosine arabinoside-blocked cells infected with 0.01-20 infectious units per cell. Electroimmunodiffusion with human serum showed that at least five of the eight early antigens gave reactions of identity with unblocked cells extracted at late times after infection.

3. Late Events

The late events are dominated by the synthesis of DNA, which begins at about 15-hr postinfection and rises to a peak after 70 hr (Davis et al., 1984; DeMarchi et al., 1980). All viral structural proteins are synthesized in this late stage (Stinski, 1976). Up to 35 virus-specific peptides have been detected in virions (Gibson, 1983; Gupta et al., 1977; Kim et al., 1976; Stinski, 1977, 1978, 1979). By analogy with a simian cytomegalovirus, which does not produce dense bodies or

NIEPs, Gibson (1983) concluded that the HCMV virion contained eight major proteins. These were designated as a high-molecular-weight protein (212×10^3), a major capsid protein (153×10^3), two matrix proteins (74×10^3 and 69×10^3) and four glycoproteins. Further studies comparing the protein species found in virions, dense bodies, and NIEPs suggested that the virion comprised seven major protein species (Irmiere and Gibson, 1983). Responses to the 153,000-major capsid protein and to the 69,000-matrix protein can regularly be demonstrated in human sera containing antibody to CMV (Landini et al., 1985; Pereira et al., 1982a). The 69,000 matrix protein is a phosphorylated protein, the nucleotide sequence of which has been detected in the HCMV genome by Davis et al. (1984) and Davis and Huang (1985). They suggest that this structural protein may have important functions, such as protein kinase activity, DNA binding, or possible transcriptional activation of immediate-early genes.

The NIEPs contain the same seven major protein species as do virions, but in addition, contain a 36,000 protein that is not found in virions. It is postulated that this protein, which is also phosphorylated and found in the nuclear fraction of infected cells, mediates DNA packaging or nucleocapsid development. Dense bodies are much simpler in construction, an estimated 90% of their protein mass comprising the 69,000 matrix protein.

Some of the late proteins are glycosylated, and because glycosylated envelope proteins are potential targets for important neutralization events, they have attracted attention and detailed study Variable numbers of glycoproteins have been described ranging from 3 (Fiala et al., 1976), 4 (Gibson, 1983), 5 (Farrar and Oram, 1984), 7 (Kim et al., 1976; Nowak, 1984b), and 8 (Stinski, 1976). The total number of HCMV-specified glycoproteins remains undetermined and the vaccine potential of any individual glycoprotein is poorly understood. Using nucleotide sequence analysis, Cranage et al. (1986) identified a HCMV gene, possessing glycoprotein characteristics, with homology to glycoproteins B (gB) of herpes simplex virus, Epstein-Barr virus, and gpII of varicella zoster virus. The protein encoded by this gene is referred to as HCMVgB. These results present some hope for the basis of an acceptable nomenclature for the glycoproteins of HCMV.

VI. DIAGNOSIS BY CONVENTIONAL METHODS

The diagnosis of HCMV infection has depended upon the isolation of virus from clinical specimens, or upon the demonstration of a rising IgG titer to the virus or the presence of virus-specific IgM.

A. Isolation of Virus

Human cytomegalovirus will replicate and produce a cytopathic effect (CPE) only in human embryo fibroblasts. Wild virus usually grows slowly and cultures have to be maintained for a minimum of 21-28 days. The CPE characteristically develops as a focal swelling and rounding of cells. Confirmation of the isolate as HCMV may be made by staining monolayers to show the large intranuclear inclusions or by using a human serum with a high titer of HCMV antibodies in an indirect immunofluorescent test. Obviously, such methods are slow and potentially nonspecific. Because virus isolation may be possible in primary infection, reactivated infection, or reinfection, the importance of virus isolation alone, particularly from nasopharyngeal secretions or urine, may be difficult to assess. On the other hand, isolation of virus from any site during the first week of life confirms congenital infection with the virus, and isolation from biopsy specimens indicates an active infection in the organ from which the biopsy was taken. Isolation of virus from peripheral blood cells is an important indicator of disseminated infection.

B. Measurement of Immunoglobulin G Antibody

Almost every possible technique has been applied to the detection of IgG antibody to HCMV in serum. A wide variety of structural and nonstructural antigens are present in different antigenic preparations, thus the observed antibody response depends upon the different reactivities of antibodies to the antigens present in each preparation.

In a comparative study of five tests for HCMV antibody in 66 human sera, Booth et al. (1982) found that the enzyme-linked immunosorbent assay (ELISA) and radioimmunoassay (RIA) systems (geometric mean antibody titers 12,139 and 6584 respectively) were much more sensitive than the anticomplement immunofluorescent (ACIF), passive hemagglutination (PHA), and complement fixations tests (geometric mean antibody titers 618, 145, and 59 respectively). When the same tests were used for screening sera, however, remarkably few discrepancies were recorded between the various methods—except PHA. Although the PHA test was the easiest to perform, antibody levels in this study were low, and the number of false-negative results were high.

Large numbers of tests for the measurement of IgG or total immunoglobulin specifically reactive with HCMV antigens are now available commercially. Five screening tests for antibodies were evaluated by Grint et al. (1985) and four by Feng et al. (1986). These include tests based primarily on ELISA and indirect hemagglutination (IHA). The ELISAs are excellent, easy to perform tests giving quantitative data. The IHA was found to be very sensitive and particularly suited to screening large numbers of donor sera for antibody (Chairez et al., 1984). A latex agglutination test (LA) is also available commercially; the test, which is completed in 8 min, had a sensitivity of 96.6% and a specificity of 100% compared with ELISA and PHA (Adler et al., 1985). McHugh et al. (1985) reported high sensitivity and specificity for both the IHA and the LA tests, thus confirming the good performance of these tests.

Indirect immunofluorescent tests have the advantage of recognizing the location and timing of antigens. Antibodies to immediate-early antigen (IEA), early antigen (EA), and to late antigen (LA) can be detected on appropriately cultured infected cells. Unfortunately, interpretation of results is rendered difficult by the production of Fc receptors in infected cells. This problem can be avoided by using a simian virus for antigen production. The detection of both IgG and IgM to EA and LA, using carefully produced antigen in an ELISA test, has given good results (Middledorp et al., 1984).

To define more clearly the immune response to individual proteins of HCMV, sera have been studied for their reactivity with HCMV polypeptides separated by sodium dodecyl sulfate-polyacrylamide gel electrophoresis (SDS-PAGE) and electrotransferred to nitrocellulose. When purified HCMV polypeptides are used as antigen, at least 15 electrophoretically distinct structural polypeptides can be detected. The number and intensity of the reactions with individual polypeptides increases with the serum titer, as measured by ELISA (Landini et al., 1985). One polypeptide, 155,000 mol. wt., was recognized by every serum regardless of antibody titer. It is likely that this polypeptide is the major capsid protein (153,000) described by Gibson (1983). Much more analytical work of this type is necessary before the complex serological responses to HCMV polypeptides are understood.

The choice of laboratory test for detecting IgG to HCMV depends upon the type of patient to be investigated and the expertise available in the laboratory. When screening for antibody is all that is required, either the IHA or the LA test may be used. The LA test also detects rising titers of antibody (McHugh et al., 1985), and this, along with a sensitive and specific test for IgM, may adequately cover the diagnosis of infection with HCMV. Indirect tests, such as RIA and ELISA, can be performed in well-equipped laboratories and will probably be preferred by specialist virology units.

C. Measurement of Immunoglobulin M Antibody

Demonstration of HCMV IgM allows a prompt diagnosis of recent infection to be made on a single specimen of serum. Anti-HCMV IgM can be detected during primary infections, in congenital infections, and in some reactivated infections in immunocompromised individuals. In view of the importance of the detection of IgM, great effort has been directed toward the production of a simple, specific, and sensitive test (Schmitz et al., 1977). Again, little information is now available concerning the individual proteins present in different antigens. Indirect methods, using an antihuman μ-chain labeled with fluorescein, enzyme, or radioactive iodine, have been described and compared. All have the disadvantage of producing misleading results when antiglobulin (rheumatoid) factors are present in the serum under test, and positive results must be confirmed after absorption of serum with human gamma globulin.

The indirect immunofluorescence test was described as long ago as 1968 but has now been shown to be less specific and less sensitive than the more recently developed tests such as RIA and ELISA (Kangro et al., 1984; Stagno et al., 1985; Yolken and Leister, 1981). The ELISA and RIA methods are equally sensitive and specific for the detection of IgM in adult sera, but ELISA appears to be less sensitive for detecting low levels of IgM in cord blood. Unfortunately, both tests are susceptible to interference by rheumatoid factor. To obviate the necessity for serum absorption with IgG, a μ-chain capture method has been used for the detection of HCMV-specific IgM (Sutherland and Briggs, 1983). This test is much less susceptible to interference by rheumatoid factor, but positive results can occur with sera from individuals recently infected with Epstein-Barr virus.

VII. PRODUCTION AND CHARACTERIZATION OF MONOCLONAL ANTIBODIES

Pereira and colleagues (1982b) were the first to publish a full report on the production of monoclonal antibodies (MAbs) to HCMV. Other reports appeared soon after (Amedai et al., 1983; Goldstein et al., 1982). Although various groups have used minor modifications, in practice, the production and characterization of MAbs to HCMV uses the well-recognized technology that has been described previously (see Chap. 1). The HCMV proteins were poorly defined at the time MAb technology appeared, with the result that MAbs were produced initially with few well-defined aims for their use.

A. Antigens and Immunization Schedules

Various antigens were used for the immunization schedules, but the production of MAbs to a particular antigen was unpredictable. AD-169-infected cell suspensions were used in initial immunization schedules (Goldstein et al., 1982; Pereira et al., 1982b). Unlike herpes simplex virus, which replicates in mice and, as a result, will stimulate an immune response to a much wider range of antigens, HCMV has to be used for passive immunization. This could be the main reason that later workers undertook partial purification of HCMV viral antigens to increase the yield of desired antibody. The MAbs against glycoproteins were produced with purified and solubilized virion envelope component antigens (Law et al., 1985). When AD-169-purified virions were used as antigens and immobilized for screening, the resulting MAbs were mainly neutralizing (Britt, 1984). All resulting HCMV MAbs were directed against a wide range of polypeptides. With no definite nomenclature or description of molecular weights, it is sometimes very difficult to make valid comparisons between the reactivity of the different MAbs.

B. The Use and Reactivity of Monoclonal Antibodies

The use of these MAbs can be divided into four main groups, as shown in the Appendix. Group 1 outlines the MAbs used primarily to study the antigenic relatedness of HCMV-infected cell and virion proteins. The MAbs listed in group 2 are useful because of their neutralizing properties. The glycoprotein complex that has been responsible for the largest percentage of neutralizing antibodies has been described by various groups (Britt, 1984; Britt and Auger, 1986; Cranage et al., 1986; Pereira et al., 1984; Rasmussen et al., 1985b). This complex, which has been assigned molecular weights of 160,000/150,000/116,000/55,000 (Britt, 1984; Britt and Auger, 1986), elicits a dominant humoral response early in infection (Cremer et al., 1985).

Coprecipitation occurs, even with single MAbs, because of disulfide linkages of these, not always antigenically related, proteins. Pereira et al. (1984) calls this complex gA, which perhaps over simplifies the HCMV glycoprotein nomenclature. The best characterized glycoproteins from this complex are the 145,000/55,000 proteins now called HCMV gB (Cranage et al., 1986). Four of ten neutralizing MAbs immunoprecipitated the gB 145,000/55,000 complex (Cranage et al., 1986). None reacted with the middle protein (116,000) associated with this complex. the main epitope capable of stimulating neutralizing antibodies must be shared between the small 55,000-mol. wt. peptide and the 145,000-mol. wt. precursor [150,000 (Britt, 1984)]. Interestingly, MAb gB reactive with the middle-range peptide from this complex did not neutralize HCMV (Law et al., 1985). One other protein, gp86 (86,000 mol. wt.), that stimulated neutralizing MAbs has been described (Rasmussen et al., 1984, 1985a). Hyperimmune sera to gp86 are independent of complement for virus neutralization (Rasmussen, 1985a).

Group 3 outlines MAbs used for rapid diagnosis (see Sect. VIII), and group 4 lists some human MAbs. One human MAb reacts with late nuclear antigen, 75,000 mol. wt. (Emanuel et al., 1984, 1986). This Mab was not suitable for direct evaluation of human clinical samples because nonspecific Fc-receptor binding gave a high background. One of two other human MAbs is neutralizing and might prove useful for immunotherapy (Matsumoto et al., 1986). The target proteins for the two latter human MAbs are unknown.

VIII. APPLICATION OF MONOCLONAL ANTIBODIES TO DIAGNOSIS

A. Culture Confirmation Test

The most widely reported method of making a successful rapid diagnosis of HCMV infection involves the inoculation of fibroblast cultures with the specimen followed, after 24-48 hr of incubation, by probing with MAbs selected for their reactivity with immediate-early major transcript 72,000 nuclear antigen (Fiaco et al., 1984; Gleaves et al., 1984; Musiani et al., 1985; Shuster et al., 1985; Swanson and Kaplan, 1985). Fibroblast cultures may be prepared on coverslips, in standard tissue culture tubes (Swenson and Kaplan, 1985), or in glass vials (Gleaves et al., 1984). The advantage of using vials or "shells" is the opportunity to centrifuge the specimen onto the prepared monolayer, thus, increasing the sensitivity (Shuster et al., 1985; Alpert et al., 1985). After centrifugation, the vials are incubated for 16-36 hr. Coverslips are then washed, fixed in acetone, and reacted with the selected MAb or antibody pool that can be traced by an immunofluorescent label or by a peroxidase-antiperoxidase (PAP) system (Gleaves et al., 1984). By combining initial centrifugation with the use of one MAb traced by a biotin-avidin label, Alpert et al. (1985) claim that HCMV excretion in urine can be recognized in 48 hr with a sensitivity equal to, or even greater than, that of conventional tissue culture methods. Whereas this may be possible in urine specimens containing $>10^3$ infectious units/ml, which would demonstrate CPE in conventional cultures in less than 10 days, we have had less success in detecting low levels of infection that take more than 10 days to become culture-positive. Monoclonal antibodies to other antigens, especially in pools, have also proved useful for tissue culture confirmation of clinical HCMV isolates (Alpert et al., 1985; Griffiths et al., 1984; Spencer et al., 1985; Volpi et al., 1983).

B. Direct Tracing of Antigen in Clinical Specimens

Direct detection of antigen, which usually employs MAbs to major late HCMV antigens (Emanuel et al., 1985; Goldstein et al., 1982; Nowak et al., 1984b), has been faced with more problems (Zuckerman, 1985). Cellular or tissue section specimens are apparently less problematic (Emanuel et al., 1986; Goldstein et al., 1982) than clinical specimens of body fluids (McKeating et al., 1986) in which low HCMV antigen concentration hampers direct diagnostic approaches. For instance, immunofluorescence has been applied to make a preliminary diagnosis of HCMV pneumonia (Goldstein et al., 1982). Volpi et al. (1983) also demonstrated the advantage of using MAbs for the rapid recognition of HCMV antigens in lung biopsy specimens from patients with interstitial pneumonia. Their cocktail of MAbs recognized 16 proteins of the virus and identified infection within 3 hr of specimen collection. Results of this IF test applied to seven specimens agreed completely with cell culture isolation of virus. Specific antigen detection in cells from fresh urine or nasopharyngeal secretions gives a rapid diagnosis of congenital infection. Detection in urine and nasopharyngeal secretions were found to be 62.5 and 71.4% sensitive, respectively, when compared with conventional virus isolation techniques (Nowak et al., 1984b).

Monoclonal antibodies bound to a solid phase may be used to "capture" antigens present in urine. The captured antigen can be detected by its reaction with a high-titer human serum which, in turn, is detected by an enzyme-labeled anti-human antibody. Although the specificity of this test (IRMA) approaches 100%, sensitivity is low (67%), possibly because of the presence of inhibiting substances in the fresh urine sample (McKeating et al., 1985). There is evidence that the interfering substance is β_2-microglobulin (McKeating et al., 1986).

C. Monoclonal Antibodies in Serological Tests

The detection of IgG can be more sensitive and specific using a competitive enzyme-linked assay, in which MAbs compete with antibodies in the test serum for binding to HCMV antigens. In one such assay (Wreghitt et al., 1986), MAb directed against an unspecified late HCMV glycoprotein antigen was labeled with horseradish peroxidase. Fifty-percent inhibition was arbitrarily chosen as the cutoff; sera giving >50% inhibition were regarded as positive, and sera giving <50% inhibition were regarded as negative for CMV antibody.

Although more sensitive than CFT or ELISA at detecting long-standing IgG and passively acquired IgG, the test is not a sensitive indicator of recent infection (Wreghitt et al., 1986). Nevertheless, the test might be a valuable addition to the screening of blood and organ donors or of transplant recipients. A comparison of this inhibition test with the IHA and the LA would help laboratories select the most economic and sensitive screening test.

Monoclonal antibodies can be used to study the serological response to individual viral polypeptides. An MAb adsorbed to a solid phase captures the specific reactive antigen from a crude preparation of infected cells. The test than can be completed as an indirect ELISA test using the serum under investigation, followed by an enzyme-labeled antihuman antibody. In studying the temporal relationship of antibody production it has been shown that there is no advantage in using the captured antigens rather than soluble cell lysate, but differences in the response to individual captured antigens are variable. A glycoprotein, designated gA but equivalent to the complex containing HCMV gB (Cranage et al., 1986), was found to elicit a dominant humoral response early in infection (Cremer et al., 1985).

Finally, MAbs can provide a standard reagent to replace the high-titer human serum required in the final steps of the μ-chain capture method for HCMV-specific IgM (Muir, 1985). Here HCMV MAbs are used as the final detection step, but the layout is very similar to the MACRIA of Sutherland and Briggs (1983) (see Sect. VI.C.).

IX. CONCLUSIONS

The increase in patient groups both at risk of, and suffering from, severe disease caused by HCMV has demanded a reappraisal of our conventional methods of diagnosis. Antiviral agents active against HCMV are under intensive investigation. In addition, our knowledge of the epidemiology and pathogenesis of HCMV infection depends upon an initial accurate diagnosis. Rapid and sensitive techniques that can clearly identify both recent and previous infection with the virus are now available, and many depend upon the use of MAbs. Monoclonal antibodies are useful in antigenic and structural analyses, neutralization studies, diagnosis, and potentially, in therapy. However, more information on their immunoprecipitation profiles and antigenic specificity is required. A HCMV protein nomenclature, similar to that of herpes simplex virus and based on good data, should be established as a matter of priority.

APPENDIX

Summary of Monoclonal Antibodies (MAbs) to HCMV

Authors	Number of MAbs	Antigen reactivity designated by authors	Interpreted antigen reactivity	Suggested uses
Group 1				
Pereira et al., 1982a	77	7 groups	–	Antigen analysis
Amedai et al., 1983	24	7 groups	–	
Chardonnet et al., 1983	5	76,000/60,000/ 54,000	–	Heterogeneity of HCMV isolates
	3	76,000/54,000	–	
	8	67,000	pp66[a]	
Kim et al., 1983	9	66,000	pp66	Epitope analysis
Nowak et al., 1984a	1	77,000	pp71[b]	Genome analysis
	1	65,000	pp66	
Pereira et al., 1984		gA	gB[c] and others	Glycoprotein analysis
Law et al., 1985	1	130,000/95,000/ 52,000	gB	Glycoprotein analysis
Mocarski et al., 1985	2	ICP 36	–	Genome analysis
Re et al., 1985	1	28,000	pp29[d]	Structure study
Rodgers et al., 1985	2	67,000	pp66	Heterogeneity of
	1	43,000/79,000	–	peptides
	1	72,000	p72[e]	
Volpi and Britt, 1985	1	90,000	–	Heterogeneity of HCMV isolates
Group 2				
Britt, 1984	6	160,000/115,000/ 55,000	gB	Neutralization

Appendix continued

Authors	Number of MAbs	Antigen reactivity designated by authors	Interpreted antigen reactivity	Suggested uses
Rasmussen et al., 1984	1	86,000	gp86[f]	Neutralization
Rasmussen et al., 1985b	2	130,000/55,000	gB	Neutralization
Britt and Auger, 1986	3	160,000/150,000/ 115,000/55,000	gB	Glycoprotein analysis
Cranage et al., 1986	4	145,000/55,000	gB	Neutralization Genome analysis
Group 3				
Goldstein et al., 1982	2	72,000 80,000	p72 –	Pneumonia diagnosis
Mazeron et al., 1983	1	68,000	p72	
Volpi et al., 1983	9	20-150,000 pool	–	Culture confirmation IF[h]
Fiaco et al., 1984	1	72,000	p72	Culture confirmation
Gleaves et al., 1984	1	72,000	p72	Culture confirmation IF and IP[i]
Griffiths et al., 1984	7	Pool	–	Culture confirmation
Nowak et al., 1984b	4	130,000/58,000 71,000 155,000 29,000	gB pp71 pp155[g] pp29	Direct diagnosis
Alpert et al., 1985	1	68,000	p72	Culture confirmation
Cremer et al., 1985	4	gA gC gD 150,000	gB – – pp155	Capture ELISA
Hackman et al., 1985	1	80,000	–	Direct diagnosis
Muir, 1985	2	68,000	pp66	IgM assay
Musiani et al., 1985	1	72,000	p72	Culture confirmation AP[j]
Shuster et al., 1985	1 1	72,000 68,000	p72 pp66	Culture confirmation IF
Spencer et al., 1985	1	80,000	–	Culture confirmation IF
Swenson and Kaplan, 1985	1	72,000	p72	Culture confirmation
Emanuel et al., 1986	6	Pool	–	Pneumonia diagnosis
McKeating et al., 1986	1	None	–	Capture ELISA

Appendix continued

Authors	Number of MAbs	Antigen reactivity designated by authors	Interpreted antigen reactivity	Suggested uses
Zweysberg-Wirgart 1986	1	72,000	p72	Culture confirmation
Group 4				
Emanuel et al., 1984	1	ILA nuclear	–	
Emanuel et al., 1986	1	75,000	–	Not diagnostic
Matsumoto et al., 1986	2	None	–	1 neutralizing
Redmond et al., 1986	5	66 000/95,000	pp66	3 neutralizing
	1	77,000	–	Not neutralizing

[a]pp66 = 64,000-66,000-mol. wt. most abundant matrix protein interfacing the virion and envelope; 70% of total viral proteins (*Source*: Kim et al., 1983; Pande et al., 1984).

[b]pp71 = 71,000-mol. wt. phosphoprotein localized inside the virion membrane (*Source*: Nowak et al., 1984b).

[c]gB = 145,000/55,000-mol. wt. glycoproteins cloned and expressed in vaccinia with nucleotide sequence homologous to gB of herpes simplex (*Source*: Cranage et al., 1986).

[d]pp29 = 29,000-mol. wt. virion-associated phosphoprotein (*Source*: Nowak et al., 1984b).

[e]p72 = an abundant immediate-early nuclear antigen predominantly transcribed (*Source*: Stinski et al., 1983).

[f]gp86 = 86,000-mol. wt. glycoprotein which is target for neutralizing antibodies (*Source*: Rasmussen et al., 1985b).

[g]pp155 = 155,000-mol. wt. phosphorylated nucleocapsid protein (*Source*: Nowak et al., 1984b) and principal abundant capsid constituent 153,000 mol. wt. (*Source*: Gibson, 1983).

[h]IF = immunofluorescence-based detection system.

[i]IP = immunoperoxidase enzyme-based detection system.

[j]AP = alkaline phosphatase enzyme-linked conjugates used for detection.

pp = phosphoprotein.

g = glycoprotein.

p = protein.

REFERENCES

Adler, S. P., McVoy, M., Biro, V. G., Britt, W. J., Hider, P., and Marshall, D. (1985). Detection of cytomegalovirus antibody with latex agglutination. *J. Clin. Microbiol. 22*:68-70.

Ahlfors, K., Harris, S., Ivarsson, S., and Svanberg, L. (1981). Secondary maternal cytomegalovirus infection causing symptomatic congenital infection. *N. Engl. J. Med. 305*:284

Alpert, G., Mazeron, M. C., Colimon, R., and Plotkin, S. (1985). Rapid detection of human cytomegalovirus in the urine of humans. *J. Infect. Dis. 152*:631-633.

Amedai, C., Tardy-Panit, M., Couillin, P., Coulon M., Cabau, N., Boue, A., and Michelson, S. (1983). Kinetic study of the development and localization of human cytomegalovirus-induced antigens using monoclonal antibodies. *Ann. Virol. (Paris) 134E*:165-180.

Blanton, R. A. and Tevethia, M. J. (1981). Immunoprecipitation of virus-specific immediate-early and early polypeptides from cells lytically infected with human cytomegalovirus strain AD169. *Virology 112*:262-273.

Booth, J. C., Hannington, G. M., Bakir, T. M. F., Stern, H., Kangro, H., Griffiths, P. D., and Heath, R. B. (1982). Comparison of enzyme-linked immunosorbent assay, radioimmunoassay, complement fixation, anticomplement immunofluorescence and passive haemagglutination techniques for detection cytomegalovirus IgG antibody. *J. Clin. Pathol. 35*:1345-1348.

Britt, W. J. (1984). Neutralizing antibodies detect a disulphide-linked glycoprotein complex within the envelope of human cytomegalovirus. *Virology 135*: 369-378.

Britt, W. J. and Auger, D. (1986). Synthesis and processing of the envelope gp 55-116 complex of human cytomegalovirus. *J. Virol. 58*:185-191.

Carney, W. P. and Hirsch, M. S. (1981). Mechanisms of immunosuppression in cytomegalic mononucleosis. II. Virus-monocyte interactions. *J. Infect. Dis. 144*:47-64.

Carney, W. P., Iacoviello, V., and Hirsch, M. S. (1983). Functional properties of T lymphocytes and their subsets in cytomegalovirus mononucleosis. *J. Immunol. 130*:390-393.

Carney, W. P., Rubin, R. H., Hoffman, R. A., Hanson, W. P., Healey, K., and Hirsch, M. S. (1981). Analysis of T lymphocyte subsets in cytomegalovirus mononucleosis. *J. Immunol. 126*:2114-2116.

Chairez, R., Schleicher, J. B., and Cesario, A. J. (1984). Comparison of an enzyme-linked immunoassay with an indirect hemagglutination assay for the detection of antibodies to cytomegalovirus. *J. Virol. Methods 9*:153-161.

Chardonnet, Y., Lery, X., and Revillard, J.-P. (1983). Identification of shared antigenic determinants of different polypeptides from Davis and Towne cytomegalovirus strains with monoclonal antibodies. *Med. Microbiol. Immunol. 172*:171-180.

Chretien, J. H., McGinniss, C. G., and Muller, A. (1977). Venereal causes of cytomegalovirus mononucleosis. *J. Am. Med. Assoc. 238*:1644-1645.

Cockerill, F. R. (1985). Diagnosing cytomegalovirus infection. *Mayo Clin. Proc. 60*:636-638.

Coetmeur, D., Delaval, P., LeDeant, P., Ruffault, A., Laurent, J. F., and Tanguy, M. (1986). Usefulness of monoclonal antibodies for the diagnosis of cytomegalovirus infection. *Presse Med. 15*:124-128.

Cranage, M. P., Kouzarides, T., Bankier, A. T., Satchwell, S., Weston, K., Tomlinson, P., Barrell, B., Hart, H., Bell, S. E., Minson, A. C., and Smith, G. L.

(1986). Identification of the human cytomegalovirus glycoprotein B gene and induction of neutralising antibodies via its expression in recombinant vaccinia virus. *The EMBO J.* 5:3057-3063.

Cremer, N. E., Cossen, C. K., Shell, G. R., and Pereira, L. (1985). Antibody response to cytomegalovirus polypeptides captured by monoclonal antibodies on the solid phase in enzyme immunoassays. *J. Clin. Microbiol.* 21:517-521.

Davis, M. F. and Huang, E.-S. (1985). Nucleotide sequence of a human HCMV DNA fragment encoding a 67-kilodalton phosphorylated viral protein. *J. Virol.* 56:7-11.

Davis, M. F., Mar, E.-C., Wu, Y.-M., and Huang, E.-S. (1984). Mapping and expression of a human cytomegalovirus major viral protein. *J. Virol.* 52:129-135.

DeMarchi, J. M., Schmidt, C. A., and Kaplan, A. S. (1980). Patterns of transcription of human cytomegalovirus in permissively infected cells. *J. Virol.* 35:277-286.

Drew, W. L., Mintz, L., Miner, R. C., Sands, M., and Kettering, B. (1981). Prevalence of cytomegalovirus infection in homosexual men. *J. Infect. Dis.* 143:188-192.

Ellner, J. J. (1978). Suppressor adherent cells in human tuberculosis. *J. Immunol.* 121:2573-2579.

Emanuel, D., Gold, J., Colacino, J., Lopez, C. M., and Hammerling, U. (1984). A human monoclonal antibody to cytomegalovirus. *J. Immunol.* 133:2202-2205.

Emanuel, D., Peppard, J., Stouer, D., Gold, J., Armstrong, D., and Hammerling, U. (1986). Rapid immunodiagnosis of cytomegalovirus pneumonia by bronchoalveolar lavage using human and murine monoclonal antibodies. *Ann. Intern. Med.* 104:476-480.

Farrar, G. H. and Oram, J. D. (1984). Characterization of the human cytomegalovirus envelope glycoproteins. *J. Gen. Virol.* 65:1991-2001.

Fazekas de St. Groth, S. and Scheidegger, D. (1980). Production of monoclonal antibodies: Strategy and tactics. *J. Immunol. Methods.* 35:1-21.

Feng, C. S. (1986). A comparison of four commercial test kits for detection of cytomegalovirus antibodies in blood donors. *Transfusion* 26:203-213.

Fiaco, V., Bryson, Y. J., and Bruckner, D. A. (1984). Comparison of monoclonal and polyclonal antibody for confirmation of cytomegalovirus isolates by fluorescent staining. *J. Clin. Microbiol.* 19:928-930.

Fiala, M., Honess, R. W., Heiner, D. C., Heine, J. W. Jr., Munrane, J., Wallace, R., and Guse, L. B. (1976). Cytomegalovirus proteins. I. Polypeptides of virions and dense bodies. *J. Virol.* 19:234-254.

Geder, L. (1976). Evidence for early nuclear antigens in cytomegalovirus-infected cells. *J. Gen. Virol.* 32:315-319.

Gibson, W. (1983). Protein counterparts of human and simian cytomegaloviruses. *Virology* 128:391-406.

Gleaves, C. A., Smith, T. F., Shuster, E. A., and Pearson, G. R. (1984). Rapid detection of cytomegalovirus in MRC-5 cells inoculated with urine specimens by using low speed centrifugation and monoclonal antibody to an early antigen. *J. Clin. Microbiol.* 19:917-919.

Goldmeier, D., Linch, D., and Mellars, B. J. (1983). Immunocompromise syndrome in homosexual men. Prevalence of possible risk factors and screening for the prodrome using an accurate white cell count. *Br. J. Vener. Dis. 59*: 127-130.

Goldstein, L., McDougall, J., Hackman, R., Meyers, J. D., Thomas, D., and Nowinski, R. C. (1982). Monoclonal antibodies to cytomegalovirus: Rapid identification of clinical isolates and preliminary use in diagnosis of CMV pneumonia. *Infect. Immun. 38*:273-281.

Grint, P. G. A., Ronalds, C. J., Kangro, H. O., Campbell-Benzie, A., Ward, F., Hardiman, A. E., and Heath, R. B. (1985). Screening tests for antibodies to cytomegalovirus: An evaluation of five commercial products. *J. Clin. Pathol. 38*:1059-1064.

Griffiths, P. D., Panjwani, D. D., Stirk, P. R., Ball, M. G., Ganczakowski, M., Blacklock, H. A., and Prentice, H. G. (1984). Rapid diagnosis of cytomegalovirus infection in immunocompromised patients by detection of early antigen fluorescent foci. *Lancet 2*:1242-1244.

Gupta, P., St. Jeor, S., and Rapp, F. (1977). Comparison of the polypeptides of several strains of cytomegalovirus. *J. Gen. Virol. 34*:447-454.

Hackman, R. C., Myerson, D., Meyers, J. D., Shulman, H. M., Sale, G. E., Goldstein, L. C., Rastetfer, M., Flournoy, N., and Thomas, E. D. (1985). Rapid diagnosis of cytomegalovirus pneumonia by tissue immunofluorescence with a murine monoclonal antibody. *J. Infect. Dis. 151*:325-329.

Handsfield, H. H., Chandler, S. H., Caine, J. A., Meyers, J. D., Corey, L., Medeiros, E., and McDougall, J. K. (1985). Cytomegalovirus infection in sex partners: Evidence for sexual transmission. *J. Infect. Dis. 151*:344-354.

Hunt, A. F., Allen, D. L., Brown, R. L., Robb, B. A., Puckett, A. Y., and Entwistle, C. C. (1984). Comparative trials of six methods for detection of CMV donors in blood donors. *J. Clin Pathol. 37*:95-97.

Irmiere, A. and Gibson, W. (1983). Isolation and characterization of a non-infectious virion-like particle released from cells infected with human strains of cytomegalovirus. *Virology 130*:118-133.

Irmiere, A. and Gibson, W. (1985). Isolation of human cytomegalovirus intranuclear capsids, characterization of their protein constituents, and demonstration that the B-capsid assembly protein is also abundant in non-infectious enveloped particles. *J. Virol. 56*:277-283.

Jahn, G., Knust, E., Schmolla, H., Sarre, T., Nelson, J. A., McDougall, J. K., and Fleckenstein, B. (1984). Predominant immediate early transcripts of human cytomegalovirus AD169. *J. Virol. 49*:363-370.

Jordan, M. C., Rousseau, W. E., Noble, G. R., Stewart, J. A., and Chin, T. D. Y. (1973). Association of cervical cytomegalovirus with venereal disease. *N. Engl. J. Med. 228*:932-934.

Kangro, H. O., Booth, J. C., Bakir, T. M. F., Tryhorn, Y., and Sutherland, S. (1984). Detection of IgM antibodies against cytomegalovirus: Comparison of two radioimmunoassays, enzyme-linked immunosorbent assay and immunofluorescent antibody test. *J. Med. Virol. 14*:73-80.

Kanich, R. E. and Craighead, J. E. (1972). Human cytomegalovirus infection of cultured fibroblasts. II. Viral replicative sequence of a wild and an adapted strain. *Lab. Invest. 27*:273-282.

Katz, P., Goldstein, R. A., and Fauci, A. S. (1979). Immunoregulation in infection caused by *Mycobacterium tuberculosis*: The presence of suppressor monocytes and the alteration of subpopulations of T lymphocytes. *J. Infect. Dis. 140*:12-21.

Kim, K. S., Sapienza, V. M., Carp, R., and Moon, H. M. (1976). Analysis of structural polypeptides of purified human cytomegalovirus. *J. Virol. 20*: 604-611.

Kim, K. S., Sapienza, V. J., Chen, C. J., and Wisniewski, K. (1983). Production and characterization of monoclonal antibodies specific for a glycosylated polypeptide of human cytomegalovirus. *J. Clin. Microbiol. 18*:331-343.

Klemona, E. and Kaariainen, L. (1965). Cytomegalovirus as a possible cause of a disease resembling infectious mononucleosis. *Br. Med. J. 2*:1099-1102.

Landini, M. P., Re, M. C., Mirolo, G., Baldassarri, B., and La Placa, M. (1985). Human immune response to cytomegalovirus structural polypeptides studies by immunoblotting. *J. Med. Virol. 17*:303-311.

Lang, D. J. and Kummer, J. F. (1972). Demonstration of cytomegalovirus in semen. *N. Engl. J. Med. 287*:756-758.

Lang, D. J., Kummer, J. F., and Hartley, D. P. (1974). Cytomegalovirus in semen. Persistence and demonstration in extracellular fluids. *N. Engl. J. Med. 291*: 121-123.

Lang, D. J. and Noren, B. (1968). Cytomegaloviremia following congenital infection. *J. Pediatr. 73*:812-819.

Law, K. M., Smith-Wilton, P., and Farrar, G. H. (1985). A murine monoclonal antibody recognizing a single glycoprotein within a human cytomegalovirus virion envelope glycoprotein complex. *J. Med. Virol. 17*:255-266.

McHugh, T. M., Casavant, C. H., Wilber, J. C., and Stites, D. P. (1985). Comparison of six methods for the detection of antibody to cytomegalovirus. *J. Clin. Microbiol. 22*:1014-1019.

McKeating, J. A., Stagno, S., Stirk, P. R., and Griffiths, P. D. (1985). Detection of cytomegalovirus in urine samples by enzyme-linked immunosorbent assay. *J. Med. Virol. 16*:367-373.

McKeating, J. A., Grundy, J. E., Varghese, Z., and Griffiths, P. D. (1986). Detection of cytomegalovirus by ELISA in urine samples is inhibited by beta-2 microglobulin. *J. Med. Virol. 18*:341-352.

Martin, W. J. and Smith, T. F. (1986). Rapid detection of cytomegalovirus in bronchoalveolar lavage specimens by a monoclonal antibody method. *J. Clin. Microbiol. 23*:1006-1008.

Matsumoto, Y., Sugano, T., Miyamoto, C., and Masuito, T. (1986). Generation of hybridomas producing human monoclonal antibodies against human cytomegalovirus. *Biochem. Biophys. Res. Commun. 137*:273-280.

Mazeron, M.-C., Berbar, T., Guillemin, M.-C., Colimon, R., Roseto, A., and Perol, Y. (1983). Production d'anticorps monoclonaux contre le cytomegalovuris humain. *C. R. Acad. Sci. III 297*:305-308.

Michelson-Fiske, S., Horodnicheanu, F., and Guillon, J. C. (1977). Immediate early antigens in human cytomegalovirus infected cells. *Nature 270*:615-617.

Michelson, S., Horodnicheanu, F., Kress, M., Tardy-Panit, M. (1979). Human cytomegalovirus-induced immediate early antigens: Analysis in sodium dodecyl sulfate-polyacrylamide gel electrophoresis after immunoprecipitation. *J. Virol. 32*:259-267.

Middeldorp, J. M., Jongsma, J., Ter Haar, A., Schirm, J., and The, T. H. (1984). Detection of immunoglobulin M and G antibodies against cytomegalovirus early and late antigens by enzyme-linked immunosorbent assay. *J. Clin. Microbiol. 20*:763-771.

Middeldorp, J. M., Jogsma, J., and The, T. H. (1985). Cytomegalovirus early and late membrane antigens detected by antibodies in human convalescent sera. *J. Virol. 54*:240-244.

Mindel, A. and Sutherland, S. (1984). Antibodies to cytomegalovirus in homosexual and heterosexual men attending an STD clinic. *Br. J. Vener. Dis. 60*: 189-192.

Mintz, L., Drew, W. L., Moiner, R. C., and Braff, E. H. (1983). Cytomegalovirus infections in homosexual men. *Ann. Intern. Med. 99*:326-329.

Mocarski, E. S., Pereira, L., and Michael, N. (1985). Precise localization of genes on large animal virus genomes: Use of lambda ft11 and monoclonal antibodies to map the gene for a cytomegalovirus protein family. *Proc. Natl. Acad. Sci. USA 82*:1266-1270.

Muir, P. (1985). Cytomegalovirus infection and immunity in homosexual men. PhD thesis, Edinburgh University.

Musiani, M., Zerbini, M., Landini, M. P., and Laplaca, M. (1979). Preliminary evidence that cytomegalovirus-induced immediate early antigens are DNA-binding proteins. *Microbiologica 2*:281-287.

Musiani, M., Zerbini, M., and Laplaca, M. (1985). Alkaline phosphatase immunoenzymatic staining for detection of antigens induced by cytomegalovirus. *J. Clin. Pathol. 38*:1155-1157.

Nowak, B., Gmeiner, A., Sarnow, P., Levine, A. J., and Fleckenstein, B. (1984a). Physical mapping of human cytomegalovirus gene: Identification of DNA sequences coding for a virion phosphoprotein of 71-kDa and a viral 65-kDa polypeptide. *Virology 134*:91-102.

Nowak, B., Sullivan, C., Sarnow, P., Thomas, R., Bricout, F., Nicolas, J. C., Fleckenstein, B., and Levine, A. J. (1984b). Characterization of monoclonal antibodies and polyclonal immune sera directed against human cytomegalovirus virion proteins. *Virology 132*:325-338.

Pande, H., Baak, S. W., Riggs, A. D., Clark, B. R., Shively, J. E., and Zaia, J. A. (1984). Cloning and physical mapping of a gene fragment coding for a 64-kilodalton major late antigen of human cytomegalovirus. *Proc. Natl. Acad. Sci. USA 81*:4965-4969.

Peckham, C. S., Chin, K. S., Coleman, J. C. Henderson, K., Hurley, R., and Preece, P. M. (1983). Cytomegalovirus infection in pregnancy: Preliminary findings from a prospective study. *Lancet 1*:1352-1355.

Pereira, L., Hoffman, M., and Cremer, N. (1982a). Electrophoretic analysis of polypeptides immune precipitated from cytomegalovirus-infected cell extracts by human sera. *Infect. Immun. 36*:933-942.

Pereira, L., Hoffman, M., Gallo, D., and Cremer, N. (1982b). Monoclonal antibodies to human cytomegalovirus: Three surface membrane proteins with
unique immunological and electrophoretic properties specify cross-reactive
determinants. *Infect. Immun. 36*:924-932.

Pereira, L., Hoffman, M., Tatsouno, M., and Dondero, D. (1984). Polymorphism
of human cytomegalovirus glycoproteins characterized by monoclonal antibodies. *Virology 139*:73-86.

Pereira, L., Stagno, S., Hoffman, M., and Volanakis, J. E. (1983). Cytomegalovirus-infected cell polypeptides immune-precipitated by sera from children
with congenital and perinatal infections. *Infect. Immun. 39*:100-108.

Quinnan, G. V., Kirmani, N., Esber, E., Saral, R., Manischewitz, J. D., Rodgers,
J. L., Rook, A. H., Santos, G. W., and Burns, W. H. (1981). HLA-restricted
cytotoxic T lymphocyte and non-thymic cytotoxic lymphocyte response to
cytomegalovirus infection of bone marrow transplant recipients. *J. Immunol.
126*:2036-2041.

Rasmussen, L., Mullenax, J., Nelson, M., and Merigan, T. C. (1985a). Human cytomegalovirus polypeptides stimulate neutralizing antibody in vivo. *Virology 145*:186-190.

Rasmussen, L., Mullenax, J., Nelson, M., and Merigan, T. C. (1985b). Viral polypeptides detected by a complement-dependent neutralizing murine monoclonal to human cytomegalovirus. *J. Virol. 55*:274-280.

Rasmussen, L. E., Nelson, R. M., Kelsall, D. C., and Merigan, T. C. (1984). Murine monoclonal antibody to a single protein neutralizes the infectivity of human cytomegalovirus. *Proc. Natl. Acad. Sci. USA 81*:876-880.

Re, C. M., Landini, M. P., Coppolecchia, P., Furlini, G., and LaPlaca, M. (1985).
A 28,000 molecular weight human cytomegalovirus structural polypeptide
studied by means of a specific monoclonal antibody. *J. Gen. Virol. 66*:
2507-2511.

Redmond, M. J., Leyritz-Wilis, M., Winger, L., and Scraba, D. G. (1986). The selection and characterization of human monoclonal antibodies to human
cytomegalovirus. *J. Virol. Methods 14*:9-24.

Rice, G. A. P., Schreir, R. D., and Oldstone, M. B. A. (1984). Cytomegalovirus
infects human lymphocytes and monocytes; virus expression is restricted to
immediate-early gene products. *Proc. Natl. Acad. Sci. USA 81*:6134-6138.

Riggs, J. L. and Cremer, N. E. (1980). Differentiation of cytomegalovirus antigens by their reactivity with various classes of human antibodies in the indirect fluorescent antibody test. *J. Clin. Microbiol. 11*:88-93.

Rinaldo, C. R., Black, P. H., and Hirsch, M. S. (1977). Interaction of cytomegalovirus with leukocytes from patients with mononucleosis due to cytomegalovirus. *J. Infect. Dis. 136*:667-678.

Rinaldo, C. R. and Debiaso, R. L. (1983). Alteration of immunoregulatory mechanisms during cytomegalovirus mononucleosis: Effect of in vitro culture on
lymphocyte blastogenesis to viral antigens. *Clin. Immunol. Immunopathol.
28*:46-55.

Rodgers, B. C., Mundin, J., and Sissons, J. G. P. (1985). Monoclonal antibodies
recognizing early and late antigens of human cytomegalovirus: Heterogeneity

of polypeptides recognized between virus isolates. *J. Gen. Virol. 66*:2045-2049.

Rook, A. H., Quinnan, G. V., Frederick, W. J. R., Manischewitz, J. E., Kirmani, N., Dantzler, T., Lee, B. B., and Currier, C. B. (1984). Importance of cytotoxic lymphocytes during cytomegalovirus infection in renal transplant recipients. *Am. J. Med. 76*:385-392.

Rubin, R. H., Tolkoff-Rubin, N. E., Oliver, D., Rota, T. R., Hamilton, J., Betts, R. F., Pass, R. F., Hillis, W., Szmuness, W., and Farrell, M. L. (1985). Multicentre sero-epidemiologic study of the impact of cytomegalovirus infection on renal transplantation. *Transplantation 40*:243-248.

Ruebner, B. H., Hirono, T., Slusser, R. J., and Medearis, D. N., Jr. (1965). Human cytomegalovirus infection. Electron microscopic and histochemical changes in cultures of human fibroblasts. *Am. J. Pathol. 46*:477-496.

Schmitz, H., Doerr, H.-W., Kampa, D., and Vogt, A. (1977). Solid-phase enzyme immunoassay for immunoglobulin M antibodies to cytomegalovirus. *J. Clin. Microbiol. 5*:629-634.

Schmitz, H., Muller-Lantzsch, N., and Peteler, G. (1980). Human immune response to proteins of cytomegalovirus. *Intervirology 13*:154-161.

Shuster, E. A., Beneke, J. S., Tegtmeier, G. E., Pearson, G. R., Gleaves, C. A., Wold, A. D., and Smith, T. T. (1985). Monoclonal antibody for rapid laboratory detection of cytomegalovirus infections: Characterization and diagnostic application. *Mayo Clin. Proc. 60*:577-585.

Spencer, G. D., Hackman, R. C., and McDonald, G. B. (1985). Immunofluorescence diagnosis of gastrointestinal herpes simplex virus and HCMV infections using monoclonal antibody. *Gastroenterology 88*:1596.

Stagno, S., Reynolds, D. W., Tsiantos, A., Fuccillo, D. A., Smith, R., Tiller, M., and Alford, C. A. (1975). Cervical cytomegalovirus excretion in pregnant and non-pregnant women: Suppression in early gestation. *J. Infect. Dis. 131*:522-527.

Stagno, S., Tinker, M. K., Elrod, C., Fuccillo, D. A., Cloud, G., and O'Beirne, A. J. (1985). Immunoglobulin M antibodies detected by enzyme-linked immunosorbent assay and radioimmunoassay in the diagnosis of cytomegalovirus infections in pregnant women and newborn infants. *J. Clin. Microbiol. 21*:930-935.

Stenberg, R. M. and Stinski, M. F. (1985). Autoregulation of the human cytomegalovirus major immediate-early gene. *J. Virol. 56*:676-687.

Stenberg, R. M., Thomsen, D. R., and Stinski, M. F. (1984). Structural analysis of the major immediate-early gene of human cytomegalovirus. *J. Virol. 49*:190-199.

Stinski, M. F. (1976). Human cytomegalovirus: Glycoproteins associated with virions and dense bodies. *J. Virol. 19*:594-609.

Stinski, M. F. (1977). Synthesis of proteins and glycoproteins in cells infected with human cytomegalovirus. *J. Virol. 23*:751-767.

Stinski, M. F. (1978). Sequence of proteins synthesis in cells infected by human cytomegalovirus: Early and late virus-induced polypeptides. *J. Virol. 26*:686-701.

Stinski, M. F. (1979). Membrane glycoproteins and antigens induced by human cytomegalovirus. *J. Gen. Virol. 43*:119-129.

Stinski, M. F., Thomson, D. R., Stenberg, R. M., and Goldstein, L. C. (1983). Organization and expression of the immediate early genes of human cytomegalovirus. *J. Virol. 46*:1-14.

Sutherland, S. and Briggs, J. D. (1983). The detection of antibodies to cytomegalovirus in the sera of renal transplant patients by an IgM antibody capture assay. *J. Med. Virol. 11*:147-159.

Sweet, G. H., Bryant, S. A., Tegtmeier, G. E., Beneke, J. S., and Bayer, W. L. (1985). Early and late antigens of human cytomegalovirus: Electroimmunodiffusion assay of numbers, relationships and reactivities with donor sera. *J. Med. Virol. 15*:137-148.

Swenson, P. D. and Kaplan, M. H. (1985). Rapid detection of cytomegalovirus in cell culture by indirect immunoperoxidase staining with monoclonal antibody to an early nuclear antigen. *J. Clin. Microbiol. 21*:669-673.

Talbot, P. and Almeida, J. D. (1977). Human cytomegalovirus: Purification of enveloped virions and dense bodies. *J. Gen. Virol. 36*:345-349.

Tanaka, J., Yabuki, Y., and Hatano, M. (1981). Evidence for early membrane antigens in cytomegalovirus-infected cell. *J. Gen. Virol. 53*:157-161.

TenNapel, C. H. H. and The, T. H. (1980). Acute cytomegalovirus infection and the host immune response. I. Development and maintenance of cytomegalovirus (CMV) induced in vitro lymphocyte reactivity and its relationship to the production of CMV antibodies. *Clin. Exp. Immunol. 39*:262-271.

Volpi, A. and Britt, W. J. (1985). Serological heterogeneity of CMV isolates with a monoclonal antibody. *J. Infect. Dis. 152*:648-649.

Volpi, A., Whitley, R. J., Ceballos, R., and Stagno, S. (1983). Rapid diagnosis of pneumonia due to cytomegalovirus with specific monoclonal antibodies. *J. Infect. Dis. 147*:1119-1120.

Weiner, D., Gibson, W., and Fields, K. L. (1985). Anti-complement immunofluorescence establishes nuclear localization of human cytomegalovirus matrix protein. *Virology 147*:19-28.

Wielaard, F., Scherders, J., Hooijmans, A., and Dagelinckx, C. (1985). Development and preliminary evaluation of two ELISAs for detection of anti-CMV IgG and IgM antibodies. *J. Virol. Methods 10*:363-369.

Wilkinson, G. W. G., Akrigg, A., and Greenaway, P. J. (1984). Transcription of the immediate early genes of human cytomegalovirus strain AD169. *Virus Res. 1*:101-116.

Wreghitt, T. G., Hicks, J., Gray, J. J., and O'Connor, C. (1986). Development of a competitive enzyme-linked immunosorbent assay for detecting cytomegalovirus antibody. *J. Med. Virol. 18*:119-129.

Yolken, R. H. and Leister, F. J. (1981). Enzyme immunoassays for measurement of cytomegalovirus immunoglobulin M antibody. *J. Clin. Microbiol. 14*:427-432.

Zuckerman, A. J. (1985). Rapid laboratory diagnosis of viral infections. *J. Virol. Methods 10*:275-281.

Zweyberg-Wirgart, B. and Griliner, L. (1986). Early detection of cytomegalovirus in cell culture by a monoclonal antibody. *J. Virol. Methods 14*:65-70.

SEVENTEEN

Miscellaneous Infections: Current Status and Future Prospects of Immunological Diagnosis

Charles S. F. Easmon and Catherine A. Ison
Wright Fleming Institute
St. Mary's Hospital Medical School
London, England

I. INTRODUCTION

This chapter deals with three very different problems: bacterial vaginosis, group B streptococcal (GBS) infection, and chancroid.

Chancroid is a sexually transmitted disease with a well-defined single causal agent, *Haemophilus ducreyi*. The problem lies in making a specific diagnosis and in understanding its etiology. Culture of *H. ducreyi* is not easy, and the media required are relatively expensive. Nonspecific microscopy is not particularly sensitive. No typing system exists to assist epidemiological studies.

Group B streptococci are not primary genital tract pathogens. However, carriage of the organism in the vagina plays a key role in the pathogenesis of both maternal and neonatal GBS sepsis. There is a need for the rapid detection of heavy colonization in mother and baby.

Finally, bacterial vaginosis. Here the etiology, pathogenesis, and epidemiology are all uncertain. If the disease is an infection no single pathogen causes it. *Gardnerella vaginalis*, nonspore-forming anaerobic bacilli (*Bacteroides* spp.), cocci, and now *Mobiluncus* spp. have all been implicated.

In each of these disorders, improved immunological methods for the detection, identification, and typing have something to offer the diagnostic microbiologist as well as those interested in pathogenicity and epidemiology.

II. BACTERIAL VAGINOSIS

A. Etiology

Bacterial vaginosis appears clinically as an increased vaginal discharge, often foul smelling, in the absence of any recognized pathogen such as *Neisseria gonorrhoeae*, *Trichomonas vaginalis,* or *Candida albicans*. The presence of a malodor, particularly after menstruation or sexual intercourse, is characteristic, and in some cases the partner is more conscious of the odor than the patient. The symptoms vary among patients from mild to profuse, but this has been attributed to differences in personal hygiene and the ability to tolerate an increased vaginal discharge.

The clinical condition was first described by Gardner and Dukes in 1955 and named nonspecific vaginitis. This term was a misnomer, and therefore, because of the strong association with certain bacteria and the lack of any inflammatory response, the condition is now called bacterial vaginosis. Gardner and Dukes originally believed bacterial vaginosis to be a specific bacterial infection caused by *G. vaginalis* (then known as *Haemophilus vaginalis*). Although many workers have confirmed the association of *G. vaginalis* with bacterial vaginosis (Akerlund and Mardh, 1974; Brewer et al., 1957; Delaha et al., 1964; Pheifer et al., 1978; Piot et al., 1982), in recent years a number of other organisms have been implicated in the etiology of this condition. Nonspore-forming anaerobes, particularly *Bac-*

teroides bivius, Bacteroides disiens, Bacteroides melaninogenicus, and peptostreptococci, have been found in greater numbers and in more patients with bacterial vaginosis than in controls (Spiegel et al., 1980; Tabaqchali et al., 1983; Taylor et al., 1982). This has led to the proposal of a mixed infection with a possible symbiotic relationship. The main evidence to support this theory is related to the characteristic "fishy" smell. This is believed to be the result of the decarboxylation of amino acids and subsequent production of diamines, preponderantly putrescine and cadaverine. Mixed vaginal bacteria, but not *G. vaginalis* alone, can produce diamines in vitro. Chen et al. (1979) have suggested that anaerobes are responsible first for the production of diamines and second for maintaining a suitable environment for the survival of *G. vaginalis.*

The theory of a mixed infection, however, may not be limited to *G. vaginalis* and nonspore-forming anaerobes. *Mycoplasma hominis* (Paavonen et al., 1983; Pfeifer et al., 1978) and *Mobiluncus sp.* have also been associated with bacterial vaginosis (Hjelm et al., 1981; Phillips and Taylor, 1982; Skarin et al., 1981; Sprott et al., 1983).

Proof of the pathogenicity of any of these organisms, alone or in combination, is still lacking. Initial experiments using human volunteers showed that inoculation with vaginal material was more successful than pure cultures of *G. vaginalis* in producing the signs and symptoms of bacterial vaginosis (Gardner and Dukes, 1955). These results suggest that more than one organism may be involved. However, further human experiments have not been ethically possible, and it has proved difficult to develop a suitable animal model (Johnson et al., 1984; Mardh et al., 1984). The approach used by Gardner and Dukes (1955) to fulfill Koch's postulates should be used with caution, because these were aimed at a single pathogen of defined virulence. In bacterial vaginosis there is strong evidence of a mixed infection with more than one organism that may also be part of the normal flora.

Although the cause of bacterial vaginosis is unclear, there is a distinctive change in vaginal ecology. The normal vaginal secretions have a pH of $\leqslant 4.5$ and a lactobacillary flora. This is replaced by a discharge with a pH of $\geqslant 5.0$ and an abundance of epithelial cells, many of which are studded by bacteria giving the characteristic "clue" cells. The primary stimulus for the change in vaginal ecology may not be microbial but rather be related to the host's physiological state or lifestyle.

B. Epidemiology

The true prevalence of bacterial vaginosis is unknown because ill-defined criteria have been used for the diagnosis. Much of the early work depended upon the presence of symptoms or of *G. vaginalis,* both of which are now regarded as unreliable indicators for bacterial vaginosis. Dunkelberg (1977) has estimated that 15%

of all childbearing women in the United States have bacterial vaginosis. However, ignorance of, or disbelief in, this condition may mean that the problem is considerably greater.

Bacterial vaginosis has been described as a sexually associated rather than transmitted infection. Different aspects of sexual activity have been linked to increased prevalence of *G. vaginalis*, such as onset of sexual intercourse (Gardner and Dukes, 1955; Gardner and Dukes, 1959; Lee and Schmale, 1973), history of pregnancy (McCormack et al., 1977), and promiscuity (Gardner et al., 1957), a greater number of sexual partners (McCormack et al., 1977; Taylor et al., 1982), and the presence of other sexually transmitted infections (Amsel et al., 1983; Brewer et al., 1957; Josey et al., 1976; McCormack et al., 1977; Ray and Maughan, 1956). *Gardnerella vaginalis* has also been isolated from the male urethra (Dawson et al., 1982; Kinghorn et al., 1982; Wentworth et al., 1978), urine (Leopold, 1953), and semen (Ison and Easmon, 1985) and has been shown to have a high prevalence in sexual contacts of women with bacterial vaginosis (De La Fuente et al., 1959; Gardner and Dukes, 1955; Gardner and Dukes, 1959; Pheifer et al., 1978). Whether the male is truly colonized or whether this just represents continued passive acquisition from the female is not known. There is evidence that the use of barrier contraceptives reduces reinfection (Pheifer et al., 1978), but there are no reports of simultaneous treatment of both partners and the resultant effect on the prevalence of bacterial vaginosis.

Many other demographic variables have been examined as potential predisposing factors, but only the use of an intrauterine device for contraception is consistently associated with increased prevalence of *G. vaginalis* and bacterial vaginosis (Amsel et al., 1983; Ison and Easmon, unpublished observation).

C. Current Diagnostic Methods

A quick, reliable diagnosis of bacterial vaginosis can be achieved by the use of specific criteria that reflect the change in vaginal ecology. The presence of three or more of the following criteria in patients who do not have a recognized pathogen is considered diagnostic for bacterial vaginosis: (1) homogeneous vaginal secretion, (2) pH of discharge >4.5, (3) presence of clue cells, and (4) production of a fishy odor on the addition of 10% potassium hydroxide. When a diagnosis was made using these criteria *G. vaginalis* was isolated from 100% and *Bacteroides sp.* from 76% (Spiegel et al., 1980). These criteria are particularly valuable in a sexually transmitted disease (STD) clinic with experienced staff. In other situations, e.g., gynecology or antenatal clinics and office practice, guidance from the laboratory may be necessary.

Direct microscopy is often used to aid in the diagnosis of an infection. Gardner and Dukes (1955) described characteristic clue cells and Gram-variable bacilli which showed a strong correlation with culture for *G. vaginalis*. However, it is clear that clue cells together with organisms that resemble *G. vaginalis* do occur in women without the characteristic signs of bacterial vaginosis (Amsel et al., 1983; McCormack et al., 1977). There is, therefore, a danger that the use of microscopy alone for diagnosis may give misleading results.

An attractive alternative is the use of Gram-stained smears to detect changes in microbial flora (Spiegel et al., 1983). A Gram smear is considered positive when small gram-variable bacilli and a mixed bacterial flora are present without any large gram-positive bacilli of the *Lactobacillus* morphotype. This approach assesses obvious changes in vaginal flora, and hence, small numbers of *G. vaginalis* that can be cultured but do not produce any major change will be classed as normal. Spiegel et al. (1983) found that this method gave good correlation with a clinical diagnosis made with specific criteria or with the semiquantitative assessment of *G. vaginalis* by culture. This simple microscopic method could be used either in a clinic setting or in a microbiology laboratory to complement or confirm the clinician's diagnosis.

Despite the controversy over the role of *G. vaginalis* in bacterial vaginosis, its isolation is still regarded by many workers as a good marker, and many requests are made to laboratories for this identification. Improved cultural techniques using selective human blood agars (Greenwood et al., 1977; Ison et al., 1982; Smith, 1975; Totten et al., 1982) have increased the sensitivity and ease with which *G. vaginalis* may be isolated. Antibiotics have been used to reduce normal vaginal flora, e.g., colistin, gentamicin, nalidixic acid, and amphotericin. The human blood (5%) gives improved growth but also allows detection of a distinctive diffuse beta-hemolysis produced by *G. vaginalis* after 48-hr incubation in 5% CO_2. The presence of typical colonies on selective agar that are gram-variable coccobacilli is probably sufficient identification for most laboratories. A full identification as described by Piot et al. (1982) is time-consuming and unnecessary. There have been identification systems described using a limited number of tests (Jolly, 1983; Yong and Thompson, 1983), but there is no agreement on an acceptable identification method.

Sensitive cultural methods have shown quantitative differences between the numbers of *G. vaginalis* present in the vaginas of women with, and without, bacterial vaginosis. The presence of small numbers of *G. vaginalis* in the normal vagina should encourage caution in the use of culture for *G. vaginalis* as a diagnostic aid. Semiquantitative methods, as described by Ratnam and Fitzgerald (1983), are a more responsible approach. Screening for anaerobes and mycoplasmas to indicate bacterial vaginosis has not been regarded as a realistic alternative because of the technical difficulties together with their presence in some normal women.

Many of the tests used to diagnose this condition are subjective. In the search for more objective diagnostic tests the biochemical changes in the vaginal contents have been exploited. Normal vaginal washings contain the nonvolatile fatty acid, lactate, whereas in patients with bacterial vaginosis, lactate is reduced and succinate increased (Spiegel et al., 1980). A succinate/lactate ratio of >0.4 is considered indicative of bacterial vaginosis. This test has been used successfully by some workers (Ison et al., 1982; Piot et al., 1982; Spiegel et al., 1980) although it is also positive in trichomonal vaginitis. It requires a relatively large sample (0.5-1.0 ml) of vaginal washings and equipment for gas-liquid chromatography.

Chen et al. (1982) described a sensitive, rapid test that requires a smaller sample to determine the presence of the diamines, putrescine and cadaverine, in vaginal washings using thin-layer chromatography. The time and expertise required for these tests have prevented them from being widely used in diagnostic laboratories.

D. Development and Use of Polyclonal and Monoclonal Antibodies in Diagnosis and Epidemiology

Bacterial vaginosis can be diagnosed quickly and reliably by clinical criteria. The need for polyclonal or monoclonal antibodies (MAbs) as diagnostic reagents is questionable. The detection of a typical microscopical appearance of the vaginal discharge in bacterial vaginosis, however, does require expertise and experience. Antibodies could be used to develop rapid objective tests that would aid diagnosis both in the clinic and in the laboratory. Fluorescent or enzyme labels would probably be the detection systems of choice.

The role of *G. vaginalis*, anaerobes, and *M. hominis* in women both with and without bacterial vaginosis still remains confused. Antibodies used in typing schemes could greatly enhance our knowledge of the epidemiology of these organisms and subsequently of bacterial vaginosis. *Gardnerella vaginalis* can be used to illustrate the potential for similarities and differences in antigenic structure to be exploited for diagnostic and epidemiological purposes.

There is only limited information on the antigenic structure of *G. vaginalis*. In 1962, Edmunds described a scheme for serogrouping *G. vaginalis*. A panel of 13 antisera, raised in rabbits using whole-cell suspensions, grouped 36 of 50 clinical isolates into seven main serogroups by a precipitin test. The remaining strains were nongroupable or gave negative or indefinite reactions. Unfortunately, no correlation could be found with either the origin or biochemical profile of the strains. Antisera raised in this way have been used to aid identification (Redmond and Kotcher, 1963; Svarva and Maeland, 1982; Vice and Smaron, 1973). Svarva and Maeland (1982) found 205 of 206 strains of *G. vaginalis* showed reactivity with antisera in an indirect immunofluorescence test. Preliminary results showed that the antisera could be used to examine smears from urogenital specimens for rapid detection of *G. vaginalis*. As these antisera were not available commercially, their use has been limited. No attempts have been reported using these antisera for detection or further epidemiological studies.

The antigenic relationship between isolates of *G. vaginalis* and related genera was studied by Smaron and Vice (1974). Antisera were raised (in rabbits) against the type strain of *G. vaginalis* (ATCC 14018, NCTC 10287). Analysis by immuno-diffusion showed that all isolates possessed a common antigenic determinant, al-though the number of precipitin bands was variable between isolates and with different cultural conditions. There was no antigenic relationship with *Coryne-bacterium cervicis, C. xerosis, Lactobacillus acidophilus,* and vaginal diphtheroids, which were biochemically distinct from *G. vaginalis.*

Smaron and Vice (1977) subsequently described three antigens (i, o, and m) which were thought to be glycoproteins and to exist on or near the bacterial sur-face.

We have raised polyclonal antibodies to *G. vaginalis* in rabbits to aid the iden-tification of both genus-specific and strain-specific immunogenic antigens. The eventual aim is to produce a rapid test for the detection or identification of *G. vaginalis* and a serological-typing scheme.

Two genus-specific proteins have been identified in whole-cell extracts of *G. vaginalis* that were electrophoresed on a sodium dodecyl sulfate polyacrylamide gel (SDS-PAGE) using a 10% separating and 5% stacking gel. The proteins of ap-parent subunit molecular weight 17,000 and 45,000 were visualized using a silver stain (BioRad). Both proteins are immunogenic in rabbits.

Nine strains of *G. vaginalis* have been used to produce strain-specific antibody in rabbits. The activity of these antisera is directed mainly against different pro-teins. Some of the antisera also contain antibody directed against a substance that is positive with periodic acid-Schiff reagent, and we believe it is a carbohydrate.

The polyclonal antibodies have been used with a dot-blotting method (Hawkes et al., 1982; Herbrink et al., 1982) to produce a typing scheme. Bacteria were grown on human blood agar before application to nitrocellulose membrane strips. Each strip was incubated with a different antisera and any specific antibody was detected by antirabbit immunoglobulin linked to alkaline phosphatase. The reac-tion was visualized by immersing strips in substrate (4 g/L 5-bromo-4-chloro-3-indoly phosphate, 1 g/L nitroblue tetrazolium, 4 mM $MgCl_2$, in 0.1 M ethanol-amine buffer, pH 9.6) giving a blue color. One hundred isolates of *G. vaginalis* isolated from patients with bacterial vaginosis have been typed. Preliminary re-sults suggest that antisera can be chosen that will give suitable discrimination be-tween strains. The antigens detected have been shown to be stable on subculture and to be present when *G. vaginalis* is grown on 5% human blood agar, with or without antibiotics, and peptone starch agar and broth.

Work is in progress to produce MAbs to those strains of *G. vaginalis* that are known to present strain-specific antigens that are immunogenic in rabbits. It is, however, highly probable that different proteins will be immunogenic in the mouse which may provide a different, but possibly a better, discrimination. To date, we are aware of no published work on the characterization and application of MAbs to *G. vaginalis.*

The approach we have used with *G. vaginalis* could easily be adapted to any of the organisms implicated in the etiology of bacterial vaginosis. *Mobiluncus* spp.

are anaerobic curved rods (ACR) that have been isolated from patients with bacterial vaginosis but whose role in the cause is unclear. These organisms can be detected by microscopy but have proved difficult to culture. In most studies, less than 50% of ACR seen in a wet preparation or Gram stain of vaginal secretions are subsequently grown. The identification and detection of *Mobiluncus* spp. have been improved by the use of DNA probes (Roberts et al., 1984; Roberts et al., 1985). However, the use of specific antibody, either polyclonal or monoclonal, may be more easily adapted for diagnostic laboratories and clinics. In addition, valuable information may be gained concerning the antigenic structure of *Mobiluncus* spp.

III. GROUP B STREPTOCOCCI

A. The Clinical Problem

Unlike most of the organisms dealt with in this book, group B beta-hemolytic streptococci (GBS) are neither primarily pathogens of the genital tract nor are they sexually transmitted. Their presence in the female genital tract, however, is central to the pathogenesis and epidemiology of serious GBS sepsis.

The organism known as *Streptococcus agalactiae* was first described in relation to bovine mastitis by Nocard and Mollereau (1887). Lancefield (1933) included *S. agalactiae* animal strains as GBS in her classification system based on group-specific carbohydrate antigens. The organism was recognized as a vaginal commensal organism and then as a maternal and neonatal pathogen (Colebrook and Purdie, 1937; Fry, 1938; Lancefield and Hare, 1935).

The GBS are known to cause neonatal sepsis and maternal infections, usually of lesser severity (Table 1). Neonatal sepsis is of two types. Early-onset disease normally occurs within 2-3 days of birth. It consists of septicemia with respiratory distress and shock. Meningitis may occur, but it is not characteristic. Mortality can exceed 50% and is highest in those infants in whom infection appears within 12 hr of birth. The portal of entry is probably the respiratory tract, and the organisms are usually derived from the mother's genital tract.

Late-onset disease occurs in the second to sixth week of life and usually presents as meningitis, although serious mortality is not as high as with the early-onset form of disease.

Table 1   Main Types of Infection Caused by Group B Streptococci

Early-onset neonatal sepsis
Late-onset neonatal sepsis
Ascending genital tract infection (amnionitis, endometritis)
Urinary tract infections

Maternal GBS infection is less serious. Ascending infections from the vagina can result in endometritis, amnionitis, wound infection following cesarian section, and in extreme cases septicemia. There is little evidence to link GBS with vaginal infection, although occasionally a pure heavy vaginal growth of GBS can be associated with an abnormal discharge. There is a similar association in men between GBS and balanitis but no final proof of cause and effect.

As an inhabitant of the lower gastrointestinal tract and perineal skin it is not surprising that GBS can cause urinary tract infections in women (Wood and Dillon, 1981).

B. Epidemiology

The primary site of GBS colonization is almost certainly the gastrointestinal tract (Anthony et al., 1981; Barnham, 1983; Easmon et al., 1981). Colonization of the genital tract is a secondary phenomenon (Kexel and Beck, 1965).

Rates of vaginal colonization vary depending upon the precise site and frequency and method of sampling. Although there is little direct evidence of sexual transmission (Jackson et al., 1982), rates of GBS carriage in the vagina are directly related to sexual activity (Embil et al., 1978). Families tend to be colonized with the same GBS strain (Weindling et al., 1981).

Overall, 20-25% of all pregnant women are colonized with GBS. Most babies acquire the organism from their mothers' genital tracts during delivery. Transmission rates depend upon the heaviness of maternal colonization and the length of time the babies are exposed (Easmon et al., 1985; Ferrieri et al., 1977). The greater the number of sites colonized with GBS, the greater the risk of infection. The main sites of colonization in the neonate are the external ear, nose and throat, umbilical stump, and rectum. Within a few weeks, respiratory tract carriage declines and the rectum and perianal area become the main sites, as in the adult.

The neonate can acquire GBS from nonmaternal sources, especially when in the hospital. Although nosocomial transmission may be common, the babies are usually lightly colonized and normally do not retain the organism for long once they have left the hospital (Easmon et al., 1983).

C. Current Diagnostic and Typing Methods

The GBS grow well on blood agar, producing a diffuse beta-hemolysis. Only a few human strains are nonhemolytic. Hippurate hydrolysis, the CAMP test (synergistic hemolysis with staphylococcal beta-toxin), and the production of an orange-yellow pigment on anaerobic incubation, can all be used to identify GBS (Christie et al., 1944; Hwang and Ederer, 1975; Islam, 1977).

The GBS have also been identified serologically using polyclonal antibodies against the group-specific antigen. The traditional method of antigen extraction (by heat, acid, formamide, or enzymes) followed by ring precipitation in capillary tubes has largely been replaced by latex agglutination (Wellcome, Oxoid) or co-agglutination (Pharmacia). These tests are sensitive and specific, only occasional cross-reactions occurring with group G streptococci. Strains can be identified from primary isolation plates using five to 10 colonies.

These methods have also been applied to the detection of GBS antigen in blood, urine, and cerebrospinal fluid. Latex and coagglutination are more sensitive than countercurrent immunoelectrophoresis for antigen detection (Baker et al., 1980; Baker and Rench, 1983).

In the genital tract rapid detection of GBS colonization would help to prevent neonatal GBS infection. Prophylactic antibiotics given to colonized women during labor will prevent transmission of GBS from mother to baby (Yow et al., 1979). This, however, requires either extensive antenatal screening to detect GBS carriers or the indiscriminate use of systemic penicillins in healthy women. The former is expensive and not fully reliable, the latter unacceptable. Rapid detection of antigen from vaginal swabs would be an alternative. This has been tried using immunofluorescence to detect GBS in smears (Boyer et al., 1981; Castle et al., 1983). Results obtained by both groups are summarized in Table 2 together with some of our more recent work with latex agglutination. Specificity is good, but sensitivity is poor. This may be the result of both sampling and the sensitivity of the detection system. When only relatively heavy vaginal samples are included, sensitivity improves. A short incubation in broth to allow bacterial growth further improves the sensitivity of antigen detection. However, there is scope for improving the sensitivity of the method with better reagents.

Whereas the group-specific antigen is useful for identification and detection of GBS, the organism is further divided into serotypes. The serotyping system

Table 2 Sensitivity and Specificity of Group B Streptococcal Antigen Detection from Anogenital Swabs

Test	Method	Sensitivity	Specificity
Immunofluorescence	Direct	49	80
Immunofluorescence	3-6 hr broth incubation	36[a]	92[a]
Immunofluorescence	7-12 hr broth incubation	81[a]	99[a]
Agglutination	Direct broth incubation	43 (73)[b]	99
Agglutination	4 hr broth incubation	62 (100)[b]	99

[a]From Boyer et al., 1981.
[b]Assessed only against samples yielding ≥ 50 colonies/plate. (i.e., moderate or heavy carriage).

Table 3 Type Specific Antigens of Group B Streptococcus

Serotype	Type antigen	
	Protein	Carbohydrate
Ia	–	Ia
Ib	Ibc	Ib
Ic	Ibc	Ia
II	–	II
III	–	III
R	R	–
X	X	–

N.B. R and X antigens can be found in combination with other carbohydrate type antigens.

shown in Table 3 depends upon both carbohydrate and protein antigens. Unfortunately, although polyclonal-typing antisera are easy to raise, GBS serotyping gives poor discrimination and is of little value in detailed epidemiological studies. A phage-typing system has been developed that overcomes this problem (Stringer, 1980), but it is more difficult to use and has not been applied widely. This is another area where improved serological reagents would be useful.

Polin and his colleagues (1985) have raised a series of murine MAbs to GBS type Ia, Ib, Ic, II, and III antigens. BALB/c mice were given three injections of formalized reference-type strains (Wilkinson, 1975) at weekly intervals and spleen cells were fused with SP2/0-Ag 14 cells.

High-affinity IgM and IgG2 antibodies were used in two systems. A sandwich enzyme assay using peroxidase-conjugated antibody and an inhibition assay with a peroxidase-labeled mouse IgG. The sandwich assay detected GBS at a concentration of 5×10^4 to 10^5 colony-forming units (CFU)/ml and GBS antigen at a concentration of 1 mg/ml. It was 10 times more sensitive than the inhibition assay and much more sensitive than CIE or latex agglutination and coagglutination with polyclonal reagents (Morrow et al., 1984). The antibodies were type-specific.

D. Future Prospects

There is clearly a place for improved immunological reagents for the detection of GBS both in body fluids and from vaginal swabs. Rapid detection of heavy neonatal colonization would also be useful. A better serotyping system combining simplicity with improved discrimination would be welcome.

To date, work on MAbs to GBS has concentrated on type-specific antigens. Polyclonal detection reagents are group-specific, and it remains to be seen whether equivalent MAb reagents would provide increased sensitivity. If not, then mixtures of type-specific reagents could be used.

The sensitivity of the system applied to swabs, however, depends upon sampling efficiency, efficiency of antigen extraction from swabs, and sensitivity of the detection method as well as the quality of reagent.

IV. *HAEMOPHILUS DUCREYI*

A. Epidemiology

Worldwide, chancroid is an important sexually transmitted disease, more common than syphilis. It is usually thought of as being restricted to tropical and subtropical regions, but there are now increasing reports of the disease in North America and Europe.

The causative organism is *H. ducreyi*. The infection is associated with poor personal hygiene and poverty. Although transmission is mainly sexual, infection can occur through accidental contamination of cuts and abrasions or by accidental inoculation.

Infection is most common in sexually active young men and women, overt infection being more common in the former.

Asymptomatic carriage of *H. ducreyi* has been shown among prostitutes (Khoo et al., 1977), and *H. ducreyi*-like organism have been seen in asymptomatic men (Brams, 1924). Kinghorn et al. (1983) also found *H. ducreyi* in the absence of genital ulcers.

The incubation period between contact and initial appearance of skin ulcers is usually short. Thereafter, the patient rapidly develops painful genital ulcers and inguinal lymphadenitis. Systemic symptoms are rare.

B. Current Diagnostic Methods

Haemophilus ducreyi can be seen in material from ulcers of lymph nodes as chains of coccobacilli. Microscopy, however, lacks both sensitivity and specificity.

The isolation of *H. ducreyi* has improved recently as a result of the introduction of better culture media. Unfortunately, these media, consisting of chocolate agar with blood or serum and vitamins, amino acid, and antibiotic supplements, are neither cheap nor easy to quality control. Their use is, therefore, limited in underdeveloped countries where most chancroid is seen. A clear hemin-based medium without serum has been suggested by Hafiz et al. (1981) but has not been widely tested in the tropics. *Haemophilus ducreyi* requires carbon dioxide, grows best between 31-33°C, and is difficult to identify, being biochemically inert.

Apart from microscopy and culture, diagnosis clinically is based on the exclusion of other causes of genital ulceration, e.g., syphilis and genital herpes.

C. Future Prospects

The lack of sensitivity of nonspecific microscopy, the lack of biochemical reactivity of *H. ducreyi*, and the relative expense of culture, all offer scope for immunological diagnosis.

Some work has already been done. Denys et al. (1978) raised antisera to *H. ducreyi* by the intravenous injection of heat-killed organisms into rabbits. The resulting antiserum when absorbed with other *Haemophilus spp.* and used at a dilution of 1:10 was specific for *H. ducreyi* from different parts of the world.

Slootmans et al. (1985) have also raised antisera to *H. ducreyi* in rabbits. They used organisms injected subcutaneously in complete Freund's adjuvant followed by intravenous injections without adjuvant. The bacteria were not killed before use. They found little cross-reaction with other *Haemophilus spp.* and with related genera including clinical isolates of *Pasteurella spp., Eikenella corrodens, Actinobacillus actinomycetemcomitans,* and *Bordetella pertussis* using indirect immunofluorescence. There were differences in cross-reactivity between strains of *H. ducreyi*, suggesting that a serotyping system might be possible as well as a diagnostic reagent. The cell proteins of *H. ducreyi* have been characterized (Odumeru et al., 1983) and immunoblot analysis should enable suitable reagents to be refined.

Hansen and Loftus (1984) have raised murine MAbs to *H. ducreyi*. Mice were immunized intraperitoneally with organisms in Freund's complete adjuvant. Most antibodies were IgG1 and showed a range of specificities. Several showed broad reactivity within the species, and two, on which further work was done, showed no cross-reactivity with either *H. influenzae* and *H. parainfluenzae* or with *Treponema pallidum* and *Neisseria gonorrhoeae*. A dot blot radioimmunoassay showed that *H. ducreyi* could be identified in clinical material.

This work is still experimental, but it does seem likely that simple immunological detection systems may soon be available for *H. ducreyi*. Typing and confirmation of the organism's identity may also be made simpler.

REFERENCES

Akerlund, M. and Mardh, P.-A. (1974). Isolation and identification of *Corynebacterium vaginale* (*Haemophilus vaginalis*) in women with infections of the lower genital tract. *Acta Obstet. Gynecol. Scand. 53*:85-90.

Amsel, R., Totten, P. A., Spiegel, C. A., Chen, K. C. S., Eschenbach, D., and Holmes, K. K. (1983). Nonspecific vaginitis: Diagnostic criteria and microbial and epidemiologic associations. *Am. J. Med. 74*:14-22.

Anthony, B. F., Eisenstadt, R., Carter, J., Kim, K. S., and Hobel, C. J. (1981). Genital and intestinal carriage of group B streptococci during pregnancy. *J. Infect. Dis. 143*:761-766.

Baker, C. J., Webb, B. J., Jackson, C. V., and Edwards, M. S. (1980). Counter-current immunoelectrophoresis in the evaluation of infants with group B streptococcal disease. *Pediatrics 65*:1110-1114.

Baker, C. J. and Rench, M. A. (1983). Commercial latex agglutination for detection of group B streptococcal antigen in body fluids. *J. Pediatr. 102*: 393-395.

Barnham, M. (1983). The gut as a source of the haemolytic streptococci causing infection in surgery of the intestinal and biliary tracts. *J. Infect. 6*:129-139.

Boyer, K. M., Gadzala, C. A., Kelly, P. C., Burd, L. I., and Gotoff, S. P. (1981). Rapid identification of maternal colonization with group B streptococci by use of fluorescent antibody. *J. Clin. Microbiol. 14*:550-556.

Brams, J. (1924). Isolation of Ducrey bacillus from the smegma of 30 men. *J. Am. Med. Assoc. 82*:1166-1168.

Brewer, J. I., Halpern, B., and Thomas, G. (1957). *Haemophilus vaginalis* vaginitis. *Am. J. Obstet. Gynecol. 74*:834-843.

Castle, D., Deeley, J., and Easmon, C. S. F. (1983). Grouping and detection of group B streptococci by immunofluorescence. *J. Clin. Pathol. 36*:463-465.

Chen, K. C. S., Amsel, R., Eschenbach, D. A., and Holmes, K. K. (1982). Biochemical diagnosis of vaginitis: Determination of diamines in vaginal fluid. *J. Infect. Dis. 145*:337-345.

Chen, K. C. S., Forsyth, P. S., Buchanan, T. M., and Holmes, K. K. (1979). Amine content of vaginal fluid from untreated and treated patients with nonspecific vaginitis. *J. Clin. Invest. 63*:828-835.

Christie, R., Atkins, N. E., and Munch-Peterson, E. (1944). A note on a lytic phenomenum shown by group B streptococci. *Aust. J. Exp. Biol. Med. Sci. 22*:197-200.

Colebrook, L. and Purdie, A. W. (1937). Treatment of 106 cases of puerperal fever by sulphanilamide. *Lancet 2*:1237-1242.

Dawson, S. G., Ison, C. A., Csonka, G., and Easmon, C. S. F. (1982). Male carriage of *Gradnerella vaginalis*. *Br. J. Vener. Dis. 58*:243-245.

Delaha, E. C., Curtin, J. A., Stevens, G., and Osborne, H. J. (1964). Incidence and significance of *Haemophilus vaginalis* in nonspecific vaginitis. *Am. J. Obstet. Gynecol. 89*:996-999.

Denys, J. A., Chapel, T. A., and Jeffries, C. D. (1978). An indirect fluorescent antibody technique for *Haemophilus ducreyi*. *Health Lab. Sci. 15*:128-132.

Dunkelberg, W. E. (1977). *Corynebacterium vaginale*. *Sex. Transm. Dis. 4*:69-75.

Easmon, C. S. F., Hastings, M. J. G., Deeley, J., Bloxham, B., Rivers, R. P. A., and Marwood, R. (1983). The effect of intrapartun chemoprophylasix on the vertical transmission of group B streptococci. *Br. J. Obstet. Gynaecol. 90*:633-635.

Easmon, C. S. F., Hastings, M. J. G., Neill, J., Bloxham, B., and Rivers, R. P. A. (1985). Is group B streptococcal screening during pregnancy justified? *Br. J. Obstet. Gynaecol. 92*:197-201.

Easmon, C. S. F., Tanna, A., Munday, P., and Dawson, S. (1981). Group B streptococci—Gastrointestinal organisms. *J. Clin. Pathol. 34*:921-923.

Edmunds, P. N. (1962). The biochemical, serological and haemagglutinating reactions of "*Haemophilus vaginalis*," *J. Pathol. Bacteriol. 83*:411-422.

Embil, J. A., Martin, T. R., Hansen, N. H., MacDonald, S. W., and Manuel, F. R. (1978). Group B beta haemolytic streptococci in the female genital tract. *Br. J. Obstet. Gynaecol. 85*:783-786.

Ferrieri, P., Cleary, P. P., and Seeds, A. E. (1977). Epidemiology of group B streptococcal carriage in pregnant women and newborn infants. *J. Med. Microbiol. 10*:103-114.

Fry, R. M. (1938). Fatal infections by group B streptococci. *Lancet 1*:199-201.

Fuente, F. de la, Rico, L. R., and Soria, F. (1959). Hemofilasis urogenital afeccion venerea? *Rev. Esp. Obstet. Ginecol. 18*:252-254.

Gardner, H. L., Dampeer, T. K., and Dukes, C. D. (1957). The prevalence of vaginitis. *Am. J. Obstet. Gynecol. 73*:1080-1087.

Gardner, H. L. and Dukes, C. D. (1955). *Haemophilus vaginalis* vaginitis. A newly defined specific infection previously classified "non-specific" vaginitis. *Am. J. Obstet. Gynecol. 69*:962-976.

Gardner, H. L. and Dukes, C. D. (1959). *Haemophilus vaginalis* vaginitis. *Ann. N. Y. Acad. Sci. 83*:280-289.

Greenwood, J. R., Pickett, M. J., Martin, W. J., and Mack, E. G. (1977). *Haemophilus vaginalis* (*Corynebacterium vaginale*): Method for isolation and rapid biochemical identification. *Health Lab. Sci. 14*:102-106.

Hafiz, S., Kinghorn, G. R., and McEntegart, M. G. (1981). Chancroid in Sheffield. A report on 22 cases diagnosed by isolation of *H. ducreyi* in a modified medium. *Br. J. Vener. Dis. 57*:382-386.

Hansen, E. J. and Loftus, T. A. (1984). Monoclonal antibodies reactive with all strains of *Haemophilus ducreyi*. *Infect. Immun. 44*:196-198.

Hawkes, R., Niday, E., and Gordon, J. (1982). A dot immunoblotting assay for monoclonal and other antibodies. *Anal. Biochem. 119*:142-147.

Herbrink, P., Van Bussel, F. J., and Warnaar, S. O. (1982). The antigen spot test (AST): A highly sensitive assay for the detection of antibodies. *J. Immunol. Methods 48*:293-298.

Hjelm, E., Hallen, A., Forsum, U., and Wallin, J. (1981). Anaerobic curved rods in vaginitis. *Lancet 2*:1353-1354.

Hwang, M. N. and Ederer, G. M. (1975). Rapid hippurate hydrolysis method for presumptive identification of group B streptococci. *J. Clin. Microbiol. 1*: 114-115.

Islam, A. K. M. S. (1977). Rapid recognition of group B streptococci. *Lancet 1*: 256-257.

Ison, C. A., Dawson, S. G., Hilton, J., Csonka, G. W., and Easmon, C. S. F. (1982). Comparison of culture and microscopy in the diagnosis of *Gardnerella vaginalis* infection. *J. Clin. Pathol. 35*:550-554.

Ison, C. A. and Easmon, C. S. F. (1985). Carriage of *Gardnerella vaginalis* and anaerobes in semen. *Genitourin. Med. 61*:120-123.

Ison, C. A., Easmon, C. S. F., Dawson, S. G., Southerton, G., and Harris, J. W. R. (1983). Non-volatile fatty acids in the diagnosis of non-specific vaginitis. *J. Clin. Pathol. 36*:1367-1370.

Jackson, D. H., Hinder, S. M., Stringer, J., and Easmon, C. S. F. (1982). Carriage and transmission of group B streptococci among STD clinic patients. *Br. J. Vener. Dis. 58*:334-337.

Johnson, A. P., Ison, C. A., Hetherington, C. M., Osborn, M. F., Southerton, G., London, W. T., Easmon, C. S. F., and Taylor-Robinson, D. (1984). A study of the susceptibility of the three species of primate to vaginal colonisation with *Gardnerella vaginalis. Br. J. Exp. Pathol. 65*:389-396.

Jolly, J. L. S. (1983). Minimal criteria for the identification of *Gardnerella vaginalis* isolated from the vagina. *J. Clin. Pathol. 36*:476-478.

Josey, W. E., McKenzie, W. J., and Lambe, D. W. (1976). *Corynebacterium vaginale (Haemophilus vaginalis)* in women with leukorrhoea. *Am. J. Obstet. Gynecol. 126*:574-577.

Kexel, G. and Beck, K. J. (1965). Untersuchungen uber die Haufigkeit der B Streptokokken im Wochenbett. *Beburtsh. Frauenheilkd. 25*:1078-1085.

Khoo, R., Sng, E. H., and Goh, A. J. (1977). A study of sexually transmitted diseases in 200 prostitutes in Singapore. *Asian J. Infect. Dis. 1*:77-79.

Kinghorn, G. R., Hafiz, S., and McEntegart, M. G. (1983). Genital colonisation with *Haemophilus ducreyi* in the absence of ulceration. *Eur. J. Sex. Transm. Dis. 1*:89-90.

Kinghorn, G. R., Jones, B. M., Chowdhury. F. H., and Geary, I. (1982). Balanoposthitis associated with *G. vaginalis* infection in men. *Br. J. Vener. Dis. 58*: 127-129.

Lancefield, R. C. (1933). A serological differentiation of human and other groups of hemolytic streptococci. *J. Exp. Med. 57*:571-595.

Lancefield, R. C. and Hare, R. (1935). The serological differentiation of pathogenic and nonpathogenic strains of hemolytic streptococci from parturient women. *J. Exp. Med. 61*:335-349.

Lee, L. and Schmale, J. D. (1973). Ampicillin therapy for *Corynebacterium vaginale (Haemophilus vaginalis)* vaginitis. *Am. J. Obstet. Gynecol. 115*:786-788.

Leopold, S. (1953). Heretofore undescribed organism isolated from the Genitourinary system. *U.S. Armed Forces Med. J. 4*:263-266.

McCormack, W. M., Hayes, C. H., Rosner, B., Evrard, J. R., Crockett, V. A., Alpert, S., and Zinner, S. H. (1977). Vaginal colonisation with *Corynebacterium vaginale (Haemophilus vaginalis). J. Infect. Dis. 136*:740-745.

Mardh, P.-A., Holst, E., and Moller, B. R. (1984). The grivet monkey as a model for study of vaginitis. In *Bacterial Vaginosis* (P.-A. Mardh and D. Taylor-Robinson, eds.). Almqvist & Wiksell International, Stockholm, pp. 201 205.

Morrow, D. L., Kline, J. B., Douglas, S. D., and Polin, R. A. (1984). Rapid detection of group B streptococcal antigen by monoclonal antibody sandwich enzyme assay. *J. Clin. Microbiol. 19*:457-459.

Nocard, D. and Mollereau, A. (1887). Sur une mammate contegreuse dos vaches laitieres. *Ann. Inst. Pasteur 1*:109-126.

Odumeru, J. A., Ronald, A. R., and Albritton, W. L. (1983). Characterisation of cell proteins of *Haemophilus ducrey* by polyacrylamide gel electrophoresis. *J. Infect. Dis. 148*:710-714.

Paavonen, J., Miettinen, A., Stevens, C. E., Chen, K. C. S., and Holmes, K. K. (1983). *Mycoplasma hominis* in non-specific vaginitis. *Sex. Transm. Dis. 10*: 271-275.

Pheifer, T. A., Forsyth, P. S., Durfee, M. A., Pollock, H. M., and Holmes, K. K. (1978). Non specific vaginitis. Role of *Haemophilus vaginalis* and treatment with metronidazole. *N. Engl. J. Med. 298*:1429-1434.

Phillips, I. and Taylor, E. (1982). Anaerobic curved rods in vaginitis. *Lancet 1*:221.

Piot, P., Van Dyck, E., Godts, P., and Vanderheyden, J. (1982). The vaginal microbial flora in nonspecific vaginitis. *Eur. J. Clin. Microbiol. 1*:301-306.

Piot, P., Van Dyck, E., Totten, P. A., and Holmes, K. K. (1982). Identification of *Gardnerella* (*Haemophilus*) *vaginalis. J. Clin. Microbiol. 15*:19-24.

Polin, R. A. and Harris, M. C. (1985). Monoclonal antibodies against group B streptococci. In *Monoclonal Antibodies Against Bacteria* (A. J. L. Macario and E. C. de Macario, eds.), Vol. 1. Academic Press, New York, pp. 37-58.

Ratnam, S. and Fitzgerald, B. L. (1983). Semiquantitative culture of *Gardnerella vaginalis* in laboratory determination of nonspecific vaginitis. *J. Clin. Microbiol. 18*:344-347.

Ray, J. L. and Maughan, G. M. (1956). *Haemophilus vaginalis* as an etiological agent in vaginitis. *West. J. Surg. Obstet. Gynecol. 64*:581-588.

Redmond, D. L. and Kotcher, E. (1963). Comparison of cultural and immunofluorescent procedures in the identification of *Haemophilus vaginalis. J. Gen. Microbiol. 33*:89-94.

Roberts, M. C., Hillier, S. L., Schoenkneckt, F. D., and Holmes, K. K. (1984). Nitrocellulose filter blots for species identification of *Mobiluncus curtisii* and *Mobiluncus mulieris. J. Clin. Microbiol. 20*:826-827.

Roberts, M. C., Hillier, S. L., Schoenkneckt, F. D., and Holmes, K. K. (1985). Comparison of Gram stain, DNA probe and culture for the identification of species of *Mobiluncus* in female genital specimens. *J. Infect. Dis. 152*: 74-77.

Skarin, A., Spiegel, C. A., Westrom, L., Holmes, K. K., and Mardh, P.-A. (1981). Demonstration of a strictly anaerobic, gram-negative, comma-shaped bacterium in females with symptoms of lower genital tract infection. *Abstracts of 4th International Meeting on Sexually Transmitted Diseases.* (Heidelberg, October 18-20), p. 9.

Slootmans, L., Vanden Berghe, D. A., and Piot, P. (1985). Typing *Haemophilus ducreyi* by indirect immunofluorescence. *Gentourin Med. 61*:123-126.

Smaron, M. F. and Vice, J. L. (1974). Analysis of *Corynebacterium vaginale* by an immunodiffusion technique. *Appl. Microbiol. 27*:469-474.

Smaron, M. F. and Vice, J. L. (1977). Immunological and chemical characterisation of the extracellular antigens from *Corynebacterium vaginale. Infect. Immun. 18*:356-362.

Smith, R. F. (1975). New medium for isolation of *Corynebacterium vaginale* from genital specimens. *Health Lab. Sci. 12*:219-224.

Spiegel, C. A., Amsel, R., Eschenbach, D., Schoenknecht, F., and Holmes, K. K. (1980). Anaerobic bacteria in nonspecific vaginitis. *N. Engl. J. Med. 303*: 601-606.

Spiegel, C. A., Amsel, R., and Holmes, K. K. (1983). Diagnosis of bacterial vaginosis by direct Gram stain of vaginal fluid. *J. Clin. Microbiol.* *18*:170-177.

Sprott, M. S., Ingham, H. R., Pattman, R. S., Eisenstadt, R. L., Short, G. R., Narang, H. K., Sisson, P. R., and Selkon, J. B. (1983). Characteristics of motile curved rods in vaginal secretions. *J. Med. Microbiol.* *16*:175-182.

Stringer, J. (1980). The development of a phage typing system for group B streptococci. *J. Med. Microbiol.* *13*:133-144.

Svarva, P. L. and Maeland, J. A. (1982). Identification of *Gardnerella vaginalis* by a fluorescent antibody test. *Acta Pathol. Microbiol. Immunol. Scand. Sect. B 90*:453-455.

Tabaqchali, S., Wilks, M., and Thin, R. N. (1983). *Gardnerella vaginalis* and anaerobic bacteria in genital disease. *Br. J. Vener. Dis. 59*:111-115.

Taylor, E., Blackwell, A. L., Barlow, D., and Phillips, I. (1982). *Gardnerella vaginalis*, anaerobes and vaginal discharge. *Lancet 1*:1376-1379.

Totten, P. A., Amsel, R., Hale, J., Piot, P., and Holmes, K. K. (1982). Selective differential human blood bilayer media for the isolation of *Gardnerella vaginalis*. *J. Clin. Microbiol. 15*:141-147.

Vice, J. L. and Smaron, M. F. (1973). Indirect immunofluorescent antibody method for the identification of *Corynebacterium vaginale*. *Appl. Microbiol. 25*:908-916.

Weindling, A. M., Hawkins, J. M., Coombes, M. A., and Stringer, J. (1981). Colonisation of babies and their families by group B streptococci. *Br. Med. J. 283*:1503-1505.

Wentworth, B. B., Bonin, P., and Holmes, K. K. (1978). Isolation of viruses, bacteria and other organisms from venereal disease clinic patients: Methodology and problems associated with multiple isolations. *Health Lab. Sci. 10*: 75-81.

Wilkinson, H. W. (1975). Immunochemistry of purified polysaccharide type antigens of group B streptococcal types Ia, Ib, Ic. *Infect. Immun. 11*:845-852.

Wood, E. G. and Dillon, H. C. (1981). A prospective study of group B streptococcal bacteriuria in pregnancy. *Am. J. Obstet. Gynecol. 140*:515-520.

Yong, D. C. T. and Thompson, J. S. (1982). Rapid microbiochemical method for identification of *Gardnerella* (*Haemophilus*) *vaginalis*. *J. Clin. Microbiol. 16*: 30-33.

Yow, M. D., Mason, E. O., Leeds, L. J., Thompson, P. K., Clark, D. J., and Gardner, S. E. (1979). Ampicillin prevents intrapartum transmission of group B streptococci. *J. Am. Med. Assoc. 241*:1245-1247.

Index

517